Injury Control

Injury Control

A Guide to the Causes and Prevention of Trauma

Julian A. Waller, M.D., M.P.H.
University of Vermont

Lexington Books
D.C. Heath and Company/Lexington, Massachusetts/Toronto

Library of Congress Cataloging in Publication Data

Waller, Julian A., 1932–
Injury control.

Bibliography: p.
Includes index.
1. Wounds and injuries—Prevention. 2. Accidents—Prevention. 3. Traumatology. I. Title. [DNLM: 1. Accident Prevention. 2. Wounds and Injuries—prevention & control. WA 250 W198i]
RD93.W33 1984 363.1 83-49520
ISBN 0-669-08232-5 (alk. paper)

Published simultaneously in Canada
Printed in the United States of America on acid-free paper
International Standard Book Number: 0-669-08232-5
Library of Congress Catalog Card Number: 83-49520

With Appreciation

To my colleagues, who fed me so well with ideas, encouragement, and data, and then waited so patiently,

To the UVM Dana Library staff, who always seem able to answer that quirky question or find that obscure reference,

To the several typists—but especially to Nancy, Andrea, Jennifer, and Estelle—for converting sinister scratches into gleaming text.

But most of all

To Elsa, who always helps just by being herself, and

To Nomi and Seth, who are the future.

Summary of Contents

With Appreciation v

Summary of Contents vii

Contents xi

List of Figures xix

List of Tables xxi

Part I Overview of Concepts, Methods, and Problems in Injury Control 1

1. **Introduction 3**
2. **Definitions of Injury Events 7**
3. **How Injury Events Occur 11**
4. **Countermeasures against Injury 39**
5. **Making Choices 47**
6. **Some Questions about Numbers 65**
7. **Evaluating Countermeasures 79**

Part II Specific Types of Injury Events 91

8. **Societal Impact of Injury 93**
9. **An Overview of Highway Injury 107**
10. **Trucks, Buses, Recreational, and Emergency Vehicles 161**
11. **Motorcycles, Mopeds, Scooters, and Minibikes 183**

12. **Bicycles 199**

13. **Pedestrians 211**

14. **Rail Transportation 225**

15. **Water Transportation and Recreational Boating 235**

16. **Air Transportation 245**

17. **Injury in the Home Environment 263**

18. **Issues in Building Design and Construction 269**

19. **The Tools of Living: Furnishings and Appliances 287**

20. **Thermal Extremes: Fire, Burns, Scalds, Hypothermia 301**

21. **Falls 321**

22. **Poisoning 331**

23. **Schools, Playgrounds, Camps, and Parks 347**

24. **Recreational Activities 361**

25. **Hospitals and Nursing Homes 405**

26. **Occupational Injury 421**

27. **Community Disasters 447**

Part III The Health and Safety Professions and High-Risk Populations 465

28. **"Accident" Proneness: Fact or Fiction? 467**

29. **Children and Youth 473**

30. **Medical Conditions and Aging 493**

31. Use of Alcohol and Other Drugs 511

32. Injury Control and the Health Professional: Preparation for the Future 525

Final Words 531

Notes 533

Index 619

About the Author 644

Contents

With Appreciation v

Summary of Contents vii

List of Figures xix

List of Tables xxi

Part I Overview of Concepts, Methods, and Problems in Injury Control 1

1. Introduction 3

2. Definitions of Injury Events 7

3. How Injury Events Occur 11

Energy as the Agent of Injury 16

People and Tasks 17

The Pre-Injury Phase 18

The Injury Phase 23

An Alternative Pathway 24
Kinetic Energy 26
Thermal Energy 30
Chemical Energy 30
Electrical Energy 33
Ionizing Radiation 35
Relationships between Acute and Chronic Energy Exposure 35

Post-Injury Phase 36

"Innocent" and Not-So-"Innocent" Bystanders 37

4. Countermeasures against Injury 39

5. Making Choices 47

Protagonistic Viewpoints 47

Why Do We Act Inconsistently? 50

Cost/Benefit Studies and The Value of a Life 51

A Scheme to Establish Priorities for Programs 57

Making Choices at the Individual Level 58

Appendix 5A An Assessment of Factors Promoting or Hindering Development of a Safety Device 59

6. Some Questions about Numbers 65

Frequency of Injury Events 65

Measurement of Exposure 69

Severity of Injury Events 73

Causation 76

7. Evaluating Countermeasures 79

OPSKARBO: What's Happening, to Whom, and for What Purpose? 79

Evaluation Strategies 82

Statistical Issues 85

Countermeasure Effect Over Time 87

Effects of Simultaneous Countermeasures 88

Part II Specific Types of Injury Events

8. Societal Impact of Injury 93

9. An Overview of Highway Injury 107

Patterns of Crashes, Injuries, and Death 109

An Overview of Crash Patterns in the United States 109

A Comparison with Crash Patterns in Developing Nations 111

Human Factors in the Pre-Injury or Pre-Crash Phase 113
- Alcohol and Other Drugs 115
- Medical Impairment and Aging 116
- Youth and Inexperience 117
- Highway Laws and the Extent to Which They Are Obeyed 118

Pre-Crash Factors Involving the Vehicle 121

Environmental Contribution to Pre-Crash Phase 125

Energy Transfer or Injury Phase 129

Post-Crash Phase 137

Appropriate Countermeasures 138

Countermeasures Directed at People 139

Vehicular Countermeasures 149

Environmental Countermeasures 155

Post-Crash Countermeasures 159

10. Trucks, Buses, Recreational, and Emergency Vehicles 161

Definitions 161

Crash Experience 162

Human Factors 165

Vehicle Factors 168

Environmental Factors 170

The Energy Transfer Phase 173

Post-Crash Phase 173

Countermeasures 1784

Emergency Vehicles 178

Causal Factors 179

Countermeasures 181

11. Motorcycles, Mopeds, Scooters, and Minibikes 183

Injury and Fatality Patterns 184

Human Factors: Pre-Injury Phase 186

Vehicular Factors 187

Environmental Factors 189

Crash Phase 190

Post-Crash Factors 191

Countermeasures 193

12. Bicycles 199

Use and Injury Patterns for Children: Human Factors 200

Injury Patterns for Children: Equipment and Environmental Factors 203

Injury-Phase Issues in Children's Injuries 205

Use and Injury Patterns for Adults 206

Countermeasures 207

13. Pedestrians 211

Injury Patterns 211

Human Factors in the Pre-Injury Phase 212

Vehicular Factors 219

Environmental Factors 220

Crash and Post-Crash Factors 221

Countermeasures 222

14. Rail Transportation 225

Collisions: Human Factors in the Pre-Injury Phase 226

Collisions: Environmental Factors 227

Collisions: Factors in the Injury and Post-Injury Phases 229

Derailment 231

Failure of Rolling Stock Equipment 232

Injuries While Coupling or Braking or Stoking the Fire 232

Injuries to Passengers Who Fall from Equipment 233

Countermeasures 233

15. Water Transportation and Recreational Boating 235

Injury Experience 236

Human Factors in the Pre-Injury Phase 237

Environmental Factors in the Pre-Injury Phase 240

Factors in the Injury and Post-Injury Phases 241

16. Air Transportation 245

Injury Experience 245

Human Factors in the Pre-Injury Phase 246

Vehicular and Environmental Factors in the Pre-Injury Phase 255

Factors in the Crash and Post-Crash Phases 258

Countermeasures 259

17. Injury in the Home Environment 263

Injury Patterns 263

Causal Factors 266

18. Issues in Building Design and Construction 269

Stairs 270

Doors 272

Windows 273

Tubs and Showers 278

Electrical Supply 283

Home Heating Systems 284

Developing Building Codes 284

19. The Tools of Living: Furnishings and Appliances 287

Furnishings 292

Appliances 294

Housewares and Containers 297

Equipment for Household Maintenance and Repair 297

20. Thermal Extremes: Fire, Burns, Scalds, Hypothermia 301

Frequency and Distribution 301

Human Factors in the Pre-Injury Phase 305

Environmental Factors in the Pre-Injury Phase 309

Factors That Increase Energy Load and/or Promote Transfer to People 311

Countermeasures 317

21. Falls 321

Human Factors in the Pre-Injury Phase 323

Environmental Factors in the Pre-Injury Phase 326

Factors in the Injury and Post-Injury Phases 328

Countermeasures 328

22. Poisoning 331

Injury Patterns 331

Human Factors in Pre-Injury Phase 336

Environmental Factors in the Pre-Injury Phase 338

Injury and Post-Injury Phases 340

Countermeasures 341

23. Schools, Playgrounds, Camps, and Parks 347

Injuries Involving Schools 347

Playground Equipment 351

Camps 355

Parks 359

24. Recreational Activities 361

Overview 361

Toys 368

Water Activities 370

Body-Contact Team Sports 377

Individual Body-Contact Sports 383

Winter Sports 387

Miscellaneous Other Sports and Recreation 393

Guns and Fireworks 397

Challenging the Great Outdoors 401

Some Additional Observations 404

25. Hospitals and Nursing Homes 405

Patient Injuries 406

Employee Injuries 416

26. Occupational Injury 421

Injury Patterns 422

Causal Factors: An Overview 425

Human Factors in the Pre-Injury Phase 427

Environmental Factors in the Pre-Injury, Injury, and Post-Injury Phases 436

Countermeasures 440

27. Community Disasters 447

Natural Disasters 449

Man-Made Disasters 459

The Aftermath: Long-Term Effects 463

Part III The Health and Safety Professions and High-Risk Populations 465

28. "Accident" Proneness: Fact or Fiction? 467

29. Children and Youth 473

Risk Factors 476

Countermeasures 478

Some Preventive Measures for Injuries to Infants 479

Some Preventive Measures for Injuries to Toddlers and Preschool Children 483

Some Preventive Measures for Injuries to Primary-School Children 488

Some Preventive Measures for Injuries to Teenagers 490

30. Medical Conditions and Aging 493

Issues Generally Associated with Normative Aging 493

Issues Involving Pathological Aspects of Aging 495

Injury Results 497

Countermeasures 499

Evaluating Medical Impairment to Driving 503

Static and Slowly Progressive Conditions 505

Seizures 506

Cardiovascular Diseases 507

Diabetes Mellitus 508

Senile Dementia and Other Disorders of Memory and Judgment 508

31. Use of Alcohol and Other Drugs 511

Metabolic and Physiologic Factors Increasing Injury Risk 511

Other Factors Affecting Injury Risk 514

Countermeasures 516

Other Drugs 522

32. Injury Control and the Health Professional: Preparation for the Future 525

Introductory Statistics and Concepts 526

Understanding and Dealing with Human Factors 526

Environmental Factors in the Pre-Injury Phase 527

Environmental Factors in the Injury Phase 527

Post-Injury Phase and Training in Emergency Care 528

Integrative Exercises on Highway and Nonhighway Injury Events 529

Organizing the Course 530

Final Words 531

Notes 533

Index 619

About the Author 645

List of Figures

3–1. Benner's Multilinear Events Sequencing Model 15

3–2. Pre-Injury Events Attributable Both to Low Human Performance and to High Task Demand 20

3–3. Relationship between Human Performance and Task Demand 22

3–4. Head Injury Tolerance: Acceleration versus Duration 27

3–5. Average Failure Loads of Thoracic (T) and Lumbar (L) Vertebrae 28

3–6. Effect of Age on Vertebral Breaking Strength (Normalized to L5 Vertebra) 29

3–7. Threshold for Various Tissue Effects from Heat and Cold 31

3–8. Thresholds to Pain and Tissue Damage According to Contact Temperature and Duration 32

6–1. Some Estimated Relative Sampling Errors for Studies of Specific Types of Highway Crashes Given Different Numbers of Survey Sites and of Crashes Surveyed Per Site 73

7–1. Conclusions and Margins of Error in Studies of Effectiveness of Passenger Restraints in Reducing Injuries and Fatalities 86

9–1. Relative Frequency of Known Sources of Major Injury to Front-Seat Occupants in Urban and Rural Crashes 130

9–2. Relationship between Velocity Change, Stopping Distance, and Injury 132

26–1. Injury Rates of Underground Miners According to Age and Years of Employment 429

List of Tables

3–1. Amount of Current (mh) at Which Events Are Postulated by Three Researchers with Reference to a 60 Hz Electric Current 34

5–1. Direct Future Productivity Loss for 1973 U.S. Highway Fatalities 52

5–2. Societal Cost Components for U.S. Fatalities 53

5–3. Injury Severity Classes in Societal Cost Study of U.S. Highway Injuries 53

6–1. Categories of Injury According to Abbreviated Injury Scale (AIS) and Its Modification through the Injury Severity Score (ISS) 75

6–2. CPSC Severity Scoring System 76

8–1. Injury and Related Disability by Age, Sex, and Type of Event, United States, 1980 94

8–2. Annual Rates of Nonfatal Injuries Per 1,000 Population by Sex, Age, and Detailed Description of Event, United States, 1971–72 95

8–3. Annual Rates and Proportions of Nonfatal Injuries by Sex, Age, and Detailed Description of Event, Punjab, India, 1959–60 96

8–4. Death Rates Per 100,000 Population from Selected Causes for Nations Reporting over 50,000 Deaths Annually 97

8–5. Age- and Sex-Specific Death Rates in 1970–74 from Unintentional Injury for Nations with over 50,000 Deaths Per Year 99

8–6. Crude Death Rates Per 100,000 Population for Specific Injury Types by Nation 104

9–1. Distribution of Automobiles, Trucks, and Buses among Populations of Selected Nations 108

9–2. Characteristics of Fatal, Injury, and Property Damage Crashes, United States, 1980 110

9–3. Types of Motor Vehicles Involved in Fatal Crashes and All Crashes, United States, 1980 111

9–4. Vehicles Per 10,000 Population and Fatalities Per 10,000 Vehicles for Developing Nations, 1971, and Developed Nations, 1970 112

9–5. Characteristics of Fatal and Injury Crashes in Kenya and Kuwait 114

9–6. Rank Order of Vehicle Components Causing Injury in Four Studies 131

9–7. Crash Distribution and Injury Rates by Crash Type 134

9–8. Distribution of Injury Rates Per 100 Occupants by Crash Severity (Delta V) in Front-, Side-, and Back-Damage Vehicles 135

9–9. Proportions of Crashes Involving Roadside Furniture and Hazards in Michigan, 1972 136

9–10. Summary of the State of Evaluation of Federal Motor Vehicle Safety Standards in the 200 Series as Assessed by Huelke and O'Day 152

9–11. Effects of Changes in Highway Design on Crashes 156

10–1. Crash and Fatal Crash Experience of Large Vehicles 164

10–2. Fatality Rates in Car/Truck Crashes According to Truck Weight, 1973 and 1974 165

10–3. Proportions of Vehicles Found Defective by Investigating Police Officer in Crashes According to Vehicle Type 170

11–1. Number of Bicycles, Mopeds, Motorcycles, and Automobiles Per 1,000 Inhabitants for Several Nations, 1973–75 184

11–2. Vehicles Involved Per 100 Million Kilometers in Property Damage, Injury, and Death by Vehicle Type 185

11–3. Causal Factors in Single-Vehicle Motorcycle Crashes Not at Intersections 189

11–4. Distribution by Body Area of All Injuries and Fatal Injuries among Motorcycle Riders and of Injuries among Helmeted and Unhelmeted Riders 192

12–1. Circumstances Leading to Event among Bicycle Injuries to Children 202

13–1. Distribution of Pedestrian Injuries by Age, United States and Nigeria 213

13–2. Blood Alcohol Concentrations of Pedestrians in Crashes and Matched Comparisons and Relative Risk of Crash Involvement 217

13–3. Distribution of Serious and Fatal Injuries in 187 Fatally Injured Pedestrians 222

15–1. Casualties and Related Deaths and Injuries, U.S. Commercial Vessels in 1975 237

15–2. Total Losses of Tankers by Vessel Age and Country of Registry 239

16–1. Event and Fatality Rates for U.S. Air Carriers, 1977–79, and Several Types of General Aviation, 1979 247

16–2. Phases of Operation in All Events and Fatal Ones for Air Carriers, 1970–79, and General Aviation, 1974–78 248

16–3. Most Prevalent Types of Events, for All Events and Fatal Ones Involving Air Carriers, 1970–79, and General Aviation, 1974–78 249

16–4. Causes and Related Factors in All Events and Fatal Ones Involving Air Carriers, 1970–79, and General Aviation, 1979 250

16–5. Relation between Flight Activities and Mishaps Involving Pilot Error in Jet Transport Aircraft, 1959–74 252

17–1. Deaths and Injuries through Various Non–Motor Vehicle Modes in the United States and Their Frequency in and around the Home 264

17–2. Home Injuries as Proportions of All Unintentional Injury Deaths and of Nontransport Injury Deaths for Men and Women in Several Nations, 1960 266

18–1. Annual Emergency Department Visits in the United States Involving Architectural Components and Building Materials 270

18–2. Most Common Injury Events on Stairs and Their Remedies 274

18–3. Most Common Injury Events Involving Doors and Their Remedies 276

18–4. Most Common Injury Events Involving Windows and Their Remedies 279

18–5. Most Common Injury Events Involving Bathtubs and Showers and Their Remedies 281

19–1. Annual Emergency Department Visits in the United States for Injuries Involving Products in and around the Home 288

19–2. Comparison of Priorities for Products Associated with Injury Based on Assumptions That All Persons in the United States Are Exposed or That There Are Fewer Users 290

20–1. Distribution of Deaths Involving Fire or Hot Substances, United States, 1975 302

20–2. Causes of Burn Injuries in and around the Home Based on 1974 National Household Fire Survey 303

20–3. Human Factors in Serious and Minor Residential Fires 307

20–4. Building Characteristics in Serious and Minor Residential Fires 312

21–1. Environmental Factors in Initiation of Falls among Elderly According to Presence of Precipitating Health Problem in Fall 327

22–1. Deaths From Poisoning by Type, Age, and Sex, United States, 1978 332

22–2. Thirty-one Products Most Often Involved in 34,653

Reported Nonfatal Poisonings, United States, July 1959–December 1961 335

23–1. Injury Rates Per 100,000 Student Days Related to School Activities by Sex and Location or Activity 348

23–2. Injury in College and University Activities by Location/Activity, Sex, and Severity 350

23–3. Distribution of Playground Equipment Injuries in Home and Public Places According to Equipment Type, U.S. 1977 Modified Estimate 352

24–1. Injuries and Deaths Per Unit Exposure for Various Forms of Recreation 364

24–2. Injury Patterns in Different Types of Competitive (C) and Noncompetitive (NC) Skiing 389

24–3. Interaction of Factors in the Initiation of Snowmobile Injuries 392

24–4. Ten Most Frequent Apparent Causes of Mountaineering Injuries in the United States, 1951–60 401

25–1. Reported Patient Incidents by Age Per 1,000 Admissions and Per 10,000 Patient Days 407

25–2. Types of Mishaps in Hospital 408

25–3. Relationships between Falls in Nursing Homes, Walking Ability, and Use of Walking Aid 410

25–4. Fall-Related Bone Fracture Rates Per 100 Persons by Age and Sex 410

25–5. Fall Rates Per 100 Persons According to Age, Prior Functional Status re Activities of Daily Living (ADL), and Contributing Factors 411

25–6. Officially Reported and Covertly Observed Medication Errors Per 10,000 Patient Days by Type of Error 412

25–7. Injuries and Their Cost among Different Categories of Hospital Employees According to Their Proportions of Hospital Work Force 417

25–8. Injury Rates Per Million Hours Worked According to Hospital Type and Employee Category 417

25–9. Employee Injury Rates Per Million Hours Worked and

Average Disability Days Per Injury by Hospital Size 419

25–10. Vehicles, Mechanisms, or Types of Injuries Reported for Two Hospital Laboratories 420

26–1. Estimated Fatal Injury Rates for Males Per 1,000 Employees by Industry, United States, 1913 423

26–2. Injuries Per 100 Full-Time Employees (200,000 Hours) Involving Death or Days away from Work by Industry Category and All Industries Exceeding Mean for Their Category 424

26–3. Disabling Work Injury Rates Per 1,000 Employed Males in California According to Age (Mean of Years 1960, 1965, and 1968) 428

26–4. Distribution of Blood Alcohol Concentrations in Nonfatal Occupational Injuries in Boston, Helsinki, and Rural Finland 434

27–1. Deaths in Catastrophic Events by Type of Event, United States, 1941–75 448

27–2. Comparison of Richter and Modified Mercalli Scales for Measuring Earthquake Intensity 451

29–1. Mean Injury Mortality by Geographic Area for Children Age 1 to 4 474

29–2. Mean Injury Mortality by Geographic Area for Children Age 5 to 14 475

Injury Control

Part I
Overview of Concepts, Methods, and Problems in Injury Control

1
Introduction

It has always been surprising to me that injury control—or accident prevention, as it is known to many—has generated so few books. Other problem conditions, such as cardiovascular disease and cancer, evoke an extensive literature, both of journal articles and of books. Certianly it could not be that the subject lacks importance, for unintentional injury is the most frequent cause of death in the United States among persons under age 45, the fourth most common cause at all ages, and has the dubious distinction of first place on the North American continent as a cause of lost person-years of productive life. Despite rampant malnutrition and infectious diseases, injury is also a serious problem in so-called developing countries.

Perhaps the answer is that these other conditions fall primarily in the purview of a single professional group—physicians and other health workers—and thus it is easier to search out and gather the papers and data about them that are the necessary ingredients of a comprehensive text. Injury control, on the other hand, has not been viewed as a separate discipline by any of the several professional groups upon which it touches. Its literature is widely scattered and uses several technical languages barely understood by persons without special training in fields such as engineering, medicine, psychology, ergonomics, law enforcement, government, sociology, or architecture.

Furthermore, for these professions injury is simply an unwanted by-product of their major professional concerns. Consequently, work in this "nuisance" area is usually aimed at solving immediate problems that are seen to have limited scope, rather than at contributing to a more generalized view of the field. At the same time, members of each of these professional groups often believe that their limited attentions represent the best and sometimes the sole useful approach to the problem, and they may be reluctant to work with others who see the problem somewhat differently.

This brings us to the several goals of this book. First will be an attempt to familiarize readers with some of the newer conceptual approaches to analyzing injury producing situations and to bringing about prevention where possible and amelioration where prevention is not possible. Second, these concepts will be applied to an examination in detail of a wider range of injury situations than is commonly considered in any one place. Attention will be given not only to injury on the highway but in various other forms of transportation as well, and to injury in other settings, including home, recreation, work, and public places and institutions. The chapters have been grouped to examine injury in a variety of activity settings, to consider unique problems that plague particular population groups, and to examine the effectiveness of specific types of countermeasures. In a few cases, such as with falls, thermal injuries, or poisoning, which take place primarily in the home, I have taken liberties with the above framework and have devoted chapters to specific mechanisms of injury that occur predominantly in certain locations. Third, and perhaps the most difficult, I have sought wherever possible to examine relevant similarities and dissimilarities of injury patterns between the North American cultural and environmental contexts and those of other parts of the world.

Although the book ranges widely and, I hope, fairly comprehensively, I do not perceive it as being exhaustive. More attention is devoted to some problems than to others, reflecting both my own biases and the vagaries of literature available. Information about injury problems and solutions outside the North American continent, Western Europe, and Australia is particularly sparse because more work appears to be occurring in these countries than in others.

Also, the book does not attempt to promote any one method as most important or most useful for reducing the toll. Until recently, the major emphasis both in word and deed was on countermeasures that attempt to alter or regulate people either by voluntary means or through coercion. Although this emphasis on changing people continues in most programs, there is now some shift toward environmental or passive countermeasures. Some individuals, in fact, have suggested that the old approaches should largely be abandoned and that most attention should be directed toward environmental countermeasures.

I admit to belonging to a middle school of thought that maintains that historically inadequate consideration has been given to environmental controls and that the balance still is weighted too heavily toward human-oriented countermeasures. Some of the human approaches, however, have been proven successful, or appear to have good likelihood for success if further developed. Therefore, a broad but selective range of efforts is warranted and will be described. This range includes both efforts that can be applied at the individual level and those that more properly should be applied across entire communities or nations or even internationally.

Finally, although the book is intended to have a scholarly base of information, I hope it is not for scholars alone. One of the major deficiencies of efforts in this field is the fact that, even more than in other endeavors, researchers and practitioners appear to be unable to communicate and often, in fact, hardly know of each other's existence. This is not primarily a cookbook of specific dos and don'ts; but it is also not intended to be a research text of use only to a limited segment of the many who are concerned with injury. In that one sense I hope that this book will be comprehensive, providing information of use both to those who are predominantly "thinkers" and to those whom circumstances require and permit to be more active "doers." Reflecting my own training as a physician, the ultimate goal of this book is not knowledge, but rather the reduction of unnecessary death and suffering.

2
Definitions of Injury Events

At first thought it hardly seems necessary to define an accident—or an unintentional injury event, as it will be called here for reasons to be explained later. Such events have plagued the human race for centuries. They seem to be unanticipated, strike quickly, leave injury or property damage, and often appear to choose their victims by chance.

According to Webster's Twentieth Century Dictionary (second edition) an accident is "an event that occurs without one's foresight or expectation, that proceeds from an unknown cause, or is an unusual effect of a known cause, and thus unexpected, or that is an unfortunate occurrence or mishap, especially if resulting in injury." Other sources state that accidents occur "by chance," and through "lack of intention or necessity."

These definitions, however, leave as many questions as they answer. Why don't we usually consider heart attacks to be accidents? They lack intention and are unexpected. Studies now suggest that many sudden deaths of infants are attributable to instability of breathing mechanisms among the newborn, rather than to suffocation from bedding. Should such deaths be considered to be accident or illness?

Should we categorize liver failure in a worker who is suddenly exposed to large amounts of chemical toxic to the liver in the same way as in another worker who has the same damage as a result of less extreme but still excessive exposures occurring over a period of ten years?

Why is it not considered an accident if people have diarrhea because a cook unintentionally stuck a finger infected by staphylococcus into food? Using the same logic, shouldn't an infection of a laboratory worker from an unexpected puncture by a dirty hypodermic needle be considered an accident? If two men are boxing and one gets killed is that an accident?

Having thoroughly muddied the waters with questions about what appear to be arbitrary decisions in classification, let us now try to describe more precisely what will be the subject of this book and then explain why the events so described will be called "unintentional injuries" rather than "accidents."

First, it must be realized that the definitions of injury and illness change over time as knowledge about causation changes and as there is new information about which problems are related that were originally thought to be dissimilar and which are now seen to be less similar than originally thought. We no longer diagnose death from a broken heart or old age, although those used to be acceptable medical diagnoses. Sometimes the changes in diagnostic terminology are logical consequences of new knowledge. At other times distinctions made between two related conditions are still purely arbitrary.

In this book *unintentional injury events* will be defined as events in which (1) injury occurs over a relatively short period of time—at most, seconds or minutes, (2) the harmful outcome was not sought, and (3) the injury resulted either from one of the forms of physical energy in the environment (kinetic, chemical, thermal, electrical, or ionizing radiation) or because normal body mechanisms for using such energy were blocked by external means (such as by drowning).

Using this definition, the questions raised above can be easily answered. Neither heart attacks, nor food poisoning, nor those sudden deaths of infants attributable to abnormal breathing mechanisns would be called "accidents" because the injuries are not generally perceived to result from physical energy. The puncture from a hypodermic needle, however, involves kinetic energy. The infection is merely a complication of the initial event. Liver failure from rapid release of a toxic chemical would be an "accidental" *injury* because of the short time interval, but arbitrarily such tissue damage over a longer time period would be classified as an occupational *illness* despite the fact that the basic mechanism is the same. Finally, a death resulting from boxing would be an unintentional injury if the goal was to defeat an opponent by outpointing and possibly injuring him, but not to the extent that such injuries would be long lasting.

This distinction, of course, is in itself somewhat arbitrary. Biochemical reactions are operational tools of all living organisms, and one could easily argue that all diseases result from alteration of patterns involving physical energy. The distinction used here, however, will follow more traditional causal concepts associated with ideas about infectious diseases, trauma, psychosocial problems, genetic manifestations, and so forth.

We now turn to one of the major differences between the dictionary definitions and the definitions used here. Webster's Twentieth Century Dictionary refers to "an event that takes place without foresight or expectation" while the Third New International Dictionary described an accident as "occurring by chance" and as "an unforeseen unplanned event or conclusion."

Throughout this book we will document that, contrary to these dictionary definitions, such events as a group are substantially *nonrandom* and that they *do not* occur by chance. While no single injury event—just as no single heart attack—can be predicted with complete accuracy, to a substantial degree its likelihood can be foreseen and even *quantitatively* predicted for specific populations and circumstances, thus permitting rate setting by insurance companies. Such events may be unwanted, but they are not or should not be unexpected.

This failure of usual definitions to describe reality is one reason why the term *accident* is not entirely satisfactory. But yet more important reasons exist. Throughout history accidents have been looked upon as acts of God, a logical consequence of sinful behavior, or primarily the result of carelessness, thoughtlessness, unawareness, or ignorance. In fact, some of these words form part of dictionary definitions of the term *accident,* and insurance policies still talk about "acts of God." Many drivers still carry St. Christopher charms and believe in their protective power. These notions of causation can be shown to be both largely inaccurate and overly simplistic.

In order to clear the mind of old and lingering connotations, therefore, we will simply use two words that describe the event without attributing causation. The event we are concerned with results in injury to people or property: consequences we wish to focus on and avoid. Furthermore, the type of injury we are referring to here occurs unintentionally, as opposed to suicide, assault, or homicide. We are thus ready to examine the circumstances and control of *unintentional injury*.

3
How Injury Events Occur

Several explanatory models for injury events are in current use, some of which are described by Benner.[1] The simplest, least accurate, but most commonly accepted is the single cause model, in which each injury event is seen as the direct and total result of a single identifiable cause. The perception of injury events as acts of God or fate is one example of this model, probably having its origin in the apparent—but not actual—randomness of such events. This "caused by God" approach is not scientifically verifiable and will not be considered further.

A more common application of the concept is seen in police and newspaper accounts of highway crashes and fatalities as being caused by excessive speed or use of alcohol. Let us examine such a crash. Two people have been traveling at ten to fifteen miles above the speed limit for the past six miles since leaving a tavern where they had too much to drink. The driver loses control on a sharp curve and the vehicle strikes a tree. The passenger is partly ejected and killed. The driver has minor injuries.

Some would ascribe this crash and its results to speed because that was the most obvious driver "error" at the moment of loss of control. Others would attribute the event to underlying impairment by alcohol, especially if the driver is in an obviously drunken state. Either choice leaves questions unanswered.

First, how does one decide between alcohol and speed as the cause—for the model permits of only a single cause? Second, if the driver was both impaired and speeding for several miles why didn't he get into trouble until this moment? Finally, why was one occupant killed while the other only had minor injuries?

The single cause model does little to resolve these issues. Its advantage—but also its overriding disadvantage—is its simplicity. It focuses attention on arbitrary and incomplete casual mechanisms that neither educate nor guide people to effective action.

The second model, which is not in common use, assumes the random interaction of multiple factors in the initiation and ultimate resolution of the event. The fact that we can both distinguish and predict frequencies of potential injury events as well as the frequencies of their ultimate outcomes if we are given enough information about contributory factors provides substantial evidence that this model is neither accurate nor useful.

The third model considers the injury event as the outcome of three phases. Human/environmental interaction during a pre-injury phase that precedes the moment of energy release or mobilization is followed by an injury phase in which the released energy may be transmitted to people and property so that physiological homeostasis is lost and damage may occur. In the post-injury phase ultimate outcome may be determined by actions aimed at regaining homeostasis.

Although this model has some apparent exceptions that require explanation (to be discussed later), it is fairly parsimonious and relates well to the common medical model of primary, secondary, and tertiary prevention (or prevention of disease, prevention of complications, and rehabilitation). It is the model preferred by this author and will be described in greater detail in this chapter and used throughout the rest of the book.

The fourth model is the so-called systems-analysis, in which an attempt is made *a priori* to identify all possible things that can fail in the design, construction, use, degradation, and destruction of a product or environment. This model is not well known to either health professionals, law enforcement personnel, or educators concerned with safety. But it is used extensively by engineers in the design or evaluation of large and complex industrial operations, such as in the aerospace industry or pipeline construction.

Three approaches to systems-analysis may be used:

> The hazard analysis addresses the total system from the standpoint of energy sources which can get out of control. . . .
>
> The logic tree or fault tree technique begins with the selection of one or more events that can not be allowed to occur as the undesired event. This event, which may otherwise be described as a postulated accident, may have to do with the public at risk, the system at risk, or external facilities at risk.
>
> As soon as the undesired events are selected, the system can be analyzed to determine the subevent that could cause the postulated accident. Analysis of the system begins with the top undesired event and spreads out in a tree-shaped diagram, proceeding down into the system to the point that the hazard is identified together with those events and conditions which can activate the hazard into the accident sequence.
>
> For each undesired event, it is necessary to reason backwards from the selected event to visualize the ways it could occur. In other words, fault paths are developed graphically through the branches of the tree

> comprising the analysis, from the top undesired event down to the least likely contributing factor. This process allows the analyst to visualize a variety of potential failures and measure the effect of such failures on the next higher level of the tree. . . . Once the probability of occurrence of each event has been determined, the relative importance of the various events becomes apparent. Further, the effects of system changes to remove hazards can be assessed.
>
> The use of the Failure Mode and Effect (FMEA) analysis method entails an examination of each component of the system on an individual basis to determine first, how it could fail, and secondly, the impact of that failure on the system. This method is strictly hardware oriented and must be applied to every component in the system. For example, select a valve. This valve can fail open, or it can fail closed. What is the impact on the system if it fails open? If it fails closed? And so on throughout the system. Those components which, by failing, can cause a catastrophic condition are identified as hazards.[2]

The system safety model has an engineering and hardware orientation and in some ways is the exact antithesis of the approaches of law enforcement and education personnel. Its important advantage is its potential completeness in exploring an entire system from top to bottom. But it is rather cumbersome and potentially rather superficial in dealing with human components of the system. Furthermore, a system analysis is no more complete than the ability of the designer of the analysis to identify accurately all of the components and potential failure modes. This problem, of course, is not limited to this particular model.

Systems-analysis may be able to identify what may go wrong, how it may do so, and with what potential effect; but it is quite incapable by itself of determining relative frequencies with which these events may happen. This determination of frequency is a task commonly undertaken through use of epidemiologic methods, a investigative area as unknown to most systems safety analysts as system analysis is unknown to most members of the health professions. The epidemiologic approach, of course, is not limited to use by epidemiologists, nor the systems approach to systems safety specialists. In some cases frequency determination, such as of exceedingly rare events, is not possible through epidemiology but can be estimated with some accuracy by means of laboratory experimentation. Examples are destructive testing of metals or other components of hardware systems, and measurement of the nature and frequency of some forms of psychological response.

Commonly, the assessment of an injury problem and the approach to its solution goes something like this:

1. Hypotheses are established based on single cases, anecdote, or nonsystematic observation.

2. The hypotheses about cause and frequency are tested through epidemiologic, sociologic, and possibly engineering analysis of real-world experience and through selected laboratory simulation.
3. Building upon initial data about frequency, severity, and causal factors so obtained, system designing then begins, identifying all possible branches that need to be considered to deal with types of failures that may occur, relative probabilities, and likely results. In some cases it may appear that the first step, rather than the third, is a systems-safety analysis: for example, in considering the injury and property loss potential for an entirely new system, such as the first nuclear power plant. Such analysis, however, probably does not arise *de novo* but is based in large part on hypotheses and previous experiences drawn from system components or somewhat similar systems (such as nuclear weaponry, nuclear physics laboratories, and conventional power plants) that have been encountered in other contexts.
4. Testing and further development of the system model takes place through additional epidemiologic, laboratory, and other studies, including simulation.
5. Priorities for countermeasures are established based on selection of those aspects of the problem that seem to be associated either with greatest frequency, severity, or both and that simultaneously have greatest likelihood of technical, economic, and cultural feasibility.
6. Finally, one or more countermeasures may be applied, preferably with arrangements for adequate evaluation.

This brings us to the fifth model, which builds on both the third and fourth models but is more amenable to the identification of serendipitous information that may be important but could be overlooked through use of the other schemes. It is clear that no one of the models in existence is perfect, and the imperfections tend to perpetuate themselves in biases of data collection that are built into each of the systems. A model, therefore, that combines the advantages of the other approaches while avoiding their limitations would be extremely useful.

Benner refers to the fifth method as "multilinear events sequencing."[3] As shown in figure 3–1 this model is based on identification of all factors that either disrupt homeostasis or that promote return to homeostasis. He notes that it permits much more accurate definition of the moment at which the event begins than do other injury event analysis models. While this model appears to complement models three and four, it stops short of considering issues commonly examined in the post-injury phase of the third model.

The emphasis on homeostasis is a comfortable approach for health

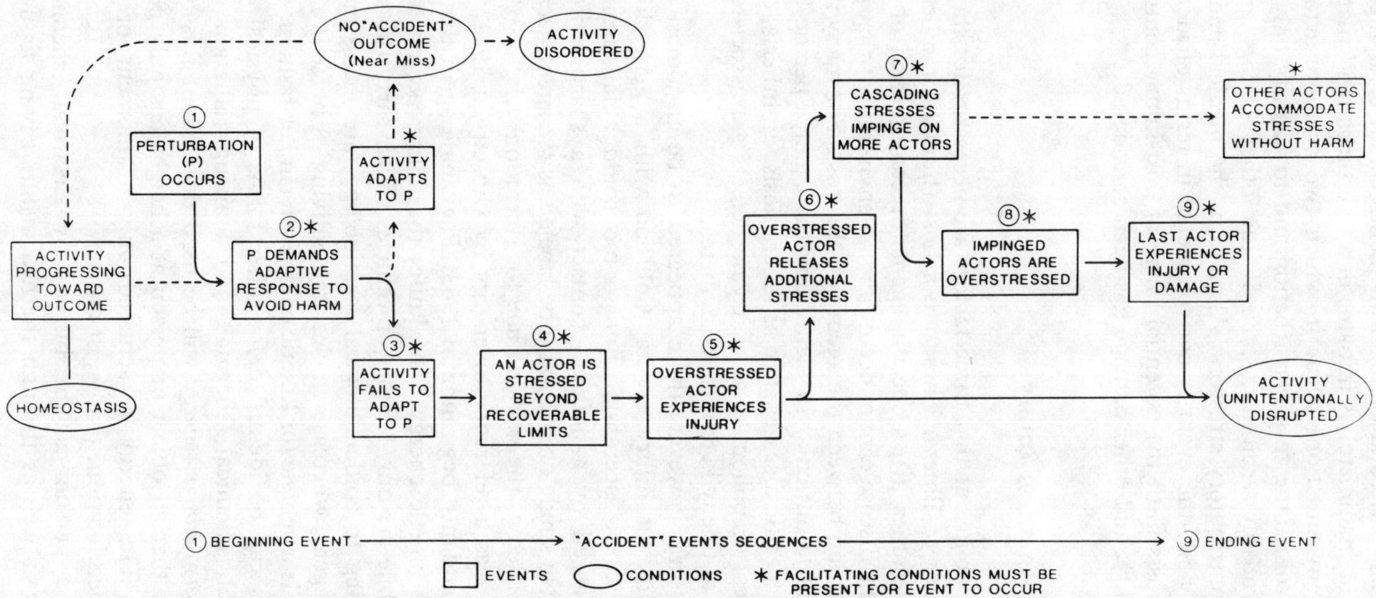

Source: Reprinted with permission from L. Benner, Jr., "Accident Investigations: Multilinear Events Sequencing Methods," *Journal of Safety Research* 7 (1975):67–73 (a joint publication of National Safety Council and Pergamon Press).

Figure 3–1. Benner's Multilinear Events Sequencing Model.

professionals. I am less comfortable with identification of a single actor (either animate or inanimate) as initiator of a "perturbation" that affects homeostasis. Many situations occur in which two or more actors may simultaneously contribute to a perturbation and to identify only one as *the* actor is probably arbitrary, even if the other factors are then considered as contributory stressors. Also, from the medical and public health point of view, the event is not completed in terms of identifying future societal costs until the potential range of post-injury contributors to death, disability, and other damage has been considered.

Energy as the Agent of Injury

Epidemiologists point out that three factors are necessary for the occurrence of an injury or illness. These are a host (human or other living organism that becomes ill), a specific agent (or combination of agents) without which the disease cannot occur, and an environment that permits a harmful interaction between the agent and the host. For many illnesses there has been little difficulty in identifying the agent. Specific bacteria or viruses cause specific diseases such as tuberculosis, diphtheria, cholera, hepatitis, measles, or poliomyelitis. Enzyme defects are associated with conditions such as phenylketonuria or diabetes.

For many years, however, there appeared to be an almost infinite number of agents for injury events. Collision with a glass door, for example, could cause laceration. But so too could a fall against the ground, being gored by a bullock, contact with a sharp knife, or a highway crash. No single object could be labeled as *the* agent because no one could be isolated as the *sine qua non* for laceration.

The answer was a reference to energy by Gibson[4] in 1961, further developed by Haddon[5,6] beginning in 1963. The single agent that causes all lacerations is kinetic energy. The knife, the falling person, and the moving automobile are only vectors or vehicles which carry this energy. Vectors, according to epidemiological terminology, are living means of transmitting an agent, whereas vehicles are nonliving. A horse is a vector, and an automobile a vehicle for kinetic energy. In similar fashion, specific types of injuries can be identified for other forms of physical energy, namely electrical, chemical, thermal, and ionizing radiation energy. (Although the term *kinetic energy* will be used throughout this book, it should be noted that an object or person at a height has only potential kinetic energy. The energy is actuated only at moment of abrupt acceleration or deceleration: that is, of impact.)

Of course, a person can be burned by electrical, chemical, or radiation energy as well as through thermal insult. Living tissues have only a limited number of ways in which they can respond to damage. One of the basic epidemiologic tenets is that a single effect (whether it be a burn or a fever) may be the result of multiple causes. What distinguishes one disease or injury from another is not single effects but rather that effects commonly are grouped into unique syndromes or combinations that we designate as specific diagnostic entities. Thus, differences in location, configuration, time of appearance, and other circumstances of a burn might help to distinguish an injury caused by contact with lye versus one that resulted from spending too much time in the sun or from falling against a floor furnace.

But why can the kinetic energy that causes a laceration break a bone instead or result only in a contusion or abrasion? One answer is that the energy may differ in quantity, in mode of transfer, or in sensitivity of tissue struck. Another answer involves a second epidemiologic tenet, the corollary to the first. Just as a single effect may be the result of multiple causes, so a single cause may have multiple effects. Measles, for example, usually brings about fever, cough, rash, and sensitivity of eyes to bright light but also can cause deafness and heart or brain damage. In similar fashion, depending on the circumstances, each of the forms of physical energy can have more than one effect on living organisms.

People and Tasks

The forms of energy surround us and are used in many ways to make life functions easier. If energy is diffuse, it can serve people only minimally, but if gathered together or massed within a limited time and space, it can be used more effectively. Examples include the massing of thermal energy in a stove, of kinetic energy in a running person or a moving motor vehicle, of electricity in a glowing light, or of specific chemical energy in a bottle of aspirin. Extreme environmental changes, such as storms, earthquakes, or tidal waves, also represent massings of energy that contribute to earth structure, climate, atmospheric transport of nutrients, and growth capabilities for plants and animals, including humans.

The safe use of energy that has been massed by humans, or the safe exposure of people to forms of energy massed by nature, depends on two generic factors: the level of functioning of the person and the demands of the tasks inherent in making the energy serve the functions we wish. A few examples will clarify the meaning of this statement. Each person has certain attributes that vary from moment to moment and from one person to another. One of these is one's knowledge about oneself in relation to different aspects of the environment. Such knowledge depends on basic intelligence, experience, education, short- and long-term memory, and attitudes and belief systems which one may bring as cultural heritage. Contributing to this is the ability to receive information about the environment through inherent senses such as sight, hearing, touch, smell, taste, vibratory sense, and vestibular or balancing function.

Another attribute is the ability to make rapid judgments about oneself in relation to the environment as a result of the combination of information received through the senses and knowledge applied in interpreting such information. Finally, there must be the capability to act in response to judgments that suggest that danger may exist. In order to act effectively to the variety of tasks that we must perform daily, a person usually must have a certain minimum of range of motion, strength, stamina, speed, and balance.

In summary, therefore, each person must have the capability to receive information correctly, process it in timely fashion, and react appropriately. Some people can put these functions together with a high degree of ability and consistency. Others may have deficits in one or more of these capabilities or may be able to combine them only on some occasions but not on others. Furthermore, a person with a given level of capability may or may not function at that particular level at any one time. That people vary from each other and within themselves over time is neither good nor bad. It is simply a fact of *all* living beings, whether human or other animal, that forms part of the equation in the occurrence of injury events.

Next we will examine task demands. Some tasks are extremely complex, requiring extensive learning, judgment, and intelligence or all three. Other tasks require use of several senses simultaneously or the ability to pay attention to multiple stimuli or signals at one time. In other cases there is a requirement for quick action, dexterity, strength, balance, or stamina. Tasks may vary in demand not only from one task to another but also for a single type of task over time. In general, the more automated the task the easier it is to perform, and the more consistent it is likely to be.

The Pre-Injury Phase

Let us now put the person with his or her capabilities and limitations together with the task and its unique set of demands. As long as the actual performance of the person exceeds the demands of the task at all times there is no likelihood that an event potentially capable of producing injury will occur from the interaction. If for any reason, however, the task exceeds the performance level, the energy being managed or controlled through the task is no longer in control and may be available to cause injury.

This moment at which task demand exceeds the performance is commonly referred to as an "accident." Here we will describe it and the immediately preceding period as the pre-injury phase of the event. It is pre-injury, since, as we shall see, simply because energy is not under complete control doesn't necessarily mean that injury has to occur. The phase during which injury occurs will be called, logically, the injury phase.

Three types of situations exist in which demands of a task may, momentarily at least, exceed the performance of the individual. In the first type what is commonly referred to as human "failure" may occur. As an example, a person who ordinarily has been functioning at a level of performance that is average for most people suddenly begins to perform at a lower level. This can happen because of an acute episode of a medical condition, such as epilepsy, diabetes, heart disease, or mental illness or because a person is temporarily under the effects of a drug, such as alcohol or carbon monoxide, of paramenstrual stress,[7] or of certain social or societal pressures. Furthermore, people have short-term natural or circadian cycles, causing specific aspects of behavior and physiology to change from hour to hour throughout the day.[8] The relationships between these cycles and injury risk appear not to have been examined, however.

As the second example of human "failure" some individuals may perform consistently below average for what people usually display to accomplish a given type of task. This may occur because a person has a chronic or long-term problem such as heart disease, arthritis, senile dementia, birth defect, poor coordination, or low intelligence. It may also reflect the fact that the person is inexperienced with the particular task and will remain so handicapped only as long as knowledge and experience are lacking, or that the person has some ongoing erroneous attitudes or beliefs about how the task should be performed.

With temporary impairment, task demands are at greater-than-average risk of exceeding performance only during the intervals when function is less than average. A person who is consistently less than average in performance, however, is also consistently more likely than average to be overwhelmed at least occasionally by usual task demands.

The same sorts of patterns apply to task demand. Given an average level of performance, the performance and task lines may cross because the task has suddenly and temporarily become substantially more demanding than usual or because the task is always excessively demanding. Some sudden increases in task demand are a tire blowout, an extensive pot hole or crater that suddenly appears in the road, or a portion of the highway that begins to slide away as one is driving over it. Less unique sudden increases in task requirements are the distraction caused by a child who demands a parent's attention or a car, person, or domestic animal that suddenly impinges on the expected path of the vehicle. An extremely winding dirt road is a task that is always excessively demanding compared to the average road in the typical developed nation.

As a task suddenly increases in demand, the performance level of the person also increases somewhat. In some cases, however, it may not be sufficient to prevent crossing of the two lines. The change on the part of the person represents utilization of some of his or her spare capacity until the person reaches maximum performance level of which he or she is capable. This occurs as an attempt to avoid what has been perceived by the person to be an impending disaster because the task is getting increasingly out of control or, to use Benner's terminology, a perturbation has occurred that is altering the person/task homeostasis. *Spare capacity* refers to the difference between the person's current level of performance and the maximum level of performance he or she is potentially able to produce at any given moment in order to prevent task demand from exceeding performance level.

We are now ready to examine the third type of failure situation, one that is commonly overlooked because people tend to think only of human failure or only of task overload. In this case (figure 3–2) both the person and the task contribute to the event. The person may be temporarily or consistently functioning at *somewhat* less than average level for most people performing this type of task, at the same time that the task is

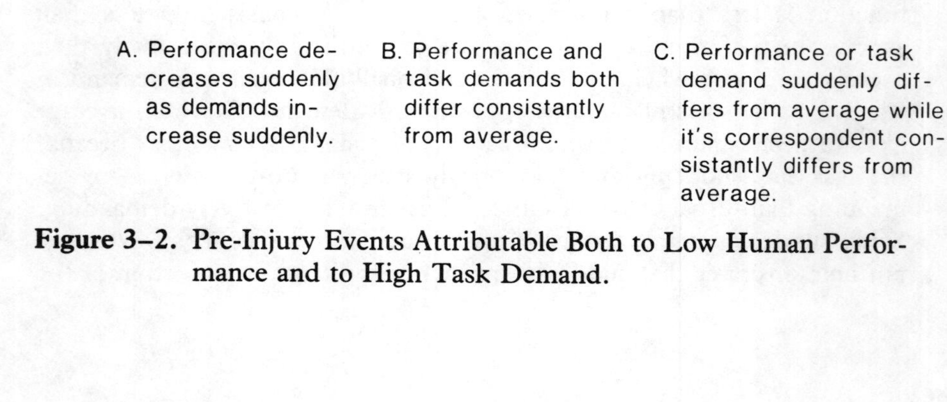

Figure 3–2. Pre-Injury Events Attributable Both to Low Human Performance and to High Task Demand.

temporarily or consistently *somewhat* more than usually demanding for this type of task. Thus, because of joint contribution the two lines are close together and have significantly greater-than-average likelihood of crossing.

Why is this sort of relationship so often overlooked when it may, in fact, be the most frequent mechanism in the initiation of injury events? One explanation is that most of us are taught to oversimplify explanations of causation. Thus, we are more likely to be trained for and attuned to seeking single causal factors than to identifying and teasing out more complex etiologies, perhaps involving several conditions acting simultaneously.

Probably equally important, many of the relative increases in task demand are so common and so subtle that most of us respond to them subconsciously, and we do not realize that it is only because we usually have sufficient spare capacity that we are able to deal effectively with sudden and sometimes unnecessary increases in task load. Fletcher Platt has estimated that in United States traffic there may be two hundred events per mile requiring twenty decisions, resulting in an error every two miles, a near collision every 500 miles, and respectively a collision, injury, and fatality every 61,000 miles, 430,000 miles and 16 million miles.[9]

In illustration of the subtleties of this human/environmental interface, a person who is driving in rush-hour freeway traffic and who wishes to change lanes may have to make quick observations, decisions, and maneuvers in order to complete the task successfully. This is a typical stress situation that most of us handle effectively most of the time despite the stress.

But if the driver owned an early 1970 automobile that was designed with a very wide rear pillar between the back side windows and the rear window, he might be unable to see around the pillar in the limited time available and might "overlook" a subcompact vehicle or a motorcycle in the blind spot.

Had any one of the factors—the heavy traffic, the wide pillar, or the small size of the other vehicle—not been present, the event probably would not have occurred. And since most of us do not usually face this combination of circumstances, do so only rarely, or somehow manage to avoid crashing despite "inappropriate responses," we and the police are likely to attribute the crash to "poor judgment," "carelessness," or "failure to observe," when in fact the individual involved may have been quite conscientious, peering very intently, and using excellent judgment based on the limited information and options available to him.

Only very few studies have begun to consider such combinations of factors, and they reach conclusions about causation that differ substantially from the official statistics that most of us—no matter what nation we are in—see in the newspapers, reports of official and voluntary agencies, and pamphlets or articles written about "accident prevention."

Varying human capabilities and spare capacity and different task demands have been combined in figure 3–3, which shows that, as the task gets more demanding, it (1) reaches a point at which it is beyond the capability of the least competent (with respect to that task) members of society and (2) reduces the amount of spare capacity that more competent members may have remaining at any given moment so that they can avert disaster if there is a sudden further increase in task demand, a sudden decrease in their own performance, or both.

Another way of describing the nature of the human/task interaction and the inevitability of at least occasional problems in that relationship has been provided by Mihalasky as follows:

> There is no sense debating whether people should make errors. The

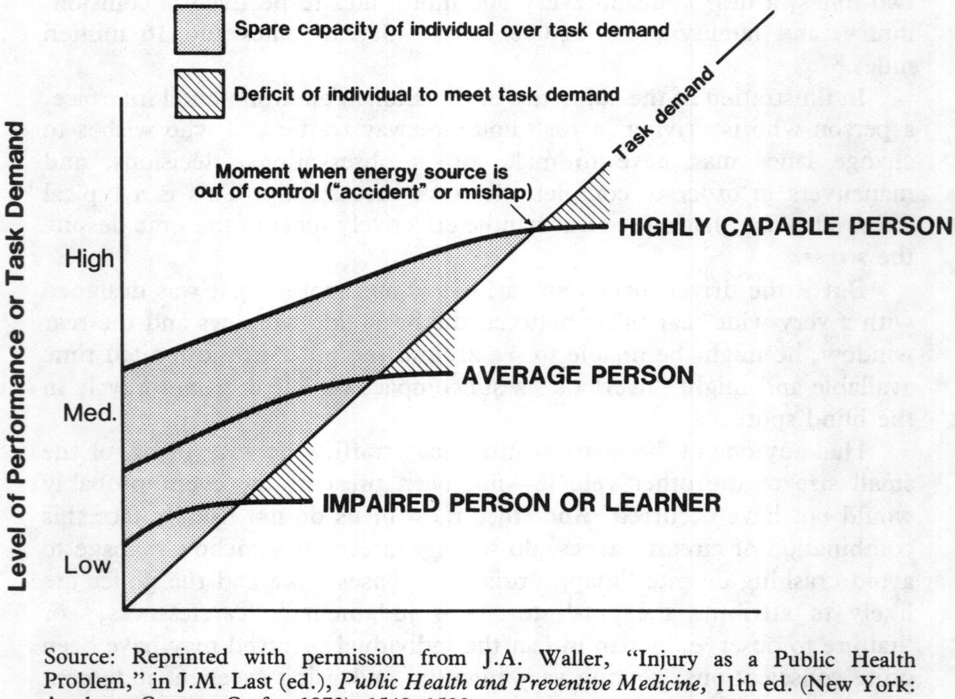

Source: Reprinted with permission from J.A. Waller, "Injury as a Public Health Problem," in J.M. Last (ed.), *Public Health and Preventive Medicine,* 11th ed. (New York: Appleton-Century Crofts, 1973), 1549–1592.

Figure 3–3. Relationship between Human Performance and Task Demand.

> fact is that they do make errors, and their error rate can be mathematically calculated and predicted just like the failure rate for equipment. . . . Error is, in fact, a function of human variability. It occurs because the human being is capable of performing so many different activities in so many different ways. There would not be errors if (a) there were no tolerance limits; or (b) the acceptable limits exceeded the variability found in human beings; or (c) the number of opportunities to commit an error was so small, that the error would not occur.
>
> Error is . . . an action that exceeds some limit of acceptability. . . . Translated into practical terms, error can be: (a) failure to perform the required activity; (b) performing the required activity incorrectly; (c) performing the required activity correctly but out of sequence; and (d) performing a nonrequired activity.[10]

Let us assume that a point has been reached at which task demand exceeds performance level and the real or potential energy that was being managed is now no longer under control. At that moment the pre-injury phase has ended and the injury phase of the event begins.

The Injury Phase

The fact that energy is out of control does not in and of itself mean that an injury must necessarily occur. Several intervening conditions determine *whether* injury will occur and *how severe* it will be.

Perhaps the most important determinant of injury occurrence and severity is the actual amount of energy that has been massed and is potentially available to injure. A cup of boiling water has more thermal energy than does one that is tepid. No matter how fast one hits a ping pong ball with the paddle its basic mass is sufficiently small so that it is not likely to "carry" a very harmful load of kinetic energy. The same cannot be said for a golf ball because its massing of energy is much greater. A single small cloud is unlikely to create much harm even if it rains its entire contents almost instantaneously. But a conglomeration of several large clouds may have sufficient energy mass to potentially create considerable discomfort and some actual harm.

What happens if the boiling water spills or if the clouds release their rain? If the hot water is released drop by drop, it may cause less of a scald than if it all is dumped at one time. The clouds will create less damage and quite possibly contribute benefit if their rain is deposited over several hours instead of in a ten-minute squall. The basic principle is that a potentially harmful amount of energy, once massed, damages less if the energy is released slowly than if released rapidly.

Assuming the energy is released rapidly enough to injure, it still may not do so if there is some means for either separating people from the energy, as in remote-control handling of radioactive materials, or if the rate of arrival of the energy is sufficiently slow because of intervening dampening effects so that the threshold for tissue damage is not reached.

Dampening also occurs if the energy is spread out not only over time but over space. The ping pong ball, if converted into the shape and size of a bullet or a dart, might conceivably contribute lethal injury simply because the energy has now been further massed. This is a principle noted by Hippocrates about 425 B.C. when he reported that brain damage is more likely to occur if there has been contact with a hard, sharp object rather than with a soft, blunt one.[11]

Finally, given a specified amount of energy, the structures impacted determine whether injury will occur and what will be the severity of that injury. For a given amount and rate of energy transfer, the femoral bone of a young child, if injured at all, will probably have a "green stick" or incomplete fracture because the bone is plaint. But an elderly person stands a much greater chance of having a fracture, and it probably will be complete, perhaps even with severe comminution, because the bone is weak and brittle and because soft tissues surrounding the bone also are less resilient. In addition, the older person may have other health problems that add to the physiologic insult of the injury itself.

The same energy, if transferred to brain tissue or heart instead of the leg might conceivably cause fatal injury, instead of simply creating repairable damage. And because of circadian cycles, there may be more vigorous and successful physiologic response if the injury occurs at certain hours of the day rather than at others.

The basic principles, then, are the following:

1. The greater the mass of energy that exists and is released, and the more rapid the release, the greater the likelihood that injury will occur and that it will be severe.
2. If the energy reaches tissues, the rate of that transfer (ideally described in units of energy per unit of body tissue per unit of time) determines the severity of injury.
3. Severity is also determined by inherent characteristics of the tissue itself and of the organism.

An Alternative Pathway

Although all unintentional injury involves damage by misapplication of physical energy, some such events occur through a mechanism other than the unintentional transfer of energy from an external source to the person. The body carries out its own internal mechanisms for energy management that permits us to maintain a balance or homeostasis with the environment. An event that interferes with this homeostasis can also cause harm through energy misapplication.

In drowning, for example, there is blockage of the normal mechanism for obtaining oxygen and removing carbon dioxide and other waste products of the chemical process known as metabolism. Poisoning may occur because there is direct tissue damage from acids or bases or because a chemical may block or overwhelm specific enzyme systems within the body that also regulate metabolism. Thermal injury can result from the direct application of excessive heat to tissue or conversely may be the effect of removing existing heat created by metabolic processes at a faster rate than the body can produce or deliver more heat. In either case, the damage may be just as severe.

In 1942 DeHaven[12] documented that people can survive falls of from 50 to 150 feet if the forces of those falls can be distributed over a broad enough surface and a long enough time. Subsequently, Stapp,[13] while wearing a four-point shoulder harness, rode a rocket sled and withstood without permanent damage a deceleration from 632 M.P.H. to zero M.P.H. in only 1.4 seconds.

These early studies indicate that, at least with respect to kinetic energy, the human body can take a lot more punishment than had previously been assumed. There now exists a large body of work concerning human tolerance to kinetic energy and to ionizing radiation, as well as a moderate number of studies dealing with injury thresholds for other types of energy.

Many unanswered questions yet remain, however. Problems arise, for example, because of difficulties in relating real world experience to mathematical models based on laboratory studies involving cadavers and animals. Commonly, age of person is not considered in determining tolerance, despite such obvious differences as fractures with greenstick patterns in children and comminution in the elderly. Nor is attention usually given in studies of kinetic energy to the contour of the impacting object. Instead, for purposes of replication most researchers tend to use a standardized blunt impacting surface. Regarding injury to head and spine, however, substantial concern has been paid to angle of impact and degree of flexion of tissues at time of impact.

Recently, studies suggest that chemical energy may act synergistically with kinetic trauma to create more harmful effects than might occur with either alone. Work by Flamm et al,[14] shows that among cats without alcohol that were impacted to the spine at 200 gm cm, none had complete permanent paralysis and 22 percent had partial permanent paralysis. In cats previously given alcohol, 86 percent and 7 percent, respectively, had complete permanent and partial permanent paralysis at this impact level. Another study[15] points to greater extravisation of blood around cerebral stab wounds in intoxicated animals. Recent work by Brodner et al.[16] suggests that potentiation may be the result of antidiuresis and fluid retention from increased tissue hydration associated with alcohol.

Attention is now being paid as well to additive effects on the total organism of several minor injuries. Work by Baker et al.[17] and by Somers[18] indicates that moderate trauma to two or more anatomic areas may have as great a harmful effect on the total organism as does a single serious injury to one area. Attempts to identify thresholds are not made any easier by the fact that a biological gradient of disease exists, with a range of severity among individuals responding to a standardized insult.

Kinetic Energy

In 1975 the diverse literature on impact trauma, complicated by nonstandard terminology for forces applied, was summarized by Carr et al.[19] (Unless specifically referenced, studies in the following paragraphs are from this report.) Most of the studies have been concerned with serious injuries and the data generally reflect this, rather than showing thresholds to minor trauma.

Deceleration forces produce several types of injury: stretching, tearing, crushing, bursting, laceration, and cytopathologic injuries (concussion). Patrick[20] identifies a total of nine factors that affect tolerance to injury. These are relative velocity, impact site, mass of the impactor, area of contact, geometry of impacted area, surface hardness, surface roughness, direction of impact, and impact duration. Altering any of these can either increase or decrease the likelihood that injury will occur or will be severe.

The occurrence of an injury reflects a relationship between the effects of impact magnitude and duration, in which the duration represents the number of milliseconds at peak magnitude. For headward impact to the whole body experimental evidence indicates that the tolerance limit for moderate injury is a pulse of about 25G maintained for approximately 0.2 sec. (*G* is the number of times the apparent weight of an object or body is increased during acceleration or deceleration. Thus, a 10-lb object at 10Gs would have an impact force equal to 100 lbs.) Some vertebral compression fractures do occasionally occur at this level. Tolerance is greatly reduced when the spinal column is in a flexed position or is misaligned laterally. For footward acceleration, the tolerance is approximately 15G for 0.1 sec, while for spineward acceleration it is 45G for 0.1 sec or 25G for 0.2 sec. Little data exist on tolerance to lateral acceleration.

Head injuries are the most dangerous type of injury resulting from impacts and are affected both by shear stresses, by head rotation, and by the impact phenomenon itself. Figure 3–4 shows tolerance data for head impact, but it is relevant only to a frontal impact on a flat hard surface.

Nahum et al. noted significant differences in skull fracture levels between men and women and that the thickness of skin and other soft tissue has an influence on fracture levels. Swearingen has reported that impacts to the cheek bones as low as 30–40G for 10–40 msec can cause unconsciousness and that with these durations fractures result to nose at 30G, mandible at 40G, cheek bone at 50G, and teeth at 100G.

The neck is reported to be sensitive to injury at relatively low acceleration levels (90–100 lb for localized impact to laryngeal cartilages), while thoracic impact tolerance appears to be in the neighborhood of 1200–1800 lbs. Failing loads for different vertebrae are shown in figure 3–5, and the effects of age on such tolerances appear in figure 3–6. It is

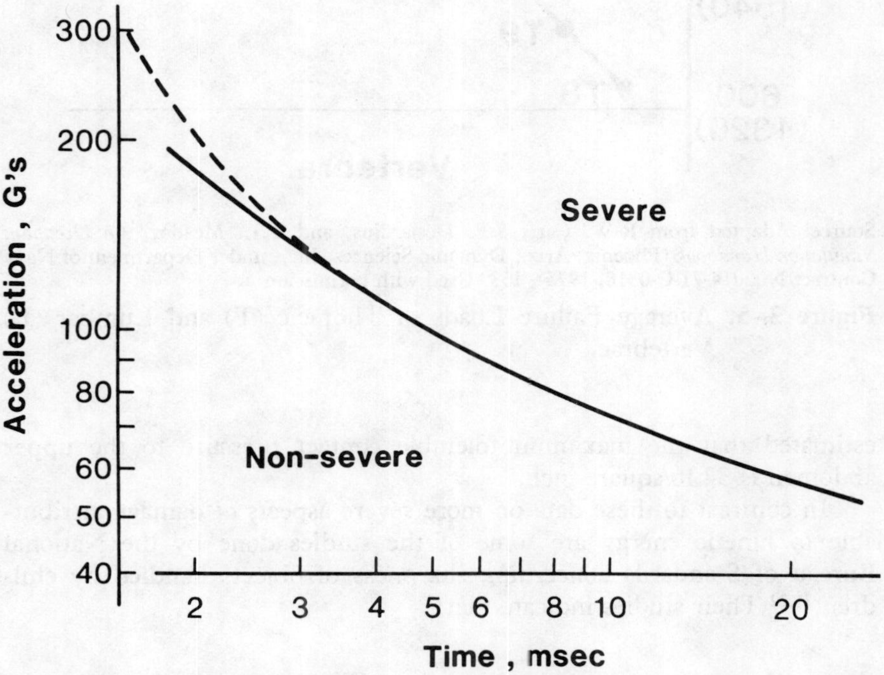

Source: Reprinted with permsision from R.W. Carr, S.P. Desjardin, and T.L. Meador, *An Occupant Simulation Handbook* (Phoenix, Ariz.: Dynamic Science, Inc., under Department of Navy Contract N00014-71-C-0318, 1975), 135.

Figure 3–4. Head Injury Tolerance: Acceleration versus Duration.

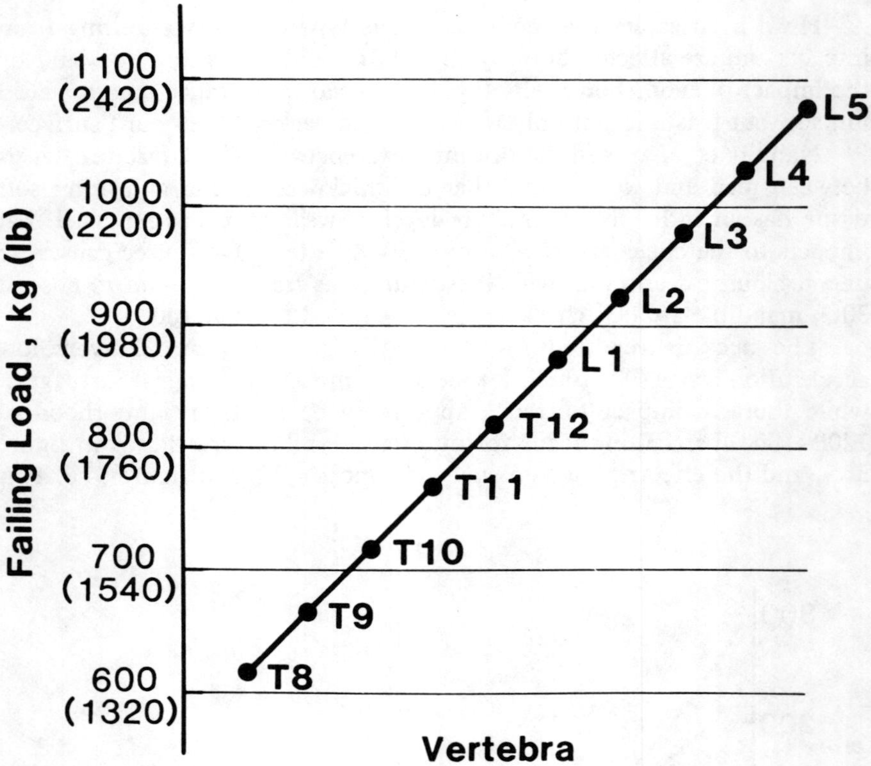

Source: Adapted from R.W. Carr, S.P. Desjardins, and T.L. Meador, *An Occupant Simulation Handbook* (Phoenix, Ariz.: Dynamic Sciences, Inc., under Department of Navy Contract N00014-71-C-0318, 1975), 153. Used with permission.

Figure 3–5. Average Failure Loads of Thoracic (T) and Lumbar (L) Vertebrae.

estimated that the maximum tolerable contact pressure to the upper abdomen is 32 lb/square inch.

In contrast to these data on more severe aspects of damage attributable to kinetic energy are some of the studies done by the National Bureau of Standards concerning sharpness of objects handled by children.[21,22] Their studies indicate that:

1. The tensile strength of human skin reaches near adult levels by age one year;
2. Children ages 5 to 8 can achieve "quick-grab" velocities of 2.1 to 2.5 m/sec with effective hand and forearm weights of 0.3 to 0.6 kg;

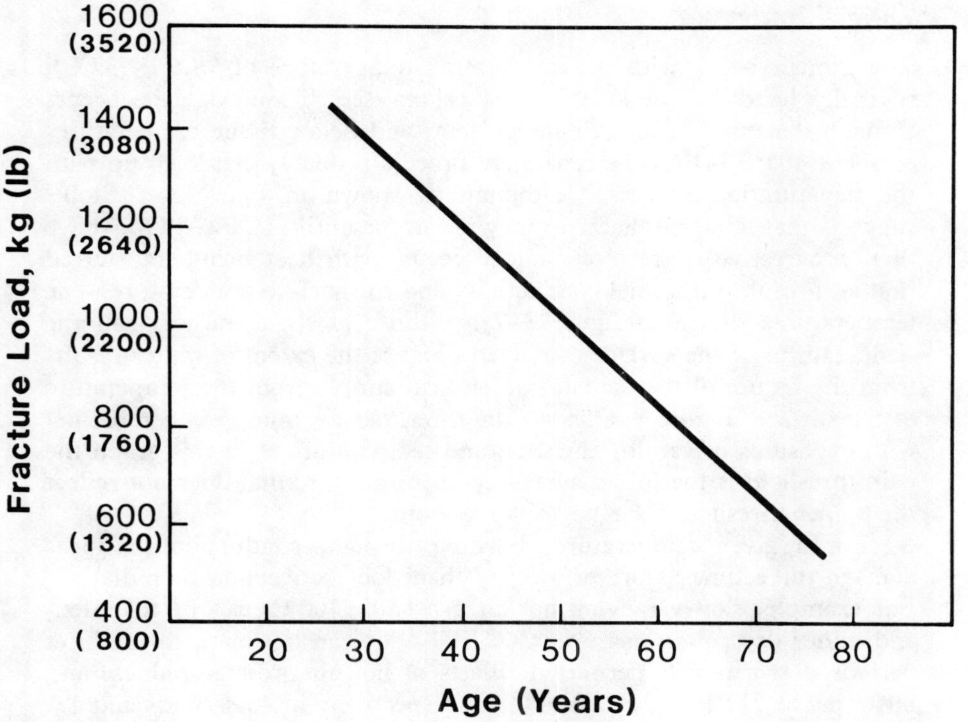

Source: Adapted from R.W. Carr, S.P. Desjardins, and T.L. Meador, *An Occupant Simulation Handbook* (Phoenix, Ariz.: Dynamic Sciences, Inc., under Department of Navy Contract N00014-71-C-0318, 1975), 156. Used with permission.

Figure 3–6. Effect of Age on Vertebral Breaking Strength (Normalized to L5 Vertebra).

3. These anthropometric characteristics are sufficient to cause injury with the average sharp metal surface, such as a knife;
4. The velocity of the knife (in the range of 1 to 10 ft/sec) is of little importance in determining severity of injury, but many edges thought to be safe assuming casual handling must be judged hazardous under impact conditions;
5. Microscopic rather than gross characteristics of sharp metal surfaces do affect injury severity.

Their studies on eye damage potential of propelled objects show that some of the relatively safer projectile toys now being sold in the United States still have enough force to cause damage to the chamber angle of the eye but not to cause peripheral damage or penetration.[23]

Thermal Energy

The human body, with usual operating temperature of 98.6°F (37°C), normally handles heat loads of .04 cal/cm^2/sec. Tissue damage occurs through denaturation of cellular protein, and below tissue temperatures of about 105°F (41°C) the reparative process probably can keep up with the denaturation process,[24] although as shown in figure 3–7 Stoll[25] suggests that failure to keep up may not occur until 111°F (44°C). Above that, progressive degrees of damage occur, with heat being transferred first as a result of thermal conductivity and the surface temperature. The temperatures shown in figure 3–7 are those of tissue rather than the temperatures of the surface contacted because the extent of injury results from the nature of the contact rather than simply from the temperature of the surface. Figure 3–8 shows the threshold for injury via conduction with exposures of varying duration and temperature.[26] In this graph the pain threshold is that of an average person, a figure that does not reflect the higher threshold for many older persons.

For a given temperature, burning through conduction produces damage three times more effectively than does convection or radiation. For example, slowly moving hot air at 212°F (100°C) can be tolerated, and under dry conditions even 300°F (149°C) can be tolerated for brief periods if sweating is permitted. Blasts of hot air produce redness and blistering at 212°F and 392°F (200°C) respectively in 45 seconds and 1.5 seconds. Exposure to a temperature of only 140°F (60°C) by conduction through a heating iron, however, produced subdermal temperatures as high as 131°F (44°C) in only 5 seconds.[24]

Injury can result from temperatures that are excessively low, as well as those that are overly hot. Figure 3–7 also shows the threshold and nature of thermal injuries that are associated with cold.

Chemical Energy

It is not possible to summarize thresholds for injury involving chemical energy because such limits are clearly a function of the mode of action of the chemical. Chemicals such as cyanide or parathion that block the action of highly localized enzyme systems may cause not only injury but fatality if administered in only minute amounts. They cannot be compared, for example, with the effects of carbon monoxide, which replaces oxygen in hemaglobin/oxygen bonds, alcohol, which poisons a wide variety of physiologic mechanisms and probably does so in several ways, or lye or acids, which may actually dissolve tissue.

As examples of this range, only a few drops of cyanide or phosphorus is a lethal dose for most people. Although some individuals are sensitive

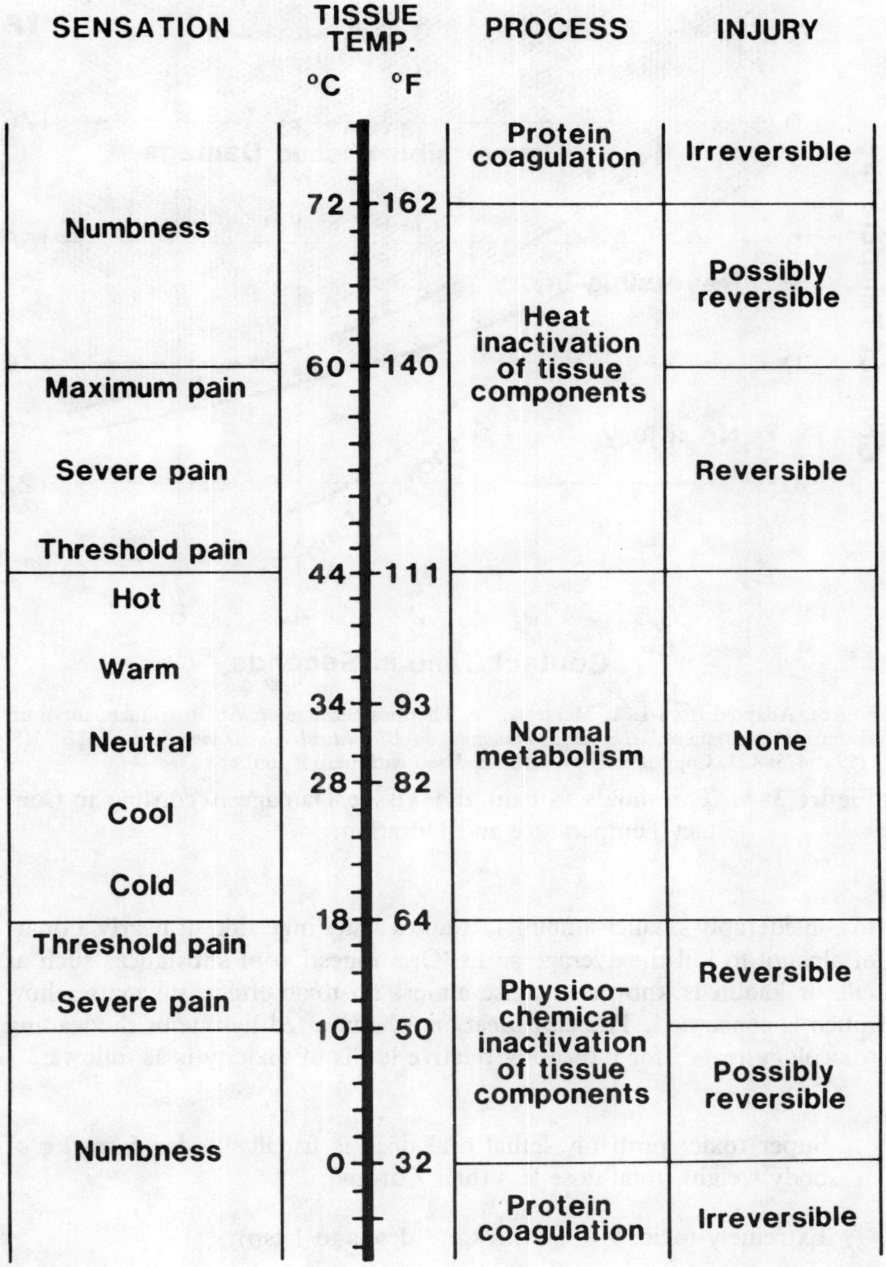

Source: Adapted from A.M. Stoll, "Heat Transfer in Biotechnology," in J.P. Hartnett and T.F. Irvine (eds.), *Advances in Heat Transfer*, vol. 4 (New York: Academic Press, 1967), 65–141. Used with permission.

Figure 3–7. Threshold for Various Tissue Effects from Heat and Cold.

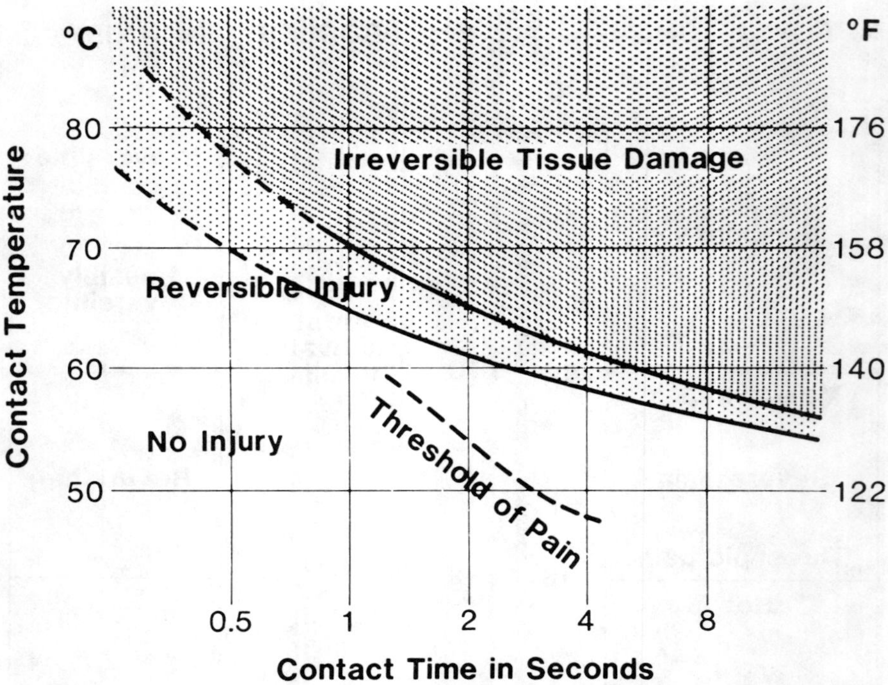

Source: Adapted from L.A. Marzetta, "A Thermesthesiometer: An Instrument for Burn Hazard Measurement," *IEEE Transactions on Biomedical Engineering,* vol. BME-21(5) (1974):425–427. Copyright © 1974 IEEE. Used with permission.

Figure 3–8. Thresholds to Pain and Tissue Damage According to Contact Temperature and Duration.

to considerably smaller amounts, it takes acute ingestion of nearly a quart of alcohol to kill the average adult. Oral ingestion of substances such as talc or kaolin is known to cause almost no toxic effect, no matter how much is consumed. The classification scheme used by one of the leading toxicology texts[27] for indicating relative levels of toxicity is as follows:

Super toxic: probably lethal oral dose is usually under 5 mg/kg of body weight (total dose less than 7 drops);

Extremely toxic: 5 to 50 mg/kg (7 drops to 1 tsp);

Very toxic: 50 to 500 mg/kg (1 tsp to 1 oz);

Moderately toxic: 0.5 to 5 gm/kg (1 oz to 1 pt or 1 lb);

Slightly toxic: 5 to 15 gm/kg (1 pint to 1 qt or 2.2 lbs);

Practically nontoxic: above 15 gm/kg (over 1 qt or 2.2 lbs.).

Electrical Energy

According to Wu[28] the extent of electrical injury is determined by four aspects of the electrical source: the electromotive force or voltage, direct versus alternating current, frequency of alternating current, and entrance and exit properties of the contact surfaces. Also determining injury are four aspects of the organism: whether it is wet or dry, its contact area and contact duration, and the resistivity or electrical characteristics of specific organs, tissues, and fluids.

Wu notes that *in vitro* data (described below) may differ from those *in vivo* and should be used only as reference values. His excellent summary of the literature on this subject is as follows:

1. The resistance of skin varies with the amount of moisture content, the temperature and the applied voltage. Dry skin could have a resistance of 50,000 ohms to 1 megohm, whereas wet skin may have a resistance of only 2,500 ohms, and during passage of current the resistance can decrease from 260 K ohms to 380 ohms. Skin resistance of cadavers at 60 Hz has been recorded as follows: at 50 V, 5,000 to 18,000 ohms; 500 V, 800 to 1,800 ohms; and 1,000 V, 800 to 1,800 ohms.
2. The epidermis is the surface most likely to contact an electrical source, and therefore its condition will affect the distribution and density of current flow and the severity of injury. The current flow for a given circuit is a function of applied voltage and takes the path of least resistance, which is the biofluids, nerve fibers, and blood stream.
3. High-frequency alternating current (A.C.) is relatively harmless. For a short duration, for example, currents up to 3 amp at frequencies from 400 KHz to 1MHz have no effect on the human body, and an alternating current of sufficient strength to light up an ordinary incandescent lamp can be tolerated at high frequency when the human body is part of the circuit. Because the current alternates, the nerve stimulation of one alternation does not have time to take effect before it is canceled by the next alternation.
4. Low-frequency alternation, however, can be quite harmful. Thus, the current required to initiate fibrillation at 1,200 Hz is about 12 times that required at 60 Hz, which is the domestic current most

commonly used today and is in the most dangerous range of frequencies.

In general, 50 to 60 Hz alternating current is more dangerous to life than is direct current because the alternations put muscles into tetanic spasm so the victim is unable to remove himself from the electrodes. Direct current, although perhaps less lethal, is more liable to cause severe local injuries.

Two types of burn situations occur. In one, resulting in a pure thermal burn, the body is struck by a spark or flash of external electrical energy but is not directly involved in the electrical network. In the second situation the body is part of the network with electricity arcing through it. Short exposures above threshold values in this latter case are likely to result only in mild tingling shock or mild involuntary muscle contraction. Exposure of longer duration or with higher current may result in neurosystem damage, ventricular fibrillation, respiratory paralysis, tissue damage or instantaneous death. As shown in table 3–1 there is some disagreement among researchers regarding the threshold values for these different effects.

When electric current flows through the body, it takes paths of least resistance causing physiological reaction (either a joulean heat effect or a direct electrical effect, according to two theories) as the injury mechanism. Again referencing Wu, "the distribution and structure of physiological entities differ at the micro level among individuals and within an individual body. Therefore, it is very difficult, if not impossible, to quantitatively evaluate the current distribution for any typical path. In addition, individual responses differ and there are no identical electrical injuries."

Table 3–1
Amount of Current (mh) at Which Events Are Postulated by Three Researchers with Reference to a 60 Hz Electric Current

Event	*Hodgkin*	*Kaufman and Michaelson*	*Keesey and Letcher*
Perception/sensation	1	1	0.1–0.5
Pain	5	—	—
Let go	—	10	5–9
Tetanic muscle contraction	15	—	—
Respiratory muscle tetanically contracted	30	—	—
Cardiac fibrillation	60–5,000	100	>10
Respiratory failure	10,000	—	—

Source: Y-C Wu, *Electrical Injuries: A Literature Review* (Gaithersburg, Md.: National Bureau of Standards, Report NBSIR 79-1710, 1979).

Ionizing Radiation

There is disagreement whether a threshold exists for chronic effects of ionizing radiation. Our concern here, however, is with acute effects: that is, clinical effects observed within minutes to days after a single exposure. According to one paper, radioactive poisons are 10^6 to 10^9 times more hazardous than chemical poisons and qualitatively must be considered a new kind of problem.[29]

The body is able to tolerate larger doses of radiation if concentrated to one organ than if the whole body is exposed. The LD_{50} (lethal dose for 50% of subjects) in thirty days for whole body irradiation in humans is about 500r. Doses of 100r or more in external irradiation from X or γ rays or by α or β emission from internally deposited material (not localized) precipitate clinically obvious effects—such as symptoms of shock and gastrointestinal symptoms—in from two to five hours. In about three hours histological evidence of bone marrow damage appears at this dose. Higher levels result in temporary loss of hair, erythema, and even a weeping eczema.[29]

Those tissues most sensitive to radiation are ones (1) in more active mitosis, (2) with a greater number of divisions before maturity is reached, and (3) with less morphologic and physiologic differentiation. The tissues would thus be listed as follows in order of decreasing sensitivity: spermatogonia, lymphocytes, erythroblasts, the rest of hemopoietic tissues, lining of small intestine, stomach, colon, skin, central nervous system, muscle, bone, and collagen.[30]

Relationships between Acute and Chronic Energy Exposure

The relationship between acute and chronic or repeated exposures of the body to energy forms also warrants discussion. In the acute exposures the body may be rapidly overwhelmed if the energy massed and reaching the body is sufficient to exceed injury thresholds. Where thresholds for acute injury are not reached no injury occurs because the body has the capability of applying mechanisms that either maintain or bring about a rapid return to physiological homeostasis.

With continuing or repeated intermittent exposures, homeostatic mechanisms may also be overwhelmed if the total body burden is great enough, but this commonly may not occur for years. With one possible exception, each of the acute energy-related traumas has patterns of chronic trauma that we commonly refer to as chronic diseases or occupational diseases. The difference in observed outcome is not a result of a different agent. Rather, in one case homeostatic mechanisms have been so rapidly overwhelmed that there has been no opportunity for reparative processes to occur, whereas with chronic diseases we are seeing the end result of a combination of agent effect plus incomplete repair repeated many times. One example is squamous metaplasia of bronchi in response to cigarette smoke.

Let us briefly note some of the chronic diseases associated with physical energy. Traumatic arthritis, deafness, and thromboangiitis obliterans are long-term effects of kinetic energy. Chemical energy can cause myocardial infarction, congenital malformations, cancer of the lung, liver, or bladder, leukemia, cirrhosis, and renal failure, to mention a few common examples. Kangri pot tumors and squamous carcinoma of the lip are associated with thermal insults, while various forms of radiation express their effects through squamous cell carcinomas of the skin, cataracts, lung cancer, leukemia, and other forms of neoplasia.

Only chronic exposure to electricity has no well-documented syndromes expressing the effects of repeated trauma and repair. Studies during the past decade have attempted to show that such a relationship does exist.[31] The results are sometimes suggestive but as yet hardly convincing. Based on the other energy/tissue patterns, however, there is ample theoretical reason to suspect that electricity-related chronic diseases exist also.

A comparison between acute trauma and chronic energy effect is particularly important because of the marked contrast in response of health professionals to prevention of these two patterns. The same physician who berates a patient for being careless or thoughtless for falling or having some other acute injury usually is much more understanding and circumspect regarding development of deafness or arthritis from years of working or playing in a stressful manner.

Post-Injury Phase

One further generic factor determines the ultimate outcome of injury. This is the entire series of actions that occur after the injury and that may result at one extreme in early rehabilitation without permanent harm or at the other extreme in either death or continuing disability. Few studies exist indicating what proportion of death, disability, and discomfort from injury need not happen were the post-injury phase more effectively handled. The limited research deals primarily with how many lives might be saved. These data suggest that somewhere between 15 and 25 percent of persons who die in highway crashes in the United States or Canada might still be alive if emergency care were more readily available and of better quality.[32,33,34] Since care on the North American continent is better or more widely available than in numerous other places throughout the world, a reasonable assumption is that internationally salvageability for fatally injured persons would probably exceed these estimates based on these studies.

"Innocent" and Not-So-"Innocent" Bystanders

The energy management model also takes into account the two types of "innocent bystander" situations: that in which the individual who is injured clearly is an inadvertent victim and that in which he or she only appears to be so. If an energy-management task is greater than the individual's capability of dealing with it, the energy may go out of control. From that point on the errant energy may be available to injure the person who was originally handling it, or it may create damage to any other people or structures that happen to be in the immediate vicinity. Thus, the driver of a bus or pilot of a plane who loses control of the vehicle may take with him not only his passengers but, especially in urban areas, many others who are only circumstantially associated.

This can be described as a random event only in a very narrow sense. One may not be able to predict which particular bystander is likely to be injured, but it may be possible to prognosticate fairly accurately how many such persons, of what types, and under what conditions. Socioeconomic, cultural, and legal circumstances, for example, determine the degree of crowding that may exist in an apartment house or on a bus and the likelihood that the particular bus or building meets specific safety codes. These issues have almost unique relevance in many developing countries where modifiction of stake trucks to serve as public transportation and overloading of all forms of public transportation are common, expected, and permitted. Federal, state, or local standards may dictate whether a plane, or a truck with high energy explosives, is permitted to travel through areas that are heavily populated or whether precautions have been taken so that even if the energy is out of control it will damage relatively few unsuspecting persons.

Let us now look at those who are not totally inadvertent bystanders. Surprisingly, there are more of these than is commonly thought. One group of not-so-inadvertent bystanders are people who stand around and observe arguments, fights, fires, and other disasters. Another group is individuals who are injured as passengers of drivers impaired by alcohol. Such persons as a rule also have been drinking and usually are as impaired as is the driver.[35]

Surely, people lost in floods, tornadoes, earthquakes, or volcanoes must be inadvertent victims? Three types of information suggest that in many instances this may not be the case. One is the long history, going back into antiquity, of houses and even entire cities that have been rebuilt at the same locations where previous ones were just destroyed by "natural events" that have high probability of recurring: for examples, houses on the slopes of intermittently active volcanoes or on top of active faults with no attention to quake-resistant design and construction or buildings still precariously located where tidal waves demolished their predecessors. This pattern, of course, is repeated year after year on flood plains in India and many other nations.

Furthermore, such redevelopment may use precisely the same methods of construction that were shown to be noneffective in the past. Flimsy dwellings may replace old flimsy dwellings recently destroyed, with the full expectation that these too will soon be demolished by nature's ravages and that additional people will be injured or killed in the process.

Finally, in contrast to this ignoring of long-term warnings, there is the deaf ear turned to notices of immediate danger. Several studies indicate that much of the loss in floods or other disasters is because people hear but do not pay attention to messages urging them to seek higher ground or more secure locations.[36,37] Thus, in the presence of natural massings of potentially destructive energy people, through all of the methods described above, do not function in a way that will limit its harmful effects on them. Such individuals cannot be called inadvertent bystanders.

4
Countermeasures against Injury

Ruby lips above the water,
Blowing bubbles, soft and fine.
Alas for me, I was no swimmer,
So I lost my Clementine.

Now you Boy Scouts heed the moral
Of this sad, sad tale of mine.
Artificial respiration
Would have saved my Clementine.
"Clementine"

For many years, the three Es—education, enforcement, and engineering—have been the traditional approach to injury control. Although involving an eye-catching phrase, this approach does not deal with the large range of countermeasure options that exist because its primary thrust is at prevention in the pre-injury phase rather than at reduction of ultimate unwanted outcome by coming to grips with aspects of all three phases.

Before describing the range of options, we need to examine first some important questions concerning relationships between what is known about the mechanisms of injury events, described in the preceding chapter, and what actions may be appropriate to reduce the frequency and severity of injury. Appropriate countermeasures to a specific type of problem—whether it be injury or illness—can be derived *logically* from what is known about the natural history of the event and its circumstances. But contrary to common opinion they do not necessarily flow *obviously* from such knowledge.

What is the difference? Poliomyelitis often results from transmission of viruses between people. One *obvious* method for prevention, therefore, was to reduce contacts between people during epidemics by avoiding public gatherings. This method wreaked havoc on social interchange but did little to stop the disease. One *logical* method of control, however, was not to prevent the infection but rather to alter host reactions to that infection through a vaccine that protects for many years.

The application of this concept to injury control comes from the observation that many factors contribute to the occurrence and ultimate outcome of injury events. A single factor—for example, alcohol—may occur with high frequency in certain types of events. It may follow obviously, but not necessarily logically, that the only or best way to reduce these events and their outcomes is to reduce use of alcohol.

An obvious solution is suggested primarily by examining relative frequencies of different factors in injury events and by attacking first the factors with highest frequency. A logical solution is one that may include information about frequency as a consideration but that is suggested primarily by examining the relative feasibility of countermeasures for affecting human losses *and* for having limited unwanted economic or social side effects. Occasionally, an obvious solution is also a logical solution, but one shouldn't count on it.

The ideal logical solution can be applied universally with a very high degree of effectiveness once applied. Examples are vaccines for smallpox, polio, or measles. Where ideal solutions do not exist, one may use logical solutions applicable to all people but under more limited circumstances or to fewer people over a wider range of events. The appropriate approach for a particular type of injury would be a network of logical solutions that have high effectiveness for limited situations or limited but acceptable degrees of effectiveness for wider situations. In combination, these partial solutions can then bring about substantial reduction in injury frequency and severity.

In the remainder of this chapter we will examine a range of countermeasures developed by Dr. William Haddon, Jr.,[1] each of which has applicability to at least some injury circumstances. Haddon's work not only provides a framework for identifying relevant countermeasures but also brushes away conceptual cobwebs that surround the philosophy of the three Es. More recently, he has expanded the context to a much broader range of hazards than those commonly associated with acute injury.[2]

Dr. Haddon uses the concept of physical energy as the agent in injury events and asks systematically what methods exist for limiting the harmful effects of that energy on people and property. Here is his list of logical solutions:

1. Prevent the initial aggregation of the particular energy form.
2. Reduce the amount of energy aggregated.
3. Prevent the energy release.
4. Alter the rate or spatial distribution of release of the energy from its source.
5. Separate susceptible structures from the energy being released by means of space or time.

6. Interpose a material barrier to separate the released energy from susceptible structures.
7. Modify contact surfaces or basic structures that can be impacted.
8. Strengthen living or nonliving structures susceptible to damage by the energy transfer.
9. Quickly detect and evaluate damage, and prevent its continuation or extension.
10. Carry out all necessary measures between the emergency period immediately following damage and ultimate stabilization of the process. Such measures include intermediate and long-term repair and rehabilitation.

This series is unique because it deals with the energy at all stages that can affect ultimate outcome, instead of emphasizing primarily how humans can be modified, and particularly doing so in the pre-injury phase, as has been so common. Changing people is not excluded per se; it is one of the methods available to prevent the release of energy. Reducing task demand is another method appropriate here.

Let us examine as mind-stretching possibilities some ways in which each of the ten options might be applied. Equally important, they are possible explanations for naturally occurring differences in injury patterns that already exist between cultures and geographic areas.

1. Prevent the initial aggregation of the particular energy form. Potential kinetic energy is massed through motion and elevation. If only shrubs and one-story buildings are available, children cannot fall from trees, down stairs, or out of second-story windows. A food preparation procedure that involves natural gelling of ingredients without mixing avoids injuries associated with use of an electric mixer.

Burns might be avoided if homemade bread and cakes generally did not require cooking. The chemical energy toxic to the liver in carbon tetrachloride fire extinguishers has been abolished and replaced by less toxic ingredients. In England hazardous natural gas or methane has been replaced with less toxic manufactured gas. In these cases the chemical energy not being massed is that capable of poisoning, rather than that capable of putting out a fire or of providing heat.

2. Reduce the amount of energy aggregated. Lower the height of hospital beds and high chairs, and reduce maximum automobile speed limits. Use regulators that limit water temperature. Small packages of aspirin and small nonrenewable prescriptions for barbiturates reduce the likelihood that children or persons contemplating suicide will swallow lethal doses. Transformers and low-voltage appliances reduce the massing of electricity at the location of customer use and possible misuse. New experimental methods for reducing stresses as they build between tectonic plates may ultimately limit the size of earthquakes to nondangerous proportions.

3. Prevent the energy release. Traditionally known as "accident prevention," this option involves efforts to improve human performance and to reduce task demand. Human performance at least theoretically (but not always in actuality) can be maintained at satisfactory levels for specific tasks by the following four means. One cannot help but be fascinated how the average person, legislator, or even safety professional thinks first or even only of these options:

1. Limit exposure to certain tasks either voluntarily or legally only to individuals who are capable of performing them. Examples are telling nonswimmers to stay away from deep water, convincing alcohol-impaired persons to take a cab home, or requiring periodic examination and licensure of airline pilots.
2. Educate people so they have necessary knowledge and skills. Driver education, skiing lessons, and boating classes are supposed to perform this function, as are some aspects of occupational apprenticeships.
3. Manipulate attitudes and behaviors amenable to conscious control through education, peer pressure, and laws and regulations. All may be applied to avoiding alcohol-impaired driving or promoting repair or construction of buildings to meet safety codes.
4. Improve physical, physiological, and psychological capabilities of handicapped persons. Treatment of epilepsy, for example, may reduce risk of injury as a driver, in falls, and from drowning.

Turning to task demands, these can be altered in the following manners:

1. Put less of a burden on single senses, and permit one to assess information using other sensory routes. A person with a gas stove can tell if it is hot either by observing the flame or by feeling the heat. A person with a ceramic top stove that changes color imperceptibly upon heating can assess the situation only by touch.
2. Require less intelligence, learning, or memory. An ignition key and automatic choke require less learning than cranking the starter and adjusting the throttle and choke.
3. Make cues more easily visible, legible, and less subject to visual confusion. Large, high contrast, simple dials, viewed head-on are easier to read than are small dials with many numbers, dimly lit, and

viewed with parallax as a factor. Adjacent dials should operate in the same direction to avoid confusion.

4. Do not require simultaneous attention to two or more cues.
5. Neither provide stimuli so quickly that the individual cannot respond to all within the time available, nor so slowly that the individual becomes bored.
6. Don't put controls of similar design so close together that they can be confused. Knobs that perform different critical functions either should not be adjacent to each other or should have contrasting shapes.
7. Make it impossible to activate a piece of equipment inadvertently while part of the body is near a portion of the equipment that can create harm.
8. Don't leave out important information that the individual needs in order to assess the environment. This concept includes sufficient repetition of information so that it is not lost entirely if it is overlooked the first time it is available.
9. Decrease the amount of strength, speed, stamina, balance, or range of motion required. A tricycle is less demanding for a young child or an elderly person than is a bicycle, and a motorized wheelchair is easier yet. A traffic light with a long walk cycle will give an elderly person a better chance to cross the road than will a shorter "walk" cycle or no walk cycle.
10. Make the task so demanding that persons not competent to perform it well will be unable even to start the activity and thus by physical means will be protected from having any exposure to the hazard. Three examples for the protection of children are child-proof closures on medicine bottles, spring actuated covers on electric sockets, and locks on doors and cabinets. The ignition lock on automobiles is aimed at teenagers who may wish to steal a car for a "joyride" but have only limited competence as thieves.

4. Alter the rate or spatial distribution of release of the energy from its source. Packaging of medications in individual units instead of in bottles slows the release of chemical energy that may be available to poison a child who is playing with and ingesting these. Flame-retardant materials that smolder and go out instead of bursting into flame are another example. Yet a third example is the safety release on home furnaces, pressure cookers, or in ski bindings, which serves both to limit the massing of energy and, if too much is massed, to moderate its release to nonexplosive proportions and to shunt the release to structures that are least susceptible to permanent harm.

5. Separate susceptible structures from the energy being released by means of space or time. For example, route trucks with hazardous materials along low-density roads or through sparsely settled areas. Separation in time occurs through use of active or passive passenger restraints in automobiles that extended by many milliseconds the time during which a given kinetic energy load is transferred to occupants, thus decreasing the peak load to the body.

6. Interpose a material barrier to separate the released energy from the susceptible structure. Use means such as hard hats, metal-toed shoes, glasses with tempered lenses, or protective hoods and clothing for both industry and sports. Insulation on electrical wires, or lead shielding around sources of ionizing radiation, are further examples.

7. Modify contact surfaces, subsurfaces, or basic structures that can be impacted. This is a commonly applied principle in boxing, where hands, floors, and posts are padded. Rounding of sharp surfaces on car interiors and exteriors is another example, as are energy-absorbing steering columns, instrument panels, and windshields.

8. Strengthen living or nonliving structures susceptible to damage by the energy transfer. Included is design and construction of buildings so they do not collapse easily during fire or earthquakes, or of fuel tanks on automobiles, tanker trucks, or ocean tankers so they do not rupture, leak, and burn in crashes. Examples involving strengthening human structure are strengthening of osteoporotic bone against fracture through incorporation of fluoride into the bone structure, immunization of laboratory workers against disease organisms from needle punctures and broken glassware, or immunization of the public against tetanus and diphtheria infection of wounds. Probably the most common method for strengthening human tissues—although not intended primarily for this purpose—is the increase of muscle mass in both athletes and debilitated individuals through exercise.

9. Quickly detect and evaluate damage, and prevent its continuation or extension. Automatic sensing devices identify the presence of fire, toxic chemicals, or radiation and sound an alarm or activate fire extinguishers, chemical evacuation fans, or shut down entire systems such as nuclear power plants.

The components of emergency care also are relevant, including crash-activated alarm devices in airplanes, pavement sensors or emergency phones on highways, and training of the public in emergency care. Recent years have also seen substantial improvement throughout the

United States in training, equipping, and organizing of an entire range of emergency personnel and services so they protect the scene from further damage and provide prompt, methodical, and appropriate evacuation and care for those who need them.

10. Carry out all necessary measures between the emergency period immediately following damage and ultimate stabilization of the process. Such measures include intermediate and long-term repair and rehabilitation. Although beyond the scope of this book, it must be noted that much disability and discomfort of injured persons exists because of:

a. Unequal access to medical and other health care for economic, geographic, and other reasons;
b. Unskilled treatment of iatrogenic (treatment-caused) illness for some who have received care; and
c. Incomplete return of function, despite adequate repair of tissues, because appropriate services for physical and psychological rehabilitation and job retraining and placement have not been used.

As noted earlier, restoration of damaged equipment, structures, and even entire cities may be carried out in such a way that the risk of further damage from injury events remains fully as great as it was in the first place.

Certain of the options discussed here place the burden of effort on people who may be at personal risk of injury, while others provide protection no matter what the person's performance level. Countermeasures can be divided into three classes based on the extent of human effort required to carry them out. Active countermeasures require either continuous or repeated and frequent human effort in order to be effective. Semipassive ones require occasional or limited effort by the individual who is to be protected. Passive measures require no personal effort by the person being protected.

Telling workers not to breath hazardous vapors when they are working with chlorinated hydrocarbons, or giving them masks they can wear, would be active measures. Arranging the work space so they can use these chemicals only under a hood but requiring them to turn on the exhaust mechanism would be semipassive. A passive approach might be an exhaust system that automatically starts through sensing devices whenever a threshold nonhazardous chemical concentration is reached.

5
Making Choices

Decisions about whether to attack a given injury problem, what methods to use, and how extensive the effort should be do not depend alone on the size of the problem or the quality of existing technology for countermeasures. In this chapter we will examine some of the many factors involved in such decisions.

By drawing on finite world and local resources we try to survive and to achieve a certain quality of life, a term that is not easily definable and that means different things to different people at different times. Just how disparate these resources and quality of life may be is demonstrated by the fact that a typical poor family in India devotes 85 percent of its income to avoiding hunger, whereas in the United States a family spends 16 percent on food.[1] Prevention of death, disability, and discomfort from injury is generally perceived to be one of the positive components of quality of life, although its relative priority varies with the situation, the population involved, and other aspects of quality of life that may come into conflict.

Protagonistic Viewpoints

Four types of arguments have most often been used to support or oppose concern about a specific type of injury event or countermeasure: arguments about feasibility, economics, convenience, and morality. Usually the first two are combined either consciously or unconsciously. Thus, the stated question, "Is it feasible to reduce highway fatalities by use of airbags, or to cut down on injuries from power lawn mowers by developing different blades or guards?" may really mean, "How much will we save in reduced death and injury for each additional dollar spent to change the product?"

Questions such as these may never even get to be asked in areas of the world where 40 percent of the male population is unemployed and would appreciate any work, no matter how dangerous. Nor may they be raised in nations where any modification of the environment other than by hand-operated tools such as scythe or machete is a luxury. Examples also can be found within the North American continent. As Lowrance[2] reminds us, in rural America, which contained most people around 1900, it was essential to deal with the hazards of axes, mules, stinging insects, boiling laundry kettles, and tetanus from rusty implements and barbed wire.

Of particular interest is who asks what questions and what assumptions and goals underlie them. At the risk of somewhat oversimplifying, the following are arguments expressed most often among the various protagonists.

1. Where the proposed safety program involves changing a product or modifying the environment, the manufacturer of that product or the person or agency responsible for the environment is likely to respond either that:

a. The problem is too small to warrant attention;[3]
b. The problem results from misaction by the consumer who must bear moral responsibility (in illustration, a study apparently done for opponents of no-fault automobile insurance questioned whether a no-fault insurance law would reduce the sense of responsibility that people might feel about driving carefully[4]);
c. The technology does not exist and cannot be developed easily for making the product safer;[3] or
d. The cost to the consumer will be too high for benefit received. The cost referred to is usually the sale price or initial cost of the product rather than the "true" or long-term cost, including depreciation, operation, maintenance, insurance, and expenses growing out of breakdown or injury. A related argument is that the consumer should be able to choose whether he or she wishes to spend money on safety. Baker[5] has documented, however, that only a minority of individuals injured in automobiles either purchased the vehicle themselves or were related to the purchaser.

Concerning the politics of safety, Merrill[6] points out that "protective, behavioral, and convenience measures are not advanced independently of one another. When proponents advocate a measure intended to increase protection of vehicle occupants in crashes, it has usually been the case that opponents of the measure seek a behavior modification remedy when such an alternative is available." The automobile industry did so, he notes, because it "stood to avoid greater costs or to incur no cost by the substitution and postponement of the protective device. A behavioral measure, moreover, shifts responsibility for compliance and blame for failure to purchase or use from the manufacturer to individuals. This strategy has been effective in delaying if not defeating protective measures." Merrill further observes that "proponents, too, frequently endorse behavioral measures when the obstacles to protective innovations seem insuperable in the short run or when they prefer to avoid conflict with in order to persuade their opponents."

2. Where the proposed safety program requires action by a community agency, typical agency questions are:

a. Is the problem in the purvue of the agency, or is it someone else's responsibility?
b. Is the problem of sufficient size to warrant attention in light of other problems the agency must deal with and given its limited resources?
c. Does the program have political feasibility—that is, capability of being funded by the legislature or of getting administrative or legislative approbation? On this issue, Merrill says that "decision making is not primarily a rational assessment of the state of knowledge with respect to the technical feasibility and efficacy of the choices at hand. It is political process in which the alignment of partisans may influence the outcome. Proponents of a measure are those who support its adoption by administrative rule making statute, or as a matter of corporate policy. In part because safety is an important social value and in part because other strategies are available to them, opponents are less likely to oppose such a measure outright than to attempt to delay its adoption or weaken it." Historically, he suggests, "behavior modification measures seem to be most readily accepted by responsible decision makers, protective measures next, and convenience measures least."
d. Will the program inconvenience the public excessively so that they will not support it? In general, the aim is to provide as little imposition as possible and yet still achieve safety goals. Again, quoting Merrill, "marginal policy changes are the norm in both public and private spheres. They reflect efforts to cope with the limited knowledge, capability, and financial resources of analysts and with conflicting values."

3. Those proposing a safety program commonly argue as follows:

a. Is it moral to continue with the current loss of life and limb when the potential for action exists and lies within the purvue of a specific industry or agency? (Waller and Klein,[7] however, asked whether injury events that arouse greatest concern are those that most often affect middle-class persons rather than those that cause the largest drain in morbidity and mortality, albeit in groups that are deviant or socioeconomically disadvantaged.)

b. Won't the benefit in terms of lives and limbs saved more than balance out any extra cost or inconvenience to manufacturers, consumers or taxpayers? This cost/benefit argument is sometimes supported by applying dollar values to deaths and injuries if the number of deaths and injuries is large enough to be imposing. Where the number is small, the appeal may be that no dollar value can or should be placed on a human life and that "to save even one life is worth any cost."

Where product development or modification is proposed the question of effectiveness is often raised. But this question is raised much less frequently regarding effectiveness of educational or enforcement programs or other attempts to modify behavior.

The general assumption is that such "common sense" programs do work and that if a program hasn't worked so far, the reason probably is that it hasn't been tried with enough resources, rather than because the basic hypothesis for action may be flawed. However, Saunders and Benson[8] note that "it is in the field of . . . behavior that the fewest cost/benefit studies have been undertaken, mainly because of the difficulty that is usually encountered in measuring the accident savings to be expected from a specific measure designed to change behavior."

Also on this point, Merrill notes that technological "protective measures have usually been shown to be effective in reducing deaths and injuries long before their adoption" but that

> behavior modification approaches, on the other hand, have been adopted in the absence of reliable evidence of their effectiveness. . . . Decision makers may institute and maintain costly policies in the presence of conflicting or absence of supportive evidence of their utility. This has been characteristic of occupant restraint measures intended to exhort, induce, or compel individuals to use available means to protect themselves. Decisions to provide means of protection other than as extra cost options to purchasers, have generally awaited the accumulation of a significant body of proof of their protective value. The evidence does not indicate whether decision makers based their eventual choices on such data, merely that they rarely acted speedily on such matters.

Clearly, the protagonists in the development of safety programs often talk past each other and the resulting actions, whether taken at a societal or an individual level, often appear to be inconsistent.

Why Do We Act Inconsistently?

In France the expenditure to save a single life is $30,000 for highway deaths and $1 million for aviation, while in Great Britain expenditures range from $10,000 for an agricultural worker to $20 million for a high-rise apartment dweller.[9] Many explanations have been given for such inconsistencies, but we will focus on three.

Joscelyn and Jones[10] suggest that both individually and on a societal level we tend to define a state known as *maximum tolerable disutility*, or the highest level of property loss and injury that we are willing to accept. Despite comments to the contrary, risk-management systems do not seek to eliminate risk, but only to keep it within acceptable levels, because society does not tolerate risk-management activities that create more negative effects than positive benefits. As they point out, however, this process of assessing negative effect and positive benefits is an imperfect one at best because of the various filters to information systems that give us perceptions of disutility, risk, benefits, and disbenefits of risk management, instead of actual values for these entities. Within any given society individuals vary both in how they perceive risk and also in how much risk they will accept. Furthermore, individuals may have very different perceptions about different risks and what should be done about them. In addition, the perception of risk is dynamic rather than static, and these changing perceptions affect societal and individual acceptance of risk-management practices.

According to Brown and Green,[11] individuals use different criteria to assess risks of different types of hazards. The risk in crossing the road, for example, is seen differently from that associated with smoking. Risks to health and safety are not evaluated in the abstract or based on pure probability estimates. Rather, such evaluations are inextricably bound up with the expected utility of the activity and the means proposed to reduce the risk.

Herbert Simon[12] deals with these problems within the "theory of limited, or bounded, rationality." Simon suggests that decision makers tend to "satisfice": that is, to choose the first management approach that is "good enough" rather than continuing to search for an ideal or optimal approach. They do so because the human has limits to memory and computer power and thus ends up as a problem solver who more often than not does not—and cannot—achieve full rationality.

One method proposed to foster rationality in decision making about safety programs is the assignment of monetary value to the losses from injury events and to the methods proposed to limit those losses. We will take a closer look at the process of assessing the value of a life.

Cost/Benefit Studies and The Value of a Life

On the one hand it is possible, albeit difficult, within very narrowly defined criteria, to come up with monetary values for lives lost or injuries incurred among individuals in different age and sex groupings. Table 5–1 shows such estimates of lost productivity from highway crashes to persons in different age groups,[13] while tables 5–2 and 5–3 summarize several types of loss data for injuries of various degrees of severity.[13] On the other hand a number of reputable researchers and administrators maintain that, claims to the contrary not withstanding, loss of life and limb cannot really be measured in dollars and any attempt to do so will always be controversial and subject to valid criticism.[14]

Speaking about the use of monetary values of lives for cost/benefit studies by the National Highway Traffic Safety Administration (NHTSA), Morganstein[15] points out that comparison of straight calculations of "present value" based on lifetime earnings for a 1- to 4-year-old child and a 55- to 59-year-old man would lead to administrative decisions that are directly contrary to what the public wants because "as NHTSA has recognized regarding School Bus vehicle standards, society values the lives of children very highly, and is willing to incur higher costs to save 100 children than to reduce the general fatality level by the same amount. Strictly monetary arguments, however, which would ascribe a lesser monetary value for a child than for a male about to retire, directly contradict this assessment."

Despite the limitation of money for usual life saving programs, we

Table 5–1
Direct Future Productivity Loss for 1973 U.S. Highway Fatalities

		Direct Productivity Loss Per Person in Age Group	
Age Group	*Number of Fatalities*	*7% Discount*	*10% Discount*
0–4	1,990	$ 47,660	$114,193
5–9	1,996	68,197	139,395
10–14	2,139	116,291	190,790
15–19	9,261	140,919	221,228
20–24	8,756	158,769	237,751
25–29	5,162	166,699	244,176
30–34	3,591	163,910	227,669
35–39	2,722	160,357	213,553
40–44	2,653	147,276	172,027
45–49	2,730	129,983	157,012
50–54	2,667	104,580	120,499
55–59	2,422	79,942	79,298
60–64	2,333	31,430	31,622
Overall average		$130,829	$189,497

Source: B.M. Faigin, "Societal Costs of Motor Vehicle Accidents for Benefit-Cost Analysis: A Perspective on the Major Issues and Some Recent Findings," *Proceedings of the 4th International Congress on Automotive Safety, 14–16 July 1975* (Washington, D.C.: National Highway Traffic Safety Administration, U.S. Department of Transportation, 1975), 155–172.

Table 5–2
Societal Cost Components for U.S. Fatalities

Component	*1971 Costs*
Future productivity losses	
Direct	$132,000
Indirect	41,300
Medical costs	
Hospital	700
Other	425
Property damage	1,500
Insurance administration	4,700
Legal and court	3,000
Employer losses	1,000
Pain and suffering	10,000
Funeral	900
Assets (lost consumption)	5,000
Miscellaneous crash costs	200
Total per fatality	200,725

Source: B.M. Faigin, "Societal Costs of Motor Vehicle Accidents for Benefit-Cost Analysis: A Perspective on the Major Issues and Some Recent Findings," *Proceedings of the 4th International Congress on Automotive Safety, 14–16 July 1975* (Washington, D.C.: National Highway Traffic Safety Administration, U.S. Department of Transportation, 1975), 155–172.

Table 5–3
Injury Severity Classes in Societal Cost Study of U.S. Highway Injuries

	Permanent Total Disability	*Permanent Partial Disability and Permanent Disfigurement*	*No Permanent Disability*
Percentage of injuries	.2	6.5	93.3
Costs			
Productivity	$191,000	$48,000	$ 350
Medical	7,800	2,800	315
Property damage	1,000	900	700
Legal and court	3,000	1,000	150
Insurance administration	4,300	4,300	800
Pain and suffering	50,000	10,000	100
All other	3,200	100	50
Total cost per injury	$260,300	$67,100	$2,465

Source: B.M. Faigin, "Societal Costs of Motor Vehicle Accidents for Benefit-Cost Analysis: A Perspective on the Major Issues and Some Recent Findings," *Proceedings of the 4th International Congress on Automotive Safety, 14–16 July 1975* (Washington, D.C.: National Highway Traffic Safety Administration, U.S. Department of Transportation, 1975), 155–172.

may spend millions to save a miner trapped underground or a person held hostage by a kidnapper. Life, in Western culture at least, is supposed to have infinite value. This issue is especially relevant to comparison of program planning in different nations and cultures in which local societal values for life in general or for specific groups in particular may differ markedly.

An even more iconoclastic view of attempts to determine monetary value of human life is present by Dyson,[16] who observes that "it is easy for the question to become subtly changed. . . . Starting as, how much per life should we spend?, it became, how much is a person worth? The first question is subjective, about attitudes and values. The second is more objective—it seeks an answer by the examination of data."

Dyson then notes that economists attempted to determine what the economic contribution of a person might be to his or her family and to society and came up with a value of approximately $200,000 per life. He continues the argument as follows:

> If life could be valued in dollars, then it was but a short step in valuing safety in dollars. The obverse of this was that injuries and deaths in highway accidents, instead of being considered (unmeasurably) as tragedies, could be viewed as *costs*. It was especially comforting that economists were the ones who had provided the figures, by estimating the average person's "contribution" to society, because this meant we weren't just using the dollar figures arbitrarily, as surrogates or benchmarks, but we were actually perceiving the *real* costs of the accidents.

Dyson then attacks the assumption that a death or injury results in economic loss to society. The national economy, he states, is not strictly the sum of its individual income earners, with the loss of any one person resulting in a reduction in the total. Rather, when people die or are disabled, they are replaced by others so that the overall economic activity of the institution is unchanged. This pattern applies not only on a national level but on the individual family level as well, with life insurance, job seeking by the surviving or nondisabled spouse, and remarriage filling the economic gap created by death and disability.

One might argue, however, that people are consumers as well as producers and that loss of too many consumers can adversely affect the economy. Furthermore, injury is only one way of losing people from the society. If this approach were applied individually to each of the health problems that by themselves affect only a small portion of society at any one time, the loss of people from unchecked injury and illness may in combination result in a rather large and measurably harmful effect on productivity, although loss from any one alone might not be important.

Surprisingly, Dyson ends on the upbeat: "Does this mean that our safety efforts . . . produce no benefits? Not at all! The benefits are the avoidance of the deaths and injuries, of the physical and psychological suffering of the victims and their intimates, of dislocation, disfigurement, dysfunction, and despair; they are the pleasures of living in a safer and therefore more civilized world."

Yet other difficulties arise in estimating costs and benefits of safety (and other health) programs. Returning again to remarks by Morganstein,

> at the most basic level, the tangible benefits of NHTSA safety programs are measured in lives, limbs and property. To this list must be added less tangible benefits, reduction of pain and suffering, prevention of lost work-time, increase of life expectancy, unburdening of emergency health-care facilities, and lowering of life and health insurance costs. To predict the savings of these resources requires accurate models of casualty causation (e.g., failure rates and potential severity for defects) and countermeasure availability, readiness and effectiveness (e.g., seat belt-usage and injury mitigation). In addition, the evaluation of the benefits of existing rules necessitates the separation of interaction effects such as the lowered speed limit and reduced driving resulting from the fuel crisis.
>
> To apply cost-benefit analysis to the evaulation of a safety countermeasure, however, the benefits must be expressed in the same units as the cost. While some of the benefits are easily measured in dollar values, most are not. No one has yet proposed a satisfactory, objective method for translating lives, eyes, or fourth degree burns into dollars and cents. Yet, it is necessary for the NHTSA to be able to choose among casualty reducing programs so as to allocate its resources wisely.

The criteria for choosing among alternatives must include an estimate of the societal cost of safety programs. O'Neill and Kelley[17] argue that motor vehicle safety standards have no cost beyond the administrative activity expended to reach a decision and communicate it to industry. They emphasize the difference between cost/benefit, which asks whether the benefits of a countermeasure are likely to exceed the costs, and cost effectiveness, which asks if the countermeasure is being applied in the most frugal (to society) manner possible.

Within this context Morganstein[15] also makes the following important points:

1. If a safety standard specifies only a level of performance it allows manufacturers choice of design options. A determination of costs and benefits, therefore, requires comparing alternative tactics over the full range of available technologies. He notes, using automotive

industry response to NHTSA bumper standard 215 as an example, that sometimes "industry design decisions are not made on the basis of *societal* cost-effectiveness, but on the basis of the free-enterprise goal of maximizing profits" (emphasis in original).

2. For this reason, costs of implementing a safety standard applicable to industry should not be estimated too quickly or by averaging the cost of options chosen by different manufacturers. "Such a procedure, if undertaken within one or two model years after the effective date of a standard, may not permit market forces (to the extent that the domestic market responds to these forces) to eliminate the more extravagant or less effective alternatives."

Saunders and Benson[8] note that program costs usually don't fall on society as a whole but rather unevenly on special segments, such as government, public or private corporations, or private individuals, while the benefits may accrue to groups different from those on whom the costs fall. Also, they note the difficulty in placing a value on restraint of freedom as a cost of some safety programs.

But in my opinion, these problems are just as relevant to *not* carrying out a specific safety program. The costs of not acting may fall on individuals who will be much more adversely affected by them than would the costs of acting represent a burden for government or industry. And what is the effect of restraint of freedom if a person who seeks a safer product is unable to get one because it is not manufactured?

Finally, all cost/benefit studies start with the assumption that the raw data they use are using for calculations are reasonably accurate. As will be documented in the next chapter, however, such assumptions all too often are just not true.

Does this mean that cost/benefit studies should be abandoned? Saunders and Benson summarize their strengths and limitations as follows:

> After such an impressive list of limitations, it may well seem reasonable to ask whether the application of cost-benefit analysis has been worthwhile. Experience justifies an unhesitating affirmative. It should not be forgotten that the technique is one among a number of tools which serve road safety policy-making. It takes its place with the statistical methods of accident analysis and all the techniques for research into means of improving vehicles and the road, and reaching a deeper understanding of road user behavior. Its great value is the capacity it gives us to make comparative evaluations of alternatives which are not in themselves comparable. . . .
>
> Cost-benefit analysis does not enable the confidence of total rationality to take the place of the uncertainties of politics. On the contrary,

it is a tool to be used in the service of the political process by which the community reaches decisions on public questions. It is in this context that it must be judged.

A Scheme to Establish Priorities for Programs

We now turn to an approach developed by Wakeland,[18] which in my opinion is useful for relative assessment of program value. In Wakeland's own words, the scheme is simply "an aid to judgment, and the overall effect relies on judgment, not scientific analysis." He observes that safety decisions almost invariably are not based on a single criterion, and he identifies eighteen different values or concerns to be taken into consideration. These can be broadly grouped into areas of economics, public image and psychological motivations, equality and fairness, deservedness of protection, critical position in a technical system, and timing.

Several steps are suggested in order to carry out an assessment. First, one needs to define exactly the action being proposed, its technical evaluation, the interest group to which it would most directly apply, other benefitting or affected groups, including those that would pay the costs, and any consumer area or portion of the economy affected.

Next, each of these concerns is to be graded from the administrator's viewpoint on a spectrum ranging from those issues that strongly favor acceptance of the action, through those that have no effect, to issues that strongly disfavor the effort. In such grading, it is important also to identify where new data may be needed and to decide whether and how much additional effort should be expanded to get new information.

Also, it is important that the administrator identify where conflicts of values might exist. In order to do this he or she should ensure that assessments are also completed from the points of view of the different groups which might be affected. By doing this, it then becomes possible to estimate which conflict areas are strongest, where support or opposition might be found, and whether and how modification of the proposal might reduce conflict (that is, increase chances of acceptance by those in opposition) without seriously impairing the proposed effort. Appendix 5A contains an example of such an assessment carried out on a Locomotive Grade Crossing Crash Attenuation Device, a protective measure recommended by the National Transportation Safety Board in 1969 and having advanced to the prototype design state at the time Wakeland wrote his paper.

Making Choices at the Individual Level

It is simultaneously both easier and harder to help individuals make safety choices at the individual level, such as is likely to exist in a physician/patient relationship. Assisting the interested and concerned health practitioner is the fact that the patient has sought his or her help as an expert on health matters. Unless other factors intervene, therefore, the patient has a bias toward following advice that is offered. The fact that there is in-person contact also adds substantially to the ease of communications. These issues will be dealt with in greater detail in the last section of the book because there is evidence that if physicians or other health practitioners know their patients well, their track record in promoting safety and health-related behaviors is reasonably good.

Unfortunately, however, many health practitioners know even their regular patients so superficially that they are unlikely to have a strong sense—or in some cases even the vaguest clue—as to what types of priorities patients are likely to have if given a choice, for instance, between greater safety and somewhat limited mobility. Consequently, these practitioners may be unable to choose the sorts of arguments that might be most convincing.

Many components of the human/environmental interaction in the pre-injury and injury phases are beyond modification by individuals either because the individual lacks sufficient financial resources or because the technology or legal mechanisms for correction exist at a societal level. These forms of modification may at first blush seem to be beyond the helping capability of the individual health professional. The truth is, however, that groups of interested professionals—in many cases through the impetus of only one or two persons—often have been successful in helping a community to make appropriate choices for safety.

Appendix 5A
An Assessment of Factors Promoting or Hindering Development of a Safety Device

The following is an example of an administrator's assessment of factors promoting or hindering the development of a locomotive grade crossing crash attenuating device recommended by the National Transportation Safety Board in 1969.[18]

Safety Measure Assessed: Locomotive Grade Crossing Crash Attenuating Device

Group Viewpoint Expressed by Assessment: Administrator

CONCERNS	← Disfavors Measure		Favors Measure →	
A. *Public Appreciation of the Economic Need for Safety*				
I. *Size of Loss Preventable*				
a. Proportion of statistical loss in field preventable				
Percentage of losses below 1%	☐			
Percentage of losses 1–5%		☐		
Percentage of losses 6–10%			☐	
Percentage of losses 11% or more.				☒
b. Proportion of field of exposure to risk covered				
Exposure field covered below 1%	☐			
Exposure field covered 1–5%		☐		
Exposure field covered 6–10%			☐	
Exposure field covered 11% or more.				☒
c. Possible loss in single accident				
Accidents never involve many fatalities	☒			
Typical single accident is catastrophic			☐	

CONCERNS	Disfavors Measure ⟵		⟶ Favors Measure
Potential large scale population loss in one accident.			☐
II. *Effectiveness in Preventing Loss Relative to Costs*			
a. Priority assessed by effectiveness relative to cost			
Low cost effectiveness relative to alternatives	☐		
Medium position in cost effectiveness relative to alternatives		☐	
High standing in cost effectiveness relative to alternatives			☒
b. Priority assessed by effectiveness relative to effort not measured by cost	NOT APPLICABLE		
Low effectiveness relative to implementation effort alternatives	☐		
Medium effectiveness relative to implementation effort alternatives		☐	
High effectiveness relative to implementation effort alternatives			☐
III. *Benefit/Cost Status and Priority*			
a. Benefit/cost status of single safety risk			
Benefits less than cost	☐		
Benefits within ± 20% of cost		☐	
Benefits up to three times cost		☐	
Benefits more than three times cost			☒
b. Priority by benefit/cost status			
Low benefit/cost status relative to alternatives	☐		
Medium benefit/cost status relative to alternatives		☐	
High benefit/cost status relative to alternatives			☒
IV. *Absolute Cost of Prevention Measure*			
a. Absolute cost in proportion to other measures in field			
Cost greater than other measures	☐		
Cost similar to other measures		☒	
Cost less than other measures		☐	
Measure produces cost saving			☐

CONCERNS	← Disfavors Measure				Favors Measure →
b. Total investment necessary					
Investment large in proportion to other forms of investment in field	☐				
Investment about same as other competing forms of investment in field			☒		
Investment small in proportion to other forms of investment in field					☐
c. Perceived cost to individuals	NOT APPLICABLE				
Cost large in relation to competing costs for other functions	☐				
Cost about same as competing costs for other functions		☐			
Cost perceived as low compared to competing functions				☐	
Measure produces cost saving					☐
d. Operational loss of time not seen as cost					
Measure perceivably loses time	☐				
No perceptible effect on time saving				☒	
Measure perceivably saves time					☐
V. *Importance of Activity in an Economy*					
a. Initial effect on U.S. vs. foreign economies					
Measure initially unfavorable to balance of trade	☐				
Measure has no apparent effect on balance of trade			☒		
Measure initially favorable to balance of trade					☐
b. Initial importance to element of national economy					
Measure initially unfavorable to portion of economy	☐				
Effects on elements of economy tend to balance out			☒		
Measure initially expands portion of the economy					☐
c. Perceived need of individuals or groups for employment					
Measure tends to reduce employability of individuals	☐				

CONCERNS	Disfavors Measure ←		→ Favors Measure
No effect on employability of individuals			☒
Measure tends to expand number of employees			☐
B. *Public Image and Psychological Motives for Safety*			
I. *Need of Activity to Demonstrate Cooperation in Safety of Public*			
a. Perceived responsibility for safety of public			
Individuals regarded as primarily responsible	☒		
Individuals and organization share responsibility		☐	
Organization which conducts operations regarded as primarily responsible			☐
b. Relative status of activity in accident losses			
Activity has low loss rates among similar activities	☒		
Activity has loss rates near median among similar activities		☐	
Activity has high loss rates compared to similar activities			☐
II. *Presence of Public Apprehension of Activity*			
Activity generates little apprehension	☒		
Sufficient apprehension to affect individuals' economic decisions			☐
High degree of public apprehension			☐
III. *Concern of Individuals for Safety of a Loved One*			
Measure does not provide for perceivable control of protection of family or loved ones		☒	
Measure places an individual in position of perceivably controlling protection of a loved one			☐
IV. *Concern that a Feasible Safety Measure is Being Withheld*			
No perception by public that feasible protective measures could be applied		☒	
Impression that feasible safety measure is being withheld			☐

CONCERNS	← Disfavors Measure				Favors Measure →
Impression that hazard is known and tolerated for self-interest reason					☐
C. *Equality of Treatment for Groups at Risk*					
I. *Degree to Which Risk or Loss is Borne by Subject Group for Benefit of Others*					
Persons at risk fully compensated	☐				
Persons at risk receive benefit of employment		☐			
Persons at risk gain benefits about same as general population			☐		
Persons at risk bear risk almost entirely for benefit of others				☒	
Persons at risk bear risk for benefit of others without compensation					☐
II. *Status of Subject Group in Benefiting from Safety Funded Effort*					
Group would receive much greater benefits than others from safety measure	☒				
Group benefits equally with other comparable groups			☐		
Group which would benefit from safety funding not receiving proportionate share of benefits					☐
III. *Change in Responsibility Required of Subject Group*					
Responsibility of subject group increased	☐				
No change in responsibility			☒		
Responsibility of subject group decreased					☐
D. *Prevention of Unfairness to Subject Group in Avoiding Risk*					
I. *Ability of Persons at Risk to Know Hazard for Possible Avoidance*					
Persons at risk fully appreciate hazard	☒				
Some appreciation of hazard, but degree of risk unknown			☐		
System tends to minimize awareness of risk or encourage unrealistic confidence					☐

CONCERNS

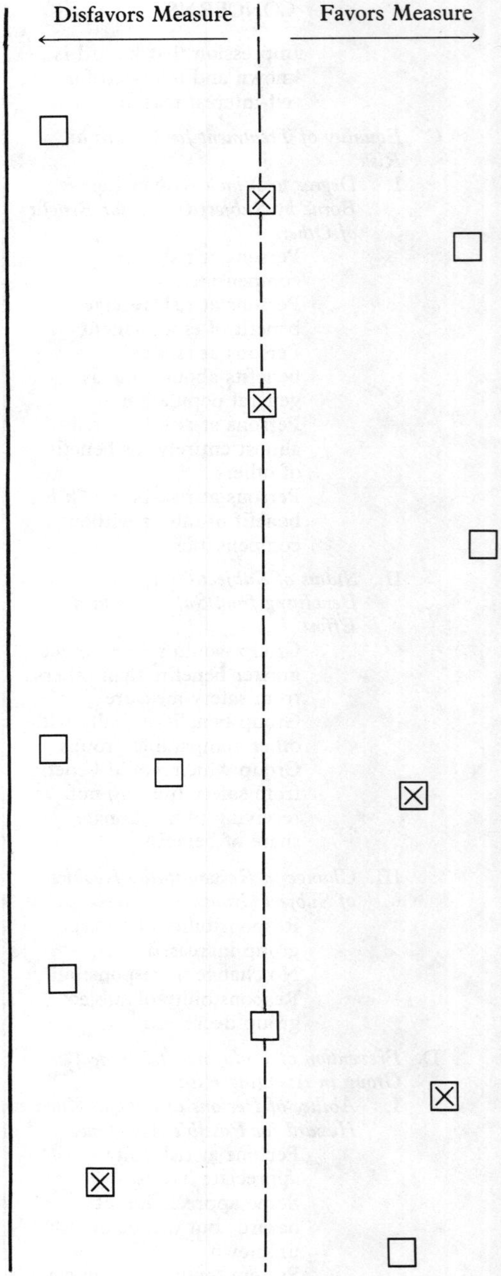

II. *Voluntary-Involuntary Status of Persons at Risk*
  - Persons at risk bear risk voluntarily
  - Persons at risk could avoid it at some cost or inconvenience
  - Persons at risk committed to risk-laden situation

E. *Status of Groups as Deserving Protection*

I. *Status by Reason of Traditional Special Consideration*
  - No special status of subject group
  - Subject group includes children, the aged, pregnant women, mentally retarded, physically handicapped, or physically ill.

F. *Technical Possibility of Safety Improvement*

I. *Technical Feasibility of Improvement*
  - Improvement presently considered not in the state-of-the-art (Awaits research or development)
  - Feasibility uncertain
  - No question of feasibility

II. *Critical-Uncritical Role of Improvement in Safety Control of System*
  - Improvement related to operation of remainder of system but not critical to complete system
  - Improvement needed but not critical
  - Improvement is critical to complete safety control effect

III. *Criticality of Timing of Action*
  - Immediate action not critical
  - Immediacy of action required to have desired effect

6
Some Questions about Numbers

One of the most crucial requirements for decision making either to initiate a safety activity or to evaluate its effectiveness is adequate information about the extent of a particular injury problem and about relative contributions of different factors to causation. Such data must accurately reflect the real world instead of being simply information of unknown validity plucked from doubtful sources in dubious manner and then subjected to questionable methods of organization, analysis, and interpretation. Unfortunately, much of the injury statistics in current use fits this sorry description. This is especially true concerning routine statistics gathered by official agencies but applies as well to some of the special research studies, in particular those that are based wholely or in part on data from such agencies.

This does not mean that statistical data should not be used, and in fact they will be used at length in the chapters that follow. Rather, they need to be used with full recognition of where and why they can be believed and where and why they must be viewed with caution or outright skepticism. This chapter, therefore, examines the various types of data being used and considers factors that determine their validity. In order to do this, we will examine closely definition, collection, analysis, and interpretation of information about frequency of events, severity of such events, and causation.

Quality of data involving countermeasure effectiveness is of equal importance to each of these three subject areas. It will be considered in a separate chapter, however, so that fuller attention can be given to appropriate goals and methods of program evaluation.

Frequency of Injury Events

According to an article from the World Health Organization,[1] about 250,000 people are fatally injured and over 7 million less seriously hurt on roads around the world each year. Furthermore, there are substantial geographic differences in death rates per 100 million passenger miles traveled. The United States had a rate of 6, the United Kingdom 13,

Kenya 55, and Uganda 65. Can these figures be believed? The answer is, barely—without substantial hedging and explanation.

The reasons for this difficulty are several: dissimilar definitions of injuries, variations in reporting requirements, incomplete reporting even where required, and in some cases no system at all for collection of data, either about exposure or about events. And these problems pale into insignificance when compared with information about injuries and deaths in the nonhighway setting.

First, let us consider definitions. Although the definitions have been becoming more similar in recent years, in one nation a death was not considered a highway fatality unless the person died at the crash site or immediately afterward, while the maximum qualifying interval between injury and death in order to be counted as a highway fatality ranged from one day in several nations through thirty days in most to one year in the United States.

And yet, according to one report[2] it is reasonable to assume internationally that only about 65 percent of highway fatalities are dead on arrival at the hospital, 88 percent within three days, and 97 percent within a month. Thus, although figures from different nations are commonly quoted in proximity to each other so as to suggest that comparisons can be made, there is no really feasible way to compare statistics from several nations in any meaningful manner without first attempting to adjust all figures to reflect expected deaths within thirty days.

To complicate matters, younger persons either are likely to die quickly from their injuries or to survive, whereas older individuals more often succumb to complications after surviving for days, weeks, or even months. Differences between nations in who gets counted according to duration of survival before death are likely to affect not only the numbers of deaths counted but also their relative distribution according to age.

If a person crashes (or is injured in other settings) as a result of a heart attack and then dies after injuries that are not in themselves very severe, such a death is commonly attributed to the illness rather than to the injury. However, it is often impossible to know what is the real cause of death unless a complete autopsy is carried out, and even in the United States such autopsies are the exception rather than the rule. This can result both in a spurious assumption that a person died of injury when the cause in fact was illness, or on the other hand that the person died of a heart attack when the cause was an internal injury that could not be identified simply by external examination of the body.

We have already noted the problem of the changing definition of sudden infant deaths, which used to be attributed entirely to suffocation. Through special studies of mechanisms of such deaths plus careful autopsies—which, as we have already noted, usually are not done—it is now possible to classify these deaths into several categories: suffocation, congenital defects, overwhelming infection, and probably developmental, congenital, or even genetic abnormalities of breathing mechanism. However, at this moment in time it is impossible to know where or how often sudden infant deaths are being correctly classified and where not so. Furthermore, even if current uniform criteria were consistently applied, there is still the problem of comparing information over time, since the number of sudden infant deaths attributed to suffocation from year to year cannot help but reflect the state of knowledge at that time as well as changes in the design and construction of bedding capable of causing suffocation. Thus, there may be difficulty in obtaining adequate information about trends even in a single community.

Consider also the classification of deaths as unintentional versus suicide. In the United States, almost 30,000 deaths a year are recorded as suicides, but it is estimated that as many as 50,000 such deaths may be occurring, many of them listed as unintentional injuries. One reason is attempts to hide the true cause for religious reasons, to avoid embarrassing family members, and for insurance purposes. Problems of under reporting and misreporting are especially serious in nations where large segments of the population have a deep commitment to religious faith that condemns this mode of death.[3] Furthermore, in most communities, investigation of the death may be quite superficial. In one city, deaths are classified as suicide only if a suicide note is left, although only about one of every three persons who commit suicide leaves a note.[4]

So far, we have considered definitions of injuries only as applied to fatalities, all of which are legally reportable. With certain exceptions, however, less serious events are not reportable. Let us now consider the definition of these events.

Highway injuries, no matter how minor, usually are reportable in the United States and Canada. So are injuries resulting from guns and occupational activities. But there is no agreement as to what comprises an injury. Back pain or minor lacerations may—or may not—be reported, depending on personal interpretation.

What little we know about unreportable injuries usually is gleaned from special studies based on either medical data about persons who sought treatment or on activities such as the National Health Survey.[5] In that program an injury is defined as whatever results in the seeking of medical care or in loss of ability to perform usual activities for a period of twenty-four hours or longer. This is probably a fairly reasonable operating definition.

Certain types of events may be reportable even if they do not result in injury, for example, highway crashes and plane crashes. Large differences exist, however, in the criteria for such reporting. In 1981, for example, in the United States and Canada one area required reporting of highway crashes only if the police investigated the crash, another only if the vehicle had to be towed. For the remainder, the criterion for reporting was property damage ranging from a minimum of $50 to $500.[6] Some adjacent areas had as much as fivefold differences in reporting criteria, and for no obvious reason.

Even this does not reflect the true diversity that exists because such criteria change over time within the boundaries of a single state or province. If we could assume that all reportable events were coming to the attention of the authorities, we still would be unable to compare statistics between geographic areas or even within one area over the years. Few public or official organizations, however, have been deterred from making such comparisons.

Most events resulting only in property damage are not reportable. A motorcyclist or snowmobiler who damages his vehicle beyond a given dollar amount on the highway would be required to report the event whether or not injury occurred. But neither property damage nor injury would be reportable if the damage occurred on a trail just a few feet to the side of the road. Again, one would learn about such events only through special surveys.

Even where reporting requirements exist, however, many such events simply are not brought to the attention of the appropriate agencies. As a general rule, the more serious the event the greater likelihood that reporting will occur. At least in most Western nations, data about number of fatalities can be considered to be reasonably reliable despite the problems already observed. However, in one study of falls among the elderly, only three of twenty-two persons who died after being hospitalized for falls had the fall noted anywhere on the death certificate.[7] This omission occurred although in most cases the illness that killed the person was a direct complication of the fall and in the remaining cases the fall was a significant other condition that should have been listed.

Checks of American, European, and Arabian Gulf hospital populations commonly identify that as many as half or even more of the individuals being treated for injuries from highway crashes have never reported these events to the police.[8,9] According to one study in California[10] the percentage of highway crashes that actually were reported to the police was only 38 percent for property damage crashes and 93 percent for events in which serious injuries occurred. When the most seriously damaged vehicle was considered beyond repair, only 86 percent were reported.

Inadequate reporting is not randomly distributed, and the resulting biases of statistics can erroneously suggest that populations or communities are either over- or underrepresented in injury events. Persons who already have recent highway crashes or citations and who might risk losing a license or insurance are less likely to report a crash than are those with previously clear records. Crashes in rural areas are overreported compared to urban crashes.[11] A self-contained rural fire might not be reported, but such a fire in a crowded urban area would probably bring the fire department.

Because of work overload, police in many jurisdictions no longer investigate crashes unless they involve injury or a vehicle so severely damaged that it must be towed, and residents of some urban neighborhoods are so hostile to the police that virtually no investigatory or reporting activities are carried out for either highway or nonhighway events unless they cannot be avoided. In some developing countries poorer people will do almost anything to avoid contacts with the police, and even relatively serious crashes may not be investigated or counted. A comparative study[12] showed that whereas in California 81 percent of reportable crashes appeared in state records, in Mississippi only 52 percent appeared, and in Illinois only 36 percent! Referring just to the Mississippi portion of this study, over 60 percent of reportable crashes of persons age 30 or under but 29 percent of those over age 30 were in the state records; 66 percent of crashes of men but 33 percent of those of women; and 71 percent of crashes to unskilled workers but 33 percent for semiprofessional or professional workers. Similar biases regarding age have been reported elsewhere as well.[11]

On the other hand, certain types of deliberate injury that are reportable may be passed off as unintentional. It has been estimated that as many as 10 percent of children treated for unintentional injuries at some hospitals may have been battered by an adult.[13] Some adults treated for injuries alleged to have occurred unintentionally in fact got those injuries in family arguments.

Measurement of Exposure

The frequency of injury events cannot be discussed without considering also the issue of exposure. It means little to say that two groups of 100 people have the same number of injuries if one group is engaged in the hazardous activity three times as frequently as the other. At least among research and evaluation personnel it is common practice, therefore, not only to present information about the number of injury events occurring (or the numerator) but also about the exposure population (the denominator) within which those events have happened. The resulting rates provide the only proper method for comparison.

The denominator most often used is the number of persons at risk. Thus, one may talk about the number of deaths from falls per 100,000 population or of crashes per 100 drivers. However, this type of denominator is appropriate only if there is reason to believe that all persons have similar exposures. But for many activities people differ both in the amount and type of exposure they have. In illustration, women have fewer crashes per 100 drivers than do men, but they drive fewer miles and perhaps on less hazardous roads and at safer times of day. With these corrections, the differences in crash rates disappear.

In the highway environment it is common practice to speak of crashes or injuries per unit vehicle miles, whereas air transport episodes are described per unit passenger miles or per unit number of landings. For ships the terminology is number of events per unit harbor entries. Occupational injuries are per unit person-hours worked and recreational injuries per unit recreational hours. For equipment, the denominator can be the number of times used or similar units of operation. The advantage of this diversity is that it permits more accurate assessment of relevant exposure. The disadvantage is that at present, because of different denominator terminology, relative risks of similar types of activity cannot be compared.

One can survey people about their exposure to various hazardous activities. This is helpful but has limitations because people often cannot easily recollect the overall extent of their exposures nor can they easily parcel exposure into subcategories such as miles of daytime versus nighttime driving and recreational versus occupational activity. Accurate prospective exposure information can be obtained for individuals engaged in specific organized athletic activities by having an observer note for each participant the number of minutes of play, number of tackles, and so forth.

Statewide overall driving exposure sometimes has been calculated based on gasoline sales. This method is crude because of unmeasurable variables that affect the outcome, despite attempts to take these into consideration. One such unknown is the proportion of gasoline used for driving versus for other activities such as boating, lawnmowers, and tractors. This may vary from one community and one season to another. Furthermore, automobiles achieve different mileage per gallon on different types of roads, in different climates and for different makes and models. Nor does this method permit estimation of mileage for specific subpopulations, such as by age, sex, or race, or in individual counties or towns.

Haddon and his colleagues[14] developed a method that controls for exposure without actually measuring the amount of exposure. Haddon's method is to interview or observe uninjured persons at the site of an injury event at a similar time of day and day of week. This method removes possible biases of interpretation attributable to inequalities of exposure, but it is useful only for activities that occur in public settings such as driving, walking, boating, or bicycling.

The "induced exposure" method for estimating the population at risk is still an experimental procedure, although preliminary data suggest that it is fairly accurate and relatively inexpensive.[15] Induced exposure is based on highway crash data. It is assumed that vehicles in single-vehicle crashes and "responsible" vehicles in two-vehicle crashes are so involved not so much because of exposure to the highway environment but because of "innate qualities" of the driver/vehicle category. The nonresponsible or "innocent" party in two-vehicle crashes, however, is presumed to be involved simply because of exposure. Analysis of characteristics of nonresponsible drivers and vehicles in crashes, therefore, should give relatively accurate information about the relative exposures of different types of drivers and vehicles not in crashes.[16]

It is generally assumed that certain types of behaviors predispose to the occurrence of injury events: for example, playing with matches by children or speeding, going through stop signs, and other forms of traffic violations. Theoretically, it should be possible to determine the rate of injury events per unit of exposure to such activities, and studies have shown that persons with traffic citations do have more reported crashes than do persons with clear records in Department of Motor Vehicle files.

But real-life problems exist in determining such exposure. How do you compare exceeding the limit by 5 miles per hour versus 15 M.P.H.? Since the violation is continuous, is the unit of exposure each mile of driving, each car met, or what? Is it important if speeding occurs when traffic is light or somewhat heavier? If one could always observe children playing with matches, do you count equally going through a whole match book and only one or two attempts?

A less theoretical problem is the existence of very pervasive biases in the issuance of citations. The traffic citation rate per 1,000 population, per, 1,000 vehicles, and per policeman and the types of citations issued vary widely depending on the philosophy of the particular police department.[17] In Dallas, for example, the rate of citations for moving violations is twenty-four times higher than in Boston, for no obvious reasons. If stopped, young drivers, men, and persons of lower socioeconomic status are more likely to be cited for a violation than are older drivers, women, or more affluent people.[12]

During the period of student unrest in the late 1960s, a sociology class in California carried out an experiment in which students whose cars and clothing ranged from "straight" to "hippy" had radical bumper stickers placed on their cars. Despite no change in driving behavior the students—all of whom had previously been determined to have clean driving records—promptly began receiving so many traffic citations that the experiment had to be stopped within eighteen days after it began![18]

A measure of exposure is useful only if it is an independent variable: that is, if it precedes rather than results from the injury event. In many cases, a citation is given because a violation is identified as a result of investigation of a crash, fire, or occupational injury rather than as a result of random or systematic observation whether or not harmful events have occurred.

Such citations are dependent variables rather than predictors, and in these cases a correlation has been automatically and spuriously built in between injury or property damage and exposure as measured by number of citations. Studies that exclude citations resulting from crash investigation show a much smaller relationship between traffic citations and crashes.[19] Furthermore, the nature of the relationship varies widely with the type of citation. Some citations—for example, for following too closely—are much more likely to be issued as a result of investigation of a crash than as an independent action of an officer who is simply observing traffic.

Finally, estimates of the frequency of particular types of injury events or of particular exposures can be affected by the type and size of the sample chosen. With the exception of data about fatalities, it is usually much too costly to try to get a complete census of all injury events (or exposures) in an area. Therefore, sampling methods are used for most research on the assumption that the sample of injury events or exposures chosen is fairly representative of all such events. Since the quality of data are fairly poor in many communities, researchers tend to collect their samples from those places where the most complete information can be obtained. The result is information that may be of high validity but often is of unknown generalizability, unless studies from a wide variety of communities come up with similar results.

Also, with small sample size and relatively infrequent events, there may be a substantial margin of difference between the real frequency as opposed to the observed frequency of the event. If 10 percent of fatalities in a sample of 200 deaths are bicyclists, two other samples of 200 deaths might show 3 percent and 15 percent bicyclists. But all three samples may differ only by chance, all reflecting the real proportion of bicyclist fatalities in that community to the degree of accuracy that might reasonably be expected for that sample size. Figure 6–1 shows how large an error might be expected in estimating the frequency of certain highway events given samples of different sizes, even when designing an expensive sampling system involving multiple sites.[20]

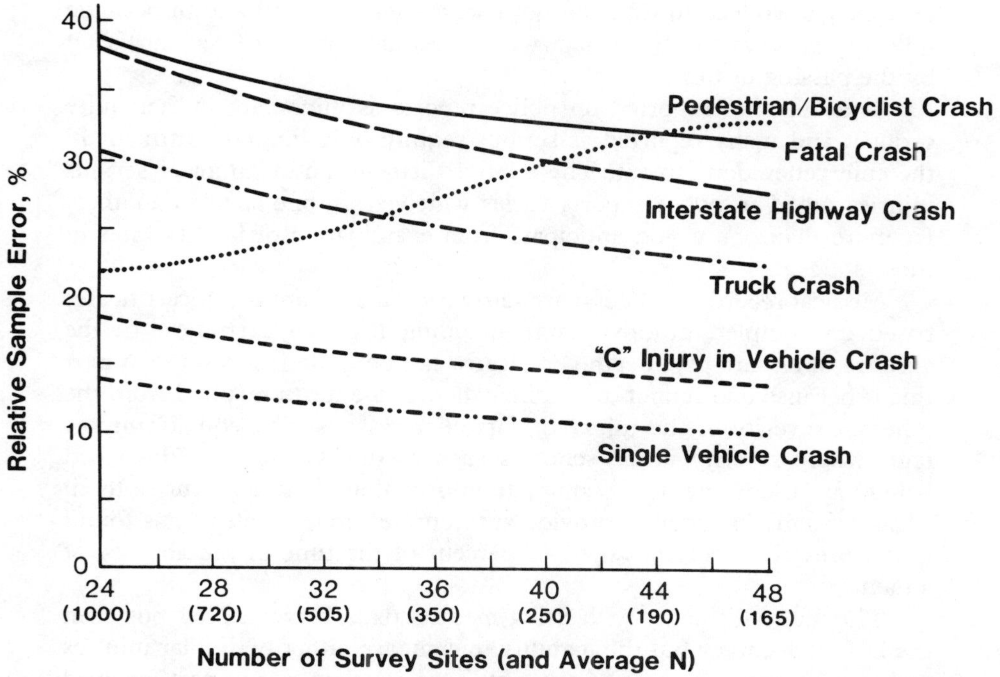

Source: Adapted from J.O'Day, A. Wolfe, and R. Kaplan, *Design for NASS: A National Accident Sampling System,* vol. 1 (Ann Arbor, Mich.: Highway Safety Research Institute, University of Michigan, Report UM-HSRI-SA-75-14-1, 1975). Used with permission.

Figure 6–1. Some Estimated Relative Sampling Errors for Studies of Specific Types of Highway Crashes Given Different Numbers of Survey Sites and of Crashes Surveyed Per Site.

Severity of Injury Events

Information about severity of injury or property damage may come from interviews of persons injured or who sustained the loss, statements on police or insurance records, medical records, autopsy reports, and information about property damage from special investigations.

People interviewed within two or three months usually are able to give fairly accurate information about time and general circumstances of the event, time lost from work or other activities, and whether medical or hospital care was needed. But they have only limited knowledge about the full nature or severity of injuries incurred.[21] For information about short-term costs, the person should be interviewed relatively soon after the event. For information about long-term costs, however, it becomes necessary to collect information both soon after the event and in periodic followup surveys to obtain data whose accuracy has not been tarnished by the passing of time.

Some injuries reported on police reports as minor are in fact quite serious, and many reported as serious require only limited treatment in the emergency department. The relative distribution of minor to serious injuries noted in police reports varies widely from one state to another, far more than one would anticipate from examination of fatality rates in those states.[21]

Medical records in general are fairly accurate, as are death certificates based on complete autopsy data, including toxicologic studies. In the absence of an autopsy, death certificates can be quite inaccurate. In part this is because one cannot determine whether the death resulted from the inherent severity of the injury or for other reasons. But equally important, where severity rating schemes such as the AIS or ISS (described below) are used, one needs complete information about all injuries to all organ systems in order to provide an accurate rating. States[22] has found that scores are incorrect up to 40 percent of the time in the absence of an autopsy.

The major difficulty with using medical data, however, has not been the lack of accuracy but the inability to compare rather dissimilar injuries and to rank them in order of severity. This problem was in part resolved with the development in 1971 of the Abbreviated Injury Scale, or AIS, which groups injuries of similar severity but involving different anatomic areas.[23]

The AIS does not take into account the fact that a person with several moderate injuries might conceivably have greater total traumatic impact than might a person with one major injury. Also, a person age 72 with a moderate injury might be in worse shape than a person age 30 with a severe injury. Initially, the AIS classified death as the most serious injury category. Some of the injuries resulting in death are not very severe, however, with death occurring because of inadequate care rather than because of the energy forces involved. Subsequent revisions in 1976 and 1980 have corrected this problem and have improved on the scaling of head injuries. Furthermore, recent work has substantially improved on the ability of researchers with varying backgrounds to use AIS as a reliable tool.[24]

In 1974 Baker et al.[25] developed a modification of the AIS known as the Injury Severity Score (ISS) in which higher scores than previously are assigned to persons with several injuries. This modified scale has now been applied by Bull[26] and others[27] to series of patients and has been shown to predict threat to life relatively accurately. More recently, Somers[27] has suggested that even greater accuracy can be obtained by scoring the two most serious injuries, no matter where they occur, instead of the three most serious injuries in different anatomic areas, as is done with the ISS. The AIS and ISS are shown in table 6–1.

The AIS and ISS define severity in terms of threat to life. But some studies are concerned primarily with less serious injuries, ranging from temporary disability or disfigurement to more lasting cosmetic defects. For this, the CPSC scale weights injury severity according to severity, body part, and disposition[28] (table 6–2) and has a hazard index for each product that represents a combination of frequency and severity.

Assessment of property damage in crashes is another problem area. Investigating police officers commonly try to assign a monetary value to vehicular losses at the scene of the crash, despite limited training in such assessment and neither equipment nor time for more than a superficial inspection. A vehicle described as a "total loss" may have incurred extensive impact resulting in total collapse of the passenger compartment

Table 6–1
Categories of Injury According to Abbreviated Injury Scale (AIS) and Its Modification through the Injury Severity Score (ISS)

AIS Code	*Severity Category*	*Illustrative Injury*
0	None	No injury
1	Minor	Headache, undisplaced nose fracture
2	Moderate	Closed, undisplaced skull fracture, loss of consciousness
3	Severe (not life threatening)	Concussion with loss of consciousness more than 15 minutes but no other neurologic signs
4	Serious (life threatening; survival probable)	Concussion with unconsciousness less than 12 hrs, other neurological signs
5	Critical (survival uncertain)	Unconscious more than 12 hrs, with intracranial hemorrhage and other severe neurological signs
6	Maximum (currently untreatable)	Massively crushed head (brain extrusion)

Calculating the ISS

1. Using AIS, grade all injuries.
2. Identify most serious injury in each of six body areas: head or neck, face, chest, abdominal or pelvic contents, extremities or pelvic girdle, external.
3. Selecting three most serious injuries in separate body areas, square each, and sum the squares (for example, $4^2 + 3^2 + 1^2 = 26$). The maximum possible score is 75 assigned either to a person with severity 5 injuries in three separate areas or one severity 6 injury.

Source: Adapted from Committee on Injury Scaling, *The Abbreviated Injury Scale, 1980 Revision* (Morton Grove, Ill.: American Association for Automotive Medicine, 1980), and S.P. Baker, B. O'Neill, W. Haddon, Jr., and W.B. Long, "The Injury Severity Score: A Method for Describing Patients with Multiple Injuries and Evaluating Emergency Care," *Journal of Trauma* 14(1974):187–196.

Table 6–2
CPSC Severity Scoring System

Diagnostic Categories	*Severity Categories (and Assigned Weights) and Examples*
Amputation	1. (10) e.g., abrasion of arm or leg
Avulsion	2. (12) e.g., foreign body in arm, leg, hand, foot, finger,
Burns	toe, eye
Cell damage	3. (17) e.g., foreign body in mouth
Concussion	4. (31) e.g., foreign body in lower trunk
Contusion or abrasion	5. (81) e.g., foreign body in head, face, ear, neck, upper
Crushing	trunk
Dermatitis	6. (340) e.g., foreign body ≥ 25% of body
Dislocation	7. (2516) any category 6 injury resulting in hospitalization.
Foreign body	Injuries in lower severity categories that result in
Fracture	hospitalization are raised to the next higher severity
Hematoma	level. (e.g., a 4 becomes a 5)
Internal organ injury	8. Death
Laceration	
Nerve damage	
Poisoning	
Puncture	
Strain or sprain	

Source: Adapted from National Electronic Injury Surveillance System, "Estimated Mean Severity" (12 April 1979); "Summary of Severity Index" (n.d.); "Priority Index for Injury Classification" (rev. October 1970) (Washington, D.C.: National Injury Information Clearinghouse, Consumer Product Safety Commission, mimeographed documents).

or may have received only moderate energy loads that make repair more expensive than total value but that have only modest injury potential for occupants.

In response, a vehicle damage scale (TAD)[29] was developed based on actual measurement of the amount of crush that a vehicle undergoes. This research tool assesses severity with reasonable success,[30] despite biases in the scaling mechanism.[31] TAD does not consider that two different vehicles may respond to similar energy loads in different ways, so that one incurs more crush than the other. Ultimately, a method is needed that assesses the actual energy loads imparted, rather than only the outcomes of that energy. The CALSPAN CRASH computer simulation model[32] attempts this. The technology is still primitive and applicable only to certain types of crashes, but for these it does provide a creditable measurement of reality.

Causation

Perhaps the greatest inadequacies of information, especially in statistics of official agencies, exist in data about the causation of injury events.

These inadequacies occur first because investigations and explanations of events commonly follow the "traditional wisdom." In some cases, those reporting on the event have been given absolutely no professionally developed guidelines about what sort of information is relevant, by excluding, for example, questions about use or presence of alcohol.[33,34] In some nations, no standard crash investigation form or system exists.

On the other hand, where investigators are given guidance, it may be so biased as to result in an entirely unrealistic picture of causal factors. We have already noted Benner's important observation that the underlying scheme of causation that guides the investigator in large part determines what will be looked for and found and how it will be interpreted and classified.

In illustration, a study identified 668 contributory factors among 104 motor vehicle crashes in Iowa.[35] Fifty percent of these factors were vehicle related, 31 percent involved the environment, and 19 percent the driver. According to the author of the study, the results contradict the prevalent concept that 85 percent of crashes result from driver error or misfunction. This widespread belief, he states, comes from the fact that individual states report their annual crash experience to the National Safety Council on a standard form, which has space for only twelve contributing circumstances, of which two relate to the vehicle, and the other ten to the driver, with no roadway circumstances included.

If the results of his investigation were tabulated on the standard summary form, the total number of contributory factors in the 104 crashes would have been reduced from 668 to 140, and 125, or 89 percent, would be driver-related. The majority of the contributory factors could not be included. In another more recent multidisciplinary investigation of highway crashes vehicular factors were identified as contributory about ten times more frequently than listed in the official statistics.[36]

Even where problems are not designed into the philosophy of investigation, those who seek to determine cause are commonly hampered by lack of training or limited availability of test procedures, time, funds, or equipment that are necessary to complete a meaningful examination and analysis. Except in rare instances, tests for alcohol or other drugs are not carried out, especially if the injury did not occur in the highway setting. Vehicles or other products and other environmental factors may be examined only superficially, if at all, and, if examined, only frank failure of parts is sought, rather than inadequate design or construction that may contribute to excessive task demand in the absence of obvious product malfunction.

The results of not observing the nature of this interaction are well described by Thorson[37] as follows: "The phrase 'the human factor' is often used to characterize the causes of accidents. The concept includes conditions that are *outside* the scope of human *influence,* as well as conditions *within* the scope of human influence. By mixing these two contrasting senses and by limiting causal analyses of accidents to ergonomic and psychological references, 'the human factor' may be put forward as especially suitable for measures, their preventive value is, however, marginal or quite fanciful."

Possible indicators of medical impairment may not be followed up or, at the other extreme, an event may be attributed to "falling asleep" despite no evidence that this is the case. The only systematic exception to such superficial investigation of which I am aware occurs in commercial airline crashes, where in a number of nations complete teams of trained investigators are available and attempt to reconstruct all aspects of each event.

In order to improve on the quality of information available, the U.S. Department of Transportation (DOT) has now established several Multidisciplinary Accident Investigation teams (MDAIs) to reconstruct specific types of crashes, and the Consumer Product Safety Commission (CPSC) has similarly sought to carry out more intensive examination of injuries involving selected types of products.

A typical MDAI investigation during the 1970s, however, cost $1,500 to $3,500, a sum far beyond the budget capabilities for routine statistics gathering of virtually all official agencies. Furthermore, both the DOT and the CPSC samples are collected in such a way that the data cannot be generalized, and in neither case has exposure information been collected, thus substantially limiting the types of conclusions about causation that can be reached. DOT, however, has recently developed a National Accident Sampling System that seeks to avoid many, but by no means all, of the current deficiencies.[38]

7
Evaluating Countermeasures

> And the earth was waste and void; and darkness was upon the face of the deep. And the spirit of God moved upon the face of the waters. And God said, Let there be light: and there was light. And God saw the light, that it was good: and God divided the light from the darkness.
>
> *Genesis*

Although the above Biblical description of the first program evaluation suggests that the subject may have divine mandate, Gordis[1] sadly observes that even this evaluation had several flaws: to wit, there was no control group, no budget, no predetermined criteria for defining success of outcome, and we must take it on faith that the program manager, in acting also as evaluator, was both unbiased and qualified for the task.

Most safety countermeasures have undergone absolutely no evaluation. In this chapter we will discuss some schemes for evaluating countermeasures and examine ways in which evaluation efforts—where they have been attempted—deviate from these schemes and what are the interpretive effects.

OPSKARBO: What's Happening, to Whom, and for What Purpose?

OPSKARBO[2] is an acronym for a method to identify the important components in countermeasure schemes and objectives. Each letter represents a separate component, and three different levels of outcome can be identified. *O* stands for organizational structure, in recognition of the often-forgotten fact that in the absence of a properly designed and applied organizational plan, countermeasure ideas become countermeasure efforts purely by chance. The organizational pattern, therefore, needs to be carefully documented and monitored.

P refers to the program elements and their process evaluation. To successfully use a portable breath tester for alcohol, it is necessary first, as part of the process of countermeasure design, to determine that the breath tester to be used is in fact capable of identifying almost all individuals with BACs above a certain point and of excluding those with lower BACs under the specific circumstances of use. An educational program should not be used until and unless there is first preliminary information from process evaluation that it at least is capable of educating in the intended manner a trial sample of the audience at whom it is aimed.

Often, however, a new safety film or poster is advertised as being successful because it has been given an award by some media-related organization or because it appeared on a certain number of TV shows or was seen by so many hundreds or thousands of people. No attention may be paid, however, to whether there has been pretesting of the theme or whether it has been documented to have a beneficial effect on the intended audience.

Whereas equipment for safety countermeasures usually undergoes extensive process evaluation before being introduced, such pretesting, even on a very limited scale, is not even thought of, much less tried, for most behavioral countermeasures. Many such behavioral modification efforts lack both a clear definition of the specific audience at which they are aimed and of the specific behavioral outcomes being sought, although they are expected to reach, affect, and alter people with a wide range of attributes.

The organization and process evaluation components of the model refer to input variables, aspects of the countermeasure itself. We now turn to three different levels of result or outcome. Level 1 outcome is covered by the letters *SKAR*. A countermeasure may bring about changes in skills, knowledge, attitudes, or resources. A campaign telling people to "drive safely" may instill appropriate attitudes toward safety but provide no knowlege about the attributes of safe driving or offer the skills in how to accomplish it with any consistency. A family with a wood-burning stove may know after a safety campaign that the chimney needs to be cleaned periodically but may be unable to do it themselves, and the appropriate resource—a competent chimney sweep—may not be available in the community.

A countermeasure that provides knowledge without the other necessary components would not be expected to be successful in bringing about a change in level 2 outcomes. One of the issues overlooked in current efforts in the United States to convince people to wear seatbelts, for example, is the fact that despite proper knowledge and attitudes, people with arthritis may be unable to reach and attach a seat belt. Inability to attach a belt may occur also for obese people or short people with heavy winter clothing who must have their seats pulled up fully so they can drive. The manufacturers, in fact, have specifically designed these people out!

The level 2 outcome is a change in behavior: the *B* in the OP-SKARBO acronym. Just because SKAR outcomes change does not *necessarily* mean that this will be accompanied by an appropriate change in behavior, as some studies of efforts to change alcohol consumption by drivers have shown. And even if behavior changes, that doesn't *necessarily* mean that ultimate or level 3 outcome (the final *O*) will change.

This final outcome may be measured by improvement in cost effectiveness of a countermeasure and/or reductions in death, disability, discomfort, dissatisfaction, or deleterious side effects of a previous countermeasure program (all summarized by the acronym CoEddddd). One deleterious side effect identified by critics of driver education programs for teenagers is that, in the United States at least, they tend to promote licensing of drivers who are only age 16 or 17 and consequently increase driving exposure, crashes, injuries, and fatalities for this very high-risk group.

Why is it necessary to go to all this trouble to tease out and examine all of these components in order to evaluate a countermeasure? Isn't it enough simply to show that a given effort either does or doesn't reduce death and injury?

Let us examine a situation where a new program to arrest and jail more alcohol impaired drivers has been found *not* to lower the fatal crash rate. Simply knowing that does not leave people with the necessary information about what to do next. Without going through all of the steps one has no idea whether the entire hypothesis was flawed (that is, reduced driving while impaired by alcohol has no effect on fatality rate), whether for organizational or other reasons the countermeasure was never really applied, or whether it was applied and changed knowledge, skills, and attitudes but not behavior.

If you only want to know *whether* a countermeasure affects death and disability, it is not necessary to evaluate all programatic aspects. But if you want to know *how* and *why* the countermeasure functions as it does (or why it doesn't function), a more complex examination is necessary.

Also important is the fact that there often must be two levels of SKARB change if a countermeasure is to succeed. In order for a countermeasure to reach its intended target—the people at greatest risk of injury—it often must be mediated by societal gatekeepers: road builders or maintainers, vehicle manufacturers or repair personnel, police, courts, teachers, physicians, city planners, and so forth. These individuals often must be reached first by countermeasure planners and must have appropriate changes in SKARB (which are also amenable to evaluation) before the intended ultimate target is even approached.

One does not have to look far for examples of altering of program ideas by gatekeepers. We already noted that a motor vehicle standard may be applied in a very cost-effective way by a manufacturer or in a manner that will be both costly and inconvenient to the public.[3] In illustration, the NHTSA proposal for airbags and other passive restraints in automobiles several years ago ended up after suggestion by representatives of the automotive industry as the infamous seatbelt interlock. This device, which prevented the driver from starting a car until the seatbelt was fastened, promptly infuriated the driving public. In Connecticut in the 1960s a law was passed requiring that drivers convicted of speeding lose their licenses for a period of time. In response, the police stopped drivers for speeding but then began to cite them with violating another section of the vehicle code that did not carry such a Draconian punishment.[4]

Evaluation Strategies

We will now consider two further issues that are essential to a successful evaluation: selection of the population to be studied and of methods for comparison. As has become very clear in the initial evaluations of driver education programs, the use of volunteers may substantially bias the outcome of a study. The first thirty or so driver education programs were all elective courses in high schools. Evaluation was carried out by comparing the crash rates after licensing of those students who had elected and taken the course and those who had not elected and not taken the course. Consistently, the course takers did better.

Skeptics questioned, however, whether the difference reflected the effects of the course, stronger prior attitudes toward safety, other characteristics of the volunteers, or a combination of these factors. Finally, Conger and his associates[5] tried to answer the question. They divided students electing driver education into two groups: those who completed the course and those who were unable to take it because of class conflicts or lack of facilities. Next, they compared characteristics and crash rates of these two volunteer groups with those of nonvolunteers who also had recently been licensed.

The results were by no means conclusive because those who completed the course, among other things, averaged fewer miles of driving exposure than did the other two groups, and the authors report that the interactions are extremely complex, involving far more than driver education alone. Two years later Asher[6] showed that student characteristics associated with electing a driver education course are the same characteristics that per se are associated with lower crash rates. Whether the issue is the injury experience of people who volunteer for driver education, who use seat belts in the absence of compulsory use laws, who purchase products with safety features, or who accept driver rehabilitation programs, any evaluation runs the risk of the volunteer bias unless some random form of treatment selection is built into the evaluation scheme.

The second important issue in evaluation strategies is the examination not only of the treatment population before and after application of the treatment but also the use of a comparison or "control" population that is similarly examined at two comparable time intervals: the so-called two-by-two study design. All too often, countermeasures are reported to be successful because a reduction in dangerous behavior or injury events has occurred in a group that had been deviant before the treatment. Without a comparison group, it is quite impossible to know whether the observed reduction occurred because of the specific countermeasure or for a totally unrelated reason (for example, reduced exposure to risk) or because of regression to the mean, a statistical concept that will be discussed shortly.

If children injured on skateboards were given lessons in skateboard safety, I would anticipate that over the next six months their injury rate would be lower. But I would also expect that a group of similarly injured skateboarders who did not have a safety lesson would have an equivalent drop in injury rate. Both had probably gained more experience in skateboarding, and highest injury rates are usually among learners. Also, because skateboarding is a fad, as are so many newly introduced recreational activities, I would anticipate that both groups would have much lower skateboarding exposure during the six months after injury than during the few months before injury.

Ideally, inferences concerning the effectiveness of a countermeasure should be drawn through a controlled experiment in which subjects are randomly assigned to either a study group that is exposed to the countermeasure or to a "control" group that does not receive the measure. Through random assignment, one hopes to achieve similar a priori characteristics for both groups and thus to rule out or weaken alternative explanations for any observed differences in outcome, as occurred with the driver education studies.

Such random asignments usually are not possible, however, in evaluation designs, and most often it is necessary to resort to quasi-experimental designs in which outcome comparisons are made between groups defined a priori, such as communities or hospital service areas. If this approach is used, careful attention must be given to choosing areas or populations that appear to have similar characteristics or whose differences at least are well documented. Cook and Campbell[7] have described in detail four basic quasi-experimental designs and consider advantages and limitations of each.

If it does not seem possible to have an "untreated" population, the "treatment" in some cases can be postponed for part of the population so that the injury event or behavior experience of the first treatment group A can be examined before and after treatment and that of the delayed treatment group B can be compared initially as a control with the first treatment group, and then with itself in a before/after mode as follows:

	Period		
	1	*2*	*3*
Group A	C	T	T
Group B	C	C	T

C = Control
T = Treatment

One then compares A_1 and B_1, A_1 and A_2, A_2 and B_2, B_2 and B_3, and A_3 and B_3. The expectation—if the countermeasure works—is that A_1, B_1, and B_2 would be equal in injury or behavior experience, as would A_2, A_3, and B_3. The latter three, however, would be less than the former three. This combination of observations documents not only that change has occurred but that it is reasonably attributable to the countermeasure and not to external factors.

Sometimes, a new product rapidly floods an entire market, or a law is applied simultaneously across an entire nation, and it is impossible to obtain either a comparison or delayed treatment population. In that case—and only in that case—it may be necessary to use a so-called time sequence technique: that is, to follow the frequency trend of the injury event or behavior in question over a sequence of months or years before the countermeasure is applied and then to observe if there is a sudden discontinuity in the trend (such as a downward displacement) when the countermeasure begins. While this method can identify *if* a shift occurs, it cannot define—although it may suggest—*why* it has occurred. If something else happened at the same time—as in 1973 with the 55 M.P.H. speed limit and the gasoline shortage in the United States—

experts may spend the next several years arguing as to what actually caused the shift.

Statistical Issues

We have already observed (figure 6–1) the extent to which the use of small samples for the measurement of a phenomenon can vastly increase uncertainty about the real size of the event. This problem also exists with respect to program evaluation. Figure 7–1 shows how the size of samples affects the conclusion reached in studies of the effectiveness of occupant restraints in reducing injury and death.[8] The high peaks represent highly believable results involving large samples that have a very narrow margin of error. The low flat peaks involve small samples and consequently have a much greater margin of error. This difference in sample size is one reason why studies have described seatbelts as anywhere from totally ineffective to over 75 percent effective in reducing injury. Another reason, apparent from this figure, is that seatbelts are more effective in reducing serious and fatal injuries than in reducing minor ones. Thus, the conclusion of "success" or "failure" depends on the care taken in initially defining the program goals and objectives. If the sought-after end point is to reduce *all* injuries, the effectiveness of seatbelts will be less (25 percent) than if the goal is defined as reducing *serious and fatal* injury (50 percent reduction) or *fatal injury only* (65 percent decrease).

One important statistical issue is the phenomenon of "regression toward the mean." During a recent year, Vermonters were upset because the number of highway deaths appeared to be rising rapidly over a period of a few months. Because this small state has an average of about 140 highway deaths a year, the total deaths in any recent year could range *purely by chance* from about 115 all the way up to about 175 or 180, if one takes into account the modest population growth over several years. Given the small size of the "samples" selected each year, variations within this wide range had absolutely no statistical significance. A death total of 170 one year could conceivably be followed by one of 120 the next year with absolutely no change in countermeasure activity. Or the figures could go in exactly the opposite direction, despite no change in circumstances.

Often, a major countermeasure activity is started in response to an initial "unacceptably high" fatality figure, and this is followed the next year by a drop back toward the average figure: so-called regression toward the mean. Unless either a two-by-two design or a time-sequence design is used, the fact that the regression is not significantly different from the high point is likely to be overlooked. This type of evaluation

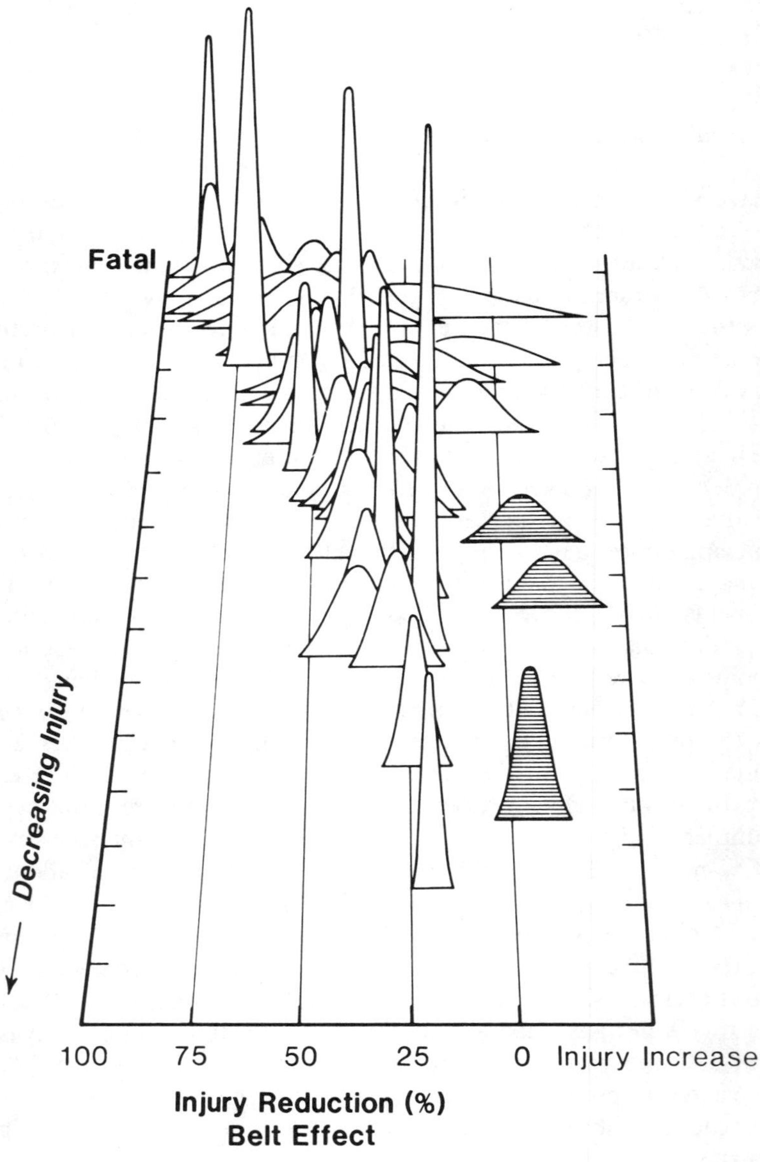

Source: Adapted from B.J. Campbell and D.W. Reinfurt, "The Degree of Benefit of Belts in Reducing Injury: An Attempt to Explain Study Discrepancies," (Warrendale, Pa.: Society of Automotive Engineers, SAE Technical Paper Series 790684, 1979). Reprinted with permission, copyright © 1979 Society of Automotive Engineers, Inc.

Figure 7–1. Conclusions and Margins of Error in Studies of Effectiveness of Passenger Restraints in Reducing Injuries and Fatalities.

error is common and results from failure to understand the random variation of all natural phenomena around a mean value.

After one such bad year in Connecticut, Governor Ribicoff was able to push through a law mandating that drivers who were convicted of speeding would automatically lose their licenses. Although the intent of the law was circumvented by police officers who stopped giving out "speeding tickets," within a year after the law went into effect the highway fatality rate dropped, and the law was described as a great success. It was, in actuality, simply a regression to the mean fatality rate of the previous several years.

Countermeasure Effect Over Time

One frustration of health and safety personnel is that a new countermeasure may show effects much more slowly than anticipated or, conversely, really "take off" with good results and then peter out. If only a two-by-two design is followed, with examination of results at one time shortly after the countermeasure is initiated, the evaluator may be wrongly disappointed in the first case and falsely elated in the second. Green[9] has described a range of responses over time to countermeasure efforts in addition to the hoped-for response of immediate and lasting improvement. Apparently all of the trends noted below occur, for reasons that are sometimes explainable and sometimes not. It is wise, therefore, in carrying out an evaluation to examine outcome over at least two (and preferably more) separate time intervals after the countermeasure effort begins.

Green's classification of outcome trends over time is as follows:

1. *Delayed impact* or *sleeper effect*, in which changes do not occur until some time after the program has been initiated;
2. *Back-sliding effect*, in which changes occur quickly but then the impact of the countermeasure decays or diminishes the longer the countermeasure is continued, until finally little or no positive effect is observed;
3. *Trigger effect*, also known as borrowing from the future, an example of which would be where people who were thinking of purchasing a safety device are finally motivated by an educational effort to undertake their purchases, but no additional individuals who were not previously interested now become motivated and make purchases. The net result would be a sudden increase in purchases followed by a decrease below the baseline level and then a return to the baseline;

4. *Contrast effect,* in which the program brings about an increase of behavior above baseline level, but then a backlash occurs upon cessation of the program so that the ultimate level of behavior is actually less than was the case during the baseline.

Green also refers to "historical events" in which change of behavior or of the phenomenon being measured occurs concordant with the countermeasure activity, but the change is simply part of a trend that was occurring already and in fact was in no way affected by the countermeasure.

Effects of Simultaneous Countermeasures

Several years ago I observed a fascinating argument between members of a state police department and the state highway engineers. The police, using the two-by-two evaluation design, had just reported that an increased enforcement effort at a specific location had reduced injury crashes. The engineers were quite upset because they had just completed a minor highway improvement at this location and had attributed the same drop in injury crashes to their program. Neither group had taken into consideration the activities of the other.

Not uncommonly, several activities occur simultaneously, whether it be the altering of medication and advice about safe and unsafe actions for the elderly patient who is having dizzy spells or the simultaneous adoption of several automobile safety standards or an entirely new building code by a governmental agency. How does one determine which countermeasure is working well, which only minimally, and which even has unwanted side effects?

At times it is impossible to tease out the individual components, and one can only speak about the overall effect of the effort because of the complexity of the interaction. How, for example, does one measure the intended positive impact on safety of various occupant protective devices in automobiles in the presence of the expected negative impact on safety of vehicle "downsizing"? At other times it is possible to examine specific types of events that appear to be unique to specific types of countermeasures. Examples would be a reduction in side impacts at night for automobiles with head and tail lights that are visible from the side, or reduction in whiplash injuries in rear-end crashes after installation of head supports.

In some cases also one can modify the two-by-two design to permit examination of different countermeasures both alone and in combination. One project in Vermont[10] compared alcohol-related behavior in a population receiving no countermeasures with those of populations exposed to an educational effort only, increased law enforcement only, and a combination of education plus law enforcement. Needless to say, such countermeasure and evaluation designs require considerable planning, extensive cooperation, and careful attention to the possibility of "leakage" of countermeasures from one population or geographic area to another.

Part II
Specific Types of Injury Events

8
Societal Impact of Injury

In part II we will explore what is known about injury events in a variety of settings, in a few cases structuring chapters instead around specific mechanisms of injury (burns, falls, and poisoning) or specific types of carriers (such as various products used in and around the home). Before starting with individual types of injury events, however, it would be useful to have a look at the whole. To what extent is injury a problem compared to other conditions that threaten health? Are there broad differences between nations? What are the relative impacts of different types of injury events?

Based on data from the National Health Survey,[1] almost a third of the population annually is injured severely enough to seek medical care or to be unable to perform usual activities for one day or longer (table 8–1). While injury rates are lowest among persons age 45 or older, days of disability requiring restriction to bed are highest in this age group. The frequency of injury involving motor vehicles is small compared to injury in the home and other nonwork activities, but its relative contribution to bed disability and, as we shall see, to death is much larger.

A more detailed categorization of nonfatal injuries is shown in table 8–2,[2] while table 8–3 shows comparable data for an undeveloped area of the world from the Gorden et al. study in rural Punjab.[3] The distributions of nonfatal injuries are quite different, with animals playing a much more important role, and falls a lesser role, in India. Representative nonfatal injury data are generally not available for other parts of the world.

Data are available more widely concerning deaths from injury, although surprising and vexing absences exist. *World Health Statistics Annual*[4] has no mortality data for most of South America or Africa, or for India, Pakistan, the USSR or China. Assuming a worldwide population of about 4.5 billion people, I would estimate approximately 375,000 fatalities per year from unintentional injury.

Table 8–4 shows mortality from injury and other specified causes for nations that reported 50,000 deaths or more annually during the mid-1970s. Although difficult to compare with accuracy, they do suggest, no matter what the state of development of the nation, that injury deaths

Table 8–1
Injury and Related Disability by Age, Sex, and Type of Event, United States, 1980

	Total	*Males*	*Females*	*<6 yrs*	*6–16*	*17–44*	*45–64*	*≥65*
Persons injured per 100 persons per yr	31.2	37.1	25.8	34.2	39.2	35.3	22.2	16.8
Moving motor vehicles[b]	2.0	2.2	0.9	0.5[a]	2.2	3.0	0.8[a]	1.2[a]
Work[b]	5.0	7.6	2.5	—	—	9.2	5.1	0.6[a]
Home[b]	12.2	12.6	11.9	22.8	14.8	10.6	9.9	10.1
Other[b]	12.9	16.2	9.9	10.9	22.8	14.1	6.8	5.2
Days restricted activity per 100 persons per yr	357.4	415.0	303.8	47.4	201.0	376.8	486.8	547.3
Moving motor vehicles	66.7	75.0	59.0	—	27.8	89.3	76.8	77.3
Work	84.7	140.6	32.7	—	—	115.8	147.9	53.7
Home	86.2	71.1	100.4	27.7[a]	51.9	55.1	133.6	223.1
Other	137.9	161.0	116.4	19.7[a]	122.0	140.2	165.3	199.5
Days restricted disability per 100 persons per yr	88.7	98.1	80.0	15.8[a]	40.8	87.8	131.5	150.2
Moving motor vehicles	16.9	17.6	16.3	—	8.7[a]	19.6	22.3	23.4
Work	19.6	31.0	8.9	—	—	23.7	40.0	13.6[a]
Home	24.4	21.7	26.9	7.4[a]	18.4	16.0	37.1	57.0
Other	32.1	34.6	29.7	8.4[a]	14.2	33.0	42.3	57.4

Source: *Current Estimates from the National Health Interview Survey: United States, 1980* (Hyattsville, Md.: U.S. Department of Health and Human Services, National Health Survey Series 10 No. 139, 1981).

[a]Because of small sample size may have more than 30 percent relative standard error.

[b]Sum of data for the four types of events may be greater than the total because the types are not mutually exclusive.

Table 8–2
Annual Rates of Nonfatal Injuries Per 1,000 Population by Sex, Age, and Detailed Description of Event, United States, 1971–72

Type of Event	*Both Sexes*		*Males*	*Females*	*0–5*	*6–16*	*17–24*	*25–44*	*45–64*	*≥65*
Moving motor vehicles	(4,722)[a]	23.2	27.5	19.3	7.0[b]	19.8	56.1	26.3	16.0	9.7[b]
Uncontrolled fire/ explosion	(93)[b]	0.5[b]	0.8[b]	0.2[b]	—	—	1.4[b]	1.1[b]	—	—
Firearms	(155)[b]	0.8[b]	1.2[b]	0.4[b]	—	0.8[b]	0.6[b]	2.1[b]	—	—
Nonmotor vehicle moving	(1,205)	5.9	7.3	4.6	10.4[b]	17.5	2.1[b]	2.0[b]	0.5[b]	1.2[b]
Operating machinery	(1,270)	6.2	11.4	1.5[b]	—	2.0[b]	13.4	9.6	7.4[b]	1.8[b]
Cutting/piercing instrument	(4,194)	20.6	24.4	17.1	14.9[b]	34.6	26.6	17.3	13.6	9.7[b]
Foreign body	(1,465)	7.2	10.9	3.8	10.9[b]	6.1[b]	12.0[b]	8.5	3.9[b]	2.9[b]
Animal	(2,682)	13.2	13.6	12.8	25.2	18.5	7.6[b]	10.9	9.0	10.7[b]
Fall from stairs/height	(4,403)	21.7	24.9	18.6	52.8	27.7	15.6	16.1	13.5	14.4[b]
Other falls	(9,208)	45.3	44.2	46.4	63.3	63.0	39.0	25.3	33.4	69.2
Bumped object/person	(5,648)	27.8	38.6	17.7	24.0	50.8	36.8	21.9	14.8	9.0[b]
Struck by moving object	(4,104)	20.2	28.9	12.1	23.5	38.1	24.8	15.6	8.5	5.7[b]
Handled/stepped on rough object	(2,309)	11.4	13.9	9.0	15.7[b]	18.5	13.2	9.2	6.0[b]	4.7[b]
Pinched/crushed	(1,203)	5.9	8.3	3.7	12.3[b]	8.4	5.2[b]	6.1[b]	3.1[b]	—
Contacted hot object	(994)	4.9	6.1	3.8	13.7[b]	2.3[b]	6.7[b]	5.5[b]	3.2[b]	0.9[b]
Lifting or exertion	(2,354)	11.6	16.5	7.0	—	2.4[b]	15.2	19.5	19.5	3.6[b]
Twisted or stumbled	(2,890)	14.2	17.3	11.3	0.9[b]	24.7	19.4	14.5	10.3	5.0[b]
Therapeutic complication	(2,455)	12.1	12.1	12.1	41.5	10.7	11.0[b]	7.8	6.6[b]	7.6[b]
Other	(3,420)	16.8	20.6	13.4	30.1	15.2	14.3	17.5	11.7	19.2
Unknown	(8,623)	42.4	42.1	42.8	47.5	30.7	65.1	52.4	28.6	36.6

Source: *Persons Injured and Disability Days by Detailed Type and Class of Accident: United States, 1971–1972.* (Hyattsville, Md.: U.S. Department of Health and Human Services, National Health Survey Series 10 No. 105, 1981).

[a]Number of injuries in thousands.
[b]Because of small sample size may have more than 30 percent relative standard error.

Table 8–3
Annual Rates and Proportions of Nonfatal Injuries by Sex, Age, and Detailed Description of Event. Punjab, India, 1959–60

Rate per 1,000	*Both Sexes*	*Males*	*Females*	*0–4*	*5–14*	*15–24*	*25–44*	*45–64*	*≥65*
All injuries	115.6	98.5	134.4	123.2	128.6	104.2	126.1	101.2	54.2
Males				139.1	136.4	85.4	64.7	68.1	62.5
Females				104.7	119.8	122.9	188.1	144.0	44.0
Proportion of injuries									
Home	43.0	22.0	60.0						
Public place	27.7	37.2	20.0						
Work	23.5	31.0	17.5						
Vehicular	5.7	9.7	2.5						
Fall	9.1	8.8	9.3						
Falling object	3.0	3.1	2.9						
Venomous animals	3.4	3.5	3.2						
Other animals	9.6	11.1	8.6						
Fire, explosion	2.6	2.7	2.5						
Hot or corrosive substance	9.1	7.5	10.3						
Cutting, piercing instrument	21.2	15.9	25.7						
Cutting, piercing object	17.0	15.5	18.2						
Striking blunt object	11.5	12.4	10.7						
Vehicular transport	6.9	12.4	2.5						
Machinery	3.6	5.8	1.8						
Unknown	3.0	1.3	4.3						

Source: Adapted from J.E. Gordon, P.V. Gulati, and J.B. Wyon, "Traumatic Accidents in Rural Tropical Regions: An Epidemiological Field Study in Punjab, India," *American Journal of Medical Sciences* 243 (1962):382–402.

Table 8–4
Death Rates per 100,000 Population from Selected Causes for Nations Reporting over 50,000 Deaths Annually[a]

	All Causes	*Infections*	*Neoplasms*	*Circulatory*	*Respiratory*	*Unintentional and Undetermined Injury*
Egypt	1,305	30	20	170	235	44
Thailand	526	54	14	24	62	28
Japan	625	13	131	270	48	29
Australia	791	5	148	426	51	50
United States	888	7	174	463	52	50
Guatemela	1,262	435	30	52	239	62[b]
Colombia	650	93	55	152	82	51
Venezuela	621	74	56	120	56	59
Chile	723	61	104	152	87	64
Austria	1,266	9	260	645	82	50
Belgium	1,218	9	256	523	86	61
Bulgaria	1,008	11	142	539	110	41
Czechoslavakia	1,169	9	231	573	113	58
Denmark	1,059	12	249	527	91	40
France	1,049	15	228	398	69	76
Germany, Democratic Republic	1,392	8	225	788	97	101[b]
Germany, Federal Republic	1,211	10	258	560	80	47
Greece	885	14	158	339	91	43
Hungary	1,247	18	248	648	61	60
Netherlands	830	4	212	376	55	39
Romania	955	12	131	510	148	58[b]
Sweden	1,102	7	241	585	63	53
Switzerland	904	8	217	434	63	47
United Kingdom	1,184	6	251	609	165	33
Scotland	1,253	8	259	661	147	47
Yugoslavia	866	23	116	358	64	60[b]

Source: Adapted from *World Health Statistics Annual*, vol. 1, 1978: *Vital Statistics and Causes of Death* (Geneva: World Health Organization, 1978).

[a]Rates are reported to the last whole number (for example, 358.8 = 358).
[b]All injury, including homicide, suicide, and war related.

represent somewhere between 3 and 10 percent of all deaths in all nations. These are crude mortality rates, not adjusted for different age distributions between nations.

National age and sex specific death rates from unintentional injury are in table 8–5. Rates for males exceed those for females and, with few exceptions, are highest among young children and the elderly. The higher death rate for the elderly contrasts with the lower injury rate in this group.

Three inconsistencies deserve comment. While young children, especially under age 1, have high death rates, there is wide variation in the extent of the excess. At one extreme Thailand, Sweden, Denmark, France, and Hungary report a very low death rate for children under age 1. Chile and Germany are at the other extreme. Although it is not possible to explain these differences definitively without more information, they may represent differences in assignment of sudden infant death syndrome (SIDS) as injury deaths. In the United States, the most rapidly increasing mortality diagnosis is sudden infant death (ICD 8 code 795), which increased sixfold between 1968 and 1977.[5] Presumably, this is a change in diagnostic preference, rather than in disease occurrence.

Marked differences also appear in overrepresentation of deaths among the elderly. Whereas persons age 85 or older usually have death rates about eight to ten times the mean, the rate is barely above the mean in Thailand and is from fourteen to twenty-one times greater than the mean in several European nations.

The low and essentially flat rate distribution across all ages for Thailand suggests an idiosyncracy of reporting rather than one of fact. I suspect that all deaths are not being reported or that they are being assigned elsewhere. Thailand has an extraordinarily high homicide rate (21/100,000), twice that of the United States, which in turn is considerably higher than most other nations. Are some unintentional injury deaths being classified as homicide in Thailand?

As we have already noted, if a person with heart disease has a dizzy spell, falls, breaks a hip, and dies from cardiovascular complications of immobility, there is considerable discretion whether the death will be attributed to the fall or to the heart disease. Perhaps in those nations with highest death rates among the elderly there is a tendency to assign such deaths to falls.

Finally, note the fairly consistent pattern, predominantly in males, in which death rates between ages 15 and 24 are modestly higher than surrounding ages. Possible explanations are entry into the job market, experimentation with heavy drinking, and initial experiences with driving.

Table 8–5
Age- and Sex-Specific Death Rates in 1970–74 from Unintentional Injury for Nations with over 50,000 Deaths Per Year[a]

	Thailand	*Japan*	*Australia*	*Canada*	*United States*
All ages	29.8	38.5	52.6	57.0	54.2
Males	43.0	58.7	72.2	81.2	77.2
Females	16.7	19.0	32.8	32.8	32.4
Age < 1	17.0	54.1	55.7	80.2	56.2
1–4	24.1	56.8–30.4[b]	44.9–22.1	34.1	30.9
5–9	17.7	19.8	17.7	25.1	19.7
10–14	15.0	8.4	15.6	23.0	20.2
15–19	27.8	32.2	73.3	43.4	63.9
20–24	41.8	32.2	73.5	77.5	69.7
25–29	39.3	26.0	45.0	52.3	52.4
30–34	34.3	25.0	37.8	46.7	45.7
35–39	34.3	29.9	38.6	46.1	44.7
40–44	37.4	35.1	38.7	48.0	45.6
45–49	38.7	36.5	43.3	52.8	48.1
50–54	35.2	43.0	47.5	55.5	50.4
55–59	35.6	51.3	52.1	58.8	55.7
60–64	34.9	61.1	57.6	66.3	62.9
65–69	32.6	77.7	66.2	75.2	69.8
70–74	33.9	101.9	92.1	87.4	92.2
75–79	32.2	144.1	161.1	127.8	134.4
80–84	38.6	197.9	297.0	208.5	203.7
≥85	34.2	294.8	638.8	496.4	402.4

Table 8–5 *(continued)*

	Venezuela	*Chile*	*Austria*	*Belgium*	*Bulgaria*	*Czechoslovakia*
All ages	50.3	37.1	79.3	65.3	41.1	57.9
Males	76.9	57.1	106.6	78.5	63.4	77.5
Females	23.6	18.0	55.2	52.6	18.9	39.2
Age < 1	61.4	105.3	71.1	93.7	75.6	49.5
1–4	31.0	26.3	40.4–25.5	25.9	28.4	28.4
5–9	22.7	14.9	20.6	19.4	18.9	20.0
10–14	24.1	12.1	18.3	17.0	13.8	13.7
15–19	46.5	18.8	75.5	51.0	28.9	40.7
20–24	67.0	30.1	74.2	61.0	40.3	51.5
25–29	65.7	37.1	53.9	42.4	38.7	40.4
30–34	61.2	41.5	49.4	41.3	38.3	38.4
35–39	56.0	43.7	54.9	40.5	38.1	40.0
40–44	53.4	56.7	58.3	40.8	39.7	41.3
45–49	54.4	52.5	50.6	40.4	44.5	45.0
50–54	59.0	57.1	57.0	47.1	44.9	49.1
55–59	59.9	62.6	71.1	55.6	48.7	59.2
60–64	76.4	69.9	79.2	67.8	48.3	66.1
65–69	68.2	70.0	102.3	84.0	57.6	86.3
70–74	93.4	100.7	149.7	127.5	74.2	133.1
75–79	121.5	}	264.3	225.2	96.6	250.8
80–84	174.5	} 154.8	522.7	433.5	147.7	459.7
≥85	319.4	}	1125.7	1027.0	208.4	819.8

Table 8–5 *(continued)*

	Denmark	*France*	*Germany, Federal Republic*	*Greece*	*Hungary*	*Netherlands*
All ages	45.2	75.8	59.7	39.8	56.0	45.6
Males	56.3	91.6	74.9	51.8	73.5	56.0
Females	34.2	60.6	45.7	28.3	39.6	35.3
Age < 1	24.7	53.2	99.7	52.9	29.4	44.8
1–4	25.0–17.7	25.5	30.3	21.9–16.0	28.4–18.3	26.1–25.1
5–9	21.1	17.0	25.2	10.3	14.5	20.2
10–14	17.2	15.2	16.3	11.5	11.7	14.8
15–19	44.3	56.1	61.4	26.9	31.1	44.6
20–24	33.5	70.4	61.0	36.6	39.7	37.3
25–29	23.2	49.8	41.8	32.7	31.7	25.7
30–34	22.5	47.3	37.2	25.5	32.8	25.0
35–39	22.8	49.8	35.5	26.5	34.7	22.5
40–44	26.3	53.5	36.0	25.5	39.3	22.3
45–49	26.3	56.3	33.8	27.5	42.0	23.8
50–54	32.4	61.2	36.3	33.5	43.3	27.2
55–59	41.2	71.2	43.7	35.6	53.4	37.5
60–64	48.4	77.4	53.7	41.9	63.7	48.6
65–69	63.7	89.8	66.8	59.4	85.6	62.1
70–74	97.0	127.7	109.5	91.5	133.0	96.5
75–79	158.0	218.6	208.1	162.7	256.2	190.1
80–84	308.7	442.7	439.9	292.9	519.5	412.1
⩾85	709.5	1164.8	1034.8	483.5	1103.8	964.0

Table 8–5 *(continued)*

	Sweden	*Switzerland*	*United Kingdom*	*Scotland*
All ages	44.5	59.0	34.0	44.5
Males	56.5	78.0	38.6	55.2
Females	32.6	40.8	29.7	34.6
Age < 1	13.5	81.7	47.9	134.7
1–4	13.2	30.3	20.5–13.9	31.4–21.3
5–9	13.6	22.3	12.5	17.9
10–14	11.3	17.5	10.1	12.7
15–19	38.0	47.2	34.2	31.3
20–24	31.3	57.9	30.4	36.3
25–29	23.3	34.7	20.5	26.8
30–34	23.6	28.3	18.2	28.3
35–39	25.3	28.9	16.8	28.5
40–44	28.4	33.8	18.1	30.3
45–49	31.3	36.6	20.2	32.0
50–54	36.3	46.4	22.0	36.8
55–59	43.0	57.6	27.7	39.1
60–64	52.8	70.6	31.4	40.8
65–69	54.8	86.7	40.3	53.2
70–74	80.5	129.9	65.4	81.0
75–79	142.1	219.0	123.2	148.2
80–84	291.1	420.3	237.9	293.4
≥85	667.1	1034.6	484.1	675.4

Adapted from *World Health Statistics Annual*, vol. 1, 1978: *Vital Statistics and Causes of Death* (Geneva: World Health Organization, 1978).

[a]Several nations listed in table 8–4 did not report data in useable form for this table, while Canada, listed here and in table 8–6, did not report data for table 8–4.

[b]Where summary rate for age 1–4 is not provided, the rates for age 1 and age 4 have been listed. With rare exceptions these represent the high and low rates for this age group.

With increasing suicide rates among adolescents and young adults, there may be some misclassification of suicide as unintentional. Again, these gross data provide only grist for hypotheses, not firm answers.

Although injuries comprise overall only about one in every twenty deaths, they are *the* major health-related cause of lost working years of life for American society because of their greater contribution to deaths of children and young men. Analyses of this type are difficult to perform and have been carried out only rarely. Hartunian, Smart, and Thompson[6] compared long-term economic costs of motor vehicle injuries in the United States with those of cancer, coronary heart disease, and stroke and concluded that costs of these injuries was exceeded only by those of cancer, despite substantially greater death rates from the other conditions.

Regarding highway injury, Thorson[7] reports from Sweden that among persons treated as in-patients, 51 percent still had after effects five years later. For most (38 percent) the sequelae were mild, but 9 percent had physical disability and 3 percent required care by others. In addition, 7 percent had ongoing psychological effects, and 18 percent had social effects of the physical injuries.

The above data are for motor vehicle injuries only. Nonhighway injuries, however, also tend to be high in children, and even a relatively low incidence of persons surviving with permanent disabilities in this age group can result in a high prevalance of disabled persons. This is why spinal cord injuries, although infrequent, are of such great social and economic importance.[8]

We have already observed that across most nations—including the developing countries—children and teenage and young adult males are at high risk of death. One can only guess whether throughout the world injury of all types represents *the* most important health-related cause of lost person-years of productivity, as in the United States and probably most other western nations, or whether it is only *an* important cause in the developing nations, competing with infectious diseases and malnutrition. Either way, it is a drain of national resources that must be dealt with.

Finally, table 8–6 shows death rates for some different types of injury events in nations reporting to the World Health Organization. Again, differences may be an artifact of reporting, rather than real differences in occurrence. Differences in highway death rates, however, probably do reflect to a large degree differences in the extent to which motor vehicles have been introduced into each nation. Also relevant is that the nations with high elderly death rates also have high death rates from falls, suggesting—but not proving—national differences in classifying such deaths.

Table 8–6
Crude Death Rates Per 100,000 Population for Specific Injury Types by Nation

	Transport	*Poisoning*	*Falls*	*Fire*	*Drowning*	*Industrial*	*Other*
Egypt	2.1[a]	0.8	0.5	9.9	0.0	1.2	3.8
Mauritius	19.2	3.8	1.7	6.0	5.3	0.8	4.1
Barbados	18.8	0.8	4.9	2.0	2.9	—	0.4
Canada	30.9	3.1	8.1	3.6	3.2	3.9	4.7
Chile	11.0	0.2	6.2	2.6	0.5	0.8	5.4
Colombia	14.8	0.8	4.3	2.0	6.4	1.7	8.6
Costa Rica	18.4	1.8	3.5	0.3	10.0	2.5	11.4
Dominican Republic	9.6	1.5	1.6	1.5	2.9	0.5	3.0
El Salvador	14.9	1.4	4.9	1.9	5.7	0.9	10.6
Martinique	10.0	1.4	1.1	2.8	4.7	0.3	11.3
Paraguay	10.9	1.2	1.6	1.2	4.2	3.3	9.8
Puerto Rico	16.7	1.3	3.4	1.0	4.7	1.2	3.5
United States	23.4	2.9	7.0	2.8	3.1	2.6	6.5
Uruguay	8.7	1.1	5.5	1.3	5.2	1.8	16.8
Venezuela	34.5	0.9	6.1	1.5	3.8	3.0	5.9
Hong Kong	9.2	0.8	3.2	0.7	3.8	1.1	2.6
Israel	19.4	0.7	8.4	1.1	1.8	1.4	11.4
Japan	12.2	0.7	4.1	1.4	3.5	2.1	3.0
Singapore	12.9	0.4	2.5	0.7	2.0	2.3	1.0
Syria	2.3	2.1	0.0	0.0	1.0	0.8	12.1
Thailand	11.1	0.5	0.7	0.6	4.3	1.5	9.5
Austria	30.9	1.3	26.3	1.0	2.0	4.4	3.9
Belgium	25.0	2.5	19.9	1.3	2.1	1.5	7.9
Bulgaria	15.7[a]	3.0	5.8	1.4	3.0	4.4	7.0
Czechoslovakia	21.7[a]	5.8	17.4	1.1	3.3	3.2	4.6
Denmark	18.3	1.3	12.1	1.3	0.9	1.0	2.2
France	23.8	1.3	26.2	1.4	2.1	1.0	16.8
Germany, Federal Republic	24.8	0.8	19.4	0.9	1.5	1.8	4.7
Greece	17.8	0.8	11.9	1.5	2.2	1.5	6.6

Hungary	20.2[a]	2.7	25.0	1.7	1.7	3.8	3.7
Iceland	16.8[a]	4.1	7.7	1.4	7.3	0.9	2.3
Ireland	19.8	1.1	14.2	2.5	2.3	1.9	3.4
Malta	4.3	1.0	8.6	0.3	1.0	3.0	2.0
Netherlands	18.9	0.7	14.2	0.6	1.8	0.9	2.2
Norway	17.3[a]	2.4	17.7	1.4	3.6	1.9	3.0
Sweden	17.0[a]	3.0	19.8	1.6	2.0	1.4	1.9
Switzerland	20.6	0.8	17.1	0.6	1.9	2.1	3.9
United Kingdom	12.7	1.7	10.5	1.4	1.1	1.2	2.5
Australia	29.6	1.1	8.7	1.2	3.2	2.3	3.0
New Zealand	24.8[a]	1.4	16.1	1.3	2.8	3.3	4.6
Northern Ireland	20.5	4.5	16.2	2.4	2.3	2.1	1.9
Scotland	17.3	0.9	14.9	2.6	1.7	1.7	3.9

Source: Adapted from *World Health Statistics Annual, Vol. 1, 1978: Vital Statistics and Causes of Death* (Geneva: World Health Organization, 1978).

[a]In all except these nations, highway motor vehicle deaths comprise at least 90 percent of transport deaths.

9
An Overview of Highway Injury

The first automobile fatality was in England thirteen years after development of the first commercially successful automobile in 1885. Originally blamed on recklessly fast driving, the primary cause soon was found to be a wheel made of poorly seasoned wood.[1] The first U.S. fatality came a year later in 1899.

Internationally, there are now at least 250,000 deaths a year. As of 1979 there were 296 million registered vehicles throughout the world, over three times as many as in 1960.[2] The United States and Canada had 42 percent of these, and Western Europe 26 percent. In some places, however, other traffic predominates. Peking, for example, has 180,000 motor vehicles, and 20,000 motorcycles and scooters, but 3 million bicycles.[3]

In many nations roads are shared not only with pedestrians, bicycles, pedalcycles, bullock carts, rickshaws, and stray livestock but also with peasants driving entire herds of animals and with produce spread on the road to dry. This is stark contrast to freeways limited only to motor vehicles and roads permitting mixing of traffic where motorists, nonetheless, resent the presence of even an occasional pedestrian or bicyclist.

This diversity is worth remembering in highly motorized nations where people may forget the past as they concentrate on current problems in current contexts. From the other perspective, in nations that still have few automobiles but many trucks, buses, two-wheeled vehicles, and pedestrian and animal traffic authorities see lower casualty rates in developed nations and may assume that the current solutions in those nations must be relevant to them as well.

The United States, for example, now has a death rate of about three per 100 million miles travelled, but around 1925 it was about eighteen and has dropped consistently since then.[4] This decline is usually attributed to various safety improvements. But it may also reflect a decreasing number of occupants per vehicle as the number of vehicles per 1,000 population has risen. Thus, there would now be fewer persons at risk of injury and death per vehicle mile traveled. Furthermore, according to Campbell,[5] about half of the U.S. decline reflects increasing urbanization and the fact that urban highway death rates are lower than rural ones.

The difference in population per vehicle is important when comparing injury and death rates of North American or Western European nations with those of places in Asia, Africa, and Central and South America, where people may literally be "packed" into and onto buses or stake trucks. This is why passenger miles or kilometers is a more useful denominator than vehicle miles.

Currently, the United States leads the world with 1.4 people per vehicle, whereas the average is 2.0 for all of North and Central America, 2.4 for Oceania, 5.3 for Europe, 14 for South America, and about 50 for Asia and Africa.[2] Table 9–1 shows comparative data for some nations, illustrating the diversity both in vehicles per population and in mix of vehicle sizes.[2] In general, the more people per car and the larger the

Table 9–1
Distribution of Automobiles, Trucks, and Buses among Populations of Selected Nations

Nation	*Number Vehicles (millions)*	*Percentage of Trucks and Buses*	*Population Per Car*	*Population Per Vehicle*
Canada	12.9	22.5	2.4	1.8
Guatemala	0.2	37.6	53	33
Mexico	4.7	29.8	20	14
United States	154.1	22.0	1.8	1.4
Argentina	4.0	30.0	9.7	6.8
Brazil	9.2	21.2	16	13
Chile	0.5	36.4	32	21
Peru	0.5	33.8	54	35
China	0.9	94.4	20,244	1,125
India	1.4	37.5	776	485
Indonesia	1.0	44.0	256	143
Japan	36.2	37.4	5.1	3.1
Kuwait	0.5	26.8	3.5	2.5
Pakistan	0.3	32.3	400	271
Australia	7.1	20.0	2.5	2.0
Egypt	0.5	23.1	108	83
Libya	0.4	18.7	9.3	7.5
Nigeria	0.8	39.7	162	975
South Africa	3.2	27.8	12	8.6
France	21.0	12.0	2.9	2.5
Germany, Federal Republic	24.1	6.2	2.7	2.5
Italy	18.4	6.7	3.3	3.1
Poland	2.8	23.4	17	13
Spain	8.4	15.6	5.2	4.4
USSR	13.5	48.1	37	19
United Kingdom	16.9	11.5	3.7	3.3

Source: Adapted from *MVMA Motor Vehicle Facts and Figures, 1981* (Detroit, Mich.: Motor Vehicle Manufacturers Association of the United States, 1981).

proportion of trucks and buses, the greater the relative density of nonmotorized traffic mixing with automobiles, trucks, and buses.

Patterns of Crashes, Injuries, and Death

Sabey[6] suggests that national road traffic and highway crash patterns go through three phases. Phase 1 involves "slow development of a mechanized transport system," a situation still existing in much of Africa and Asia. In phase 2 there is an "explosion into rapid growth," such as in Kuwait.[7] Phase 3 nations are experiencing "a slowing down to saturation point," as in the United States, with Canada, Western Europe, and Australia close behind. Between 1975 and 1979, for example, U.S. vehicles increased by 15 percent, while going up by 25 percent in the rest of the world (including other phase 3 nations).

Sabey believes that the crash and fatality rate increases throughout phases 1 and 2 and then decreases as nations enter phase 3. This view appears to be contradicted by Haight's data.[8] In the United States, for example, the crash rates per unit vehicle miles were highest during the earliest years—equivalent to phase 1—and dropped continuously until the present day. Generally, he says, highest rates are in the developing countries, followed respectively by Eastern Europe, Western Europe, and the United States. These data suggest that crash rates per unit of travel are highest in phase 1 rather than in phase 2.

Sabey, however, doesn't clarify whether she means crash rates per unit of travel (as with Haight) or per unit population. Her description would apply in the latter case, with few vehicular deaths per 100,000 population when few vehicles are around, a marked increase in death rate as vehicles become an important mode of transportation, and finally a downturn as vehicle use pattern stabilizes and safety efforts catch up.

In the United States the death rate per 100,000 persons rose from 0.5 around 1905 to about 11 in 1920, 27 in 1930, and a peak of 31 in 1937 and then began declining to the low 20s until the early 1960s. It climbed again to 28 in 1969 and then dropped to about 22 with the gasoline crisis and 55 M.P.H. national speed limit in late 1973, where it has remained.

An Overview of Crash Patterns in the United States

During 1980 the United States had 52,600 highway deaths and an estimated 4.8 million injuries (substantial reductions in deaths have occurred since 1980). Seventy-seven percent of drivers in fatal crashes were males, and 23 percent females. For all crashes, however, 67 percent are male. The distribution of fatalities according to age is as follows for crashes not involving pedestrians or pedalcyclists: 1,500 (3 percent) age 0 to 4, 3,100 (6 percent) age 5 to 14, 19,000 (37 percent) age 15 to 24, 4,100 (27 percent) age 25 to 44, 8,000 (15 percent) age 45 to 64, and 5,800 (11 percent) age 65 or older. The economic costs for 1981 were estimated to be about $39 billion.

Table 9–2 shows the distribution of crashes involving fatality, injury, and property damage by population density and type of event.[4] Fatal crashes are seldom an urban phenomenon (38 percent), while nonfatal injuries more often are urban (67 percent), and property damage crashes are urban even more often (72 percent). The death rate per 100 million miles is 2.2 for daytime driving and 6.5 at night, with 54 percent of fatal crashes but only 32 percent of all crashes occurring between 7 P.M. and 6 A.M. Whereas 46 percent of all crashes occur Friday through Sunday,[9] 53 percent of fatal ones are then.

Crashes and registrations by type of vehicle are compared in table 9–

Table 9–2
Characteristics of Fatal, Injury, and Property Damage Crashes, the United States, 1980

	Deaths	*Injuries*[a]	*Property Damage*
Total	*52,600* *(47,400 crashes)*	*2,000,000* *(1.4 million crashes)*	*(16.5 million crashes)*
Urban	19,500 (17,500)	1.12 million (.94 mil)	12 million
Pedestrian	6,900	105,000	
Bicycle	800	50,000	
Train	500	2,000	
Two-vehicle	5,300	820,000	
Fixed object, noncollision, animal	6,000	143,000	
Rural	33,100 (29,900)	880,000 (460,000)	4.5 million
Pedestrian	2,700	15,000	
Bicycle	400	10,000	
Train	400	2,000	
Two-vehicle	15,900	560,000	
Fixed object, noncollision, animal	13,700	293,000	

Source: Adapted from *Accident Facts, 1981 Edition* (Chicago, Ill.: National Safety Council, 1981).

[a]Data from the National Health Survey suggest that a more accurate figure is about 4.9 million injuries annually, whereas initial data from the National Accident Sampling System estimate that there were 4 million injuries just in those 7.3 million crashes that are police reported.

3.[4] Semi-trailer trucks, buses, and motorcycles and scooters are over-represented in fatal events.

Although highway injury and fatality generally results from collision involving vehicles or vehicle rollover in noncollision events, it must not be overlooked that each year about 350 people are killed as a result of jumps or falls from noncrashing vehicles.[10] This occurs more often in nations where people are packed into public transportation vehicles.

A Comparison with Crash Patterns in Developing Nations

In many phase 1 and phase 2 nations, important questions are never asked in crash investigation and analysis. Jacobs et al.[11] note that a good crash investigation form may have as many as 188 questions covering administrative details and records of immediate actions, details of injuries, characteristics of drivers, vehicles and passengers, site and statistical information, and space for statements. Forms in Cypress and Great Britain have over ninety questions. In Sarawak only five questions are asked, followed by Botswana (seven), St. Helena (eleven), Fiji (eighteen),

Table 9–3
Types of Motor Vehicles Involved in Fatal Crashes and All Crashes, United States (1980)

Type Vehicle	*Percentage in Fatal Crashes*	*Percentage in All Crashes*	*Percentage of Vehicle Registrations*	*Percentage of Occupant Fatalities*
Passenger cars	65.3	76.5	74.7	69.1
Trucks	24.2	18.4	21.2	16.3
Truck or truck tractor	15.3	14.8	20.4	?
Truck tractor and semi-trailer	7.0	2.3	} 0.8	?
Other truck combination	1.9	1.3		?
Farm tractors, equipment	0.2	0.1	—	0.3
Taxicabs	0.7	0.8	0.2	0.8
Buses, commercial	0.4	0.5	0.1	0.2
Buses, school	0.2	0.3	0.3	0.1
Motorcycles	6.6	1.7	} 3.5	9.6
Motor scooters and bikes	0.8	0.2		1.1
Other[a]	1.6	1.5	?	2.5

Source: Adapted from *Accident Facts, 1981 Edition* (Chicago, Ill.: National Safety Council, 1981).
[a]Fire trucks, ambulances, special vehicles.

Sri Lanka (twenty), and India (twenty-six). When studied, Indonesia and Nigeria had no organized system for reporting crashes, and several of the thirty-four nations queried had no analysis form.

The data that follow, therefore, are from nations where data can be found comparable to those presented for the United States rather than from nations that are known to be "representative" of the phase 1 or 2 nations. Overall highway fatality burdens for several nations are shown in table 9–4.[12] Jacobs and colleagues[12,13,14] point out that as a general rule rates of fatal and severe injuries per 10,000 vehicles are inversely proportionate to the number of vehicles available per 10,000 persons, and the number of vehicles per 10 km of road but are directly proportionate to the population per physician and per hospital bed and to the

Table 9–4
Vehicles Per 10,000 Population and Fatalities Per 10,000 Vehicles for Developing Nations, 1971, and Developed Nations, 1970

	Vehicles Per 10,000 Persons	*Fatalities Per 10,000 Vehicles*
Ceylon	141	38
Chile	359	58
Ethiopia	17	207
India	26	89
Indonesia	74	36
Iraq	127	62
Ivory Coast	223	39
Kenya	116	77
Malagasy	124	28
Malawi	51	71
West Malaysia	823	21
Morocco	146	83
Nigeria	24	83
Pakistan	20	80
Syria	94	137
Thailand	235	29
Tunisia	225	45
Turkey	111	92
Zambia	243	76
Britain	2623	5.3
United States	5245	4.8
Australia	3981	7.6
Canada	3680	6.4
France	3888	9.2
Netherlands	3834	6.4
Italy	2559	8.1
Germany (Federal Republic)	2570	12.1
Spain	1309	9.5

Source: Adapted from G.D. Jacobs and P.R. Fouracre, *Further Research on Road Accident Rates in Developing Countries* (Crowthorne, Berkshire, U.K.: Transport and Road Research Laboratory, Department of Environment, TRRL Supplementary Report 270, 1977).

numbers of motorcycles per population. The cost of highway crashes in developing nations as a percentage of the gross domestic product is at least equal to that in Great Britain,[15] ranging from about 0.5 to 1.5 percent of the G.D.P.

Table 9–5 compares highway crash data in Kenya,[16] a phase 1 nation and Kuwait,[17,18] a phase 2 country. In Quatar, 44 percent of casualties and 50 percent of fatalities are pedestrians, motorcyclists, and pedal cyclists, and over 90 percent of casualties are males.[19] A third of the population are laborers, who often are crowded in trucks and lorries, and 2.4 percent of the casualties were individuals who had fallen from a moving vehicle. (The U.S. proportion is 0.7 percent.)

Compared to the United States each of these nations has a much higher proportion of fatalities and injuries to pedestrians and bicyclists, more involvement of occupants of commercial and passenger service vehicles, fewer occupants of vehicles in solitary crashes, and far more male drivers among casualties. North American women probably have many more activities outside the home than in many other cultures.

In Kenya 15 percent of the fatalities and 11 percent of all casualties are under age 15, but no further age information is provided. Among Kuwait fatalities, 12 percent are under age 5, 14 percent are 5 to 14, 12 percent 15 to 24, 35 percent 25 to 44, 19 percent 45 to 64, and 6 percent age 65 or older. Only among children under age 10 do females represent more than about 10 percent of all fatalities. In this youngest group they comprise about 40 percent. Among drivers in fatal crashes, 27 percent are under age 24, 58 percent ages 25 to 44, 11 percent age 45 to 64, and less than 1 percent older. This differs from the United States, with more children among fatalities in developing nations, and fewer fatalities among persons age 15 to 24 and age 65 or older.

Human Factors in the Pre-Injury or Pre-Crash Phase

We now turn to causal factors in the pre-crash phase. The discussion in this chapter will be limited as far as possible to consideration of crashes involving only automobiles, since large vehicles, two-wheeled vehicles, and pedestrians are subjects of separate chapters.

The driving environment, although appearing simple, is extremely complex and involves interaction in the pre-injury phase alone of at least a dozen driver attributes, three major vehicular systems (handling and stability, visibility, and driver environment), and five roadway systems (informational, visibility, geometrics, user separation, and road surface characteristics). In discussing driver contribution to initiation of crashes,

Table 9–5
Characteristics of Fatal and Injury Crashes in Kenya and Kuwait

	Kenya (1972)			*Kuwait (1977–78)*		
	Fatal	*Serious Injury*	*Slight Injury*	*Fatal*	*Injury*	*Property Damage*
Total number	1,198	2,413	4,805	380	2,459	16,482
Urban (%)	31	35	45	—	—	—
Rural	68	64	53	—	—	—
Car occupants (%)	22	39	41	41[a]	66[a]	—
Pedestrians	45	29	20	55	29	—
Motorcyclists	2	5	5	2	3	—
Pedal cyclists	9	6	8	2	2	—
Occupants of passenger service vehicles	6	4	5	—	—	—
Occupants of commercial vehicles	12	16	18	—	—	—
Others	3	2	1	—	—	—
Single vehicle (%)		27		13	14	
Vehicle versus pedestrian		39		58	38	
Vehicle versus cycle		12		3	3	
Vehicle versus motorcycle		3		—	—	
Two-vehicle		18		27	45	
Daylight (%)	73	78	79	—	—	
Darkness	27	22	21	—	—	
Male (%)	—	—	—	93 (of drivers)	92 (of drivers)	

Source: Adapted from G.D. Jacobs and I.A. Sayer, *An Analysis of Road Accidents in Kenya in 1972* (Crowthorne, Berkshire, U.K.: Transport and Road Research Laboratory Department of Environment, TRRL Supplementary Report 227 UC, 1976); A. Bayoumi, "The Epidemiology of Fatal Motor Vehicle Accidents in Kuwait," *Accident Analysis and Prevention* 13 (1981):339–348; A. Bayoumi, "The Epidemiology of Injury Motor Vehicle Accidents in Kuwait," unpublished paper (Kuwait: Department of Community Medicine, Kuwait University Faculty of Medicine, 1979).

[a]Some of the percents for fatal injuries are based on 726 fatalities for 1977 and 1978. Numbers are for 1978 only.

four types of factors will be emphasized that cut across these system components. These are alcohol and other drugs, medical impairment and aging, youth and inexperience, and highway laws and the extent to which they are obeyed.

Alcohol and Other Drugs

In the United States alcohol is the single most frequently found human factor in fatal crashes.[20,21] Its important role in fatal crashes has been well established in Canada, Britain, Australia, and the Scandinavian nations and is strongly suspected elsewhere. (For a fuller discussion of alcohol see chapter 31.)

Very little "hard data" regarding alcohol are available for the developing countries. Only anecdotal information exists from many phase 1 countries, but it suggests as much alcohol abuse in fatal crashes in some of these areas as in the phase 3 nations. In some Moslem nations alcohol is reported in only 1 or 2 percent of fatal crashes.[22] Without systematic testing the extent of underreporting is unknown, but the strong religious prohibition suggests that in these nations alcohol abuse might be less.

In the United States about half of drivers who die within six hours after a crash have alcohol in their blood, and over 40 percent have blood alcohol concentrations (BACs) of 0.10 percent by weight or higher.[20,21] In contrast, about 15 percent of drivers not involved in crashes but exposed to similar circumstances of time and place have alcohol, and only 2 percent have high BACs.[20] In order to reach 0.10 percent a 150 lb person drinking between one and two hours after an average meal would have to consume five shots (7.5 oz or 225 cc) of 80 proof liquor or a full six-pack of beer (72 oz of 4 percent alcohol) in one hour.

The risk of crashing increases as blood alcohol concentrations exceed 0.05 percent by weight[20,21] and the percentage of drivers responsible for initiating crashes also goes up.[23] At BACs of 0.10 percent or higher, over 90 percent can be designated as the "responsible" driver. The risk of crashing for young drivers increases with even one drink and thereafter rises at a faster rate than for persons over age 25 or 30.[24,25]

Minor crashes involve alcohol less often. Thus, in one study[26] 16 percent of drivers in noninjury crashes had any alcohol, and 5 percent had BACs of 0.11 percent or higher, whereas 22 percent and 11 percent respectively of those involved in "serious injury" crashes had BACs in these ranges. Among noninvolved drivers 11 percent had any alcohol, and 1 percent had 0.11 percent or higher. A majority of alcohol-impaired drivers either have no passengers or have passengers who are as impaired as the driver.[27]

Two groups appear to comprise the vast majority of drivers who get into trouble after drinking. Over half are heavy drinkers with patterns of problem drinking or frank alcoholism.[20,21] Most of the rest are teenagers and men in their early twenties who are experimental or heavy social drinkers.[20] Studies have identified such patterns in the United States, Canada, Germany, and Denmark. But drinking patterns vary between nations, and cross-cultural generalizations should be made only with caution. In Australia, for example, over half of males—far more than in the United States—are heavy drinkers.[28] But alcoholism may be less common among impaired drivers in that country.[29]

Much less is known about other drugs in crashes. Despite data from laboratory studies suggesting that some of the psychoactive drugs impair functions relevant to driving there is little or no epidemiological evidence as yet to suggest that these drugs by themselves are implicated other than rarely in the initiation of crashes. This may reflect the fact that these drugs are seldom a problem or that all of the epidemiologic studies to date have been beset with very serious difficulties of design and implementation.[30,31]

Nonmedical use of drugs, such as barbiturates, tranquilizers, amphetamines, opiates, LSD, PCB, Quaaludes, and cannabinols (THC) has also been suggested as a driving hazard, and anecdotal data indicate occasional contribution to crashes. In some nations, there are few restrictions on use of hashish or other drugs illicit in the Western world, and there are undocumented stories of truck drivers who are impaired and crash because of them; but no data exist whether this constitutes a serious problem.

Attention has been focused particularly on the effects of marihuana and other forms of THC. In general, it has not yet been possible to document whether THC increases crash risk. This may reflect difficulties in study design, such as comparing crash and control drivers and identifying the presence and amount of THC at a time when it is causing psychoactive effects.[30,31] Laboratory data suggest that impairment of driving may occur but the nature of the impairment may differ from that with alcohol.[30,31]

In the Western world, where the limited epidemiologic research is occurring, the heaviest users of other drugs are also likely to use alcohol simultaneously in impairing amounts. Most crashes with other drugs also involve alcohol and BACs of 0.10 percent or greater.[32]

Medical Impairment and Aging

Theoretically, many medical conditions may impair driving ability, and some have proposed requiring elderly drivers to undergo special licensing procedures because of serious medical conditions at this age. Some nations require all drivers to pass a medical examination.

At the other extreme, physicans and associations concerned with epilepsy, diabetes, and other conditions state that these conditions are associated with no increase in crash risk. Based on crashes per 100 drivers, elderly persons do not present unique hazard. In some states, licenses are renewed by mail and visual acuity is not checked at any time after the initial license is obtained.

The facts will be presented briefly here, and in greater detail in chapter 30. Less than 5 percent of crashes are attributable to obvious clinical episodes of illness such as heart attacks, seizures, or diabetic reactions.[33] However, persons with these and other medical conditions that are associated with rapid fluctuations of sensorium or judgment have been shown in some studies to have twice as many crashes per unit miles as do drivers without these conditions.[34] But few of their excess crashes involve clinical episodes, suggesting that subclinical impairment plus moments of increased driving demand bring about greater risk.[35] Persons with stable medical conditions, such as amputations, have normal risk.[36] In one interesting study, half the crashes of young women occurred during the approximately eight paramenstrual days per month.[37] Elderly persons have higher crash rates than middle-aged persons per unit mile of driving; but this excess, according to one study, exists only among those older drivers who have cardiovascular disease, or signs and symptoms of senility.[38]

Youth and Inexperience

Persons under age 25 comprise 22 percent of licensed drivers in the United States but 39 percent of drivers in all reported crashes and 36 percent of those in fatal crashes.[4] This is true in many other phase 3 nations as well. Several explanations have been suggested for this substantial overrepresentation, and to some degree all seem to apply. One explanation is that young drivers are new and inexperienced drivers. The crash rate per 100 drivers and per exposure unit is somewhat high among drivers age 16, then rises markedly among those age 17 to 19, and from there decreases progressively with increasing age.[39] Studies partly support this hypothesis of inexperience but suggest also that for any given level of experience age per se may be a factor as well.[40]

Another explanation is that, although not having greater exposure overall, young drivers are more frequently exposed at hazardous times and locations. Klein[41] points out that teenagers temporarily are members of a deviant society who may consequently use the motor vehicle in deviant ways, and for reasons that reflect more on adult society than on the group that has been labeled as deviant.

In illustration, he notes seductive advertising of high-performance cars with the specific intent of attracting young adult purchasers. Many young drivers are economically precluded from owning cars, and some turn to auto theft for joy riding. This elicits high-speed police chases, which substantially increase the risk of crashing.[42]

Higher crash risk is not uniformly distributed among all young drivers but is most closely related to feelings of hostility and rebellion and to acting out of these, especially among male drivers.[43] Also, as noted earlier, young drivers are more sensitive to even small amounts of alcohol than are older and more experienced drinkers. Despite this, heavy alcohol use is more frequent among persons under age 25.[20,21]

Regarding inexperience, consider also driving in unfamiliar territory, a situation faced by most drivers at least on occasion. Dr. Robert Hess of the University of Michigan has commented to me that preliminary studies there showed overrepresentation of collisions in which drivers resident to the area crash into the rear ends of cars driven by nonresidents who slow down at intersections, apparently because they are unfamiliar with directional cues.

Highway Laws and the Extent to Which They Are Obeyed

With certain important exceptions, there is suprisingly little evidence in the phase 3 nations to support the contention that very many crashes are a result of either conscious or repeated deviation from rules of the road. Furthermore, the wide variation from one state or community to another in traffic laws for similar types of environments suggests that the lawmakers either disagree about best ways to achieve safety through legal means or consider other issues more important: for example, promoting vehicular flow, instead of for both pedestrians, bicyclists, and vehicles.

The police goal in crash investigation is to show the person who "caused" the crash that he violated the law, thus helping him avoid future crashes.[44] It is not known how many of traffic citations issued after crash investigations are for actions truly avoidable through conscious effort and how many are for actions forced by subtle human/environmental discrepancies or that violated some local law but not the concept of safety. Several studies may offer some insight.

One study showed that even after removal of so-called spurious citations (that is, citations issued after a crash and consequently possibly a dependent variable) persons with one or two traffic citations have twice the likelihood of crash involvement than do persons without citations.

The risk increases respectively to 3, 4, 5, and 7 for those with 3, 4, 5 to 8, and 9 or more citations.[45] This suggests that persons who do not obey the law are at greater risk of crashing.

A second study found that few persons with crashes in one time frame have subsequent crashes. This suggests that despite the findings of the first study, crashes are widely distributed among the entire driving population rather than limited *predominantly* to certain high-risk groups. Such high-risk groups account for only a small proportion of all crashes.[46]

A third study explains why this may be the case. In reporting why a television campaign to reduce eleven types of driver errors had only limited effect, a group of investigators stated that a major part of the responsibility for these "driver errors" rests with inadequate roadway design rather than with driver "fault."[47] They note, for example, that at seven of eight intersections observed traffic capacity was so inadequate that it encouraged certain types of driver errors and that design and operational changes at three of the intersections resulted in increases in some types of errors while drivers were adjusting to the changes. At least part of the improvement of drivers depends on the extent to which local conditions encourage driver adjustment related to specific errors.

Some drivers disobey the law simply because they are unskilled. Drivers who do poorly on licensing examinations have somewhat higher crash rates than do those with better test scores, although there is disagreement which parts of the test are predictive.[48,49] A study of cab drivers showed that 36 percent of drivers with slow reactions to traffic lights had been struck from the rear in the previous five years, whereas 10 percent of drivers with normal reactions had such crashes. But those with slow patterns had fewer front-end collisions.[50]

The same study that found that *in general* persons do not continue at high risk of crash involvement from one time frame to the next also documented that this is not true for persons with crashes involving alcohol.[46] Those with alcohol crashes continue at high risk. As we have shown, ingestion of alcohol is much more often associated with fatal crashes than with minor ones. Robertson and Baker reported that drivers involved in fatal crashes, especially if under age 20, more often had previous traffic citations than did all drivers of similar age and sex.[51] Only 2 percent, however, could have been labeled as "habitual offenders" based on the laws of a neighboring state, and the majority had no conviction for violations in the previous three years.

The data from these two studies suggest that to a certain degree deliberate (but not necessarily correctable) violation of laws may be associated with fatal crashes to a greater extent than with minor crashes, again emphasizing the fact that to some extent these two types of crashes may be different phenomena.

A more recent study, however, dealt with behavior that by and large is deliberate (and correctable to the extent that people can be convinced to change behavior).[52] Individuals observed in a traffic survey to leave a headway of less than one second between themselves and cars immediately in front had higher crash rates than did persons who permitted greater headway. This study is one of the few examples of such correlation between independently observed driving behavior and crash experience. The difference in crash experience, although statistically significant, was a modest 6 percent.

A study by Solomon showed that the likelihood of crash involvement rises as the difference in speed (either slower or faster) increases between a given vehicle and the general traffic flow.[53] The association between speed and fatal crashes may be as much a reflection of what happens in energy transfer after the crash is initiated as it is an indication that cars going at high speed are more likely per se to crash. One reason why cars may go at unduly high or low speed is because their drivers are impaired by alcohol.

Regarding driver behavior in developing nations, it is impossible to make real comparison with phase 3 countries either currently or in the past. Roads may have been similar in the early 1900s in what are now phase 3 nations with what they are now in phase 1 and 2 areas. But the vehicles certainly behaved differently, and the populations of road users may also be different. The literacy rate, for example, probably was not the same for the United States, England, or Western Europe in the 1920s as it is now in many phase 1 countries.

In Sudan drivers may go around the wrong side of a traffic island simply because they don't know any better.[54] In some nations drivers not only take tests of driving skill and knowledge but also of ability to do vehicle repairs. In other nations, however, driver education is given by friends or relatives who themselves are not very knowledgeable or capable drivers, and licenses are purchased through bribes.[55] Many nations have substantial mixes of persons from neighboring countries who are unfamiliar with both the language and the rules of the road of the nation in which they may be driving.[56]

I have seen a number of reports from phase 1 and 2 countries that describe frequencies for various "driver errors" in crashes. Unfortunately, as explained in chapter 6, it is impossible to know the biases of collection, analysis, and interpretation of these data, and I can not present them as valid.

On the other hand, a careful study compared driver behavior at red and amber signals, zebra crossings, and priority junctions in several developing nations with similar locations in Britain.[57] Whereas in Britain, Jamaica, and Kenya in 1977 fewer than 7 percent of drivers did *not* stop at red signals, figures for cities in Turkey, Thailand, Indonesia, and Pakistan, and for Kenya in 1975, ranged from a low of 17 percent to as high as 50 percent in several places. Similar discrepancies were observed concerning response to an amber signal. Based on data such as these, I suspect that deliberate failure to obey traffic laws—whether because of lack of knowledge or for other reasons—is more often a factor in crashes in phase 1 and 2 nations at this time than in more developed countries.

Pre-Crash Factors Involving the Vehicle

Almost seventy years after the first automobile fatality was shown to be caused not by reckless driving but by a fracture in improperly seasoned wood on a wheel, Ralph Nader pointed out the crashes because drivers shift into "drive" gear when intending to shift into "reverse" or vice versa, should be attributed to a design defect.[58] His argument was met with incredulity by the American automotive industry and by many of the traditionally trained safety experts. Nader's rationale, shared by human factors engineers, was that if the drive and reverse gears had been separated by the neutral or parking gear, such an error would be less likely.

Within the first ten years after passage of the Motor Vehicle Safety Act of 1966 a total of thirty million vehicles sold in the United States had been subject to recalls for possible safety-related defects. Yet the frequency with which vehicular design, defect, or outright failure contribute to crashes is still largely conjecture.

As noted earlier, complete crash investigation is difficult, time consuming, and expensive, and even a routine check of all except the tread depth in tires is beyond the usual activity, and perhaps even the capability, of most police officers who fill out crash investigation forms. Some answers about outright vehicle failure come from a research project in Indiana.[59] For each crash the study team examined the crash site, interviewed persons involved, and for a representative sample examined the vehicles at a garage facility with the assistance of vehicle diagnostics consultants and special testing equipment. According to the authors of the report, in examining for vehicular contribution, definite causal involvement was established in at least 6 percent of crashes investigated, and possible vehicular involvement may have been as high as 13 percent.

Inadequate braking systems represented 43 percent of the vehicular contribution, usually with total failure of all or part of the brake system or side-to-side imbalance. Inadequacies of tires and wheels (usually involving inflation or tread depth) were contributory in 26 percent of vehicle-initiated crashes, with problems of vision, lighting, or steering comprising most of the remainder.

Frequency of defects was compared for crash vehicles and for a sample of vehicles in the general population. Although not reaching the level of statistical significance, the safety condition of vehicles in crashes was worse than that of the general population, and among crash vehicles inspected, the safety condition of the "most-at-fault" vehicles was worse than that of less culpable ones.

Some defects occur because drivers let their tires become bald or underinflated or do not keep a vehicle in good repair. Perhaps more often than generally considered, however, the person who tries to maintain a vehicle in good repair may also be at risk of vehicle failure. Investigations consistently show that in a very high proportion of cases service station personnel either cannot or will not make correct diagnoses and that they carry out repairs inadequately, in excessively costly manner, or both.[60,61] At risk particularly are the young and the poor, who are most likely to have vehicles that are old and need repairs.[62]

In developing nations, the problems are twofold. In many such nations the cost of an automobile or any other vehicle is far beyond most incomes. As a result, second-hand vehicles may be imported, refurbished, and kept until they literally fall to pieces despite repeated repairs and replacement of parts.

Studies as complete as the Indiana research have not been carried out in phase 1 or 2 nations, but in several such nations, despite limitations of investigative capability, the police have identified vehicle failure in substantial proportions of crashes (for example, 16 percent in Ghana and 12 percent in Botswana).[57]

In Israel, mechanical failures are a factor in nearly half of all crashes because drivers cannot afford the exorbitant cost of replacement parts.[63] At the time of the study the cost of a clutch disc, for example, was $7.50 in West Germany but $39.00 in Israel, with half of the extra cost coming from taxes and import duties. In a spot inspection program of 8,500 vehicles, one in every eight had such serious defects that the vehicle was ordered off the road immediately.

Vehicular contribution in the absence of "defect" or failure is almost never considered in police crash investigation. The rare exception—at least in phase 3 nations—is that involving cars overloaded in the rear so that the center of gravity is shifted or the driver cannot see traffic without an outside mirror. Even when actively seeking human/vehicular mismatch, it may be easier to identify that such discrepancies exist than it is to show how often they contribute to crashes.

In illustration, during the early 1970s American-made automobiles often had a wide rear pillar so that it was often impossible to see a vehicle approaching from behind in an adjacent lane. Such vehicles conceivably would have an excess of "two vehicle/same direction" crashes during lane changes. To my knowledge, epidemiologic study comparing crash patterns of wide-pillar and narrow-pillar models has never been attempted. Consider also the potential crash implications of the following observations:

> Studies of the placement of driver controls in automobiles manufactured during the early 1970s showed that, when wearing seatbelt and shoulder harness, drivers in the top and bottom 20 percent of height either had difficulty or could not reach or see all necessary controls.[64] This may be relevant to crash rates in other nations that import American vehicles because average size of both males and females in many of those nations is smaller than in the United States.[65] Furthermore, as more elderly women enter the U.S. driving population, the U.S. vehicles may become less suitable to our own drivers as well.
>
> In several 1971 model American vehicles total visibility that the driver had of the surrounding environment varied from 69 percent to as low as 39 percent of the ideal.[66]
>
> A driver needs 50° of vision to both left and right in the rear view mirror in order to meet 98 percent of his or her visual needs behind the car. Current mirrors provide 15° in each direction, or 52 percent of needs.[67]
>
> A consumer-aid document concerning 1976 passenger cars indicates that the reserve load capacity for tires recommended by auto manufacturers for specific vehicles varies from a high of 25 percent to as little as 0 percent.[68] For 97 of the 180 models listed, the reserve capacity is under 5 percent. No data were presented for the reserve capacity if a driver uses tires not recommended by the manufacturer or not maintained at recommended pressures.
>
> Data from another consumer-aid booklet about the capacity of a vehicle's brakes to stop the car without locking the wheels from a speed of 60 miles (97 km) per hour show that the necessary stopping distance ranged from 159 feet (48 meters) for the best vehicle to 250 feet (76 meters) for the worst.[69] Similar differences were found in passing ability.[70]

As pointed out by concerned members of the National Highway Safety Advisory Committee in 1979, the National Transportation Safety Board ten years previously had already noted four examples of driver/vehicle incompatibility and had shown how these could lead to crashes through no fault of the driver, although in each such case usual crash investigation techniques would conclude that the driver was culpable.[71]

As some recent examples of incompatibilities involving downsizing, they note that downsizing probably affects vision of the driver over and around other vehicles and places drivers of small cars in the glare range of lights from many vehicles.

Regarding all vehicles, no matter what the size, they observe that "rear vision requirements for vehicles are not defined in such a way that adequacy in relation to multi-lane highway situations can be determined and assured. Vehicles vary widely in capability, but the differences are undeterminable. Driver failure is thus blamed in many cases because an inadequate mirror is hard to prove. Mirrors of superior performance have no market because their superiority can't be related to operations. Mirrors which cause blind spots are not considered inferior."

What do these data mean? It is reasonable to assume that subtle vehicular contribution to crashes is occurring more often than even the multidisciplinary crash investigations can identify because the tools for such identification are not part of their armamentarium. How much more often? At this point in time no one knows.

Does overall vehicle design contribute to crash occurrence? Nader stated that the Corvair and the Volkswagen were excessively involved in crashes, and this problem has been attributed to other small vehicles as well.

Small vehicles do have greater involvement in fatal crashes, but this results from problems in the energy transfer phase. There is little evidence that specific models of vehicles are overrepresented in the initiation of crashes.[72,73] Such overrepresentation, if found, could reflect vehicle characteristics, different driver population, or both. The data do support Nader's contention that the Corvair was a hazard to drivers because of leakage of carbon monoxide from the heating system into the passenger compartment.[74] Fatalities have resulted from carbon monoxide in other models of cars as well, in this case because of trapping of the gas under vehicles as a result of short tailpipes.[75]

More difficult to assess is the psychological/performance axis involving vehicle design. The automobile is not only transportation but a means of ego gratification. The automotive industry has always been aware of this and has used this fact to promote sales, in particular with promotion of "muscle cars": high-performance vehicles attractive to young men. These vehicles and their drivers have been substantially overrepresented in injury and fatal crashes and in traffic citations. To what extent the overrepresentation represents driver behavior per se probably cannot be determined.

An important hidden vehicular factor that sometimes contributes to crashes in high-speed police chases with young males driving such vehicles is the fact that a rapidly moving vehicle commonly outdistances its own siren or other warning devices. The siren of a vehicle traveling over 50 M.P.H. may be heard for only one or two car lengths in front of the vehicle if the windows of other automobiles are closed. Even where drivers hear a siren, they often cannot determine its direction. Yet the fault in crashes with emergency vehicles is often placed on the driver of the other vehicle because "he should have paid attention to the siren."

Environmental Contribution to Pre-Crash Phase

As with the vehicular contribution to the pre-crash phase, the environmental one ranges from blatant to exceedingly subtle. Blatant examples are higher crash rates in construction zones because of poor or absent warnings about roadway or traffic discontinuities[76] and crashes because of poor roadway maintenance, rockslides, or weather.

While these factors are more common in some geographic areas, they are rare compared to more subtle issues of roadway geometry, signing, and the contribution of specific construction materials. When a driver skids on a wet or icy road, for example, the police blame the driver for going too fast for conditions or not being sufficiently alert and skilled. However, certain states have much higher crash rates in such weather than do neighboring states, and this correlates directly with the density of the materials used to build the road.[77]

Furthermore, according to Olsen,[78] not only do people usually drive without paying conscious attention to details of their behavior, but they can initiate caution only after they perceive that a hazard exists. Any system designed to train drivers in skid control will not succeed unless it also informs them when there is an impending skid. This is not possible, however, because the vehicle and the environment have not been designed to provide adequate premonitory knowledge or feel in advance of skid situations through visual inputs from road surface and edges, steering torque feedback, engine and tire sounds, and road noises and vibrations. In vehicle skid crashes Olsen concludes that the driver often is victim rather than cause.

Regarding informational cues, signs must meet several criteria. First, they must exist where information is needed. Drivers often are given absolutely no cues by those responsible for building and maintaining the environment. Second, signs must attract sufficient attention to alert the driver. Many signs, however, are hidden, too small, inadequately lighted, or do not stand out against competing commercial or other signs or during the nighttime.

Third, signs must be legible at all times of day and night. Letters that are too small or too close together or that lack sufficient contrast with the background make for an illegible sign.

Fourth, the message must not confuse either people quite unfamiliar with the area or those who are somewhat familiar. Also, it should help those who seek advice about how to get to distant locations as well as drivers trying to get to intermediate points or to places close at hand. One reason why signs may be confusing is that too many messages are grouped too close together. If the messages can be separated and repeated, individuals have a chance to avoid or to sort out confusion.

A message must give a driver sufficient time to react. A sign that first appears within a few yards of a decision point cannot fulfill this function. Finally, signs should be placed and built so as not to obstruct vision, be struck by cars, or if struck, substantially increase crash severity.

In 1968 Congressman John Blatnick summarized this environmental contribution to crashes that all too often is assigned as *caused by driver error* when, in fact, it is environmental inadequacy that *results in driver error:*[79]

> Traffic signs and markings are supposed to regulate, warn, or guide motorists. They are supposed to supply a primary source of information which the driver needs to safely adjust his actions to highway conditions. Hesitation or confusion, particularly on high-speed highways, can create chaos and contribute to traffic accidents. Yet in one recent nationwide survey more than 60 percent of the respondents complained about confusing and inadequate signs. . . .

This brings us to roadway geometrics and related issues. The scientific literature is consistent and voluminous in documenting that characteristics of the environment are major determinants of crash frequency, as well as of crash outcome. These characteristics include, among others, the road and shoulder width, number of lanes, surface, markings, curves, and other aspects of road geometry, separation of roads, and lighting.[80,81] Again, loss of vehicle control because of these problems often—in fact, usually—is attributed to driver error, with little or no attention to the environment with which the driver must interact.

In illustration, drivers do not usually enter freeways heading in the wrong direction unless they are confused by factors related to old age or alcohol. But *despite* the old age or alcohol, they do not get confused if entrance and exit ramps are separated spatially and are clearly marked to alert the driver who chooses the wrong ramp.[82] Alcohol and old age may be facts of life. The associated errors need not be. The full extent of the interaction is summarized by Clayton in an analysis of driver errors in 210 crashes involving 348 road users.[83] Among the 249 drivers, the errors identified were as follows: failure to look, 10.8 percent; misperception, 11.2 percent; excessive speed, 13.7 percent; panic reaction, 5.2 percent; and other error of decision, 10.4 percent. There was no driver error 48.6 percent of the time. Why did the errors occur? The reasons listed were these:

Distraction	13.5%
Alcohol	5.2
Fatigue	2.1
Incorrect mind set	4.7
Visual deficiency	1.6
Emotional disturbance	1.6
Miscellaneous road-user factors	6.3
Sight restriction	15.6
Restriction in road width	8.8
Actions of other road users	7.8
Weather conditions	6.8
Lighting deficiencies	5.2
Defects in signs, markings, or alignment	6.3
Problems of skid resistance/skidding	3.6
Vehicle defects	10.9
	100.0%

Clayton states,

> "for errors of failure to look, the prime causal factor was distraction of the road users at the critical moment. The causes of this distraction varied widely and included signposts, side roads, and other landmarks. Sometimes the hazard was a sudden restriction of the road width caused, for example, by a parked car which the road user failed to see. Other causes of this error occurred at junctions with major roads. Here, it is possible that some road users were incapable of monitoring two sources of stimuli (that is, two traffic flows) virtually simultaneously. They may have sought to simplify the task by waiting for one lane to become free,

> assumed that it would remain clear, and then moved out when a gap appeared in the other traffic flow.
>
> For errors of misperception, the adoption of an incorrect set or perceptual expectancy appeared to be more prevalent than a visual defect. There were, however, several cases of the presence of alcohol and fatigue which other research has shown to reduce visual acuity. Many of the misperception errors were found to occur under either unfavorable or inadequate lighting or where the signs, markings, or design of the road had created an ambiguous situation. The road users who committed errors of excessive speed have been shown to be younger and to have less driving experience than non-error road users. Few road-user factors were associated with these errors. Rather, the errors tended to be related to restriction of the available sight distance, usually at bends or crests, and to vehicle defects such as inadequate brakes or steering. These environmental causal factors were assessed according to current official codes of practice.
>
> Errors of panic reaction were primarily caused by one road user suddenly infringing or threatening to infringe the intended path or travel of another road user. A possible explanation of this phenomenon is that the reacting road users, because of their lack of driving experience, may have found it impossible to process all the available perceptual information accurately and quickly. Thus, instead of responding rationally to the situation, they merely tried to stop as quickly as possible. In doing so, they tended to lose control of their vehicles."[83]

There is substantial anecdotal information to conclude that environmental factors contribute far more to crashes in developing countries. Regarding Nigeria, Owosina[55] reports narrow one-lane earth roads, subjected to deterioration and erosion by torrential rains. Even at best, they are usually so narrow that wide vehicles cannot pass without brushing against each other or one of them skidding off the road. Such roads have no shoulders, no facilities for separating road users, and usually no road signs. Trees often fall across them.

Most state roads are two-lane with dressed surfaces, but most of them are riddled with potholes and bumps, and many have dangerous bends and curves. Bridges usually are very narrow, allowing only a vehicle to pass at a time, and often have lost their side railings. While federal highways and express roads are better, some of them deteriorate with potholes and other problems within a short time after their completion.

Sabey says that in the phase 1 and 2 countries there is greater potential for remedies through low-cost engineering than in the phase 3 countries. In the latter, such remedies have been estimated as likely to bring about a 20 percent saving in crashes.[6]

Yugoslavia has yet other problems.[56] Its roads join major east/west traffic arteries of Eastern Europe, and large numbers of Greeks and Turks use them on their way to and from jobs in Western Europe. Except for a thirty-three-mile stretch of four-lane divided highway, there are no modern roads but rather truck routes crowded with slow-moving traffic.

Sharp curves are rarely banked and no parking places exist, requiring disabled vehicles to stop in the middle of the road and put up triangular danger signs. Cars often run out of fuel because only major towns many miles apart have filling stations. Horse-drawn wagons and bicycles are prohibited, but they also clog main highways and only rarely display lights at night.

Theoretically, the speed limit is 60 miles an hour on open roads. But almost everyone ignores it because enforcement is ineffective. A driver's license examination includes complicated mechanical tests, a driving test, and a rigorous physical examination. Officials consider improved driver education a more pressing need than improved roads. The discrepancies between needs and proposed solutions, I believe, speak for themselves.

Energy Transfer or Injury Phase

The contribution of the driver to the energy transfer phase can be documented but not modified very easily. The elderly are more sensitive to moderate injury and less likely to survive than are younger persons.[84] For a given energy load, tissue trauma may be more severe if the injured person has alcohol.[85]

But the major and most correctable contributions to injury severity in this phase involve the vehicle and the roadside environment. Until about 1950 conventional wisdom said that ejection promoted survivability in crashes. Studies showed just the opposite to be the case.[86] An ejected person impacts the car interior, then the ground, and may also have the vehicle roll on top of him. The death rate for ejection is high, and immediate deaths are six times more frequent than for persons who remain inside the vehicle.

Two solutions are occupant restraints and improved door locks so that doors do not open as often during crashes. As noted earlier, Ralph Nader labeled the Volkswagen Beetle as an excessively hazardous car. One reason is that it rolled over more often than other makes and ejected occupants.[87]

Although deaths from ejection have decreased since door lock improvements in the late 1950s, contact with the windshield, steering column, and dashboard continue to present a source of death and disability. Figure 9–1 shows the relative frequency of contact between

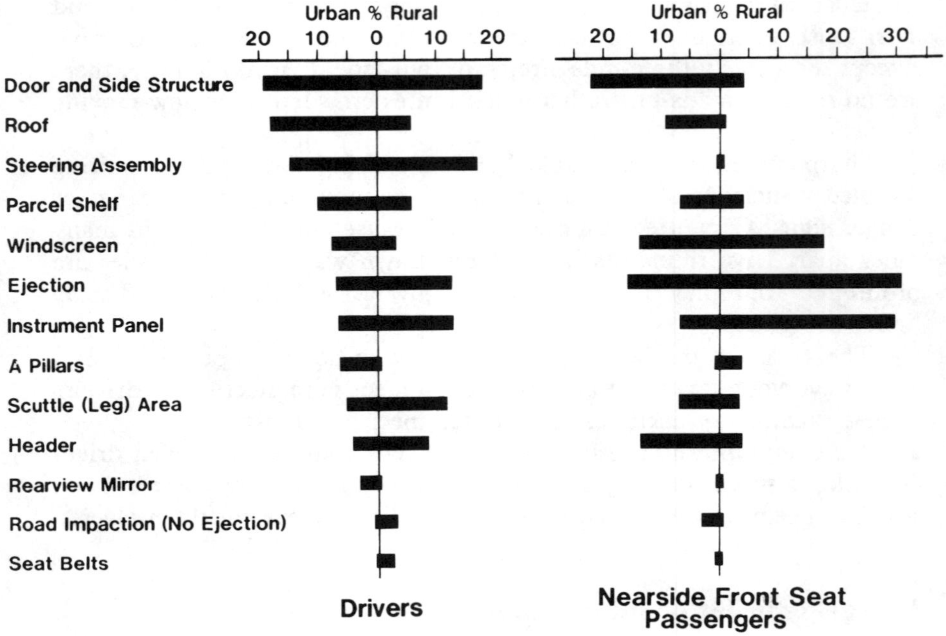

Source: Reprinted with permission from G.M. Mackay, "Some Features of Traffic Accidents," *British Medical Journal* 4 (1969):799–801.

Figure 9–1. Relative Frequency of Known Sources of Major Injury to Front-Seat Occupants in Urban and Rural Crashes.

driver and front seat passengers and various interior fixtures in urban and rural crashes in England.[88] Table 9–6, on the other hand, compares the causes of major injuries in two studies in urban areas (England and Australia) and two in rural areas (England and the United States).[89]

Typical of the problems faced in such reconstructive research is that in two of these studies injuries with cause unknown exceed those with known cause. As the authors observe, this research shows that the priorities for improvements must vary with the particular environment, and a detailed knowledge of the crash circumstances in each country is required for design changes to have maximum effect. The patterns of contact and injury differ in rollover, frontal-impact, side-impact, and rear-impact crashes, and the frequency of these crashes varies with the environment.

Regarding vehicle weight Mela says, "In two-car crashes, the chance of serious or fatal injury to an unbelted driver decreased about 5% for

Table 9–6
Rank Order of Vehicle Components Causing Injury in Four Studies

	Area 1	*Area 2*	*Area 3*	*Area 4*
Average speed (M.P.H.) (KmP.H.)	43.8 (70.5)	26.5 (42.6)	21.9 (35.2)	21.7 (34.9)
Cause known (number of injuries)	19,745	117	126	603
Cause unknown	Unknown	206	179	266
Rank: all injuries				
1	Instrument panel (4,610)	Instrument panel (35)	Door (33)	Instrument panel (169)
2	Steering wheel (4,130)	Ejection (23)	Instrument panel (28)	Door (157)
3	Windshield (2,950)	Windshield (16)	Header (25)	Windshield (63)
4	Door (2,410)	Door (13)	Other (11)	Header (56)
5	Ejection (2,210)	Header (11)	Windshield (9)	Steering wheel (45)
6	Front seat (1,660)	Steering wheel (10)	Ejection (7)	Ejection (40)
7	Top structures (760)	Front seat (4)	Steering wheel (6)	Front seat (34)
8	Corner post (510)	Other (4)	Corner post (5)	Other (27)
9	Rear mirror (505)	Corner post (1)	Front seat (2)	Corner post (12)
Rank: minor injuries excluded				
Cause known	6,056	44	34	152
1	Steering wheel (1,292)	Instrument panel (15)	Door (13)	Door (50)
2	Ejection (1,214)	Ejection (9)	Header (8)	Windshield (21)
3	Instrument Panel (1,179)	Door (7)	Instrument panel (4)	Instrument panel (19)
4	Windshield (775)	Windshield (5)	Ejection (4)	Header (17)
5	Door (681)	Steering wheel (5)	Windshield (2)	Ejection (15)
6	Front Seat (389)	Header (5)	Other (2)	Other (13)
7	Top Structures (217)	—	Steering wheel (1)	Steering wheel (11)
8	Corner Post (207)	—	—	Front seat (4)
9	Rear Mirror (102)	—	—	Corner post (2)

Source: Adapted from G.A. Ryan and G.M. Mackay "Comparisons of Car Crashes in Three Countries" *Proceedings of the 13th Stapp Car Crash Conference, Boston, Mass.: 2–4 December 1969* (Warrendale, Pa.: Society of Automotive Engineers, 1969), 336–352.

each hundred pounds additional weight in his car, and increased about 2 percent for each hundred pounds increased in the weight of the other car in the collision."[90]

Vehicle size relates closely to frequency and extent of injury because in larger vehicles occupants have more room to decelerate before impacting the interior. Because lighter vehicles also tend to have less "ride down space" for occupants, one would expect their occupants to do poorly in single vehicle collisions, not because the vehicles are light but because they are small. Figure 9–2 shows this relationship and indicates the importance of speed (measured as change in velocity) as a contributor to severity.[91]

One of the most extensive and detailed studies of the crash phase is the National Crash Severity Study (NCSS) involving crashes requiring towing or where someone was injured.[92] Twenty-three percent of occu-

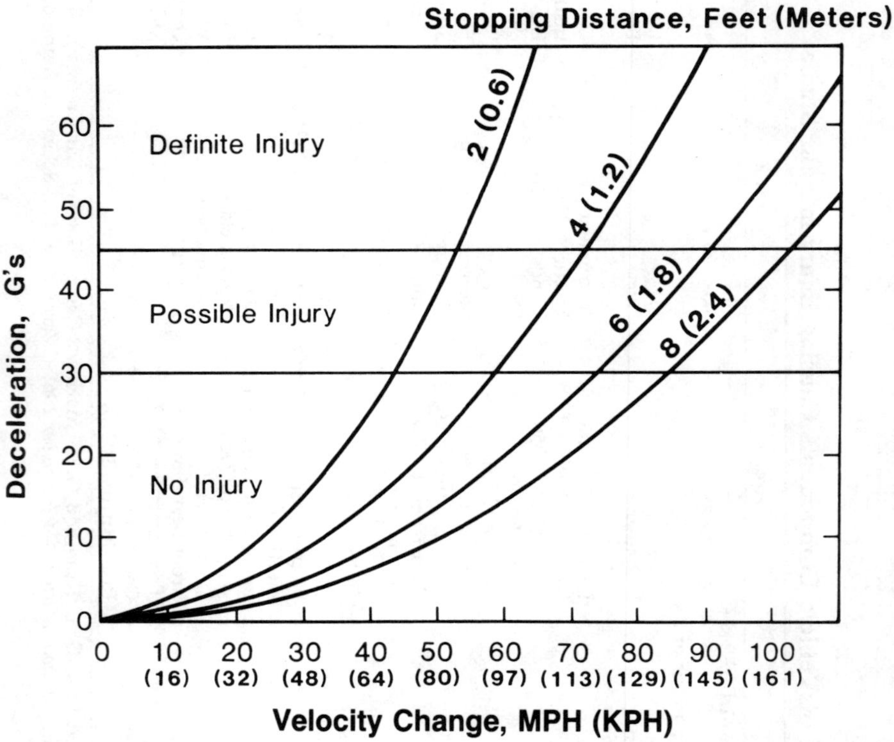

Source: Adapted from W. Haddon, Jr., "Reducing the Damage of Motor-Vehicle Use," copyright © *Technology Review* 77(8) (July/August 1975):1–9. Used with permission.

Figure 9–2. Relationship between Velocity Change, Stopping Distance, and Injury.

pants in all crashes, but 41 percent of those in fatal crashes, were in a single-vehicle crash. Crashes involving three or more vehicles affected 13 percent of occupants for all crashes but 6 percent of those for fatal crashes. The vectors for these crashes and relative injury rates appear in table 9–7 while table 9–8 shows injury rates for different crash severities (as measured by change in velocity) in all crashes and in frontal, right-side, and left-side impacts.

In the United States a quarter to half of fatal collisions involve contact with unnecessary or unyielding roadside "furniture"[93,94,95] (see table 9–9). The problem is greatest in rural areas. Although data are sparse, I suspect, based on personal observation, that the problem of roadside hazards is much worse in many other nations. Despite higher average speeds of travel, freeways have crash fatality rates per unit miles that are from one-half to one-third those of primary and secondary roads, largely because their sides are usually cleared of trees, rocks, and similar hazards for at least thirty feet from the road edge.[96] (Absence of intersections is another reason for this low rate.)

Ideally, roadside environment should be flat, even, and clear enough of obstacles that can cause damage so that a driver who, for whatever reason, goes off the road is able to regain control before the vehicle and the occupants suffer injury. A driver may wish to leave the road to park a disabled vehicle or to avoid a pedestrian or another vehicle that encroaches or may go off the road despite wishing to stay on it either because he loses control or because he continues off the road after being in an on-road collision.

Damage can be caused by cliffs, gullies, or bodies of water that make the vehicle overturn, by natural objects or manmade "furniture" (such as trees, stumps, rock outcroppings, signs, protruding drainage covers, telephone and lamp poles, and bridge piers), or by objects placed to protect vehicles and occupants. If improperly designed and constructed, these may be capable of causing very serious damage. Examples include bridge railings, guard rails whose ends are not protected, and lane separators.

The same principles that apply to vehicle interiors are relevant here. Damage will be more severe if there is little ride-down space and if the surface struck is firm and pointed. While cars may be more likely to skid off the road in winter weather the resultant crashes are often very minor because snow banks provide a ride-down cushion that does not exist in summer, when a car might hit a tree, sign, or lamppost that doesn't break away easily.

A study of fatal crashes in Georgia emphasizes both roadway geometry factors that help initiate a crash and the roadside factors that make it more severe than necessary.[97] This study found more than 26 percent of

Table 9–7
Crash Distribution and Injury Rates by Crash Type

		Occupants						
			AIS[a] *2 +*		*AIS 3 +*		*Fatal*	
Type of Impact	*Percentage of Crashes*	*Percentage of Total*	*Percent*	*Injury Rate*[b]	*Percent*	*Injury Rate*	*Percent*	*Injury Rate*
One vehicle								
Fixed object	24.9	19.4	31.2	9.4	30.4	4.5	28.7	1.2
Rollover	4.2	3.6	7.5	12.1	9.2	7.3	13.1	2.9
Undercarriage	1.6	1.2	0.9	4.2	0.7	1.7	0.6	0.4
Two-vehicle								
Head-on	7.5	8.9	15.6	10.2	17.1	5.5	20.1	1.8
Rear-end	15.4	14.0	4.8	2.0	3.8	0.8	2.9	0.2
Angle	32.4	37.2	29.2	4.6	29.3	2.3	27.5	0.6
Sideswipe	1.5	1.9	0.5	1.4	0.2	0.3	0.0	0.0
Three-plus-vehicle	4.6	4.7	1.4	1.8	0.6	0.4	0.2	0.0
Unknown	8.0	9.1	8.9	5.7	8.7	2.7	7.0	0.6
Total	100.0	100.0	100.0	5.8	100.0	2.9	100.0	0.8

Source: Adapted from L. Ricci, *National Crash Severity Study Statistics* (Ann Arbor, Mich.: Highway Safety Research Institute, University of Michigan, Special Report on National Highway Traffic Safety Administration Contract DOT HS-8-01944, 1979).

[a]Abbreviated Injury Score.

[b]Per 100 occupants.

Table 9–8
Distribution of Injury Rates Per 100 Occupants by Crash Severity (Delta V) in Front-, Side-, and Back-Damage Vehicles

Location of Damage and Delta V	*AIS*[a] *2+*	*AIS 3+*	*Fatal*
All crashes combined			
1–10 M.P.H.	1.9	0.7	0.1
11–20	8.5	3.3	0.3
21–30	21.7	12.3	3.2
31–40	47.0	34.6	13.3
41–50	60.3	49.2	25.4
> 50	57.8	47.7	37.6
Total	7.1	3.5	0.8
Frontal			
1–10 M.P.H.	1.9	0.7	0.0
11–20	8.7	2.9	0.3
21–30	22.3	11.8	2.2
31–40	41.5	30.5	9.6
41–50	57.9	45.6	24.6
> 50	75.0	59.4	46.9
Total	7.4	3.4	0.8
Right side			
1–10 M.P.H.	1.9	0.7	0.0
11–20	8.0	4.1	0.5
21–30	30.0	19.8	8.1
31–40	67.9	55.4	33.9
41–50	80.0	80.0	20.0
> 50	100.0	92.3	76.9
Total	7.3	4.3	1.4
Left side			
1–10 M.P.H.	2.3	0.9	0.1
11–20	11.3	5.9	0.6
21–30	13.8	9.2	3.9
31–40	80.0	53.3	22.2
41–50[b]	100.0	100.0	100.0
> 50[b]	100.0	100.0	50.0
Total	7.4	4.0	0.9
Back			
1–10	0.7	0.0	0.0
11–20	2.4	0.6	0.0
21–30	13.6	9.1	2.3
31–40	11.1	5.6	0.0
41–50[b]	0.0	0.0	0.0
> 50	0.0	0.0	0.0
Total	1.8	0.5	0.1

Source: Adapted from L. Ricci, *National Crash Severity Study Statistics* (Ann Arbor, Mich.: Highway Safety Research Institute, University of Michigan, Special Report on National Highway Traffic Safety Administration Contract DOT HS-8-01944, 1979).

[a]Abbreviated Injury Score.

[b]Each of those categories had fewer than two persons at risk. All other categories had from 10 to 9,340 persons at risk.

Table 9–9
Proportions of Crashes Involving Roadside Furniture and Hazards in Michigan, 1972

Object Hit	*Total*	*Fatal*	*Injury*	*Property Damage*	*Urban*	*Rural*
Guard rail/post	10.6%	12.3%	9.7	11.1	10.8	10.3
Sign	9.3	6.9	6.2	11.3	8.4	10.5
Pole	15.9	13.3	19.7	13.7	8.6	26.3
Culvert, ditch, embankment	19.1	10.9	21.1	18.0	28.4	5.7
Bridge	2.0	8.5	2.5	1.5	2.0	2.2
Tree	13.7	34.1	18.1	10.6	16.0	10.4
Other object	29.4	14.0	22.7	33.8	25.7	34.5
Total objects						
%	100.0	100.0	100.0	100.0	99.9	99.9
(N)	(63,726)	(649)	(23,968)	(39,109)	(37,411)	(26,315)
Percentage of total crashes	17.7	32.5	13.8	16.0	34.8	10.4

Source: Adapted from J.F. Fitzpatrick, M.M. Sohn, T.E. Silfen, and R.W. Wood, *The Law and Roadside Hazards* (Charlottesville, Va.: Michie Co., 1974).

fatal crash sites, but only 8 percent of comparison sites, had curvature greater than 6 degrees combined with a downhill gradient of 2 percent or steeper at or approaching the sites. Half of the fatal crashes, but only 23 percent of comparison sites, involved curves greater than 6 degrees. Over 80 percent of fatal crashes into fixed objects were on nonlocal roads, although such roads comprised only 33 percent of all the roads in the state. Finally, 98 percent of the objects struck were located less than 50 feet (15 meters) from the pavement edge.

Post-Crash Phase

Emergency medical services for highway crashes will be covered later, but it is noteworthy that especially in developing nations substantial delays may occur in finding crashes on rural roads and the injured may be brought to the hospital by automobile or by police vans unequipped for emergency care. In some Arabian Gulf nations utilizing such transportation, virtually every highway fatality occurs within the first few minutes after arrival at the hospital.[3] In such nations there is an inverse correlation between number of doctors and beds per population and highway fatality rates.[13]

Alcohol again assumes importance in the post-crash phase because fully 70 percent of drivers who die when their cars go into bodies of water have BACs of 0.10 percent or higher.[98] Were they not so befuddled by alcohol, some of these drivers and their passengers probably could have extricated themselves and survived.

Regarding post-crash fires, controversy exists about how many fires are occurring, how often they contribute to death, what are their causes, and what can or should be done to prevent them. Much of the concern has been associated with the documented fact that gas tanks sometimes leak, even on abrupt noncrash maneuvers of the vehicle, and often rupture and leak in crashes.

One literature review[99] concluded that each year about 17,000 fires result from motor vehicle crashes and that between 450 and 1250 fatalities result directly from these fires. *Leakage of fuel* most often resulted from severe damage to the rear ends of the vehicles, especially of small or intermediate size. However, at least half of *fires* were associated with front-end collisions involving engine damage, and only a minority involved rear-end collisions. It was concluded that improving the rupture resistance of the fuel tank might save 180 to 200 lives a year.

Appropriate Countermeasures

In a presentation in 1971, C.F. Scheffey[100] shared his frustrations as follows:

> An investment of $1 billion by the American public, either in tax funds or in private outlays, for instance, represents a very limited attack on any one of the three components in the system.
>
> 1. It could provide an investment of only $1000 per mile or about $0.20 per foot for a new feature if incorporated into the entire primary highway system. It could purchase an item such as an improved guardrail system type for only about 10 percent of the length of the primary system where such guardrails are warranted.
> 2. If invested in improvements to the vehicle, it could provide for a device costing a mere $10 per vehicle, if all vehicles were to be so equipped, for a more elaborate device such as a passenger restraint system costing $100 per automobile for only 10 percent of the motor vehicles now on the road.
> 3. If we choose to invest the $1 billion in driver education it could provide a 20-hour retraining course for approximately 10 percent of our driving population.
>
> Perhaps even more frustrating . . . is the time required to implement a change . . . in the system after all research and development has been carried out. A device required by Federal regulations on all new vehicles will not appear on two-thirds of the vehicle population until after a period of perhaps 5 to 6 years. If driver education is restricted to the young, it could conceivably take from 25 to 30 years to get two-thirds of all active drivers retreated. Investments in the highway system can be made at whatever rate resources permit, but the design, construction and operation sequence takes something on the order of 3 years for major changes. Minor modifications such as the replacement of sign supports with frangible device are limited primarily by available resources.

With these sobering thoughts as background, I would like to briefly explore some of the more common and some of the more promising countermeasures applied to reduction of crashes involving passenger cars. Before discussing ways to improve upon the driver, vehicle, or environment, let us examine a different perspective about countermeasures by David Klein, a sociologist, who makes the following observation about highway researchers and practitioners:[101]

> This highly diverse group of parochials is unified in only one respect:

an unquestioning acceptance of . . . the present system of highway transportation by privately owned vehicles. This loyalty to the status quo is either caused or reinforced by the fact that most research funding comes from sources that are committed to the present system. . . .

The use of an exposure rate rather than a population rate produced . . . considerable satisfaction . . . over the *reduction* in fatality rate per million miles when in fact . . . an *increasing proportion* of the United States population was being killed in highway crashes. From a social or a public health point of view, this would not be grounds for self-satisfaction; on the contrary, efforts would be made to reduce the exposure.

In short, their loyalty to the status quo tends to keep research investigators searching for the "better mousetrap" in terms of their organization's definition of mousetrap, whether or not an improved mousetrap has either relevance or cost effectiveness.

This argument deserves more serious attention than it usually gets. Development of highway systems in the United States and elsewhere is typically accompanied by a cutting back of tram, bus, and train service, which provided and could still continue to provide quite satisfactory transportation. The Highway Users Federation for Safety and Mobility (HUFSAM) continues to urge that the only acceptable changes for highway safety are modest incremental efforts that will improve upon the driver, vehicle, or environment. Such changes are needed and will now be discussed, but only with an awareness that at the same time the context and the solutions must be broader.

Countermeasures Directed at People

Over the years the thrust of highway safety programs has predominantly been directed at changing people. Although there has been some shift in emphasis, this statement continues to hold true today, especially if one takes an international perspective. In the October 1975 issue of *World Health,* for example, the need to improve upon either the vehicle or the environment was mentioned only in passing, with virtually the entire emphasis going to what is wrong with people and how to change them. The following is the distribution of the $640 million in federal funds expended from 1966 to 1975 for the U.S. Highway Safety Standards program established under the U.S. Department of Transportation[102]: for changing or regulating people, 49 percent, for environmental change, 13 percent, and for programs in vehicle inspection and registration, 2 percent. Fully 35 percent of the funds went to two programs: police traffic services and driver education. Twelve percent of funds were for emergency medical services, and 24 percent for activities relevant to all above categories.

In addition, of course, some funds were expended under the Motor Vehicle Safety Act to improve upon the vehicle, but the lion's share still went for people-oriented countermeasures. Large amounts of state and local government funds were spent for educational, licensing, and law enforcement activities and traffic records, with much smaller amounts for emergency services, crash investigation, and environmental activities for safety (as opposed to environmental activities to promote mobility). Most, if not all, of the expenditures for vehicle safety are passed by manufacturers to the public.

We now consider four areas of countermeasures involving the driver: namely, educational efforts, licensing, laws and their enforcement, and particular alcohol programs. Educational efforts assume most crashes result from human errors, deriving from inadequate knowledge or skills or wrong attitudes, and can be improved through education, with a consequent reduction in errors and of crashes.

An educational program must meet three criteria:

1. It must teach what people don't already know or are not currently sufficiently skilled to perform.
2. What is taught must play a sufficiently major role in safe driving so that its effect cannot be substantially washed out or negated by other factors, such as environmental contributors. That is, behavioral change must deal with volitional causes of crashes rather than with involuntary human errors.
3. The knowledge or skill must remain over time and across an appropriate range of circumstances with high crash risks.

As we have already noted, these criteria may be met in some phase 1 nations. One reason for the high crash rate in Sudan, for example, is that people do not yet know on which side of a traffic island they should travel.[54]

As the system matures, however, and after gross and more easily correctable educational and environmental changes have been made, educational efforts are much less likely to have value because the basic hypotheses may no longer apply. Thus, in the United States, studies of the benefits of individualized driver education programs either for new drivers or for purposes of reeducation have been consistently discouraging.[103,104]

Two studies in fact have even more negative import. In response to the argument that teaching driving skills reduces crash risk, critics have shown that highly skilled racing drivers have above average non-racetrack crash rates.[105] Driver education in schools simply increases the number of young, high-risk drivers on the roads and therefore results in higher injury and death rates for this age group. Shifting the age of first license from 16 to 17, for example, reduces fatal crashes of 16 year olds by 65 to 85 percent without increasing fatal crash rates at older ages.[106]

Public information programs, such as are carried out through radio and television spot announcements, posters, and so forth, generally—but not always—have had similarly disappointing results. One important and successful role for such efforts is to inform the public of changes in laws or in application of laws: for example, compulsory seat belt use, routine stopping of drivers to test for alcohol, or, as in Sweden, shifting the side of the road on which everyone is expected to drive.

But much more often, public information programs simply consist of signs or posters that tell people to "drive safely," "be courteous," or offer some similarly noninformative instructions. And it would appear that the more these efforts lack in specific information, the greater seems to be the corresponding level of naive expectation of the sponsors.

The problem with driver licensing as a countermeasure is summarized by Williams.[107]

> One of the most dangerous myths that still haunts highway safety efforts is the notion that 5 or 10 percent of the drivers cause 90 percent of the serious accidents. According to this logic, we could eliminate 90 percent of the serious accidents if we could identify and remove from the highway the guilty 5 or 10 percent of the drivers. . . . The idea . . . simply does not hold up under the light of research.
>
> One of the problems is that [drivers] don't always fit the classifications or stay classified after we put them in what we think are their proper pigeonholes. . . . There are tests for screening out potentially bad drivers, but the best test ever devised to date has such a low validity . . . that in eliminating even a small number of poor-risk drivers, it eliminates a large number of good ones also. To reduce accidents from, say, 15 million to 10 million . . . would mean the unfair and meaningless removal of 18 million safe drivers along with the 5 million poor drivers. Drivers would never tolerate this type of trade-off in the name of safety, nor should they.

I doubt, however, that Williams is asking for cessation of all licensing efforts. There are two different levels of screening drivers. The initial screening—the knowledge, vision, and driving tests—seeks to ensure that people do not use the roads until they have achieved a certain minimum level of knowledge and skill. This screening functions reasonably well in meeting its limited expectations. Of course, since by definition all persons who fail this screening are precluded from driving, there is no way to completely evaluate this countermeasure, although among persons who do pass, those with lower scores have higher crash rates.[49]

Psychologists have sometimes recommended that new drivers should be given psychological screening tests as well to weed out those who are psychologically unfit. As Williams noted, this system identifies a changeable phenomenon and one with very tenuous relationship to safety.

Medical examinations for drivers have also been recommended and are required in some nations. Some obvious impairments can be identified either with or without the help of a physician: severe visual deficit, extreme levels of mental retardation or advanced senile dementia, and severe arthritis or cerebral palsy. Many other conditions are more subtle and harder even for a physician to identify, and there is disagreement about the extent to which persons with these conditions can be screened and/or should be limited from driving. This issue will also be discussed in a later chapter.

A system for issuing new or renewal licenses must have three components: periodic renewal of licenses with personal appearance by the applicant; periodic vision testing; and requirements for drivers to report to the motor vehicle authorities if they have specific medical conditions. Such drivers are then screened to restrict or remove licenses for less than 25 percent.

The second screening level in driver licensing deals with those individuals who have gotten into trouble on the highway. This includes surviving drivers in fatal crashes and persons with certain types or more than a certain number of crashes, traffic citations, or both in a stated time. These drivers are easy to identify, but as noted before, their excess of crashes still comprises only a minority of all crashes. Any effort to control them, therefore, must start and end with the realization that, at best, only a small portion of the problem is likely to be dealt with.

That was the good news. The bad news is that in general methods to deal with these identified individuals often do not appear to be successful in preventing recidivism. The majority of those whose licenses are suspended or revoked continue to drive anyway *and* to get into trouble.[108]

This does not necessarily mean that screening efforts should be abandoned entirely. Several official agencies have tried and carefully evaluated a range of activities to deal with these deviant drivers, including the problem of deviant drivers who fail to complete or even begin a rehabilitation program to which they have been assigned.[109] Examples of their results are described below.

1. Warning letters to drivers beginning to show an excess of viola-

tions or crashes are commonly sent as a first step in driver rehabilitation. One evaluation compared letters with low, medium, and high threat of punishment, and with low through medium to high intimacy of writing style.[110] All of the approaches resulted in lower average crash and citation experiences when compared to the control group, with the low-threat letter showing significantly fewer crashes in a seven-month followup; but these effects appeared to diminish after seven months. There was evidence that low threat and high intimacy reinforced each other.

In a later program two types of letters plus an informational pamphlet were used to reduce subsequent crash and conviction records of "pre-negligent drivers," with a followup reinforcement letter to drivers who were crash and conviction free. Six months after treatment no significant effects were found on convictions, but there was a positive pamphlet effect on crashes. The followup reinforcement analysis for crash and citation free drivers showed no significant treatment effects on crashes. But for citations, there was an effect attributable to type of warning letter, as well as an interaction between type of warning letter, pamphlet, and followup reinforcement. Results showed no significant influence by subject characteristics.[111]

2. Where warning letters do not work, "negligent drivers" may be called in for an interview. The Oregon interview program was found not to be effective in an initial evaluation.[112] Tapes of interviews at that time revealed rambling, moralizing, and excessive use of slogans, statistics, and stereotypes. Subsequently, the interviews were restructured to respond to four areas of individual need: faulty self-perception, inadequate knowledge of traffic laws, unhealthy driver attitudes (such as excessive competitiveness and aggressiveness), and serious personality problems. In addition, interviewers received extensive training.

After this restructuring drivers who had been interviewed were compared with those who had not (excluding, however, persons with alcohol offenses). Interviewed drivers had substantially fewer citations and somewhat fewer "avoidable" crashes during the first year than did drivers not interviewed. The differences disappeared entirely during the second year after interview.[113]

3. If such interviews are not effective the next step may be a Defensive Driving Course (DDC), such as developed by National Safety Council (NSC), or some sort of driver clinic or school. An NSC evaluation claiming the course is effective has been challenged because it is based on research methods incapable of showing cause-and-effect relationships.[114]

Regarding clinics or schools, Harano and Peck[115] state that for males only, the Uniform Driver Improvement School was associated with 12 percent reduction in crashes and a 6 percent reduction in convictions. But they found that the effectiveness of the new school varied with the type of driver treated and that the subject's prior driving record had a major influence. Females showed no evidence of positive treatment effect.

Prothero compared a course using group discussion, role playing, and other experiential activities to help problem drivers become aware of their driving behavior with the Defensive Driving Course and a control group, the problem drivers being randomly assigned to the three treatments.[116] Mean numbers of collisions and of violation points respectively before treatment were 0.49 and 10.39 for the clinic group and 0.14 and 1.44 during the year with treatment. For the DDC subjects respective means before treatment were 0.40 and 9.17 and after were 0.23 and 2.15.

Both groups show substantial drops in crashes and citations, but so did the control group, whose initial means were 0.35 and 8.22. After a year they were 0.26 and 2.75, probably reflecting a regression toward the mean. (Coppin[117] points out that whereas 90 percent of persons who attended driver improvement meetings had clear records during the year, so did 83 percent of negligent drivers not attending meetings.) Overall, Prothero concludes that while no significant improvement occurred between the groups in driving knowledge or in attitudes, the experimental group had a greater reduction than the DDC group, and a significantly greater reduction than the control group, in traffic citations and crashes during a one-year followup.

4. What about drivers who continue to get into trouble despite treatments? Persons in North Carolina with several major moving violations in seven years are defined as habitual offenders (HO) and are eligible for mandatory license revocation. But many district attorneys are not interested in prosecuting these cases. For those that were prosecuted, no evidence was found that the HO cases processed through the courts subsequently had better driving records than did HO cases not processed.[118]

Opinions regarding traffic law enforcement range from arguments that it is an inherently hopeless practice to the equally untenable argument that if only the laws were strict enough, with enough police officers, and judges who gave stiff sentences, even the most recalcitrant scofflaws could be changed and crashes would decrease.

Laws themselves do appear to set basic patterns of behavior. Thus, while many people exceed the speed limit, most do so at less than 5 to 10 miles per hour.[119,120] In phase 3 nations, few people ignore stop lights, while ignored stop signs are passed at substantially lower rate of speed than if signs were absent. And in phase 1 areas fewer people ignore stop signals if a police officer is present.[57]

But what about the 10 or 15 percent of drivers who deviate substantially and often? For at least some of them it would appear that no matter how rigorously the laws are enforced, the message does not get through because they are marching to a different psychological or sociological drummer. Persons arrested for DWI are similar to other drivers in their assessment of the seriousness of other crimes, but differ substantially in feeling that alcohol-impaired driving is not a very serious offense.[121]

Even the largest police force cannot be everywhere all the time. Police officers are estimated to be able to identify and arrest only one of every 100 to 200 drivers with illegally high BACs who pass them.[122] Equally important is the wide variation in the intensity of enforcement by police departments of similar size because of attitudes by the officers or their superiors.[123]

This diversity has two aspects. First, the largest proportion of citations for moving violation is for speed. Beyond this, officers and departments develop specific patterns, with distinct preference for issuing certain types of citations but avoiding other types. But there may be little correlation between the types of unsafe driving acts (UDAs) most often involved in crashes and those most often cited.[124] In illustration, of five different UDAs, following too closely was the single most common one reported in crashes and the third most hazardous act (hazard being defined by crash risk per number of times done) but was virtually never cited by officers.

Speed was the least risky of the six UDAs but was the most frequent behavior cited by officers. Although this suggests a mismatch between enforcement attention to violations and their relative risk, part of the reason for the low risk of speeding comes from violations at lower speeds. When only high speeds (70 M.P.H.) were considered, this UDA was associated with very high risk of crashing.

Second, police enforcement behavior reflects a balance between the public's wish for safety and its willingness to be inconvenienced. As Streib notes, there is not *a* traffic law system in the United States but *many* systems, all nominally similar in functions, duties, and responsibilities.[125] At one extreme is the laissez-faire system, which seeks noninterference with driver activities, next the traffic flow-oriented system, third the safety-oriented system, and most stringent, the legalistic system. With respect to highway safety, laws regulating traffic can thus be considered either a limited success or a limited failure.

This estimate of the effect of laws applies as well to other nations. Scandinavian laws concerning driving after drinking seem to be an effective deterrent for social drinkers but not so for problem drinkers. Until recently most European nations have had no laws regulating speed, but such laws were introduced in several nations after 1973, and they appear to be accompanied by reduction in fatality rates.[126] The reduction in maximum speed in the United States at that time also was accompanied by a lower fatality rate, reflecting several factors (such as reduced mileage and effects of passenger restraints and other vehicular safety devices), but lower speed was one of the most important reasons.

A qualified solution to these dilemmas of enforcement exists in a study by Lawrence Ross of the effectiveness of legal countermeasures for alcohol safety.[127] People more often obey laws, he says, if they perceive a high likelihood of apprehension and conviction. Severity of the punishment is largely irrelevant. The deterrence comes mostly from perceived rate of punishment. Unfortunately, however, the results of successful programs are not long lasting.

How can *perceived* rate of apprehension be increased if there are so few police officers around? And how can conviction rates be improved? Regarding the second question, when punishment is Draconian, plea bargaining and other post-arrest adjustments occur that undermine police morale. As a result, police stop citing drivers for violations with poor conviction and punishment rates. And in response to this may come cries that the laws be made harsher yet.

The anguish is quite understandable. What is often needed, however, is a less harsh punishment coupled with simpler arrest or citation procedures. The police officer then feels surer that a citation, once issued, will probably lead to conviction and reasonable punishment.

It is difficult to be sure what will be acceptable to the community, but surveys of public opinion ask people only about their thoughts concerning specific punishment. To my knowledge, no one has ever linked questions about likelihood of apprehension and conviction with those about severity of punishment to determine what combination the public and the law enforcement personnel (who should be surveyed too) would find most acceptable.

Regarding public perception of risk of apprehension, there must be linkage of enforcement with public education efforts. Each reinforces the other. Ten criteria are relevant to changing behaviors that are likely to reduce morbidity and mortality from behavior-related injury.

1. The behavior to be changed must be a *primary and modifiable* cause of injury events, rather than being an effect of environmental pressures.
2. The effort must be aimed at a specific, easily understandable, and achievable behavioral change. Exhortations to "remain alert," to "be courteous," or to "avoid excessive speed for conditions" are vague admonitions that meet neither the criterion of primary cause nor that of specificity and achievability. Telling people to maintain maximum speed under 55 M.P.H. or to wear a helmet or seat belt meets both criteria.

3. Intermediaries, such as police, must be convinced that the effort is beneficial and must have necessary knowledge, skills, and resources to carry it out.
4. The target population must be at high risk of precipitating injury events because of the behavior to be changed. Most safety programs are diffuse and reach low-risk populations. On the other hand, data about anticrime programs suggest that they work best on populations that have no serious commitment to long-term deviant lifestyles. But if, as with alcohol abuse, a large part of the problem involves those with deviant lifestyles, standard approaches to education or motivation, even if aimed at the high-risk population, may have limited effect. Approaches tailored to the perceptions and motivations of the deviant segment may achieve greater success.
5. Preferably, the population to be reached is relatively circumscribed by size or geographic area for easy identification and monitoring. Laws aimed at small groups, such as manufacturers, are easier to implement than those aimed at the entire population.
6. The target population must sense that a safety problem really exists, that the behavior to be changed is a serious threat to safety, that they have a high risk of being penalized through sanctions if the behavior is not changed, and that the behavioral change is not a serious inconvenience and ego-threatening departure from usual behavior patterns.
7. The intermediary urging change must have high credibility with the target population, and that population must not have important conflicting influences, especially affecting economics or ego. In occupational safety, for example, management interest in safety is necessary for success but may be overwhelmed by the economic pressures of piecework contracts even though behavioral changes sought are clear, specific, circumscribed, and beneficial.
8. Behavioral change is easier to achieve if the behavior is subject to deliberation, rather than a spur of the moment act requiring quick judgment and decision (such as overtaking and passing in traffic).
9. True legal alternatives must exist to the proscribed behavior. Illegal parking, for example, may reflect poor city planning for legal parking, while driving at a hazardous but still legal BAC may reflect a governmental decision to license road houses that can be reached only by private motor vehicle.
10. Finally, sufficient time and intensity of program effort must be provided. Short-term efforts, such as "safety weeks," have little demonstrable effect, or result in evanescent changes that do not warrant the effort involved.[128]

Countermeasures against alcohol-impaired drivers cut across licensing, education, and road behavior enforcement efforts. The major efforts through the years to reduce alcohol crashes have had little documentable effect. These have been:

1. *Prohibition*. Crashes with alcohol were as common during Prohibition, and continue as common in areas that still proscribe alcohol, as in times and places where alcohol is permitted.[20] This pattern could conceivably differ, however, in Moslem or other nations with strong public support for religious and legal prohibition of alcohol use.
2. *Other laws that control circumstances of drinking*. Teenagers below the age of legal consumption consume alcohol in large amounts[24] and then drive. Raising the minimum legal age for alcohol consumption, however, may be associated with a decrease in alcohol-related fatalities in the newly excluded age group.[21] Changing the hours of service, type of drink permitted, or method of sales have little or no effect on alcohol crash rates.[20]
3. *Passage and implementation of laws imposing heavy fines or jail upon arrest and conviction for drunken driving*.[20] One reason why this has had only limited effect is that those most likely to get into trouble are problem drinkers, most of the social drinkers already being deterred both by the laws and their lack of need for heavy drinking.

Until about 1970 virtually no judge in the United States would refer a person arrested for DWI to undergo evaluation and treatment for a drinking problem except in the most blatant case of alcoholism. The Department of Transportation subsequently developed an Alcohol Safety Action Program (ASAP), a major component of which is the identification and rehabilitation of problem drinkers and alcoholics in highway crashes or arrested for DWI.

Although important questions have been raised about the evaluation methods used for this effort,[129,130] the fact is that for perhaps the first time evaluation was designed as an integral part of the ASAP projects. The absence of evaluation is one reason why it has been so difficult to learn from previous efforts. The results of ASAP projects suggest that:

1. Some of the education efforts have brought about modest changes in behavior;[131]
2. Law enforcement efforts have increased dramatically, but with mixed results;
3. Referral of people with documentable drinking problems to alcoholism treatment facilities has also increased many fold; and
4. Such referrals may have brought down the recidivism rates, but the poor quality of the evaluation research does not permit any firm

conclusion on this.[132] In keeping with the earlier observation by Ross, greatest effect appears likely to occur where arrest and conviction has been followed by actual suspension of driving privilege (seen as punishment) rather than just by referral to treatment in lieu of suspension.

Vehicular Countermeasures

Many vehicular changes that promote safety have occurred over the years: for example, improvement of vehicle suspension systems, replacement of the crank starter, and development of the windshield wiper. These changes, however, were carried out as much—or even more—for comfort and convenience as for safety. Improvement of doorlocks in response to the ACIR data in the 1950s represents an important and reasonably successful exception.

Beginning with ACIR, data about crash injury causation began to be gathered more methodically. It rapidly became apparent that there was substantial room for vehicular improvement, predominantly to reduce crash severity. It also became apparent that the automotive industry at that time was largely nonresponsive, opposing even the installation of inexpensive fittings so people could put seat belts in their cars: all this at a time when vehicular deaths were climbing.

This led to increasing frustration among segments of the U.S. public and the U.S. Congress. First came legislation requiring some safety components in automobiles purchased by the federal government, and finally the Highway Safety and Motor Vehicle Safety Acts of 1966. The latter of these acts affects automobiles manufactured throughout the world that are sold in the United States. The vehicular countermeasures emerging from this Act in some cases came as a result of well-documented problems, in other cases more because of a common-sense approach to needs and solutions.

Six types of vehicle countermeasure programs result from the Motor Vehicle Safety Act, and one other came as a result of the Highway Safety Act. These are:

1. A series of standards ("100" series) for vehicle and component construction was aimed at reducing the *frequency of crashes*.[133] These include the following for passenger cars (marked[a] if also applicable to trucks or buses and [b] if also applicable to trucks, buses, and motorcycles):

[a]101. Proper labeling and placement of vehicle controls for easy and correct access by drivers

[a]102. "Neutral" shift lever positions on automatic transmissions shall be between the "drive" and "reverse" positions
[a]103. Requirement for windshield defrosters and defoggers (front windshield only required)
[a]104. Requirement for windshield wiping and washing systems (front only)
[a]105. Requires improvements in braking system aimed at increasing performance and reducing likelihood of failure
[b]106. Establishes minimum standards for brake hoses and assemblies
[a]107. Reduces likelihood of visual glare in the driver's eyes from horn rim, windshield wipers, and so forth
[b]108. Improves lights, reflective devices, and signaling equipment
109. Requires greater performance for tires
110. Improves performance of tire rims
111. Sets minimum performance requirements for rearview mirrors
112. Reduces likelihood of malfunction for headlamp concealment devices
[a]113. Sets minimum standards for hood latch performance so hood won't fly open while vehicle is in motion.
114. Requires a key-locking system that will retard auto theft, reducing one important cause of serious crashes involving young males. Not all manufacturers have been equally ingenious in designing a key-locking system, and some cars remained relatively easy to steal.[35]
115. Requires each automobile to have a unique vehicle identification number (VIN) to promote ease of recall and for research and program evaluation.
[b]116. Sets minimum standards for hydraulic brake fluids.
117. Sets standards for retreaded tires.
118. Minimizes injury from use of power-operated windows.
[a]124. Reduces likelihood of accelerator sticking in open position.

2. A series of standards ("200" series) for vehicle and component construction was aimed at reducing *injury* in the crash phase.[133] Standards include:

201. Requirements for energy-attenuating design and construction of instrument panels, seat backs, sun visors, arm rests, and glove compartment doors
202. Requirements for head restraints to reduce neck injury in rear-end collisions
203. Requirements that steering columns yield forward in crashes, reducing chest injury to drivers

204. Limitation of rearward displacement of steering column in crashes, again to reduce chest injury to drivers
205. Improved glazing materials
206. Improved door locks and hinges to decrease ejection
207. Sets minimum standards for integrity of seating system in crashes
208. Requirements for active and passive restraining systems. At one point this included a starter interlock so that vehicles couldn't be started until the belts were buckled. This was repealed by Congress. For several years there was an extensive argument whether this standard should require installation of passive restraints such as airbags. In 1981, however, the Secretary of Transportation opted not to require passive restraints, preferring instead to carry out educational programs to promote voluntary use of restraint systems.
209. Sets minimum standards for seat belt webbing and hardware
210. Sets minimum standards for seat belt anchorages
212. Reduces likelihood of windshields popping out in crashes, thus ejecting occupants
213. Sets standards for child seating systems
214. Increases strength of side doors to resist deflection on impact
215. Reduces exterior damage to vehicle in low speed impacts. This standard is aimed at reducing property damage rather than injury
216. Sets roof standards to reduce collapse in rollovers
219. Aims at preventing intrusion of hoods and other external objects through the windshield in crashes

3. Standards ("300" series) were promulgated for vehicle construction to reduce severity attributable to *post crash* events,[133] as follows:

301. Sets standards for fuel system integrity to minimize fuel spillage and fire hazard in collisions
302. Sets burn resistance requirements for fabrics and other materials in vehicle compartments

How effective have these standards been in reducing crash frequency and severity? One study compared occupant fatality rates per 100,000 registered cars for three sets of vehicles: pre-1964 models, cars manufactured in 1964–67 that had seat belts and (in 1966–67) met some General Services Administration (GSA) safety requirements, and post-1967 cars that met standards listed above.[134] The post-1967 cars averaged 23 percent fewer occupant deaths per 100,000 registered cars yearly than did 1964–67 models and 39 percent less than pre-1964 models. The report also notes that the experience of these cars reflected their inherent qualities when new and cannot be attributed to their ages or to driver characteristics that may be associated with older cars.

Examination of specific standards has demonstrated effectiveness of the collapsible steering column (#203 and 204),[135] improved glazing (#205 and 212),[135] and head restraints (#202).[136] On the other hand, in critique of the "200" series, Huelke and O'Day have vigorously attacked the entire program because evaluation was not designed into it, most evaluation to date having been completed outside of DOT jurisdiction.[137] Their summary of what is known about the effectiveness of the "200" series is shown in table 9–10.

Personal experience in citizen advisory groups to the NHTSA leads me to substantial agreement with this criticism. At present, little is known about effectiveness of the "100" series, the "300" series, substantial components of the highway safety program, or of other aspects of the vehicle countermeasure program.

4. A program to monitor in-use performance of vehicles was established so that hazardous component failures can be identified and vehicles can be recalled for correction if other similar failures are likely. Recalls involving some 30 million vehicles had been initiated in the first ten years. The effectiveness of this program is totally unknown because DOT has no truly organized and consistent way of learning about failures and owner response to a recall often is low. Thus, many vehicles needing

Table 9–10
Summary of the State of Evaluation of Federal Motor Vehicle Safety Standards in the 200 Series as Assessed by Huelke and O'Day

Standard	*Title*	*Effectiveness*
201	Interior impacts	Insufficient data available
202	Head restraints	Partially effective
203–204	Steering control system	Partially effective
205	Glazing materials	Effective
206	Door locks	Partially effective
207	Seating systems	Insufficient data available
208	Passive restraints	Insufficient data available
209–210	Seat belt assemblies	Insufficient data available
211	Wheel nuts, hub caps	Insufficient data available
212	Windshield mounting	Insufficient data available
213	Child seating systems	Insufficient data available
214	Side door strength	Conflicting data
215	Exterior protection	Insufficient data available
216	Roof crush	Insufficient data available

Source: D.F. Huelke and J. O'Day, "The Federal Motor Vehicle Safety Standards: Recommendations for Increased Occupant Safety," *Proceedings of the 4th International Congress on Automotive Safety*, San Francisco, Calif., 14–16 July 1975 (Washington, D.C.: National Highway Traffic Safety Administration, U.S. Department of Transportation, 1975), 275–292.

inspection are never checked. Furthermore, DOT has never designed program evaluation into this activity.

5. A program of labeling and booklets was developed to inform the public about minimum performance standards for vehicles and components or about differences in performance between makes and models. The effectiveness of this program also is not known, but there is evidence that these materials often are not displayed as required in automobile showrooms and the public, therefore, is not even aware that they exist.

6. A highway safety standard initially required that each state establish a vehicle inspection program to ensure that vehicles in use are properly maintained. Such programs do not exist at all in many of the developing nations where, for reasons stated before, they would probably be most useful.

Critics find little correlation between low crash fatality rates and geographic areas that have compulsory inspection programs. The lack of such an association exists, they believe, because in most crashes it is the driver, not the vehicle, that is at fault and because many inspection stations have neither the proper equipment nor the necessary skills to undertake necessary repairs in a proper manner. They point also to corrupt inspection stations resulting both in unnecessary repairs at unnecessary cost to unsuspecting consumers (and possible danger, if done improperly) and in fraudulent sales of inspection stickers for cars that have not been inspected or have failed an inspection.

Advocates, however, observe that crash fatality rates are a function of several variables, one of the most important being the degree of rurality of a state. When these confounding variables are taken into consideration, inspection programs do appear to have benefit.

There is now strong evidence that vehicle populations that have periodic inspection are in substantially better mechanical condition than are populations without such inspections, that the greater the frequency of inspection the better the mechanical condition of vehicles, and the fewer the number of defects per rejected vehicle.[138] In one study, states with vehicle inspection programs had lower crash fatality rates than did states without periodic inspection. These differences held up even after a variety of potential intervening variables other than inspection were considered[139] and have been confirmed elsewhere as well.[140]

One program long overdue is certification and regulation of garage repair and service personnel to help ensure that they can meet minimum standards for mechanical knowledge and skill. Lobbying activity by the industry to be regulated has killed such proposals in the past.

7. Promotion of legislation has been carried out to require compulsory use of seat belts and shoulder harnesses. Although the Department of Transportation has gone on record as supporting such legislation

within the individual states, it has not acted forcefully to date on such support.

The issue of occupant restraints is an important one to highway safety. One of the earliest and most important findings of the ACIR analyses in the 1940s and 1950s was that ejection markedly increased the likelihood of severe injury or death in a crash.[86]

Two solutions seemed apparent and both were undertaken. One was improvement of door locks so that doors could not spring open as easily on impact. The other was the use of seatbelts, and by the mid-1950s lapbelts could be purchased if one knew how to install them. Lapbelts reduced serious injury and death by preventing ejection but were less successful in reducing minor injury because occupants could still strike the interior. For this purpose, a lapbelt/shoulder harness combination was required.[141]

A majority of people now know the benefits of passenger restraints, understand that alleged drawbacks—fire, submersion, pregnancy—in fact are not reasons to avoid use, and favor the use of such systems for safety. Unfortunately, despite repeated and extensive educational programs the proportion of vehicle occupants actually using restraints has never gotten very high except in vehicles that had an interlock that prevented the driver from starting the car until he or she buckled up. In recent years seat belt use has hovered around 10 to 15 percent in the United States because belts have been uncomfortable or inconvenient.[142] This pattern remains, despite evidence that wearing such of restraints reduces all injury about 25 percent, serious injury about 50 percent, and fatal injury approximately 65 percent (see figure 7–1).

Given this impass of "proper" knowledge and attitudes but "improper" behavior, one option was legislation to require use of restraints, and this has been passed in twenty-four nations as of 1981.[143] Compliance rates in some cases are 85 to 90 percent, accompanied by substantial reductions in fatalities (such as 27 percent in Australia),[144] but not to the extent anticipated, and use rates have often dropped after an initial surge.[145] Earlier studies were based on voluntary users who were probably less likely to drive at high speeds or to be heavy consumers of alcohol. Those least likely to use restraints despite a law probably include the alcohol abusers and speeders, two groups particularly associated with increased crash severity. An argument that when people wear restraints they feel safer and therefore are willing to take more risks has been shown to be incorrect.[146] In fact, persons who, despite a compulsory use law, remained nonusers were more likely to be risk takers than were users.

Except for infant restraints, however, the compulsory use approach has not been seriously accepted in the United States, and passive restraints, such as airbags, have been recommended instead. The airbag, when not in use, resides in the steering wheel, the dash board on the passenger's side, or the back of the front seat for rear passengers. If a threshold level of deceleration occurs, the bags automatically inflate and then deflate over a couple of hundred milliseconds. The interval is long enough to prevent collision with vehicle interior for most crashes, but short enough to permit the driver to retain control of the vehicle.

Critics complain that airbags are costly, not effective except in frontal collision, likely to "go off" at times when the vehicle is not in a crash, likely to harm young children, to be a hazard to service personnel, and to make people deaf. Few, if any, of these arguments really seem to hold up. Airbags are somewhat less effective across a range of crash situations than are lap/shoulder restraints, but this deficit is more than made up by the fact that they are always ready for use, whereas an unbuckled active restraint is not. In balance, active restraints and airbags seem to offer equal protection. Cost is an issue, with a set of bags adding up to $250 in 1976 dollars to the cost of an automobile.[147]

Unfortunately, in the absence of passive restraints, I see little further progress toward protection in the United States. The downsizing of vehicles threatens to add an additional 5 percent in fatalities by 1995 to the U.S. toll.[148] Compulsory seatbelt-use laws do not seem likely in the United States, and purely educational efforts appear to have hit a dead end, especially since current belt design precludes or fiendishly aggravates many would-be users.

Environmental Countermeasures

If properly carried out, environmental modification and maintenance can reduce both the frequency and severity of crashes. Particularly cost-effective has been the "spot improvement" program in which limited high-risk segments of highway are upgraded at relatively low cost, instead of building entire new roads. Quoting one review, "4.78 lives could be saved and 86.96 injuries could be avoided for each $1 million spent for highway safety improvement work. . . . The cost-effectiveness of the highway safety improvement work, in terms of lives saved, was shown to be about five times greater than that of regular highway construction work."[149] An evaluation of 381 safety projects in California showed a 31 percent reduction in fatal crashes, 8 percent reduction in injury crashes, and 14 percent fewer crashes involving property damage only.[150] Some examples involving crash frequency and severity appear in table 9–11.[150,151] Of particular value have been activities that remove roadside hazards such as nearby trees and rock outcroppings, that guide vehicles

Table 9–11
Effects of Changes in Highway Design on Crashes

Type of Project (N)	*Percentage Reduction All Crashes*[a]	*Percentage Reduction Fatalities*	*Percentage Reduction Injuries*	*Percentage Reduction Property Damage*	*Benefit/Cost Ratio*
Channelization					
(39)	28	25[b]	24	24	1.02
(13)	65				
(27)	30				
Guardrail					
(11)	24[b]	300[b]	0	0	1.35
(?)	40–60				
Pavement grooving or antiskid treatment (4)	62	100[b]	58	64	5.67
Flashing beacons					
(15)	56	200[b]	50[b]	57	2.27
(45)	20–80				
Safety lighting					
(6)	12	40[b]	7[b]	15	2.85
(41)	60 (night)				
New signals					
(8)	53	0[b]	75	35[b]	0.61
(94)	15				
Modified signals					
(27)	13	43[b]	25	7[b]	0.32
(18)	10				
New signals and lighting (15)	43	200[b]	48	37	0.53
Signals, lighting, and Channelization					
(12)	28	200[b]	14[b]	33	0.11
(46)	20				
(42)	35				
(13)	15				

Signing					
(22)	37	45[b]	32	41	5.60
(?)	20[b]–75				
Delineation					
(26)	24	70	23	23	5.88
(32)	2[b]–65				
Reconstruction					
(widening, etc.) (51)	20				
Miscellaneous (36)	13	73	11[b]	11[b]	1.57

Source: Adapted from "Annual Evaluation of California's Traffic Safety Program," *FAWA Notice* 1 February 1971 (Washington, D.C.: Federal Highway Administration, U.S. Department of Transportation); R.N. Smith and T.N. Tamburri, "Direct Costs of California State Highway Accidents," *Highway Research Record 225* (Washington, D.C.: Highway Research Board, 1968) 9–29.

[a]Studies with data on crash types and benefit/cost ratios are from source 1. Those with data on all crashes only are from source 2. Ranges of results in these latter studies reflect substudies of specific subcategories within project type (such as flashing beacons at intersections versus as advance warning).

[b]Results not significant at 10 percent level using chi square.

away from hazards that cannot be removed (for example, guardrails to guide cars away from bridge piers), or that convert obstacles causing high-energy impact into ones with lower energy transfer (such as break-away signs or lamp posts to replace ones of more rigid construction).

The simultaneous trend toward smaller automobiles and toward larger trucks and buses is a problem. Guardrail and other roadside furniture systems that only three or four years ago were quite adequate for most vehicles but were inappropriate for vehicles at both extremes of size are now causing trouble because those extremes represent much larger proportions of the total.[152]

Unfortunately, many guardrails and other safety devices are constructed so they spear vehicles or guide them into obstacles instead of away from them. Despite strong recommendations and written guidelines for widespread use of safer design and construction,[153] highway departments have implemented this program only grudgingly, in part because federal matching funds have not been as extensive for this activity as for building new roads.

Factors limiting implementation of safe highway design can be categorized into six areas as follows:[154]

1. scarcity of sound research findings;
2. highway department organizational patterns within a state;
3. lack of a statewide design manual;
4. lack of funds for safety because of competition from construction needs;
5. lack of communication among officials; and
6. lack of adequate training for engineering personnel.

In some phase 1 and 2 nations the road environment may be so inadequate that the most appropriate step may be to build new roads rather than to initiate spot improvements. A report from Israel, however, documents the benefits of spot improvement programs in developing countries also.[155] Such roads must include separation of different categories of road users and space for parked and disabled vehicles. As this is done attention can be turned as well to signing, signalization, removal of roadside booby traps, improvement of road geometry, and so forth. Another early step that is commonly overlooked in the phase 1 and 2 nations is the necessity for developing a good traffic records system that includes attention to the road environment as well as to other aspects of crash investigation.

Post-Crash Countermeasures

In order for post-crash countermeasures to be effective the following criteria must be met:

1. An organizational system must ensure that necessary police, fire, health care, and environmental protection services will be available to respond quickly and with appropriate resources to all geographic areas and at all times of day and night.
2. There must be capability for mobile communication between base hospital, fire station, and other headquarters and all rescue vehicles at the scene. Communication capability should also exist between these bases and regional centers, such as trauma centers.
3. Especially with the trend toward downsizing of vehicles, resources must be at hand to support rapid but careful extrication of occupants who have become trapped.
4. All personnel at the scene or enroute to the hospital must meet minimum training specifications. In the United States in recent years this usually means at least the EMT-A certification.[156] Operators handling the base communications system need similar training.
5. Personnel should work with agreed upon protocols both regarding patient care and concerning relationships among different groups of rescuers.
6. A system should be in place for periodic review of crashes responded to, and for refresher training, to identify and correct errors or problems in management and to ensure minimal decay in skills and knowledge. This is especially a problem in rural areas, where personnel may get insufficient experience.[157]
7. Ambulances should be specifically designed and constructed to have adequate working space[158] and should carry a designated set of equipment in good operating condition.[159] Some ambulances and base hospitals now have equipment exchange programs so that vital equipment, such as MAST trousers, can remain at the hospital with the patient and the ambulance crew can leave immediately with replacement equipment.
8. Hospitals should be well identified by directional signs placed at key locations on roads throughout the service area, and there should be easy access to the emergency department.
9. The emergency department should be staffed at all times of day and night by personnel specifically trained in resuscitation techniques, maintenance of airway and of blood volume, and stabilization proce-

dures.[160] In rural areas such personnel will often be nurses or physician's assistants. These personnel should be in contact—preferably by voice—with appropriate physicians if the hospital does not have physicians in the emergency department or in the hospital at all times.

10. Hospital staffs need appropriate protocols, designated equipment in good working condition, periodic review of cases, and refresher training.
11. Agreement should exist as to which hospitals have greatest capability for handling patients requiring specialized treatment. There also must be a system for ensuring that patients with these problems can be identified quickly and transported to the designated trauma centers either directly from the crash scene or after initial stabilization at a less fully equipped facility.
12. A disaster plan needs to be in place and to be tested periodically.

The United States has seen extensive concern and effort to deal with all of the above prehospital and in-hospital recommendations over the past fifteen years. There is now ample evidence that the national effort has paid off in more generally available emergency care of a quality far better than previously.

Preliminary evaluations of a hospital categorization system also suggest that these improvements are associated with lower case fatality rates among patients.[161] Unfortunately, because of problems in the design of the evaluation program it is not yet possible to determine whether the reductions are brought about by the program itself or by other possible intervening factors.

There can be little question that inadequacies of the prehospital and often the hospital phase of care exist widely in many of the phase 1 and 2 nations. Recent work in Egypt, however, suggests that these inadequacies can be overcome with substantial reductions in morbidity and mortality.[162]

10
Trucks, Buses, Recreational, and Emergency Vehicles

This chapter deals with several types of four-wheeled vehicles that have special uses and task demands. The largest group is trucks. The trucking industry in the United States provides 49 percent of total transportation for manufacturers and up to 95 percent of the transportation for some industries.[1] In phase 1 and 2 nations, trucks and buses may be the single most important motorized means of transportation for people, as well as for goods.

Conflicting patterns of growth seem to be occurring between places such as the United States and the phase 1 and 2 nations. In the latter, the early predominance of commercial vehicles is gradually replaced by larger proportions of automobiles. The United States, however, is now seeing a reverse pattern. Between 1970 and 1978, for example, there was a 3.4 percent annual growth in registered automobiles, twice that rate for trucks, but half that rate for commercial buses.[2] Also, associated with affluence, has been the rapid growth in registration of recreational vehicles (RVs) in the United States.

Definitions

While this chapter groups vehicles that to some degree share size, weight distribution, and operating characteristics, such grouping overlooks substantial dissimilarity, for example, between a pickup truck and an 80,000 lb eighteen-wheeler or between the almost continuous daily use of a "double bottom," the once-a-year vacation trip for a recreational vehicle, and the emergency trips of a fire truck.

According to Pierson, vehicles defined as trucks should be limited to commercial vehicles having more than four tires on the pavement, more than 10,000 lbs GVW (gross vehicular weight), and used for commerce.[3] The American Association of Motor Vehicle Administrators identifies three classes of vehicles (other than motorcycles) for purposes of licensing drivers.[4] These are:

Class C. Any single vehicle not in excess of 24,000 lbs GVW or any such vehicles towing a vehicle not in excess of 10,000 lbs GVW, except buses. This category would include as light trucks such vehicles as pickup trucks and vans weighing about 5,000 lbs, stake trucks weighing about 15,000 lbs, and van trucks weighing about 20,000 lbs. It would also include self-powered motor homes and campers, pickup campers, and vehicles pulling travel trailers, boat trailers, and some livestock trailers.

Class B. Any single vehicle weighing over 24,000 lbs GVW or any such vehicles towing a vehicle not in excess of 10,000 lbs GVW and any bus. This would include as intermediate trucks a 40,000 lb dump truck or other large unarticulated vehicle.

Class A. Any vehicle or combination of vehicles. All articulated or heavy trucks would be in this category, ranging from the 40,000 lb three-axle combination through a 70-80,000 lb five-axle combination to a "double bottom" combination of a tractor and two trailers that in some special cases might even exceed 100,000 lbs.

The Fatal Accident Reporting System (FARS), however, defines *light* trucks as pickup, van, and truck-based station wagon body types, *medium* trucks as single-unit trucks between 10,000 and 26,000 lbs and *heavy* trucks as vehicles that exceed this weight, whether or not they are articulated.[5] The various studies referred to in this chapter often do not make clear what definitions they use, although I sense that in general they use the FARS definitions.

Crash Experience

In 1980, according to FARS, there were 41,913 occupant fatalities in the United States.[5] Sixty-five percent of those were in passenger cars, 15.7 percent in light trucks, 0.7 percent in medium trucks, 2.3 percent in heavy trucks, and 0.1 percent in buses. Such fatalities in part reflect number of occupants per vehicle. Among all occupants of passenger cars in fatal crashes 4.1 percent died. By contrast, 20 percent each died among occupants of heavy and medium trucks, but 35 percent of those in fatal crashes involving light trucks.

Occupants of medium and heavy trucks in two-vehicle crashes are personally less at risk of death per crash, but those they hit are at much greater risk because of the discrepancy in weight. Parsons says that "in fatal collisions involving a large truck and a car 97% of the deaths are to car occupants,"[6] and Baker et al. have shown similar results in fatal collisions between cars and tractor-trailers.[7] In that study no truck occupant died unless in addition to striking the car there was another major impact. Since truck drivers spend most of their working hours on the road, Karlson and Baker have asked what is the risk of death per 100,000 workers for this occupation as compared to other occupations.[8] The derived risk of 65 fatalities per 100,000 is one of the highest occupational fatality rates in the United States. Table 10–1 shows relative crash and fatal crash involvement for several different vehicle categories[9,10,11] and table 10–2 examines fatality rates for reported crashes between cars and trucks.[12]

Of course, it has been pointed out—and correctly so—that trucks, and especially the largest ones, travel many more miles per year than do virtually all other vehicles except taxicabs (which have three times as many crashes and two times as many fatal crashes as expected based on their percentage of all registered vehicles).[10] However, at least in the United States, these same large trucks are driven by the most carefully selected and regulated drivers in the nation, and they do more of their mileage on freeways, which are the safest driving environment. Despite this, large trucks do have more crashes per unit miles. In Kenya, however, cars have 7.1 crashes per million kilometers compared to 3.1 for buses and 2.2 for trucks.[13]

Crash rates of trucks exceed those of other vehicles on all types of roads, including freeways,[14,15] and when heavy truck traffic reaches a level of 25 percent of the traffic volume on an expressway system, a 3 percent increase in truck traffic produces a 23 percent increase in crash frequency per mile.[16] Recreational vehicles, especially trailers, have much higher crash rates than do other vehicles on freeways.[17]

Large trucks are somewhat more likely than passenger cars to be involved in single-vehicle crashes and are also more prone to rollovers.[4,18] When trucks and cars do collide in *nonfatal* crashes, 60 percent of such crashes are rear-end contacts, 15 percent head-on, and 25 percent at an angle, as compared to 50 percent rear-end, 13 percent head-on, and 37 percent angle for car/car crashes.[18] The rear-end, head-on, and angle crash figures for *fatal* car/truck collisions are 28 percent, 38 percent, and 34 percent, respectively. In fatal car/car crashes only 13 percent are rear end, and 57 percent head-on.[18] Thus, rear-end crashes between trucks and cars are only slightly more common than between cars and cars overall but over twice as common for fatal crashes.

An analysis of school bus crashes showed 30 percent rear-end, 1 percent head-on, 14 percent side-swipe in opposite direction, 15 percent side-swipe in same direction, 25 percent angle crashes, and 14 percent single vehicle crashes, and 1 percent contact with pedestrian.[19] One study of 405 crashes involving car/trailer combinations showed 13 percent rear-

Table 10–1
Crash and Fatal Crash Experience of Large Vehicles

Type of Vehicle	*Fatal Crashes* Number	*Fatal Crashes* Percent	*In All Crashes* Number	*In All Crashes* Percent	*Percentage of Total Vehicle Registrations*	*Relative Fatal Involvement Per Unit Vehicles Compared to Car Involvement (set at 1.0)*
Truck or truck tractor	7,300	12.6	2,730,000	10.9	17.6	0.8
Truck and tractor semi-trailer	3,300	5.7	444,000	1.7	} 0.8	} 10.0
Other truck combinations[a]	900	1.6	230,000	0.9		
Commercial buses[a]	350	0.6	150,000	0.6	0.1	6.6
School buses[a]	160	0.3	43,000	0.2	0.3	1.1
Mobil homes[b]	?	?	?	?	3.6	>1.0
Car/trailer combinations[c]	?	?	?	?	?	4.0

Source: Adapted from (a) *Accident Facts, 1981 Edition* (Chicago, Ill.: National Safety Council, 1981); (b) R. Lindsey, "Risk Factor Cited in Mobil Homes," *New York Times*, 2 September 1973; (c) *Arizona Safety Sad-istics* (Phoenix, Ariz.: Arizona Department of Highways January/February 1973), 2.

Table 10–2
Fatality Rates in Car/Truck Crashes According to Truck Weight, 1973 and 1974

Truck Weight (in pounds)	*Number of Crashes*	*Number of Crashes in Which ≥1 Others Killed*	*Fatality Rate*
1– 5,000	200	4	0.020
5,001–10,000	551	15	0.027
10,001–15,000	958	57	0.059
15,001–20,000	905	36	0.040
20,001–25,000	1,875	142	0.076
25,001–30,000	2,667	250	0.094
30,001–35,000	1,087	89	0.082
35,001–40,000	803	79	0.098
40,001–45,000	811	78	0.096
45,001–50,000	769	76	0.099
50,001–55,000	888	88	0.099
55,001–60,000	1,042	109	0.105
60,001–65,000	1,257	117	0.093
65,001–70,000	2,190	212	0.097
70,001–75,000	3,124	360	0.115
Over 75,000	573	73	0.127

Source: T.N. Herzog, *Injury Rate as a Function of Truck Weights in Car-Truck Accidents* (Washington, D.C.: Office of Statistics and Analysis, National Highway Traffic Safety Administration, U.S. Department of Transportation Report DOT-HS-801-472 Technical Note N43-31-7, rev. 1976).

end collisions, 17 percent head-on, 13 percent side-swiping another vehicle going in the same direction, 4 percent right angle collisions, 45 percent single vehicle, and 8 percent other crash types.[20]

Human Factors

According to police reports only 3.8 percent of drivers in single-vehicle crashes of large trucks and 0.6 percent in other large truck crashes had been drinking.[4] Comparable figures for drivers of interstate trucks were 6.5 percent and 1.1 percent. However, tests for alcohol were administered in only 1 percent of these crashes.

In routine testing of fatal truck crashes 36 percent had alcohol.[21] A spot check of trucks entering Delhi, India, found one in every four drivers was impaired by alcohol.[22] Only anecdotal data are available, but in one study, 37 percent of long-haul drivers queried said they knew drivers who use pep pills occasionally and 23 percent knew several using them regularly.[23] What this means in terms of crash risk is not clear.

The role of aging and medical impairment in truck crashes is also unknown. Where personnel are carefully screened, illness-related crashes appear to be rare.[24] Also, elderly drivers are probably somewhat underrepresented among truck and bus drivers. About half of the states in the United States, however, require no special licensing or screening for drivers even of heavy or articulated vehicles,[25] a probable pattern in other nations as well. Furthermore, even where drivers are screened, some lie about conditions such as alcoholism or epilepsy or, as suggested by Owosina,[26] obtain licenses through bribes. The data about alcohol supports such suspicions, since 20 percent of the tractor trailer drivers in fatal crashes had BACs of 0.15 percent or higher.[21] Truck driving can cause medical impairment, such as deafness from noise and back trouble from vibration.

Recreational vehicles may require no special licensing and are particularly likely to be used by older individuals, including some with medical impairment and many with reduced vision. The roles of aging and of health problems in such crashes is unknown, however.

Fatigue is probably more of a problem among commercial drivers than among drivers in general. Owosina[26] points out that purchase agreements for taxis in Nigeria may involve such high interest rates that drivers are forced to take chances, including excessive speed, too many trips per day, and so forth. One hears similar problems regarding economics of truck operation in the United States.

What are the actual facts involving fatigue as a crash cause? One study collected performance and physiological data during 1,550 hours and 62,000 miles of truck and bus driving.[23] Some conclusions of the study follow:

1. Significant increases in performance errors and significant decreases in driver arousal occurred within the current DOT 10-hour limit on driving time. Differences appeared among drivers and different kinds of operations, but these effects began to appear by the fourth hour and increased throughout the rest of the trip except for some recovery as the driver approached the terminal under more arousing conditions.

   Crash frequency increased disproportionately after about seven hours of driving—equal to eight to nine hours of total duty time—and remained higher than expected per unit of exposure for all driving times above seven hours. Decrease in driver subjective feeling of well-being became more prominent after six to seven hours of driving.
2. The first rest break, after about three hours, usually produced physiological recovery and reduced driver errors. An increasing trend in driver errors, however, was not affected by the second rest break

at about six hours. A further decline in psychophysiological arousal followed a third rest break at nine hours for those drivers who took one. Sleeper drivers (who may be on the road from forty to 100 hours or more) recovered less from breaks. Bus drivers (whose runs usually were seven hours or less) did best.

3. A cumulative effect was noted on the drivers' level of psychophysiological arousal over several successive days on duty. Relay drivers who had more than four runs in a particular driving cycle without extended time off had an earlier decline in psychophysiological arousal and also a lower absolute level of arousal after only five hours of driving than did drivers with fewer runs. They also failed to show the typical "recovery" at the end of the trip that was shown by other drivers.
4. Adverse effects of prolonged driving were more pronounced for drivers age 45 or older, who generally showed an earlier decline, and dropped to a lower absolute level of arousal than did younger drivers. Older drivers had a larger proportion of their crashes after five hours on the road than did the younger drivers, although the absolute crash rate of younger drivers was higher.
5. There are marked diurnal variations in arousal level, with the lowest level occurring between about 2:00 A.M. and 7:00 A.M. Most drivers in this study had irregular schedules requiring them to drive frequently, not regularly, at these hours. For many whose runs ended at this time, the diurnal effect accentuated the fatigue effect. As a probable consequence, over 50 percent of crashes in which the driver was reported to be "sleepy or inattentive" occurred between midnight and 8:00 A.M.

Young drivers and those with fewer years of inexperience have higher crash rates, particularly with avoidable crashes than do older and more experienced drivers.[23] Among schoolbus drivers, those under age 17 have the highest rates and those over age 25 the lowest.[19]

Brown found that trainees who failed a bus-driving course had considerably less reserve capacity to simultaneously handle a primary and subsidiary task than did successful trainees.[27] Possibly young drivers with limited experience might also have less spare capacity. In Nigeria 18 percent of public transport drivers are under age 18.[26]

Inexperience may be an important issue with trailers and mobile homes.[10] In the United States most users of the 4.5 million recreational vehicles purchased them recently, use them infrequently and in unfamiliar terrain, or rent them. About 500,000 trailers are available for rent in the United States,[11] commonly to people with little or no previous experience.

Finally, let us consider deliberate violation of rules of the road. Since licensing is done by individual states in the United States, there is no single driving record for any truck driver engaged in interstate transport. Drivers often have multiple licenses.[25] For economic reasons drivers often overload their vehicles, and they exceed posted speed limits more often than do car drivers.

The implications seem clear. In low-speed areas (where over three-quarters of rigid and articulated heavy trucks exceed their posted speed limits) trucks are overrepresented in rear end collisions. "For vehicles in the traffic stream, trucks hit cars more frequently than cars hit trucks, which might indicate a truck braking problem. . . . In rear-end accidents in the [high speed] region, cars hit trucks more frequently than trucks hit cars, but the frequency of these accidents is small."[28] (Quoted with permission.)

In support of this conclusion, 64 percent of car drivers had no violation in collisions between large trucks and cars, whereas only 49 percent of the truck drivers were violation free.[4] The most common type of violation for the truck driver was a "safe movement violation" (17 percent) followed by speeding (10 percent). For these two violations and for following too closely and improper turns, the truck drivers exceeded the car drivers at least twofold.

Mention should again be made of the substantial overloading of trucks and buses for passenger transport in phase 1 and 2 nations. Jacobs and Sayer state that Kenya has a much higher proportion of casualties involving commercial vehicles than do European nations and that this might be due to the fact that such vehicles are used in Kenya to transport workers.[13] It is common, they note, to see open lorries carrying up to thirty men. Malik and Hakim refer to deaths of occupants who fall off such vehicles in Sudan.[29]

Vehicle Factors

Size per se contributes to crashes involving large vehicles. The longer the vehicle the greater the radius of curvature necessary for turns and the greater the distance required for passing.[30] Lengthening a truck-trailer combination from fifty to fifty-five feet requires at least a 27 percent increase in the radius of curvature for a 90° turn on twenty-four-foot wide pavements in order to prevent the truck from encroaching on opposing lanes of traffic. A five-foot increase in truck length also requires *under ideal conditions* a 282-foot increase in minimum passing sight distance.[30] Furthermore, the larger the vehicle the greater the requirement for articulation and the greater the likelihood of "jackknifing" whenever differential brake action or a weight shift occurs. However, Waller and Li[25] suggest that double-bottom (tractor double trailer) trucks might not have excessive crash experience.

The larger the vehicle the greater the aerodynamic turbulence it creates for smaller vehicles passing it,[31] and the longer the period that it will splash rain and mud onto the windshields of passing cars. Because large vehicles carry greater weight loads they move much more slowly on even small upgrades and have greater difficulty in stopping once in motion, with much greater likelihood of either skidding or jackknifing.

In thirty rear-end collisions between tractor-trailers and other vehicles, seventeen occurred on a grade and the tractor-trailer was the lead vehicle in seven of eight known collisions on upgrades.[7] Among the thirty-one rear-end collisions not on an upgrade, the tractor-trailer was the striking vehicle in twenty-three, or 74 percent. Almost two out of every three of the multivehicle crashes involved situations in which the tractor-trailer's braking ability may well have played a role. And yet, prior to Standard 121 to reduce stopping distance and prevent locking of wheels, a tractor-trailer's stopping distance was 350 feet from 60 M.P.H. compared to 250 feet in the worst performing passenger car.[32]

In rear-end collisions on the interstate system, vehicle types with the longest average stopping distance are also the vehicles with the highest rate of involvement in fatal crashes.[33] One study showed that, of 453 crashes involving one or more vehicles, more than three-fourths involved skidding, and loss of control occurred following application of the brakes in more than half of them.[33] When the tractor rides "bobtail," or without load, it may again be mismatched with its braking capacity, resulting in serious crashes.[7]

Instability is also a problem with larger vehicles. There may be sudden shifts of liquid loads as vehicles stop or turn, and these sometimes cause drivers to lose control, with disastrous results.[7] In other cases, portions of loads may be dropped onto the road or extend past the end of the trailer, creating a hazard for other users.[30] Live animals present a problem because of movement and noise.

Heavy commercial vehicles have four types of unintended responses to braking and steering.[34] These are (1) loss of control during braking, (2) directional instability during cornering, (3) roll instability, and (4) amplified directional motions occurring with full trailers. Erwin states that the dynamic maneuvering capabilities of heavy trucks limit both the options available to the truck driver in braking or in steering to avoid conflicts produced by other vehicles, and the tolerance available to compensate for any inattentiveness or misfunction by the truck driver himself.[34]

The threshold of roll instability is so low for loaded heavy trucks that rollover can easily occur in medium-stress maneuvers on paved surfaces. An example is a steady-turning maneuver of approximately 0.4g lateral acceleration, such as might occur if a problem came up while a tractor-trailer was negotiating a freeway exit ramp. The inability of tires to maintain traction adds greatly to the hazard of such maneuvers.[35]

Particularly unstable are campers placed on pickup trucks or automobiles pulling trailers. Despite heavy-duty additions, automobiles and pickup trucks have not been designed to carry this added weight, a situation that at least should have been foreseen by the truck manufacturers. Furthermore, there are dangerous dislocations in the center of gravity. Instability of the vehicle/trailer combination may have been a factor in 43 percent of 405 crashes involving towed trailers, often with more than one stability factor involved. In 20 percent the trailer overturned.[20]

The U.S. Army's M151 quarter-ton truck had 3,538 crashes, with 1,858 injuries and 104 deaths during 1967.[36] Designed for use over rough terrain—for which it is well suited—it nevertheless is widely used on highways, for which it isn't suited. The independent rear-wheel suspension makes it dangerous on such roads unless driven by a skilled driver. As a result, 36 percent of its crashes involved overturns without collision, compared to less than 2 percent for all vehicles in domestic crashes.

The best mirror systems currently on trucks are no better than the worst systems on passenger cars,[37] which as we observed in the last chapter is rather inadequate. About 30 percent or 900,000 of 2.7 million truck crashes in the United States annually are related to difficulties in rear vision, and over 500,000 of these could be prevented by improved systems.[37] McFarland and colleagues documented truck crashes because placement and design of gear shift controls, brake pedals, and so forth, did not permit the driver to maneuver the vehicle as quickly and easily as road conditions required.[38]

Component malfunction because of aging and other reasons is the last vehicle area to be discussed. Larger vehicles log many times more miles annually than do passenger cars. Manufacturers of large trucks commonly produce "glider kits," which permit a truck to be "rebuilt" with new axles, engine, drive train, and/or cab while retaining the original chassis. Depending on the extent of component replacement, new safety standards can thus be avoided.[32]

School buses purchased by financially hard-pressed educational institutions may be kept for many years with only minimal maintenance. After that, they may be sold to church groups for even more tenuous service with untrained drivers operating decrepit equipment. Such equipment is common in many developing countries.

And yet, as we observed before, data about mechanical failures and other problems are difficult to get because of the inadequacies of crash investigation. As minimum estimates, in North Carolina[4] vehicle defects were reported in 8 percent of crashes of large trucks, 11 percent among intermediate-size trucks, and 5 percent for small trucks, with failures from two to four times as often for single-vehicle crashes. Brake problems comprised over half of the failures for large and intermediate-size trucks.

The distribution of defects in Texas according to type of truck appears in table 10–3.[18] Tire failures account for almost 5 percent of truck crashes on turnpikes and 1 percent of all truck crashes in Texas, and less than 1 percent of truck crashes in several other data sets. Less than one in every 1,000 to 2,000 tire failures results in crash.[39]

Vehicle defects were reported in 2.4 percent of school bus crashes, usually involving brake failure.[19] Fifty (12.5 percent) of 405 crashes involving car/trailer combinations occurred because of mechanical failures (tire failure 9, coupling failures 13, wheel, axle, or suspension failures 10, and brake defects 8.)[20] Coupling failures were reported in 20 percent of trailer crashes.[11]

Environmental Factors

It would appear that many crashes occur because of a discrepancy between the size and operational dynamics of heavy trucks and the capability of roads that are available. Some states in the United States

Table 10–3
Proportions of Vehicles Found Defective by Investigating Police Officer in Crashes According to Vehicle Type

Type of Vehicle	*Percentage Defective*
Passenger cars	1.5
Pickup trucks	2.2
Panel trucks	2.4
Average of 12 heavy trucks	6.7
Bobtail	4.8
Dump	8.0
Fire	2.1
Flatbed	7.6
Float	9.2
Transit-mix	7.8
Pole (log)	14.1
Refrigerator	6.8
Stake	7.3
Tank	5.9
Vans	5.5
Wreckers	7.1

Source: J. O'Day and R.E. Scott, "An Analysis of Truck Accident Involvement," *HIT Lab Reports* 4(8) (April 1974):1–16 (Ann Arbor, Mich.: Highway Safety Research Institute, University of Michigan). Reprinted with permission.

currently permit unarticulated trucks as long as fifty-five feet, and under special circumstances articulated trucks as much as 108 ft long, 108 in wide, 14 ft high, and 129,000 lbs gross weight may be permitted.[40] (In most cases the maximums are respectively 40 ft, 65 ft, 96 in, 13 ft 6 inches, and 80,000 lbs). Brown states that a 65 ft double-bottom truck represents a serious mismatch of vehicle and highway design. The total truck length determines the necessary radius of curvature for negotiating highway curves, and only the latest highways have been designed to accommodate units as long as 55 ft.[41]

Greater sighting distance, not commonly available on many roads, is required for other traffic to pass longer trucks. And Brown says that one heavy truck driving over a high-grade pavement does as much pavement damage as do 6,000 passenger automobiles. If this is correct, the operation of heavy trucks (and larger buses) on roads creates an environmental hazard not only for trucks but for all other vehicles as well.

One study concluded that "based upon limited research and operating experience available, there appears to be no evidence that increased sizes and weights will result in increased commercial vehicle accident involvement."[42] This study, however, had several serious limitations. As one critic noted, the data "suggest that the statement . . . that all is well appears to be a very premature one in light of some of the very limited but nevertheless disquieting data about what happens to large trucks on the nonfederal aid system."[43]

Because of the limited braking capacity, large trucks often outdrive their visual capabilities, especially in inclement weather. Cassidy has reported an overrepresentation of fatal crashes involving heavy trucks during such weather, but this may simply reflect the fact that trucks often travel regardless of weather conditions in order to meet delivery schedules.[25]

Referring to other types of vehicles, it was hypothesized that very young school bus drivers, being less experienced, would experience difficulty more readily in less than optimal driving conditions.[19] Analyses of crash data support this hypothesis, since sixteen-year-old drivers tend to have more crashes on loose surface roads, roads with defects, and roads that are not straight and level. Crashes of car/trailer combinations and campers commonly occur under conditions of heavy cross winds, which accentuate the instability of these vehicles.[10,20]

In Nigeria, Owasina comments about one-lane earth roads that force heavy vehicles to brush against each other on passing or to skid off the road.[26] Data do not exist on the frequency of interaction of human, vehicular, and environmental factors in crashes of these large vehicles in phase 1 and 2 nations, but it is clear that the three are so closely intertwined that anyone who considers only one is deluding himself.

The Energy Transfer Phase

A large truck in a crash at freeway speeds may have the inertial equivalent of a 4,000 lb vehicle traveling at 250 miles per hour. Little wonder then that fatalities in other vehicles that collide with trucks so vastly outnumber the truck occupant fatalities.

Truck design that permits automobile underride adds markedly to the severity of crashes because tops of cars that crash into the sides or rears of trucks commonly are crushed or ripped open.[44] The trucking industry has opposed a design standard to prevent such occurrences.

Truck drivers in single-vehicle crashes fare no better than do drivers of other vehicles.[4] Contrary to common opinion, development of the cab-over-engine tractor was not to give the driver more sighting distance, but to increase payload (that is, trailer) length by reducing the tractor length, while remaining within the forty- or fifty-five-foot total legal length. As a result, the crashworthiness of tractors has decreased since extra distance between the driver and the front bumper are now gone.[32] And, as noted in the last chapter, with increasing truck size, standard guardrails and similar protective roadside furniture are now less suitable for large vehicles.[45]

Crash-attenuation design of buses, trailers, campers, and motor homes is almost nonexistent.[10,46] All these vehicles have little resistance to buckling or crush when they roll over: which they commonly do. Objects or occupants can be tossed around freely because there is inadequate tie-down in trailers and motor homes and low seat backs in buses, which permit occupants to catapult. In buses, seats tear loose on impact. Seats also are lethal because occupants hit bare metal pipes with no cushioning. In fact, after one fatal bus crash involving extensive crush the National Transportation Safety Board accused the Department of Transportation of using such crashes, instead of vehicles with instrumented dummies, for its safety research program.

Post-Crash Phase

Extrication is a problem in crashes of large vehicles because of rollover, crush resulting from override of cars by trucks, and unreinforced construction of buses and recreational vehicles.[3,46] Fire is often a problem in crashes of large trucks because of greater forces involved, exposed fuel tanks, rollover, and carrying of high-energy fuels or other flammable cargoes. The trucker often has little control over cargo packaging and may not know what the contents are or how to deal with spills. Each year sees truck crashes involving leakage of noxious gases, spillage of pesticides or, in some cases, massive explosions.

Countermeasures

Clearly, there is ample reason to be concerned about the contribution of large vehicles to the highway toll throughout the world and considerable room for improvement regarding operation, vehicle design characteristics for crash prevention and attenuation, and environmental steps for prevention and crash attenuation.

Who should drive and how should they be licensed and followed? Currently, in the United States no standard pattern exists outside of the relatively small proportion of vehicles and their drivers in interstate commerce, which are regulated to some extent by the Federal Bureau of Motor Carrier Safety (BMCS). In nine states, for example, the minimum permissible age for driving a school bus is 16, in five others 17, and in twelve additional states it is 18. There is no maximum age requirement in thirty-five states.[46]

The following countermeasures would seem appropriate for most nations:

1. For vehicles above 10,000 lbs in size, or articulated combinations, special licensure should be required, with demonstration of sufficient general driving experience plus specific knowledge and skills, with an on-road skill test involving a vehicle of the size and type for which the person is to be licensed. These requirements should apply as well to operation of recreational vehicles.
2. In the United States there should either be a single federal license or sufficient cooperation among states so that a driver meets similar standards throughout the nation and has a single identifiable driver's record throughout the nation.[25]
3. The higher the class of vehicle being driven the more stringent should the health requirements be for operation. The rationale is that:

    a. The consecutive hours of operation and loading or unloading duties for commercial drivers may exacerbate health problems such as diabetes or heart disease.
    b. The greater total mileage logged by these drivers, and in vehicles with larger potential for lethality because of weight and instability, means that this exposes other road users to hazards far more than does the average driver of a passenger car.

c. Many unregulated trucks carry hazardous materials, while all buses carry large numbers of passengers.

4. The ten-hour stretch for long-haul drivers currently permitted by the BMCS creates a hazard both to the driver and to the public. This should be reduced to no more than eight hours, and perhaps even less, and enforced with an appropriate logging system.

Regarding the vehicle itself, at least ten countermeasures are possible that deal with the pre-crash phase, as follows:

1. As Gustafson suggests, work could "improve speed maintainability of trucks to reduce disparate speed differences between trucks and cars on upgrades" because speed differential leads to increased risk of crash.[32]
2. He also recommends uniform national weight and size limits commensurate with safety, specifically omitting the tractor from overall length limits. Establishment of limits commensurate with safety potential of existing roads is extremely important in all nations.
3. Integrated with the above must be improvement of brakes. Until the mid-1970s there was no requirement that certain trucks have brakes on more than two wheels. DOT standard 121 was adopted requiring antilocking brakes, but technical problems prevented successful application of this standard, and it was withdrawn.[47] Improvement of braking systems to prevent lockups, skidding, and jackknifing still represents one of the more important possible pre-crash countermeasures. In 1974 the U.S. trucking industry had supported its request for increased federal weight allowance by arguing that MVSS 121 permitted heavier weights of vehicles to function safely. Subsequently, however, the industry asked that the standard be amended, delayed, or abandoned.[48] The net result has been a greater discrepancy between maximum truck weight and braking capacity.
4. Work is needed to reduce instability of large vehicles by reducing sway in suspension systems, by lowering center of gravity, and by altering loading and tie-down processes. Relatively inexpensive solutions may exist to the sway problem,[49,50] and better compartmentalization of liquid loads could reduce the problem of surging of fluids during cornering maneuvers. Labeling of camper tops to indicate maximum safe combinations for trucks and campers (now required under U.S. Motor Vehicle Standard 126) may help reduce discrepancies between height and weight of camper and truck brake and suspension capability.
5. Part of the solution for overloading trucks or buses with passengers comes from sufficient availability of public transportation and en-

forcement of laws to prevent overloading. But, particularly with buses in phase 1 and 2 nations, part of the problem of people hanging onto the outside of vehicles probably also results from vehicle design that gives people places to hang onto.

6. Turning to visibility, the sides of large trucks are not well illuminated so that other vehicles crash into them while the trucks are in the process of backing into driveways or loading areas. Although not frequent, these crashes are severe because of car underride and are unnecessary because the corrective technology is available and the costs are low.
7. The truck driver is unable to see adequately to the sides and rear of most large vehicles, and there is substantial room for improvement. At least one existing commercial system indicates technological feasibility, and standards should be required in this area.[51]
8. Improvement also appears feasible and warranted in the hitching mechanism for recreational vehicles to reduce frequency of failures.
9. Motor Vehicle Standard 119 specifies performance and labeling requirements for new pneumatic tires designed for highway use on multipurpose passenger vehicles, trucks, buses, trailers, and motorcycles. It also requires tread-wear indicators in tires to reduce likelihood of tire failure because of excessive wear. Rim-matching information is also required concerning these tires.
10. It is necessary to prevent vehicular failures. Especially in phase 1 and 2 nations adequate systems for periodic motor vehicle inspection and/or enforcing correction of any defects found must have high priority among possible countermeasures in the pre-crash phase.
11. One unique problem for school buses is that while waiting for students in winter, vehicles may line up with the nose of one bus near the exhaust of the one in front. If motors are kept running for warmth, all except the first bus may suck in high levels of carbon monoxide.[52]

Some roads present problems only in certain weather, such as fog or sandstorms. In these areas, warning systems can be installed to prohibit larger or less manageable vehicles at such times. Separation of larger vehicles from other traffic is sometimes essential and feasible. In one phase 1 nation bridges are often so narrow that when two trucks try to pass each other pedestrians are forced to jump into the water and sometimes drown.

One component of roadway design particularly successful in preventing crashes is the runaway truck escape ramp.[53] At downgrades large vehicles sometimes slip gear in down-shifting, lose their brakes, or otherwise lose control, with disastrous results. Escape ramps that remove the runaway vehicle from the traffic stream and that bring it to a safe and gentle stop have cut down markedly on the slaughter.

The following countermeasures are appropriate in the crash and post-crash phases.

1. It is both feasible and not unduly expensive, either initially or through retrofit, to prevent underriding by smaller vehicles in car/truck crashes. A barrier can be installed along the vulnerable portions of the truck.[44] Industry objections to this countermeasure appear to be substantially self-serving and to totally ignore responsibility to the public interest.
2. Countermeasures to reduce jackknifing and rollover also decrease the severity of truck and bus crashes, being particularly helpful to occupants of the truck or bus itself. Attention also must be paid to improved escape from these vehicles.
3. Relatively few of the 200 and 300 series motor vehicle safety standards required for automobiles have been applied to larger vehicles. As a result, not only are larger vehicles more likely to roll over, but when they do so, they are much more likely to have devastating and unnecessary crush and to have contents thrown about within the vehicles. One exception has been MVSS 217, which sets minimum standards for retention and release of most bus windows to reduce passenger ejection in crashes and to enhance passenger exit in emergencies. Also an exception are standards applicable to school buses that strengthen the shell against crushing, increase the height and strength of seats, provide anchorage for seatbelts, and improve upon the padding of seats. In my opinion, they are a sufficient response to a very small aspect of the highway safety problem since, among the 20 million children carried to and from school each day, few are injured each year, and about 100 are killed, mostly as pedestrians near buses.
4. Capability of fuel tanks and truck vans to rupture and to release either flammable or toxic materials must be limited through cellular fuel tanks that reduce leakage and double walls for compartments containing hazardous materials.[54]
5. Appropriate evacuation, cleanup, and disaster plans need to be in place in all communities where particularly hazardous crashes could occur, to prevent or to deal with large numbers of injuries. Placarding or external warning is essential on trucks carrying hazardous materials. But in one study, 41 percent of vehicles requiring placarding were in violation of the law, limiting its effect.[55] In phase 1 and 2 countries there often seems to be an inverse relationship between the number of people jammed into stake trucks or other vehicles not

meant for passenger transport and the adequacy of plans and facilities for dealing with the consequent disasters.

Recommendations such as these are likely to be countered with the argument that they will adversely affect the contribution of trucking to the economic health of nations. In the United States, the industry contributes a third of state road-use taxes. There is reason to believe, however, that the importance of that contribution has been overestimated.

Trucks are the most costly in terms of lives lost of all freight modes, four times more costly than railroads, the next highest on the list.[32] Furthermore, according to Brown, a pavement that requires replacement after ten million 2,000 lb axle loads would have to be replaced after only five 18,000 lb single-axle or 32,000 lb tandem-axle loadings.[56] For the pavement to withstand ten million typical truck loadings one must quadruple the thickness index (combination of subbase, base, and surfacing) needed for 1,000 lb axle loads. If truck mileage is calculated based on damage potential, heavy trucks should pay $11.46/mile in road-use taxes instead of 7.35¢/mile. A thirty-ton truck thus is being subsidized at a rate of 4.6¢/ton mile.

Currently, according to one source, one-quarter of the road-use taxes that each and every driver in the United States pays go to subsidize the trucking industry.[30] If these figures are correct, there is good reason to make demands for greater industry contribution to highway safety.

Emergency Vehicles

Emergency vehicles are used in ways or under circumstances that place the driver and the vehicle under considerable stress. About 36,500 emergency vehicles were involved in crashes in the United States in 1974, of which 200 were fatal crashes with 950 fatalities.[57] Police vehicles overall averaged 18.86 crashes per million miles during 1972–74, as compared to 7.49 for passenger cars.[57] There were wide differences in rate, however, among police vehicles, as follows: municipal patrol cars 5.63, two-wheel motorcycles 37.14, and three-wheel motorcycles 32.51.

Among almost 12,000 truck crashes in Texas, 143 involved fire trucks, with a fatality rate of 4.2 per 100 crashes (in every case the fatality was in the other vehicle struck).[18] This was a higher fatality rate than for most other trucks. The injury rate was 49.7 per 100 crashes, twice that of other truck types, with a slight majority (27.32 versus 22.38) occurring in the other vehicle.

In a study of 61 percent of total ambulance travel in Denmark, emergency runs were less than 4 percent of total distance.[58] The crash rate was 5.3/million kilometers during emergency driving and 0.4 in ordinary driving, with injury rates of 8.9 and 0.7/million km, respectively. In one year 61 persons were injured in 41 crashes. The severity of 17 injuries on emergency runs was 8 light, 9 serious, 0 fatal. On ordinary runs 9 injuries were light, 23 serious, and 4 fatal, for a total of 41. Among those injured during emergency runs 8 were ambulance personnel, 1 passenger, and 8 other parties. No patients were injured. Of 10 emergency crashes, 6 involved intersections (5 with stop lights), 2 other vehicles not giving way, and 2 loss of control on slippery roads (in one case while overtaking another vehicle).

In a two-year period in New York State 617 ambulance crashes occurred, killing 7 and injuring 750.[59] Fifty-one percent occurred at intersections and in about half of those (25 percent of total) the ambulance was going against a stop signal.

Causal Factors

Four related human factors are relevant in most crashes: training, judgment, difficulty in hearing or locating the siren, and the nature of local laws and ordinances. Most personnel driving emergency vehicles have not received formal behind-the-wheel training in how to deal with the special driving tasks involved. Consequently, many do not know how to approach an intersection, under what circumstances or how they should engage in high-speed chase, what constitutes a real medical emergency, how to avoid skidding, or how to drive effectively while in a skid.

Only 2 or 3 percent of all ambulance runs require high speed, a figure rather close to the experience of the Danish ambulances. As noted above, 152 (25 percent) of the New York crashes involved an ambulance going against a traffic signal.[59] In 71 of these the driver of the other vehicle said he or she didn't see or hear the ambulance. Contrary to what the general public and many drivers of emergency vehicles believe, a rapidly moving ambulance or police car may almost outrun the noise of its own siren.

In illustration, on one occasion I observed a police car coming behind me with its light flashing and a closing rate of between 10 to 15 M.P.H. (16 to 24 K.P.H.). Not until the cruiser was within two car lengths could I first hear the siren and, by the time it was two car lengths past, the siren could no longer be heard. And most of the time people cannot correctly identify the location of the siren unless they also have visual cues.

Laws governing emergency vehicle operation may affect crash rate. There was a 70 percent decrease in the number of crashes of ambulances in New York City after sirens were removed and drivers were given orders to obey normal traffic regulations.[60] In many communities there is such a diversity of lights and warning equipment on cars of volunteer fire or ambulance personnel that other road users may get confusing and in some cases hazardous cues.

Of the 617 New York crashes, 167 involved excessive speed by the ambulance, 30 head-on collisions, usually in attempted passing, and 35 collisions with pedestrians.[59] Two ambulance drivers among the 617 were cited for driving while under the influence of alcohol!

Apparently in many cases formal arrangements have been made for periodic maintenance and repair of emergency vehicles, which are often under governmental jurisdiction or ownership. Thus, despite higher and stressful usage, vehicle failure would not be anticipated as a common problem. In the fire truck study[18] 2.1 percent of crashes involved identified defects, compared to 6.7 percent for twelve different types of trucks.

Police vehicles have been subject to recalls because of design hazards. One involved failure of lower control arms on Fords, making wheels suddenly fall out of place. One police department had six such failures among 116 vehicles.[61] Although Ford repaired 85,000 police cruisers NHTSA ruled that no defect existed, a decision not supported by the data.[62] Chrysler vehicles had leaking power steering hoses, with 13 failures in one fleet of 400 police vehicles.[63] Again, recall was made for police vehicles only.

In a third case carbon monoxide seeped from excessively short tailpipes that did not clear car bumpers, thus permitting exhaust fumes to accumulate under vehicles, especially if—as is common police practice—they stand still for a long time with motor running.[64] The problem was not specific to police vehicles but generic to all similar vehicles of the same manufacturer.[65]

Problems generic to fire trucks and ambulances contribute both to the pre-crash and crash phase and involve obvious tradeoffs in order to make quicker and easier the tasks of fighting fires or caring for patients en route to the hospital. Squads commonly hold on to the outside of fire trucks. Unless strapped on they may fall off, and they are unprotected in crashes. This is one explanation for the large number of injuries per crash in the fire truck study noted earlier, although the number of occupants per fire truck is higher than for other trucks.

Current modular or van type ambulances have a high center of gravity. This provides more headroom for patient care but promotes loss of control and rollover. Also, equipment may break loose in crashes.

All of the environmental problems noted previously apply to emergency operation, in particular intersections with blocked vision, winding roads, and roads that do not permit safe and easy passing.

Countermeasures

Improved training and operating rules, uniform traffic rules, better vehicle design and improved control of intersections appear to be relevant measures to reduce the toll of crashes under emergency conditions. All persons doing emergency driving should be required to have special training in criteria for and methods of emergency operation, and a review mechanism should ensure that these are being properly applied. This is especially needed for volunteer personnel, who may lack sufficient experience to maintain skills.

Police departments must have specific written protocols for high-speed chase. Two-way communication systems—and adequate training in their use—together with well-trained dispatchers can reduce the need for high-speed operation by bringing in additional help for police officers, by identifying in advance whether a call for medical help really is an emergency, and by providing medical advice for ambulances that are en route to the hospital with patients.

All emergency vehicles should be required to follow rules of the road for vehicles of this type, such as spelled out in the Uniform Vehicle Code. Fewer than half of states currently comply. Light and siren systems should be standardized, especially for private vehicles owned by volunteer squads. Current modular ambulances represent substantial improvement upon earlier designs in room for patient care. But the van body needs strengthening to minimize crush in rollovers.

Finally, one method of dealing with emergency vehicles in urban areas is to use preemptive traffic control devices that automatically give emergency vehicles right of way. According to Lewis,[66]

> Several cities have purchased and installed these systems with mixed results. In some instances the fire or police had the capability but not both departments. Commercial ambulances were not so equipped and, therefore, did not have the purported advantages offered by the gear. The cost of these systems is roughly $5–10,000 per intersection. A city of 50,000 inhabitants could easily require the instrumentation of 200 intersections for complete coverage . . . and, obviously, a minimum number of intersections must receive the installation before a recognizably favorable effect can be achieved. If one assumes that emergencies, irrespective of type, are distributed equally in any section of the city, then it follows that a large number of instrumented intersections are

required. Hospitals are notoriously poorly distributed and, geographically, represent the final destination of ambulances. In the "ambulance only" application, therefore, a relatively large number of intersections must be outfitted. If the community is served by commercial private ambulance firms, the question of who pays for equipment installed on the vehicle arises. The maintenance costs associated with these systems are reportedly high.

Reports on the use of these devices describe "clumping" of traffic along the intended path of the emergency vehicle. This phenomenon occurs even without the pre-emptive devices, as motorists try to pull to the right and stop, particularly on four or six lane streets. Problems also arise at complex intersections and traffic circles . . . There is frequently a need to drive on the wrong side of the street to clear halted vehicles. . . .

From a strictly ambulance safety benefit point of view, their use is not feasible on a sufficient scale; nor have they been proven effective.

11
Motorcycles, Mopeds, Scooters, and Minibikes

The motorcycle is generically as old as the automobile, having been invented by Dailmer in 1885.[1] By 1941 the unique hazards of this transportation and the potential protective value of helmets were already being documented.[2]

A motorcycle is a two-wheeled vehicle with a 50 to 1,000 cc motor. The rider sits between the two wheels. A moped has a motor smaller than 50 cc and a heavier frame than a bicycle. (It is sometimes erroneously called a motorized bicycle to avoid motorcycle vehicle and use standards. A real motorized bicycle has a much lighter frame.) A scooter has a shield on the front, and the rider sits atop the rear wheel, as if on a stool. A minibike is a smaller version of a motorcycle designed for recreational use by children.

In 1954 there were almost 1.1 million motorcycles in Great Britain, nearly one-fifth of motorized traffic.[3] In that year there were only 405,000 motorcycles in the United States, and the major growth pattern there began in the 1960s.[4] The pattern in Britain was similar to that of several other European nations. Around 1959, when seven European nations had a total of 17 million machines, the population per motorcycle ranged from 9 to 15 for the other nations but was still only 19 for Britain.[5]

Mopeds did not begin to increase in popularity until after World War II. They have now exceeded motorcycles—but not bicycles—as a form of transportation in several European nations (table 11–1).[6] In the United States there are now about 4 million motorcycles (about 17/100 inhabitants) and an estimated 500,000 mopeds (about 5/1,000) as of 1978.[6] Mopeds are also immensely popular in the Far East, India, and the Caribbean, with a worldwide total of about 30 million.[6]

Throughout most of the world these vehicles are used as transportation throughout the year, especially for less affluent individuals, such as students. In the United States, however, they are used largely for recreation,[6] with most use, especially in northern climates, being during warmer months.[7,8]

Table 11–1
Number of Bicycles, Mopeds, Motorcycles, and Automobiles Per 1,000 Inhabitants for Several Nations, 1973–75

Country	*Bicycle*	*Moped*	*Motorcycle*	*Automobile*
Austria	—	63	11	209
Belgium	296	45	9	242
Canada	—	—	—	353
Denmark	590	89	8	249
Finland	522	47	10	200
France	218	112	7	280
Germany (Federal Republic)	419	20	4	275
Italy	214	51	21	247
Ireland	—	—	—	161
Japan	382	71	7	145
Netherlands	550	130	4	240
Spain	—	—	34	109
Sweden	491	50	4	308
United Kingdom	202	8	12	248
United States	—	—	—	482

Source: W. Hunter and J.C. Stutts, *An Analysis of Mopeds as a Potential Safety Problem in the United States, vol. 1, Review of the Literature and Data Search. Final Report* (Chapel Hill, N.C.: Highway Safety Research Center, University of North Carolina, Report DOT-HS-805-035, 1979). Reprinted with permission.

Injury and Fatality Patterns

Two-wheeled motorized vehicles have much higher injury and fatality rates than do automobiles per unit registered vehicles and per unit miles or kilometers traveled. Less data are available about relative crash involvement, whether or not injury occurs. Information from Finland (table 11–2)[6] suggests that motorcycles, but not mopeds, have higher crash rates than passenger cars. But the data are not controlled for type of exposure, such as traffic density or occupants per vehicle. In a London study, where traffic density was probably more evenly distributed, casualties (not overall crash risk) per 100 million kilometers were 49 for drivers of cars and taxis, 42 for drivers of other four-wheeled vehicles, 1,391 for motorcyclists and their passengers, 1,323 for scooter riders, 615 for moped riders, and 539 for pedal cyclists.

Hunter and Stutts have conservatively calculated that the actual rate of crashes or falls involving mopeds is about 3.5/10,000 miles while the reported crash rate is 1.0 and the "near miss" rate is 43.[8] The reported crash rates of mopeds, according to their estimate, is 27 times higher than the rate for all vehicles.

Two-wheeled vehicle crashes almost never involve property damage only. Hurt's monumental study of 900 motorcycle crashes found only 12

Table 11–2
Vehicles Involved Per 100 Million Vehicle Kilometers in Property Damage, Injury, and Death by Vehicle Type

	Death	*Injury*	*Property Damage*	*Total*
Passenger cars	3.7	64	142	210
Delivery vans	2.9	41	105	149
Lorries	7.1	46	127	180
Buses	8.1	91	211	310
Motorcycles	11.8	213	64	289
Mopeds	16.8	156	41	214

Source: W. Hunter and J.C. Stutts, *An Analysis of Mopeds as a Potential Safety Problem in the United States, vol. 1, Review of the Literature and Data Search, Final Report* (Chapel Hill, N.C.: Highway Safety Research Center, University of North Carolina, Report DOT-HS-805-035, 1979). Reprinted with permission.

percent without injury, 9 percent with first aid at the scene, 36 percent and 9 percent respectively with emergency department care or outpatient care only, 28 percent requiring hospital care, and 6 percent fatal,[9] in contrast to 0.8 percent fatality rate for automobile occupants.[10] In 1981, with motorcycles and mopeds covering 2 percent of all vehicle mileage, their riders were 10 percent of all U.S. highway fatalities.[11]

National Health Survey studies indicate twice as many persons injured on motorcycles as suggested by data using police statistics (420,000 to 540,000 persons versus 250,000 annually for 1968–70).[12] In one study only 39 percent of crashes resulting in treated injuries were in police statistics, the remainder being identified through hospital reports and death certificates.

Distribution of single-vehicle as compared to car versus cycle collisions among the unreported events is not known. However, among those reported to police, 63 percent were collisions with cars, 12 percent single-vehicle crashes in which the motorcycle ran off the road, 15 percent overturning of the cycle on the road, and 5 percent each collision with a fixed object (such as a parked car) or another object (bicyclist or pedestrian). There is little information about frequency of injuries in off-road or trail biking. One study suggests about 21 treated injuries per 1,000 minibikes annually, and half involve rider loss of control.[13]

Because these are low-cost vehicles they are often used by young persons with greatest productive life expectancy (although this was not found in one moped study[8]). In a California study, 91 percent of those injured were males, and 88 percent were under age 35.[12] Almost three-quarters of those injured reported disability, with a mean duration of 72.7 days and a median of 29.4 days.

Further documenting the lethality of these two-wheeled vehicles, in phase 1 and 2 countries there is an inverse relationship between number of vehicles per 10,000 population and fatality rate; but the greater the percentage of motorcycles and scooters among all vehicles in these nations, the higher the severity index.[14]

Human Factors: Pre-Injury Phase

The majority of motorcycle crashes involve inexperience, failure of another driver to perceive the two-wheeled vehicle, or use of alcohol. Barry found that 23 percent of crashes involved persons who had borrowed the machine, although only 2 percent of all motorcycle mileage involved borrowed vehicles.[15] Borrowers in two-vehicle crashes tended to be travelling slower than were owners in such crashes and were cited for a traffic violation more often. In single-vehicle crashes they were reported more often than owners to have crashes while attempting to execute a turn.

In New South Wales, 60 percent of fatally injured riders had ridden less than one year, a figure three times greater than the annual increase in licensed motorcyclists.[16] Supporting similar results, Harano and Peck note that among motorcyclists youth and inexperience are better predictors of crash involvement than is previous number of traffic citations.[17] Operators with less than six months experience are twice as likely to crash as are more experienced riders.[5] In another study 70 percent of those injured had borrowed or rented the cycle, and 20 percent had ridden a motorcycle less than three times previously.[18]

Because it is poorly protected against weather, the motorcycle is used mostly during warmer months, requiring the rider to reacquaint himself with his vehicle each year. In a Michigan study 75 percent of fatal crashes occurred during an eighteen-week summer period.[7]

Failure of another driver to observe (or if he observes, to perceive) the motorcyclist has been listed as a human factor, although it is clearly a human/vehicular interaction, which will be discussed under vehicular factors. Patricia Waller says regarding North Carolina crashes that about two-thirds were multivehicle and in 62 percent of those the car driver was at fault.[19] Most often the car made a left turn or pulled out in front of the motorcycle. The motorcyclist was at fault in only 29 percent of the multivehicle crashes, most often "following too closely." In 9 percent of the multivehicle crashes, culpability could not be assigned.[19] Car drivers appear to ignore motorcycles because these vehicles are small in size and currently comprise only a small proportion of all vehicles.[20] Thus, the motorcycle either is not seen or is misperceived.[12]

In Australia lack of visibility accounted for 16 percent of injury crashes but fewer fatal ones.[21] The major problem was reduced frontal visibility.[18] Hurt et al. report that motorcycle conspicuity (ability to be seen) was low or absent in 46 percent of those crashes where conspicuity was critical (such as where the other vehicle violated motorcyle right of way).

The data on alcohol in crashes is scanty because most information available comes from police reports, which tend to be incomplete or even fallacious concerning this variable. Graham found that 46 percent of motorcyclists who survived less than six hours had alcohol in their blood, 35 percent with BACs of 0.10 percent or higher and 11 percent with 0.20 percent or more.[22] In a second study 38 percent of fatalities had alcohol, 20 percent with BACs of 0.10 percent or greater.[23] Baker and Fisher report that two-thirds of fatally injured motorcyclists had alcohol and half had 0.10 percent or higher, in sharp contrast to police reports that only 20 percent of these same drivers had been drinking.[24]

Questions have arisen about characteristics of motorcycle users that might predispose them to crashes because early users in the United States tended to be black-leather-jacketed stereotypes of Marlon Brando movies. Nicholi describes a small group of frequently injured patients whose motorcycle preoccupation represents a "motorcycle syndrome."[25] In recent years, however, this vehicle is primarily an inexpensive means of transportation. A study on one U.S. college campus showed few differences between motorcycle owners and car owners.[26]

Little is known, however, about persons who use trail bikes or minibikes for recreational purposes. Little Leagues exist for racing minibikes and larger vehicles.[27] Members start riding as young as age 3 to 4, and are racing by age 6, with all of the parental frenzy and encouragement that occurs in Little League baseball. Riders at three race tracks experience about twelve to fifteen broken collar bones and similar numbers of arm or leg fractures per season.

In one three day series of races involving 400 child and teenage riders, major injuries included a severely lacerated lip and concussion in one boy, three broken collar bones, a fractured tibia and fibula, plus many lesser injuries not requiring hospitalization. The father of the boy with the broken leg said it was much safer than football but more dangerous than Ping-Pong. This description of persons at organized activity may apply as well to other users of minibikes but probably not to the larger population of motorcycle, moped, and scooter riders.

Vehicular Factors

The two most important vehicular factors in the pre-crash phase seem to be the size and instability of the two-wheeled vehicle. As we already observed, other motorists tend not to be aware of the motorcycle, scooter, or moped because of its smaller size and unanticipated profile. I would hypothesize—but lack documentation because it has never been studied—that wide rear pillars in cars and narrow visual fields in car and truck mirrors contribute to the motorcyclist's difficulties. Because of vibration, the cyclist himself has limited use of his rearview mirror.

Almost by definition, a two-wheeled vehicle is less stable than a four-wheeled one. Factors determining stability are complexly interwoven and include the following:[5]

1. wheel size, spin capability, gyroscopic stability;
2. wheel base;
3. frame rigidity;
4. balance factor, related to contact area available for knee and leg pressure;
5. steering geometry and suspension characteristics;
6. skid resistance, including tires—high hysteresis tread patterns, non-lock operation braking, and brake distribution (front versus rear);
7. aerodynamics;
8. engine flywheel effects;
9. rear suspension, controlled geometry; and
10. center of gravity, including engine location, rider position, and passenger position.

In order to turn, a motorcyclist must first shift the weight and direction of the vehicle briefly in the opposite direction and only then bank and turn the vehicle toward the intended route. This takes time to learn and may help explain why novices get into trouble. Furthermore, some machines have inadequate clearance between pedals or kickstands and the ground when the vehicle is banked sharply.

The presence of a passenger also affects the center of gravity and vehicle stability. P. Waller reports that passengers were present in 11 percent of all crashes and 30 percent of fatal ones and were more likely to be in single-vehicle than multivehicle events.[19] This overrepresentation remained even after considering the fact that the presence of a passenger doubles the candidates for a fatality. The passenger increases the driver's risk of fatality as well.

Munden examined crash rate per unit of exposure according to vehicle size and age of machine and rider.[28] He reported that young drivers, especially under age 25, had higher rates than older drivers and that for each age group crash rates rose as vehicle weight increased. He found no increase in crash rate with age of machine for the first ten years of life, but an increase was noted for machines older than ten years.

In contrast to Munden's conclusions are those of Hurt based on comparison of characteristics of injured cyclists with those of uninjured cyclists having similar location, time of day, day of week, and weather.[9] In that study, machines under 250 cc engine size are 1.5 times overrepresented in crashes, those 251 to 500 cc 1.4 times overrepresented, and larger machines 0.7 times underinvolved.

Component failure, although rather seldom listed in police reports,[2] has been identified as an important cause of crashes by staff of the National Highway Traffic Safety Administration.[29] Lights may not be powerful enough with small generators, and some brake cables are not made to resist normal expected grip pressures even when the cable is straight. They may be installed with sharp angles, adding to their inadequacy. Brake failure is suspected in 16 to 17 percent of motorcycle crashes, with cable failures occurring in some cases within two months after installation. In one study 16 percent of motorcyle crashes resulted from tire failures, although the causes of these failures were not disclosed.[30] Hurt's study notes motorcycle vehicle failure in 9.1 percent of single-vehicle crashes (usually because of tire failure) but 0.4 percent of multivehicle crashes.[9]

Environmental Factors

Table 11–3 shows the relative contributions of human, environmental, and vehicular factors in single-vehicle nonintersection crashes in rural and urban Maryland.[31]

Hurt lists "roadway defects" as factors in 6.5 percent of single-vehicle crashes and 0.4 percent of multivehicle events, with animals contributing another 3.9 percent in the single-vehicle crashes.[9] However, visibility obstructions existed for the motorcyclist in 23 percent of all

Table 11–3
Causal Factors in Single-Vehicle Motorcycle Crashes Not at Intersections
(percentage)

Causal Factor	*Urban*	*Rural*
Motorcycle operator	44	36
Other vehicle	15	10
Vehicular	12	20
Environment	27	33
Operator and environment	2	0

Source: Adapted from M.L. Reiss, W.G. Berger, and G.R. Vallette, *Analysis of Motorcycle Accident Reports* (Falls Church, Va.: Biotechnology, Inc., 1974).

crashes and for the other vehicle 32 percent of the time. Note that the Maryland study is limited to nonintersection crashes and thus is not totally comparable to the Hurt report. Greater environmental contribution might be expected with off-road riders of trail bikes, who not only must contend with obstacles at ground level but also poorly visible hazards, such as fence wires or cables, that can sever the windpipe or trachea.[32]

Buchanan[30] has cogently described the diversity of hazards facing the motorcyclist, including patches of sand and gravel, parts and debris that have fallen from other vehicles (especially a problem at night), steel bridge grating and highway grooving, poor maintenance of road surface, especially with puddles that conceal pot holes, speed bumps, heaving of pavement joints, washboard pavements, and freeway exit ramps that a motorcyclist may enter at an appropriate dry weather speed only to find in the middle of the curved ramp that the pavement is wet due to sprinkling systems used for watering foliage. He particularly faults highway departments for inadequate cleanup of spillage and for ignoring the needs of motorcyclists, who, because of the inherent instability of their vehicles, require special warnings about the existence of the above hazards, which usually present less problem for automobile drivers.

To what extent is there interaction of human, vehicular, and environmental factors in two-wheeled vehicular crashes? The interrelationship that often exists between rider inexperience and necessity to respond to environmental threat, given a vehicle that has unique characteristics, stands out clearly in Hurt's analysis.[9] Sixty-one percent of the time the cyclist had two seconds or less between the precipitating event and the crash itself. Often, I suspect, this extremely short interval was because of the visual obstructions noted earlier. A third of riders took no evasive action, and where an evasive action was taken, it was either the improper one or was improperly executed 76 percent of the time. Riders who did not have specific motorcycle training and licensing were substantially overrepresented in crashes when compared to the trained population.

Crash Phase

Bothwell attributes the lethality of two-wheeled vehicles to three factors:[5]

1. At impact or in skids the machine does not remain upright.
2. On impact the rider receives little or no protection from the machine. Unlike the automobile occupant, he is like an egg riding outside the carton.

3. The rider is usually ejected from the vehicle, making him vulnerable to further injury.

Vehicles with greater power may be associated with serious crashes, as described by Munden,[28] both because they can achieve higher speeds and thus greater kinetic forces on impact (and are owned by persons who wish to take such risks) and also because the machine itself is likely to be larger, heavier, and thus more to contend with in a crash. A large Harley-Davidson may weigh ten times as much as a moped and can go several times as fast. This same fact of an additional heavy obstacle to collide with may explain why the presence of a passenger appears to increase about threefold the risk that the driver will be killed if a crash occurs. The difference in results between the Munden study and the Hurt one may simply reflect that larger vehicles may be driven in different locations and in different ways, factors that the latter study somewhat controlled for.

When a motorcycle goes out of control the occupants either catapult over the machine or skid along the ground, commonly with the machine on top of them. In either case head injuries are an expected outcome. As long ago as 1941, Cairns identified head injuries as contributory to death in two-thirds of a series of 149 motorcycle fatalities.[2] In 1957, before extensive use of helmets, Bauer compared the distribution of 1,001 injuries among 686 persons with injuries of all degrees of severity and that of fatal injuries in 101 deaths.[32] These appear in table 11–4 together with more recent data on injury rates for helmeted and unhelmeted riders.[33] Clearly, less serious injuries tend to be distributed among head, legs, and arms, while those resulting in fatality overwhelmingly involve the head, with most of the remainder affecting the chest and abdomen. Just as clearly, helmeted riders have fewer injuries to head, face, and neck than do unhelmeted riders.

Among persons with "serious" (but usually not fatal) injuries in the northern California study, 77 percent had trauma to one anatomic region (31 percent lower extremity, 22 percent upper extremity, 19 percent head, and 6 percent trunk), 14 percent to two regions (with 9 percent involving head plus an extremity), and 4 percent with three or four regions (always involving the head).[12] No data were available for 5 percent of cases. However, it is relevant that 32 percent of persons in this study were wearing helmets, an issue to be discussed shortly.

Post-Crash Factors

The motorcyclist faces three somewhat unique problems in the post-crash phase. First, the likelihood of gas tank rupture or leakage is

Table 11–4
Distribution by Body Area of All Injuries and Fatal Injuries among Motorcycle Riders and of Injuries among Helmeted and Unhelmeted Riders

Location	*Percentage of All Injuries*[a] *(1,001 in 686 persons)*	*Injury Rate Per 1,000 Riders*[b]		*Percentage of Fatal Injuries*[a] *(101 persons)*
		Helmet	*No Helmet*	
Head	50	129	369	79
Neck	2	28	38	1
Face	—	105	161	—
Chest	6	128	144	8
Abdomen	3	61	53	7
Pelvis	—	83	85	—
Upper extremity	13	} 790	} 742	1
Lower extremity	27			4

Source: Adapted from (a) K.H. Bauer, *CIBA Symposia* 5(1957):148, as quoted by P.W. Bothwell, "The Problem of Motorcycle Accidents," *Practitioner* 188(1962):474–488; (b) C.E. Dare, J.C. Owens, and S. Krane, *Impact of Motorcycle Helmet Use in Colorado: Executive Summary* (Denver, Colo.: Division of Highway Safety, Colorado Department of Highways, Final Report DOT-HS-803-679, 1978).

greater, usually abetted by an inadequate gas cap. But despite leakage 62 percent of the time, the frequency of fires is only 2 percent.[9]

Second, in single vehicle crashes along side the road, especially at night, the motorcycle and its occupants may disappear from view, discovery, and treatment.

Finally, the motorcyclist who arrives in the emergency department faces an entirely new, unanticipated, and unwarranted obstacle: the sometimes open hostility of physicians and nurses, who often view the motorcycle and its riders as a menace to the public health. This attitude derives both from the higher injury rate and from prior images of counterculture, drugs, and rebellion.

Countermeasures

Some people feel that nothing can be done to make motorcycles and mopeds even a bit safe, and on occasion it has been suggested that motorcycle use be abolished or severely restricted. At the other extreme, motorcycle users commonly feel that they are being singled out for application of laws that abridge constitutional freedoms. Just what can be done and what are the limitations to improvement? In 1963 Bothwell proposed the following six-step program to deal with the problem:[34]

1. Provide training in school to improve motorcycle handling.
2. Test drivers for vision and handling ability.
3. Provide nonlocking brakes and high-hysteresis tires.
4. Improve stability.
5. Require wearing of crash helmets.
6. Design machine to be crash resistant, with packaging of the rider.

1. Training and proficiency testing for special licensing will be considered together. Hurt noted that persons with no license or a revoked license were 2.4 times overrepresented in motorcycle crashes, while those with a driver's license but without motorcycle endorsement were 2.0 times overrepresented. In contrast, the risk for persons with a motorcycle endorsement was 0.7. Whereas 54 percent of all crash-involved riders had endorsements, only 46 percent of rider errors were in this group.

Wagar suggests that training would be of benefit primarily during the first few months of driving, noting that in Japan, where such training is required, a peak of crashes during the first year of riding is not seen, as in the United States.[35] Training unique to this special driving task does indeed have merit. But even with such training, excessive crash and injury risk exists. Some fear, therefore, that if training becomes available in high schools, with the aura of school approval, the net result would be a sufficient increase in motorcyle use, especially by high-risk young drivers, to more than outweigh the advantage of training, thus resulting overall in more injuries and fatalities.

In the United States as of 1974 in-traffic tests either alone or in combination with other tests were required by twenty states and the District of Columbia, off-road tests only by seventeen others, and no special test by thirteen states.[36] All states required a driver's license of some sort for on-road operation of a motorcycle but not necessarily for trail bikes, minibikes used off road, or mopeds used on road. In the United States four states did not require any license to operate a moped, while most of the remainder required a license but no special endorsement.[6] Most European countries require only a written test on rules of the road for this vehicle.

Recently, California tested two special programs for motorcyclists.[37] The first was an improved licensing program requiring more knowledge and more rigorous skill testing than previously. The second program required all who failed the test to take Remedial Skills Training. Both programs were associated with a statistically significant reduction in motorcycle crash rates during the year after the program, with reductions ranging from 15 percent to 21 percent. Persons who took the programs did not differ in motorcycle and automobile convictions, automobile crashes, and in total crashes and convictions but did show a significant reduction in injury and fatality. I believe the risk data support a requirement that similar training and licensing standards should be applied for moped use as well.

2. Use of these vehicles should be limited only to circumstances that would reduce their hazard. In the United States motorcycles are not permitted on a few high-speed roads.[30] Ironically, however, mopeds—which are much slower than motorcycles—are permitted on expressways in twenty-seven states and on interstate highways in twenty-five states.[38] In my opinion, mopeds should be limited only to roads with maximum speeds of 30 M.P.H. or less. Most European nations have maximum speed limits of 30 to 40 K.P.H. (25 M.P.H.) and require use of bicycle paths.[6]

3. Improve upon the conspicuity of two-wheeled vehicles. Use of front and rear lights during the daytime is required in seventeen states[39] and appears to have brought about 4 to 5 percent reduction in daytime crashes (projected to 7,100 crashes nationally) at an annual cost of $3 per machine for more powerful vehicles and $7 to $14 for ones with marginal electrical systems.[39,40] Hurt reports that in daylight, only 32 percent of

motorcycles in crashes but 68 percent of the time/site controls had lights on, while at dusk 44 percent of the crash cyclists but 71 percent of the control vehicles were illuminated.

Manufacturers of mopeds, however, have sought to be permitted to meet less stringent lighting standards than do motorcycles because their smaller electrical systems are inadequate to meet the existing standards. I personally find such a request quite irresponsible with respect to safety. Within current U.S. rules that permit use in a wide range of environments, the moped is likely to have a much greater speed differential from surrounding vehicles than does the motorcycle. At such high closure rates, having a vehicle that *by design* cannot be seen until the last moment is asking for trouble.

Use of properly placed reflective materials for helmet, clothing, and tires can increase conspicuity also, having the advantage at night of making the rider and machine visible to cross traffic.[41,42]

4. Regarding brakes, stability, and improved vehicle design for occupant packaging,[43] modest—but not substantial—improvement in stability appears possible, anti-locking brakes may be feasible within a few years, but only meager improvements can be expected in crash resistant packaging of riders.

It is possible, however, to improve upon performance of brake cables and other aspects of existing brake systems, to improve the location, operation, identification, and illumination of controls, and to prevent stands and footrests from striking the ground when the vehicle is banked moderately. Motor vehicle safety standards 122 and 123 now apply to these issues.

5. The greatest controversy in the United States, but not especially in other nations, has been over the requirement that cyclists wear helmets that meet minimum standards for crash attenuation. Helmets for moped riders have been ignored in the United States but not in other countries. The issues are identical for both vehicles.[6] Other protective clothing such as goggles or face shield, shoes, jacket, and so forth are also relevant.

a. The major cause of death and permanent disability from motorcycle crashes is head injury, which can be prevented entirely or markedly reduced through helmets. Since 1959 standards have increasingly ensured that this equipment meets adequate performance specifications,[44] and table 11–4 shows how effective this countermeasure can be. According to a California study, the risk of serious head injury doubled from low-speed to high-speed crashes but at each speed the risk of such injuries was 50 percent less for helmet wearers than for nonwearers.[45] In Colorado, Oklahoma, South Dakota, and Kansas respectively, fatal head injuries per 1,000 crash-involved riders were 9, 11, 13, and 6 for helmeted riders but 23, 63, 38, and 41 for riders without helmets.[46]

b. Typically a young person with serious head injury does not have sufficient financial assets to cover his extensive and prolonged medical care and social services. These may go on for many years, particularly if the person becomes a mental vegetable, as happens all too often. While the person may injure only himself, the costs of that injury fall upon the entire community, which should have some way of reducing its financial risks.

Bothwell points out that in 1960 in England the cost attributable to motorcycle crashes was much more than the value of machines produced. Recent data on hospital bills for seventy-one motorcyclists in Colorado indicates that 32 percent of the cost was unpaid and another 30 percent was paid from government sources.[46] Billing losses for unhelmeted riders in Kansas exceeded those for helmeted ones by a ratio of five to one.[46]

Those who oppose compulsory laws argue that helmets restrict hearing and vision and thus are a safety hazard. With the exception of one brand of helmet, however, the reduction in visual field ranged from 0.4 percent to 7.3 percent, scarcely enough to be meaningful.[47] The alleged reduction in hearing is actually shielding from extraneous street noises that commonly mask important sounds. One legitimate complaint is that helmets do get warm in hot weather.

Opponents also argue that compelling the wearing of helmets is an abridgement of civil liberties. This is a philosophic issue, as is the issue of the public protecting its interests, and the question of which is the more compelling argument can be answered only by the courts and the legislature, and only in the context of a particular time and place. The U.S. Supreme Court has upheld the right of the public to protect its interests by compelling helmet use.[46]

The third argument of opponents is that helmets increase the incidence of neck injuries in crashes. Table 11–4 refutes this completely.

Between 1966 and 1969 laws requiring compulsory use of helmets became effective in forty states, and the U.S. fatality rate per 10,000 motorcycles dropped from 13 to 7. Between 1976 and 1979, however, twenty-seven states repealed or weakened their laws, and the national fatality rate rose again to 10, the increase being in those states that had changed their laws.[46] Muller estimates that such repeals may generate between $16 to $18 million of unnecessary medical care costs annually in the United States.[48]

Where laws exist, at least 95 percent of riders comply. When laws do not exist or are repealed, only about 50 percent wear helmets despite the widespread belief even among nonusers that helmets are useful.[46] Therefore, it is reasonable to conclude that public information programs to increase use voluntarily would yield little results but high cost.[46]

Asogwa has documented, however, that it is not enough simply to require that motorcyclists wear helmets.[49] In Nigeria, passage of a compulsory use law was not followed by a reduction in serious injuries. The reason for this, he believes, is because almost 40 percent of users did not know how to wear their helmets properly and 9 percent wore the wrong type of helmet. Therefore, little or no protection resulted because helmets were inadequate or flew off in crashes. In cases such as this, education can play an important role.

In a Swedish study[50] persons with protective leather clothing had fewer injuries overall than those without protection, but the differences were statistically significant only for back and lower extremities. The reductions were in soft tissue injuries only, although Feldkamp had previously reported that riders with protective clothing had three times fewer compound fractures.[47] Regarding hands and wrists, 18 percent with protection had injury versus 48 percent without gloves. Fifty percent of those with trousers and 74 percent of unprotected persons had leg injuries. For upper extremities the figures were 49.5 percent versus 58 percent, while foot and ankle injury occurred in 27 percent with boots but 35 percent without boots. This is one area where I suspect most riders, in the United States at least, are less knowledgeable than they are about helmets and, therefore, where education may have some degree of success.

12
Bicycles

In the United States, Canada, and a few other nations, the predominant use of the bicycle has been for children's recreation and as limited transportation for children until they are able to obtain access to a motor vehicle during their late teen years. Only since the 1970s has it become more than occasional transportation for adults. Throughout most of the world, however, the bicycle is an important—and in many nations the most important—mechanized means of transportation. The annual worldwide production of 35 to 40 million bicycles substantially exceeds that of all motorized vehicles.

The earliest prototype of the bicycle first appeared about 1816.[1] Improvements followed throughout the mid-1800s, until by the latter part of the century cycling became a major fad on both the North American and European continents, to be replaced eventually on both continents by new loves, the automobile and motorized two-wheeled vehicles. But extensive use of the bicycle for practical, inexpensive transportation remains in much of the rest of the world, where the initial and operating costs for automobiles are far beyond what many can afford.

As transportation for adults, the issues involved in the design and use of the bicycle are basically the same from one nation to another. An exception occurs in those nations, predominantly Asian, where bicycles serve as transportation not only for people but for quantities of cargo as well.

As combined recreation and transportation for children, other issues are also relevant: for example, special seat, wheel, and handlebar designs that are promoted as fad, for specific types of play, or both. Also relevant is the question of the appropriate age at which children have sufficient neuromuscular and judgmental maturity to permit safe use of this vehicle.

According to *Accident Facts,* a total of 1,200 bicyclists were fatally injured and 60,000 nonfatally injured involving collision with motor vehicles in the United States during 1980.[2] In addition, an estimated 100 bicyclists died as a result of falls or similar single-vehicle events.[2]

About 550,000 injuries annually are estimated requiring emergency department treatment (plus others treated in doctors' offices), for a rate of 258 per 100,000 population.[3] The peak rate is 907 for persons age 5 to 14, with 255 to 270 for persons under age 5 and age 15 to 24, and then a rapid drop to 60 and 16, respectively, for persons age 25 to 64 and 65 or older. The rate is twice as high for males (365) as for females (156). Of these injuries, 97 percent result from solo spills or other problems of bicyclists, rather than from collision with automobiles.[4]

One estimate is that there are about 80 million bicycle riders in the United States.[5] Another places the number of pedalcycles at 62 to 65 million in 1981.[6] Using this latter figure, there would be about two deaths per 100,000 bicycles and 85 to 89 nonfatal injuries per 10,000 bicycles annually. The rates involving contact with motor vehicles would be 1.8 to 1.9 deaths per 100,000 bicycles and 9.2 to 9.7 injuries per 10,000 bicycles.

As with automobile trauma, the death rate per 100,000 vehicles has dropped over the years, from 12.8 in 1935, 9.6 in 1940, and 5.6 in 1945.[2] Until 1973 the majority of these deaths had been among children, but this has shifted markedly. Persons age 15 and older comprised over three-fifths of the deaths in 1980, compared to one-fifth in 1960.[2] The shift in age distribution of deaths—which are almost entirely associated with bicycle versus motor vehicle crashes—is not necessarily reflected in the age distribution of less serious injuries, which are still predominantly among children and do not involve motor vehicles.

Use and Injury Patterns for Children: Human Factors

Because of the important age-associated differences in patterns of use and injury, and in factors involved in the causation of injury events, the discussion will be divided into the experiences of children, which are predominantly nonhighway related, and those of adults, in which injury usually results from contact with other vehicles. Five major studies in recent years have examined use patterns and injuries among youthful riders,[7,8,9,10] or among late teens and young adults (age 16 to 30).[11] While all have methodologic limitations, they probably present a reasonable overview of bicyclist injury in the United States.

Waller examined all 107 treated injuries among children age 3 to 12 in a four-month period among 6,000 children in Burlington, Vermont, but did not estimate mileage travelled.[7] By kindergarten age, two-thirds of children own bikes, and this increases to 80 to 90 percent between age 7 to 12. Mean age for learning to ride was 5.9 years, consistent with Thorson's observation that in Stockholm 43 percent of boys own bicycles by age 5[12] and Vilardo and Andersen's estimate that in the United States 93 percent of youths age 6 to 16 ride bikes.[10] One-third of bikes owned were high rise (small wheel, large flared handlebars, and long "banana" seat), with boys much more likely than girls to own this style (48 percent versus 23 percent). In kindergarten about 20 percent of children reported using their bikes at least occasionally after dark, but this rose rapidly to about 60 percent for boys and 35 to 40 percent for girls by age 12.

Injury rates over four months were 11.2 per 1,000 owners (estimated to be half the annual rate), but were over twice as high for boys as for girls (15.0 versus 6.9). It was not clear from this study whether the higher rate for boys reflected greater exposure, different use patterns or other factors. Children age 5 to 9 had somewhat, but not significantly, higher injury rates than did older ones. Nor was there overrepresentation (compared to uninjured neighboring children of similar age and sex) of injured children who learned to ride at a very early age. Those who learned at a very young age usually had athletically inclined parents who closely supervised their learning.

Over two-thirds of injuries were minor, with 21 percent fractures, 5 percent concussions, and 2 percent avulsions. Multiple injuries occurred a third of the time, with most frequent single trauma being to leg and foot (28 percent), head and face (20 percent), and shoulder, arm, or hand (17 percent). Thirty-seven percent of injuries were on borrowed bikes, and passengers were present in about one-sixth of injuries.

Over three-quarters of injuries involving passengers occurred on borrowed bikes. In many cases, the owner was sitting behind the borrower as a passenger. This required the driver not only to handle an unfamiliar bike but to do so while carrying additional weight. The end result commonly was that the owner got injured.

The immediate mechanisms of the events appear in table 12–1. Some vehicular and environmental factors that underlie these mechanisms will be discussed later. However, relevant human factors are the frequency of horseplay, distraction, panic in presence of a car or other hazard, and riding too close to stationary objects. All suggest limited skills, judgment, or both, which are hardly surprising behavior for young children. Not one event occurred after dark, perhaps because the study was carried out during summer.

Regarding bicycle versus motor vehicle collisions, Williams says that the cyclist was probably responsible in 94 percent of such collisions to children under age 10, in 86 percent involving children age 10 to 14, in 55 percent with all cyclists age 15 or older, but only 34 percent of those with cyclists over age 24.[13] This suggests that the maturation process for some aspects of bicycling may extend all the way into teen years. Williams's study indicates that, especially with older children and adults, the motorist is responsible more often in collisions at dusk or after dark than in daytime collisions.

Table 12–1
Circumstances Leading to Event among Bicycle Injuries to Children

Circumstance	*Percentage*
Lost control, no apparent reason	7
Lost control while attempting to turn	6
Lost control while attempting to stop	7
Hit obstruction	17
Horseplay	19
Distracted	7
Foot caught in bike	11
Part of bike broke	3
Rode too close to stationary object	9
Panic in presence of car or other hazard	6
Car initiated event	4
Other	6
Total	
%	102
(N)	(104)

Source: Adapted from J.A. Waller, "Bicycle Ownership, Use and Injury Patterns among Elementary School Children," *Pediatrics* 47(1971):1042–1050.

In a study by Pascarella, odometers were attached to over 300 bicycles (unfortunately, a nonrandom sample of volunteers).[8] Boys, predominantly age 7 to 12, averaged 313 miles per year, while girls accumulated only 159 miles. As a result, the higher injury rates per person for boys converted to lower rates per unit exposure (1.49/1,000 miles for boys versus 1.79 for girls). Children with one and two years respectively of riding exposure were overrepresented in mishaps by 39 percent and 22 percent, while those with three years or more of previous riding were underrepresented.

Most injuries were relatively minor, with 72 percent resulting from noncollision falls. Nine percent involved contacts with motor vehicles. Two of every five injuries were to the leg, about 30 percent the arm, and 20 percent the head.

The study by Chlapecka et al. covered over 23,000 school age children in eighty cities and thirty-four states, unfortunately with only a 31 percent return of questionnaires.[9] The authors allege no bias toward excessive returns by persons with injuries or mishaps. Overall, 21 percent of students reported at least one such event in the previous year.

Based on recentness and number of hours per day of bicycle use, at an estimate of 5 miles per hour, they calculated about 500 to 550 miles annually for girls, with no age-related variation. Among boys, it ranged from just under 700 for seven-year-olds, up to slightly over 800 for twelve-year-olds. According to this study, mishaps per 1,000 miles increase from 0.58 at age 7 to 0.84 at age 13, with a mean of 0.72 and no substantial sex-associated difference. Children with two or less years of experience, however, had a rate of 0.89, while those with more experience averaged 0.68.

The fourth study—by Vilardo and Andersen—also suffers from inadequate questionnaire return (33 percent), thus again raising questions of biases of response.[10] In that study also, young children had higher injury rates per unit of exposure than did older children.

One important analysis should be referenced even though it is limited to collisions between bicycles and other motor vehicles and does not distinguish between events involving children and those involving adults.[14] Half the riders in both fatal and nonfatal collisions were under age 15. Overall bicyclists had suboptimal pre-crash courses in 52 percent of fatal crashes and 69 percent of nonfatal ones, while motorist course was suboptimal in 21 percent and 11 percent respectively. Much of the suboptimal behavior of cyclists, however, involved darting out, sudden turns, and similar behaviors characteristic of youthful riders.

The authors identified seven categories of interaction:

1. The bicyclist rode out of the driveway, alley, or other midblock location. This accounted for 15 percent of fatal collisions and 14 percent of nonfatal ones.
2. The bicyclist rode out at a controlled intersection: 12 percent of fatal and 17 percent of nonfatal events.
3. The motorist turned, merged, drove through a controlled intersection or backed out of a driveway: 2 percent fatal and 19 percent nonfatal.
4. The motorist overtook the bicyclist while travelling in the same direction: 38 percent of fatal and 11 percent of nonfatal collisions.
5. Bicyclist suddenly swerved or made an unexpected turn: 16 percent and 14 percent respectively.
6. Motorist made unexpected turn: 2 percent and 15 percent, respectively.
7. Miscellaneous or nonclassifiable other actions: 14 percent and 11 percent.

Injury Patterns for Children: Equipment and Environmental Factors

While some of the equipment and environmental issues involving the occurrence of bicycle mishaps are similar to those with motorcycles and mopeds (such as stability of two-wheeled vehicles in the presence of road discontinuities, and conspicuity, especially at night), several of the issues differ substantially. These different issues result in large part from the fact that bicycles are often used by children, whereas motorcycles and mopeds usually are not. The associated problems are that (1) a parent often will buy a child a bicycle that for the moment is too large, (2) "fad" bicycle designs and equipment have been created to attract more purchasers, (3) two children often ride a bike that was designed for only one person, and (4) in the United States, at least, many bicycles are sold unassembled and are put together by the purchaser.

Brezina and Kramer have labeled the first of these phenomena "disaccommodation."[15] In a study of urban collisions between bicycles and motor vehicles they reported that among riders age 8 to 10 years old, those who could not reach their pedals comfortably when seated had a fivefold increase in crash risk. Waller noted that of children who learned to ride at age 6 and who still had their first bikes, 22 percent had bicycles with 26-inch wheels.[7] The seat should be no higher than the rider's hip so that his or her feet can touch the ground without making the bicycle lean.

Based on anecdotal data, high-rise or spider bicycles were originally thought to present an unusual hazard.[16] Crude data on high-rise bikes do, in fact, show overrepresentation in injury events per 100 vehicles.[7] Taking into account, however, the fact that this style is owned and used predominantly by boys, who have substantially greater exposure and more injuries than girls, no difference can be found in injury rates for an exposure-corrected population.[7,8,9] This style may be somewhat more difficult to handle at low speeds, making it a less appropriate choice as a first bicycle for an inexperienced rider. That most high-rise bicycles also have elongated seats, which more easily permit the bike to carry two people, is also important.

Several studies have noted the high frequency—and probably substantial overrepresentation—of riding double in bicycle injuries to children. The proportion is 17 percent, for example, in each of two reports.[7,17] A two-wheeled, pedal-powered vehicle provides what often becomes an unmanageable task for the energy output and tracking capabilities of a child when the weight of a second child is added, especially if the driver is borrowing the bike and is less familiar with its idiosyncracies than is the owner-passenger.[7] Furthermore, the brakes of the average bicycle were not designed for this additional load. And with two people on a bicycle, the passenger is likely to get his feet tangled in the exposed spokes.[18]

The problem with at-home assembly of bicycles is that, with use, parts important for maintaining control may loosen. Such loosening is encouraged by the fact that these parts are made of rounded (rather than flattened or ridged) stock at the point where adjustment and tightening occurs. Maneuvers such as "popping wheelies" (or rearing back suddenly on the rear wheel) that are possible with newer bicycle designs seem particularly likely to place stress on the handlebars and other adjustment points. Some episodes have occurred in which the frame has broken, but the relative frequency of these is unknown, since the method by which injuries from this cause were identified contained substantial biases of selection.[5]

Regarding stability, Gonski et al. report, for example, that 10 percent of a series of 139 treated injuries to child bicyclists in Australia involved striking potholes and another 4 percent were from spills while taking a turn.[16] Other studies also indicate the importance of striking obstacles, skidding during turns, and riding on gravel or dirt surfaces in the initiation of falls from bikes.[7,9] Hazards can also result if drainage grates on roads have parallel bars that are placed so that it is possible for a bicycle wheel to get caught between the bars.

While collisions between child cyclists and motor vehicles are not common, the fact that these vehicles do share the roads sometimes leads to injury because a young rider becomes frightened and loses control. Brezina and Kramer also note the many obstacles to visibility in urban neighborhoods that are not well understood by the child who has learned to ride but is not yet "streetwise."[15] Bicycles that lack reflectors and lights may be all but invisible to other road users at night. For this reason, even the relatively few nighttime collisions that occur are over-represented with respect to the amount of nighttime exposure and tend to be more severe than are daytime injuries.[19,20] Problems of poor visibility for both cyclists and motorists, especially at night, have also been extensively documented by Cross and Fisher.[14]

Injury-Phase Issues in Children's Injuries

The object struck by the majority of children is the road or ground, a logical result of the fact that the bicyclist, like the motorcyclist, has no protective packaging. The most important equipment-related source of injury appears to be the bicycle wheel and spokes. These spoke injuries at first seem to be relatively minor but often turn out to be more serious, both because of the twisting motion that a moving wheel imparts and because broken spokes may leave a long tract of trauma that may not be suspected on examination.[21] On some bikes, genital injuries have occurred because of enlarged gear shifts placed on the frame, rather than on the handlebar.[22]

Use and Injury Patterns for Adults

Although adult bicycling has increased dramatically in popularity in the United States, there has been very little research effort either to examine use patterns or injuries of adult bicyclists.[11] To correct this deficit, Schupack and Driessen surveyed adults age 16 to 30 on twenty-seven college campuses.[11] Again, the problem is a low return rate (24 percent), but currently no better data are available.

Overall, men averaged 705 miles annually and women 456. About half of this was for transportation, and almost half of all riding was in the presence of moderate to high-density motor vehicle traffic. Thirty-nine percent of women, but only 21 percent of men, owned single-gear or single-speed bikes, a type that was used more often for recreation, that averaged less mileage (287 versus 882 for six-to-fifteen-speed bikes), and that had higher reported mishap rates (0.72 per 1,000 miles driven versus 0.54 for three-speed bikes and 0.48 for five- or more speed models). In contrast to children, adult riders far more often had bicycles with hand brakes, rode on the road and in the presence of traffic, and far less often carried a second rider.

Males averaged 0.45 mishaps per 1,000 miles and women 0.67. Except for single-gear bicycles, women always had higher mishap rates than men. Six percent of adult riders reported having fallen on the most recent day they used a bike, but unlike children falls represented only a third of mishaps. Among all mishaps, 85 percent resulted in injury and 15 percent did not. One mishap in every five involved contact with or avoidance of a motor vehicle. Another 46 percent were collisions with other bikes, hitting or falling off a curb, or hitting a hole, bump, or obstacle.

A more recent study was a randomly distributed survey of 1,200 Wisconsin college students, 71 percent of whom responded.[23] Among the two-thirds who were bicyclists, 13 percent reported a mishap in the previous year, 62 percent resulting in injury, 32 percent requiring medical attention, but only 8 percent being reported to the police. Almost nine of every ten persons who sustained injury had trauma to the extremities, with 30 percent and 18 percent, respectively, reporting injury to trunk or head. Half of the events were felt to have resulted at least in part because of road conditions, 26 percent because of an automobile, 15 percent from personal inattention or conflict with a pedestrian or other cyclist, and 10 percent because of equipment defects, especially brakes.

Cross and Fisher[14] report that alcohol was known to be present in 0.8 percent of nonfatally injured bicyclists and 0.6 percent of fatalities in bicycle/vehicle crashes. Half of the bicyclists were children, and they note that the figures presented probably represent an understatement.

Among the motorists in these crashes 3.5 percent had alcohol in nonfatal collisions, and 17 percent in fatal ones.

More recently, Lind and Wollin[24] found 13 percent who admitted to alcohol use prior to injury among 520 Swedish bicyclists. Eleven percent were felt to be moderately or severely impaired. Based on a substudy of persons who denied alcohol use but who had positive BACs, however, they estimate 20 percent of their injured sample had ingested alcohol. Alcohol-impaired riders, in similar fashion to young children, were more likely to topple off their bikes without protective reflex action and to incur head injury. Sober adults and older children, on the other hand, were more likely to stretch out their arms on falling and to injure these. Also from Sweden, Thorson[12] reports intoxication in 29 percent of injured male bicyclists and 5 percent of injured women.

Particularly a problem in many of the phase 1 and 2 nations are collisions that occur at night when trucks or other vehicles overtake bicyclists who are using narrow, unlit rural roads. Often the bicyclist is not discovered until daylight arrives, by which time it already may be too late to provide care. Many of these may also involve alcohol in the vehicle driver, the bicyclist, or both, although data are not available to validate this impression. As already noted, the use of bicycles by adults in some phase 1 and 2 nations may be not only for transportation of people but of goods as well. Without modification to provide stability, this use of the bicycle for a purpose for which it was not originally intended cannot but increase the rate of injuries both by requiring the individual to engage in a more difficult balancing act and sometimes by reducing visibility for the rider.

Countermeasures

Since many of the injuries among children appear to be related to immature skills and judgment, two potential countermeasures are to delay the learning process until age 6, 7, or even later, when these abilities are more developed, and to provide specific formal training. In a study of a Cycling Proficiency Training program, children who failed a proficiency test had higher injury rates than did those who passed the test.[26] With the exception only of boys age 10 and 11, however, those who took the training showed no difference in injury rates from children who did not receive training. Possible intervening variables were, who volunteers for testing and training, and extent and type of exposure before and after training, which were not controlled for.

To my knowledge, licensing only of bicyclists who show ability to meet minimum proficiency requirements has not been attempted. The above data suggest that children unable to pass a test are at special risk, but they represented only 6 to 7 percent of those tested and fewer than 10 percent of those injured. Furthermore, in nations where bicycles are used primarily for transportation and consequently where the majority of users are adults, there is no compelling reason to believe that proficiency tests relevant for growing children would also be applicable to adults. Nor is there reason, however, to believe that they definitely would not be appropriate. The issue simply has not been put to the appropriate test. In the United States, attempts to "license" or register bicycles have not been successful.[7]

In theory, traffic laws apply to bicyclists as well as to motor vehicles. However, cyclists often ignore rules of the road and almost never are cited for infractions.[26] On the other hand, motor vehicle operators often show disregard or even hostility for cyclists using the roads. Better enforcement of existing laws as they pertain to driver/cyclist interactions would appear to be one approach that has not been seriously tried. Any attempt to try this approach, however, should be tied to well-designed evaluation of the method and results and should include consideration of alcohol impairment in bicycle injuries to adults.

Can public education campaigns work? Dewar's observation of riding behavior of 2,200 bicyclists indicated that 32 percent made important riding errors and that many bicycles were poorly equipped from the safety viewpoint.[27] He concludes that educational efforts might be warranted. My own impression is that if, despite safety campaigns, very few people are willing to register their bikes to increase chances of recovery if stolen, the overall success of campaigns to improve rider behavior can hardly be counted on.

High priority must be given to use of reflective materials on moving parts of the bicycle, such as wheels and pedals.[28] Incorporation of this countermeasure on all new bicycles in the United States during the past several years has substantially increased nighttime conspicuity for these vehicles, but I am not aware of any evaluation of the results. It is, however, a countermeasure that should be particularly amenable to the dark roads and low incomes of many phase 1 and 2 nations, as well as to more developed ones.

Handbrakes appear to be more effective than pedal-operated brakes. The data suggest that multispeed bicycles have fewer mishaps than single-gear styles, but it is not clear how much this reflects the number of gears or that the multispeed styles more often have handbrakes. Handlebar, seat, and fork design could be modified to lessen the likelihood of loosening, and wheels should be covered so that feet cannot get entangled.

Is there much to be gained from avoidance of faddish equipment such as small wheels, high-rise style, and banana seat? No clear answer is forthcoming. Children appear to play games more actively with the so-called gimmicky styles, but this may be because children who already like to play such games seek out this equipment, rather than because the equipment suggests the risk taking. In fact, the modified equipment may conceivably permit these games to be played more safely than would be the case with standard style. Clearly, however, parents should be advised not to buy a first bike that is too large for the child at that stage of development.

Whether children have banana seats available or not, there appears to be little difference in the likelihood of riding double. If one assumes that children will continue to ride double no matter what they are told by adults, injury risks can be reduced by improving braking capability and covering the wheels. And given the fact that many people in developing countries will need to continue to use bicycles for transportation of goods, bicycles in these areas should be designed to permit this activity to be done with less hazard.

Over 90 percent of fatalities are from contact with motor vehicles. One solution is design and construction of roadways to permit separation of motor vehicles and other traffic. In Davis, California, separate bicycle lanes were associated with a 31 percent reduction overall in motor vehicle versus bicycle crashes and a 53 percent reduction in collisions where lanes would be expected to be beneficial.[29] In nations with large numbers of both pedestrians and cyclists, however, attention must be paid as well to protecting pedestrians from being struck by bicyclists. And we have already observed that gravel, potholes, and similar surface irregularities must be dealt with if they are not to remain a real hazard for persons on two-wheeled vehicles.

Three limited options seem possible to reduce severity in the injury phase. One is not to place gear shifts on the bicycle frame where genitalia can be struck. A second is further development and wider use of effective helmets or other protective clothing. According to Cross and Fisher[14] in bicycle/motor vehicle collisions *body surface* injuries might be reduced 14 percent by knee padding, 11 percent by helmets, 9 percent by elbow pads, 8 percent by face guards, 7 percent each by shin or foot/ankle protection, and 6 percent each by gloves and hip padding. It is difficult enough, however, to get people to wear head protection. As yet, there is no good agreement as to what is adequate head protection, and many helmets on the market do not meet those standards that have been established.[30]

Lind and Wollin,[31] however, report that 70 percent of head injuries fall within the area covered by most helmets designed for bicyclists, and that another 8 percent would be covered by helmets that come down to neck level. Only 1 percent of injuries involve pointed objects, supporting their argument that airholes in helmets to make them lighter and more comfortable do not compromise safety.

The third option, at the moment more theoretical than accomplished, is the design of automotibles to cause less trauma to pedestrians and cyclists who may be struck.

13
Pedestrians

Walking is the original and still almost universal means of transportation, being used some of the time by virtually all people, and virtually all of the time by some people, especially in phase 1 and 2 nations. It is small wonder, then, that pedestrians are an important part of the highway injury and fatality problem in every nation. Very interesting differences exist between nations, however.

Injury Patterns

In the United States in 1980 a total of 9,600 pedestrians were fatally injured, representing 18 percent of the highway toll.[1] There were 120,000 injured, or 6 percent of the 2 million reported injuries[1] (and as few as 3 percent of all highway injured, whether reported or not).[2] But, in Kuwait pedestrians were 38 percent of the injured and 58 percent of fatalities,[3,4] in Nigeria 24 percent of the injured and 36 percent of the fatalities.[5] Malaysia reported 22 percent of casualties as pedestrians.[6] In stark contrast is Sweden, where 10 percent of highway casualties are pedestrians.[7]

Because little is known about walking habits in different nations, most exposure-based injury estimates for pedestrians are calculated using miles or kilometers of vehicle travel rather than pedestrian travel. Haddon and Baker estimate that daily pedestrian travel per U.S. resident is 0.25 to 0.5 miles, while in Britain it is 1.25 km/day.[8] They calculate that pedestrian death rates *for those nations* may be 20 to 40 per 100 million person miles, compared to 17 for motorcycles, 1.4 for car occupants, and 0.15 for occupants in bus transportation.

Smeed states that pedestrian injuries do not necessarily increase with increases in motorization and that after an initial rise in injuries further increases in vehicles sometimes result in a reduction in pedestrian injuries.[9] He observes that the ratios of pedestrian plus pedal cycle fatalities and casualties to total fatalities and casualties decreased in seventeen out of eighteen developed countries over a ten-year period. In developing nations where this ratio does not decrease, the overall highway fatality rate does not decline.[10]

International differences exist as well in the distribution of casualties and fatalities according to age (table 13–1). In Rio de Janeiro, Brazil, 65 percent of the pedestrian fatalities were between age 20 and 59, compared to 27 percent in Baltimore, Maryland.[11] Fatalities under age 10 were 6 percent in Rio and 24 percent in Baltimore.

More important, the age-specific annual death rate per 100,000 population in Baltimore was highest under age 10 and age 70 or older, peaking at about 10/100,000 for children age 5 to 9 and at about 20 for those age 80 or older. In Rio it rose progressively with age, peaking at about 120 for the very old. Rates in Baltimore for black males was 14.0 and for white males 7.3. In Rio the rate for males was 41. Regarding females, the Baltimore rates were 2.7 and 2.3 respectively for blacks and whites and the Rio rate was 14.

Smeed describes a U-shaped curve according to age for pedestrian injuries per unit distance walked, with a minimum for the age 30 to 39 group.[9] Pedestrians age 65 or older have a rate three times the minimum for all injuries but about twenty times the minimum for fatal ones.

In the United States 72 percent of pedestrian fatalities are urban, and pedestrians represent 35 percent of all urban fatalities but 8 percent of rural ones.[1] Smeed has observed that the risk of a pedestrian becoming a casualty increases with population density, the rate of increase being greater for minor than for serious injuries and for serious than for fatal ones.[9] Thus, although the risks of injury are greater in high-density areas, the proportion of crashes with fatal or serious injuries is greater in low-density areas.

Human Factors in the Pre-Injury Phase

We will examine youth and inexperience, old age and disability, alcohol use, and risk-taking behavior by both drivers and pedestrians as human factors in the pre-injury phase. Havard notes that injuries are the leading cause of death under age 15, with highway deaths, especially to pedestrians, as the most important cause.[12] Even babes in arms or on backs may be at risk. In phase 1 nations where mothers carry small infants with them as they do their chores, these infants often become casualties as well if the mother is struck.

The time of highest risk, however, is shortly after the child begins to walk and is permitted to move away from the house (or moves away unpermitted) but as yet lacks concepts of risk, experience, the speed of an adult, and the visual field or the conspicuity that a taller person is

Table 13–1
Distribution of Pedestrian Injuries by Age, United States and Nigeria

	<5	*5–14*	*15–24*	*25–44*	*45–64*	*65–74*	*≥75*	*Total*
U.S. injuries	7.5%	30.8	21.7	20.8	12.5	3.3	3.3	99.9
Fatalities	7.0	13.1	18.1	21.1	19.6	8.3	12.6	99.8
Nigeria injuries	3.7	26.0	18.7	42.3	6.3[a]	3.0[a]	—	100.0

Source: Adapted from *Accident Facts, 1981 Edition* (Chicago, Ill.: National Safety Council, 1981); S.E. Asogwa, "Deaths and Injuries on Nigerian Roads," *Journal of Traffic Medicine* 6(1978):52–54.

[a]Age 45–59 and 60 or over.

afforded, especially in the presence of obstacles. Thus, Havard shows that age specific pedestrian casualty rates per 100,000 inhabitants are highest between age 6 and 9[12] (for example, for England, 239 under age 6, 441 age 6 to 9, and 277 age 10 to 14). Similar patterns exist for fatalities as well. A Swedish study places the age of greatest risk at age 3 to 8.[13] The difference may either reflect the method of grouping or some national difference in the age at which children are permitted certain activities. In the United Kingdom by age 8 all but 14 percent of children are allowed to go to sweet shops unaccompanied and all but 26 percent are permitted to go on errands, visits, and so forth on their own.[12]

Ability to obtain and deal with visual cues is particularly important. Vinje's review of the literature[14] shows that:

1. the child is hampered by limited field of view because of lower eye level;
2. even without obstructions children still have less ability to deal with peripheral cues because they take longer than adults to react to movement in the peripheral fields; and
3. in scanning a visual field young children do not plan their search but are directed by conspicuous parts of the visual field, such as something new, surprising, or emotionally involving. Until age 5, they lack control of attention. From then on control grows but still is not effective in ignoring irrelevant information. At about age 6 or 7 they learn to differentiate situations requiring more systematic search. But a real focusing on relevant information occurs only in children of about 11 years old. This is reflected in observations of 150 children whose mothers were waiting for them on the other side of a street.[15] Most children age 4 to 5 crossed the street quickly without looking around. The children age 6 to 7 looked around but then ran across, as did the younger children. The majority of children age 8 to 9, however, walked across the street, looking around before and during crossing.

One common pattern involves a small child who suddenly darts into the road from between two cars or other obstacles. Until the last minute the child—usually under age 7—is not visible to the motorist, nor is the motorist visible to the child. The Skandia Report explains that stationary vehicles restrict vision in one-fifth of all pedestrian injuries.[13] Small children prefer to cross the street on straight stretches because they see traffic more easily there than at street corners where too many things happen at once.

One of the most graphic examples of pedestrian problems involving aging and medical impairment is provided by Haddon et al., who observed clustering of fatally injured elderly pedestrians in a small area.[16] The reason was that residents of a home for the elderly were forced to cross a busy intersection in order to make purchases at a neighborhood store.

In attempting to cope with traffic as pedestrians, the elderly often are hampered by reduced vision and hearing, slowed locomotion, and difficulty in dealing with stress of multiple stimuli requiring rapid decision. In addition, some elderly must deal with transient ischemic attacks, dizzy spells, or other acute signs and symptoms of chronic diseases that may occur while they are exposed to traffic. Once struck, they are more likely to have serious trauma and because of medical complications are less likely to survive even moderate trauma. This is why the elderly show a modest overrepresentation among injured pedestrians but a marked overrepresentation among the fatalities.

Because many handicaps are subtle (such as reduced visual acuity, visual fields, or hearing) and not likely to be picked up in usual crash investigation, it is difficult to estimate their contribution to pedestrian crashes. Snyder and Knoblauch state that pedestrian old age was a factor in 3.6 percent of 1,500 cases on which they have health interview data.[17] Drawing from data elsewhere in the report, it appears that 13 percent of injured pedestrians were age 60 to 80. If so, impairment associated with old age may have been a direct factor in over a quarter of the injuries in this age group.

In a Bako et al. study, among 153 pedestrians who contributed to their fatal crashes, 32 (21 percent) were under age 15 and 41 (27 percent) were age 60 or older.[18] By contrast, 18 percent and 16 percent respectively were under age 15 and age 60 or older among 50 pedestrians who did not initiate their crashes.

Overall, 63 (41 percent) of the "responsible" pedestrians failed to yield to an oncoming vehicle. Forty-five of these were persons age 15 or older and 23 (51 percent) of this adult group were elderly but not impaired by alcohol. The unanswered question here is why these elderly people failed to yield. I suspect impairments related to aging played a role.

The classic work of Haddon et al. in 1961 left no questions about the role of alcohol among pedestrians in fatal pedestrian/vehicular crashes.[19] In that study 74 percent of adult fatalities who died with six hours had alcohol, as compared to 27 percent of the site-matched controls, but 42 percent versus 7 percent had BACs of 0.10 percent by weight or greater. Other U.S. studies as well have shown 30 percent or more of fatally injured pedestrians with BACs in this high range,[20] and a note on pedestrian injuries in Moscow states that half of the fatalities were "drunk."[21]

Persons age 60 or older have alcohol and high alcohol concentration less often than do younger persons. In one study, 68 percent of adult pedestrian fatalities under age 65 had been drinking, whereas 22 percent of elderly fatalities had positive BACs.[22] Since elderly persons are more likely than younger persons to have delayed deaths and therefore not to have BAC testing, there is a modest bias in all of the alcohol studies toward estimating that more people had alcohol than probably is the case.

The only other study comparing injured and fatally injured pedestrians with pedestrians not involved in crashes was completed in New Orleans, Louisiana, in 1975.[23] Whereas the risk of crash involvement clearly rises with BAC, it does not rise as quickly for pedestrians as for drivers; in other words, an alcohol-impaired pedestrian appears able to maneuver safely at a higher BAC than can an alcohol-impaired driver; but even at BACs under 0.10 percent both groups have measurable increase in crash risk. In one study at least 10 percent of drivers who struck pedestrians were known to have been drinking and all of these drivers were felt to have been "responsible" by independent assessors who did not know their BACs.[22]

Waller examined the relationship between pedestrian BAC and responsibility for the pedestrian/vehicular crash.[24] Among pedestrians age 15 to 59 with no alcohol in their blood, 23 percent were "responsible" for the crash, whereas 61 percent of those with BACs of 0.10 percent or higher were "responsible." The New Orleans study showed that alcohol-impaired pedestrians were particularly likely to be involved in crashes in which they darted out from between parked vehicles, dashed into an intersection, struck a vehicle that was already passing, or were involved in otherwise nonclassifiable activities, such as lying in the roadway.[23] Some injured pedestrians are individuals whose cars have stalled or been damaged on freeways and who consequently step out of their vehicles.[25] A fair proportion of these are believed to be under the influence of alcohol and are too impaired to protect themselves. As with alcohol-impaired drivers, a majority of alcohol-impaired pedestrians have stigmata of alcohol abuse or frank alcoholism.[26]

So far we have been examining the pedestrian injury primarily in terms of characteristics and behaviors of the pedestrian. We next consider interactions between pedestrians and drivers and the processes that lead to a decision by either or both to take risks.

Snyder and Knoblauch note that in urban collisions five different behaviors account for slightly over half of all pedestrian crashes.[17] These are: "dart out" between intersections in which the pedestrian is struck when less than half-way across the street (24 percent), dart out in which the pedestrian gets more than half-way across before being struck (9

Table 13–2
Blood Alcohol Concentrations of Pedestrians in Crashes and Matched Comparisons and Relative Risk of Crash Involvement

BAC (percentage by weight)	*Fatalities*	*Injured*	*Comparisons Matched for*			*Risk Based on*		
			Age/Sex	*Site*	*Random*	*Age/Sex*	*Site*	*Random*
0.00%	49%	51%	} 84%	87%	93%	1.0	1.0	1.0
<0.05	2	9						
0.05–0.09	4	4	3	5	4	2.1	1.5	1.9
0.10–0.14	11	6	6	4	3	1.7	2.6	4.5
0.15–0.19	8	7	4	2	0	2.1	4.5	} 37.7
0.20–0.24	9	10	3	1	0	5.2	10.3	
≥0.25	18	13	1	2	1	37.9	13.2	
N	80	143	155	967	80			

Source: Adapted from R.D. Blomberg, D.F. Preusser, A. Hale, and R.G. Ulmer, *A Comparison of Alcohol Involvement in Pedestrians and Pedestrian Casualties* (Norwalk, Conn.: Dunlap and Associates East, Final Report on Contract DOT-HS-4-00946, 1979).

percent), pedestrian dash across an intersection (9 percent), multiple threat to the pedestrian (3 percent), and a vehicle turn or merge with an attention conflict (7 percent).

In commenting about this type of terminology, Haight and Olsen tartly argue that "dart out" is described as a pedestrian appearing suddenly from the roadside.[27] It is described from the viewpoint of the driver. For the pedestrian, it is the car that appears suddenly. An "intersection dash" is defined as a person running across an intersection, again reflecting a bias toward the driver; a car driving across an intersection could as easily be said to engage an "intersection dash." The entire taxonomic system, they note, is gravely flawed, being oriented toward classifying pedestrian rather than driver behavior.

Jacobs et al.[28] examined behavior of drivers and pedestrians at crosswalks in several nations. About three-quarters of drivers stopped for pedestrians who entered zebra crosswalks in London and Reading, England, during 1967. The London figure was only 40 percent ten years later. By comparison, the proportion of drivers willing to stop for pedestrians in crosswalks was only 0.2 percent in Indonesia and ranged from 10 to 17 percent in Cyprus, Kenya, Thailand, Turkey, Pakistan, Sri Lanka, and Jamaica.

Whereas average delay times in getting across the street were 0.5 seconds in England, they were 19 seconds in Indonesia and 6 seconds in Bangkok, where pedestrians commonly experienced long delays at crossings because few drivers would stop for them.

How did pedestrians respond? In Britain, almost nine out of every ten pedestrians near a crosswalk used it, whereas in other nations the proportion was less than half. Why should they use crosswalks if drivers ignore the requirement to yield?

Baker et al. have shown that drivers who strike pedestrians often are individuals with large numbers of previous citations, including license revocation or suspension, that a majority of those convicted for killing a pedestrian receive a total punishment of less than a $50 fine, and that many are subsequently in trouble on the highway within a few months.[22]

Returning to fatalities in Rio and Baltimore, Baker found that in Rio the pedestrians being killed often are healthy young men who are *not* under the influence of alcohol and who have been struck while crossing a freeway.[11] Why? Since adequate access for pedestrians from one side of a freeway to another is necessary but wasn't provided, pedestrians are forced to take risks that they can avoid in places such as Baltimore, where pedestrian access is given greater consideration. Even in the United States, Haight and Olsen observe that, with few exceptions, pedestrian safety laws are not enforced because officials believe enforcement would be unpopular and not worth the effort.[27]

Given an environment that often forces pedestrian/vehicular interaction, risk-taking behavior often occurs because both parties have assumptions that fly in the face of physical reality. Pedestrian injury rates in San Diego, California, are twice as high per unit users in marked crosswalks as in unmarked ones, perhaps because of assumptions about safety that pedestrians have in the delineated areas.[29] Drivers in crashes with pedestrians often express surprise that the pedestrian thought the driver could stop quickly and therefore risked stepping into the street. The implication is that the pedestrian lacks a basic knowledge of practical physics.

On the other hand, pedestrians are surprised that drivers make no attempt even to slow down when they have ample time to see pedestrians. The driver, it turns out, often assumes that a pedestrian is capable of seeing more and of stopping faster than is the case, especially as we have identified regarding young children. Allen et al., in fact, have shown that, at least in dusk and darkness, pedestrians commonly believe that they can be seen further than is really so.[30]

In many cases, therefore, drivers and pedestrians take risks, not because they don't care but because they believe their behavior is not risky. Often they are wrong. Unfortunately, also, official attitudes as expressed in laws and law enforcement do not give pedestrian traffic any degree of equity with vehicular traffic.

Vehicular Factors

Although the environment appears to play a more important role than the vehicle in the pre-injury phase, four vehicular issues can be identified. Given the fact that both pedestrian and driver often have little advance notice of each other's presence or actions, the fact that brakes vary widely in capability suggests that some impacts are occurring because even at low speeds the driver has exceeded braking capabilities of the vehicle.

At night the driver can easily outride both the headlights and the braking capabilities of the vehicle. Smeed says that the number of adult pedestrian injuries per million kilometers walked is about one in midday but about ten during midnight hours.[10] Alcohol use by both drivers and pedestrians increases in late night hours, and at least some of the increase should be attributed to this fact.

Wet roads seem to increase pedestrian injuries by about 5 percent in daylight and by about 90 percent in darkness.[9] Darkness and wetness also increase the severity of pedestrian injuries, which are least severe on dry roads in daylight (when 4.1 percent of injuries are fatal) and most severe on wet roads at night (when 7.8 percent are fatal).

Inadequacy of mirror systems on all vehicles, but especially on trucks and buses, is also an issue. Thus, a small but constant proportion of pedestrian impacts involves vehicles that have backed into or onto pedestrians.[17]

The fourth situation involves specific types of vehicles that attract pedestrians (such as ice cream trucks) or that take on and discharge passengers (such as buses).[17] The first motor vehicle fatality in the United States was a person getting off a trolley car, and half of U.S. school bus fatalities each year are children just about to get onto a bus or who have just stepped off.

Environmental Factors

Nighttime and wetness, described above, cannot be altered. Other aspects, however, can be modified. The most important of these is that in virtually every nation the pedestrian is forced to interact with vehicles but without equity. In many nations they get pushed off or struck on bridges or narrow roads by trucks and cars.

Disabled vehicles in Yugoslavia are unable to pull off the road because there is no "off" to pull to. In the United States and elsewhere shoulders are often so narrow that even on freeways a person who gets out to change a tire is still close to or partly in the travel lane. Consequently, especially in slippery weather, pedestrians dealing with disabled vehicles often get hit and killed.

At intersections pedestrians have trouble seeing and coping with vehicles that turn into their paths during crossing. This is now more difficult in the United States with laws that permit vehicles to make right turns at intersections when the light is red.

A typical pattern in Rio de Janeiro is that the pedestrian needs are completely overlooked, forcing them to take extreme risk that may kill even the quick and the able.[12] As Baker reports, traffic lights are rare in many places where pedestrians have to cross heavily traveled routes. In a ten-block stretch of busy beach-side road, there was not one traffic light to help pedestrians reach the popular Copacabana beach. She also notes that 27 of 115 pedestrians killed were on a single high-speed highway fifteen miles long that divides a densely populated area. The highway can be safely crossed only by widely separated overpasses that are difficult to climb, forcing pedestrians to take chances by dashing across six lanes of traffic, sometimes with bicycles and children.

Differences between the two cities in overall pedestrian death rate and age distribution suggests that the pedestrian's task is far more difficult in Rio than in Baltimore. In Baltimore, pedestrians have an easy test that is failed only by the weakest or least capable; in Rio, the test is failed by capable persons as well. Pedestrians should not be forced to decide between an easy or quick way and a safe way. They should be the same.

Considering needs of very young children, Preston found that boys have higher injury rates than girls, especially while playing in or at the edge of the street, and that rates are higher in neighborhoods where there is more overcrowding. Lack of safe play spaces may be the main reason why some areas have high rates, and provision of attractive play areas would reduce injuries to young boys in the worst areas.[31]

Finally, there is the small but unnecessary number of workers who are injured as pedestrians in construction or maintenance areas.[25] As with other vehicular problems in these areas, these events often reflect the fact that inadequate warnings and lane delineators and barriers have been set up by construction or maintenance crews who know or care little about how to alert the driver so that he may have sufficient time to react.

Crash and Post-Crash Factors

During the 1960s Wakeland graphically documented the extent to which sharp hood ornaments and protrusions on automobile bumpers were causing unduly serious trauma to pedestrians.[32] Young children tend to go under an automobile after being struck, whereas taller persons are thrown onto the hood (and hood ornament) or, with faster moving vehicles, into the windshield. The pedestrian then falls and contacts the road surface where additional serious injuries may be incurred. The nature of the injury depends on the configuration of the front of the vehicle.[32,33] Table 13–3 shows typical injury patterns for pedestrians.[34] Heavier vehicles create more serious injury, as does higher speed. Adoption of the 55 M.P.H. speed limit in the United States in 1973 was therefore associated with a reduction not only in occupant deaths but in pedestrian fatalities as well.[27]

Regarding the post-injury phase, if the crash occurs at night, and especially if the driver is guilty of hit-and-run behavior, the pedestrian may be tossed to the side of the road and not be found for several hours. When the injured pedestrian is found, whether immediately or after a delay, the elderly may receive less strenuous attention than do younger persons.[35] Since the elderly comprise such a large proportion of injured pedestrians, this problem is particularly relevant.

Table 13–3
Distribution of Serious and Fatal Injuries in 187 Fatally Injured Pedestrians

	Serious and Fatal	*Fatal*
Number of body areas injured	639	306
Head	22%	34%
Neck	12	26
Thorax	16	25
Upper extremity	5	0
Abdomen	10	12
Pelvic	14	3
Lower extremity	21	0

Source: Adapted from D.F. Heulke and R.A. Davis, *A Study of Pedestrian Fatalities in Wayne County, Michigan* (Ann Arbor, Mich.: Highway Safety Research Institute, University of Michigan, HSRI Report Bio-9, 1969).

Countermeasures

As Snyder and Knoblauch have identified, a wide range of pedestrian crash configurations exist.[17] It is difficult, therefore, to focus on any single countermeasure or group of countermeasures that will affect a large portion of the problem.

Given the limited capabilities of children, education would seem to offer little in prevention. On the other hand, this age group is most impressionable, most eager to learn, and most likely to emulate behavior of adults. Television programs such as Sesame Street in the United States have considerable educational impact. With respect to pedestrian safety, young children are more responsive to an authority figure than to an animated comic book character,[36,37] and they respond to demonstrations of real rather than simulated traffic situations.[38]

With this in mind, a film and TV spot effort, entitled "Willie Whistle," was developed and tried in California.[39] Its goal was not necessarily to guide children to intersections and crosswalks, where they are often overwhelmed with stimuli, but rather to prevent "dart-out" and "dash" behavior, no matter where they decide to cross. The method, therefore, was to offer steps to be followed on starting to cross the street. Preliminary evidence indicates that this program is being seen and internalized by children and is associated with about a 20 percent reduction in dart-out impacts in the age group at whom it was directed.

It is far more difficult to change hazardous behaviors of persons impaired by alcohol and of the elderly. Members of the first group commonly are too impaired to cope, while the latter often are too set in their ways. Weiner observed that a substantial proportion of elderly pedestrians who had just been warned by a police officer for jay walking promptly repeated the same violation in the next few minutes![40]

Education and enforcement of laws regarding driver behavior is another possible approach. Drivers take their cues from the fact that little official attention is paid to the rights of the pedestrian as a road user. Where government authorities indicate a concern that drivers stop when a pedestrian steps off the curb—as in Britain and the state of California—the proportion of compliant drivers rises markedly. Blomberg et al. have developed a series of model regulations aimed at improving pedestrian safety.[41]

One approach to help pedestrians get safely across intersections or crosswalks is to ban parking of cars near these locations so that a broader visual field is afforded to both drivers and pedestrians. This will work only if it is strongly enforced and, equally important, if drivers have enough parking space elsewhere so they aren't tempted to park despite the enforcement.

A second approach is to place a barrier on the sidewalk so that pedestrians are unable to cross where particularly hazardous contacts between pedestrians and turning vehicles are likely to occur. Avoiding right-turn-on-red legislation is another countermeasure, as is use of signals that stop all vehicular traffic during part of the cycle. Since many elderly persons have poor vision, linking the pedestrian part of the cycle with an audible signal, such as a bell, will give people an additional cue as to when it is safest to cross. Of course, traffic lights themselves are an important countermeasure.

In the United States it is assumed for signal timing that pedestrians walk at a rate of four feet per second. This probably is excessive for some elderly and impaired persons, especially if they have to cope with vehicles turning into their paths.

Risk can be reduced for some impaired persons by having a healthier person do shopping for them, therefore removing them entirely from the roads. The meals-on-wheels program for the elderly serves such a function. Where large numbers of elderly persons are clustered, placement of shopping and other services on the same side of the street or in other ways accessible without contact with vehicular traffic will also limit exposure to risk.

In 1967 Bartholomew examined pedestrian injury rates in seven highly congested neighborhoods before and after playgrounds were constructed.[42] Their construction was followed by a significant decrease in injuries. This was more pronounced in the one quarter-mile zone around the playgrounds, and very few pedestrian injuries occurred immediately adjacent to the recreational facility.

Reflectorized clothing markedly increases conspicuity of pedestrians even for alcohol-impaired drivers,[43] and when crosswalks are illuminated they have a marked reduction in nighttime pedestrian impacts, whereas there is no change in daytime impacts, or in crashes at unilluminated crosswalks.[44]

Separation of road users is costly but in some places is worth it. Wide shoulders and pull-off areas for disabled or parked vehicles are needed. Freeway crossovers that are too widely separated and that require people to climb steps with bicycles, baby carriages, and packages get little use and force people to choose more risky modes of crossing.[11]

It may be better but in the short run more costly for highway departments to have pedestrian crossovers at grade level and to lower the freeway at these spots. If the total cost to society of injured people and medical and other emergency services is considered, the higher cost to highway departments may more than balance out.

Turning to vehicular countermeasures, standardization of color and warning devices on school buses is appropriate, as is use of pop-up stop signs and flashing lights on ice cream trucks. Such devices on ice cream trucks resulted in an average reduction of vehicle speeds near the trucks from 29 M.P.H. to 16 M.P.H. and a 77 percent reduction in child pedestrian injuries at these locations.[45] Improvements of vehicular braking and lighting systems and improvement of mirrors for trucks and buses have already been mentioned. Many trucks are now fitted with audible warning devices to alert pedestrians when the vehicle is backing up. This should be required on all such vehicles. Limitation of maximum weights for trucks, removal of sharp exterior components on vehicles, and use of energy absorbing materials for bumpers are all potentially useful countermeasures in the crash phase. Reducing maximum speed limits is another documented way to reduce crash severity for pedestrians.[27]

14
Rail Transportation

Just as the automobile and airplane have become the modes of transportation in developed nations during the late twentieth century, so the train was the major people mover over longer distances during the century preceding. It is still an important transport medium for materials throughout much of the world and remains more important for carrying people in Europe, Japan, and several other nations than it is in the United States and Canada.

Relatively speaking, deaths and injuries involving rail transportation are not common, and most involve collisions at automobile crossings. In years past deaths were far more common to railroad employees and passengers. The reduction in these deaths reflects fewer people exposed and especially newer and safer technology.

From 1947 to 1973 the average death rate per 100 million passenger miles traveled in the United States for rail transportation remained around 0.16, compared to 2.5 to 3.0 for motor vehicle travel during the earlier years and declining to about 1.9 during the early 1970s.[1] The ten-year rail death toll from 1969 to 1978 was 19,185, of which only 128 were passengers, 1,505 employees, 13,091 nontrespassers, mostly at crossings, and 5,461 trespassers.[2] In the late 1930s there were 6,000 to 9,000 untoward events per annum. This increased to between 10,000 and 16,000 during the 1940s and early 1950s and then declined rapidly to under 4,000 by 1958. It then rose again to about 10,000 at present.[3,4] At the same time the number of collisions between two or more trains was decreasing from an average of 200 between 1936 and 1940 to less than 80 during recent years,[3] and the number of deaths was dropping from about 5,000 in the 1930s and 1940s to 1,400 in 1980.[5] Passenger deaths declined from an early average of over 50 to fewer than 10 over the past several years, and all other categories of death (employees, trespassers, and nontrespassers) have also declined.

Grade crossing collisions also decreased, as have grade-crossing fatalities and total fatalities. (A change in 1975 in the definition of a reportable grade crossing collision resulted in a sudden increase from about 3,200 such events to about 11,000 per annum. The statement about a declining trend is based on pre-1975 patterns. There is no way to compare that with the post-1975 years.) The 1930s and 1940s saw an average of 30,000 to 60,000 reportable injuries per year. This declined to 18,000 to 20,000 in the early 1970s, but with a change in the definition of a reportable injury in 1975, the figure went up over the next five years to between 54,000 and 74,000 injuries annually. Again, there is no way to compare the pre- and post-1975 data.

Collisions: Human Factors in the Pre-Injury Phase

Overall, human factors and equipment defects account for less than a quarter of all train mishaps, with track defects comprising about 40 to 45 percent of causation.[4] At present, collisions are the most important source of deaths and injuries. Periodically, anecdotes appear of crashes caused by alcohol-impaired train personnel, but no documentation on overall frequency is available.[6,7] In one English study, over a three-year period forty-two drivers were so impaired that they had to be removed from their trains.[6]

Another human factor involving personnel was perhaps more of a problem in the past. In the absence of a regulatory or scheduling system, railroad management selected individuals who could move trains quickly and who were willing to take risks in order to keep their jobs. The legendary Casey Jones in fact died while taking such a risk, and the songs about this crash are a romanticized example of this policy.[8]

Similar risk taking occurs among drivers of trucks and automobiles that approach grade-level railroad crossings and among trespassers on railroad rights of way. At open crossings drivers approach the track more slowly if vision is obstructed but even when they know a train is scheduled to come, are unlikely even to look up and down the track.[9] Some studies have shown that at least one driver in twenty—and sometimes many more—are willing to drive a vehicle across the tracks after a warning signal or even a mechanical barrier has been activated by an approaching train.[10]

Waller reported that 30 percent of automobile drivers and 64 percent of adult pedestrians had been drinking in fatal collisions with trains.[11] Eighty-seven percent and 73 percent, respectively, of crashes between the hours of 6 and 11 A.M. and noon to 5 P.M. did *not* involve alcohol, whereas 65 percent and 73 percent between 6 and 11 P.M. and from midnight to 5 A.M. *were* alcohol related, often with extremely high BACs in persons with histories of previous alcohol arrests. Elderly persons in crashes appeared to be confused or unaware of the trains, and younger persons without alcohol were attempting to outrace trains at crossings.

Wigglesworth, however, reports that only 10 percent of drivers had alcohol and in most cases a law-abiding citizen had momentary decrement in performance, unrelated to breach of any regulation.[12] Frequently, there was lack of conspicuity of the train, made worse by wet weather, diverted attention, and sun dazzle.

Similarly, Green states that 13 percent of fatalities in rail/vehicle collisions in Michigan had alcohol compared to 27 percent of all vehicular fatalities.[13] He attributes the difference to the fact that collisions with trains more often occur during the daytime when use of alcohol is less. His data, however, are incomplete and in some cases may represent simply police impressions.

Collisions: Environmental Factors

Several environmental factors in collisions are now only of historical relevance in the United States. Jones notes that collisions between trains in the United States declined from an average of 220 between 1936 and 1940 to about 80 during the 1960s.[3] In part, this reflects fewer train trips. But in large part, he points out, it also reflects seven environmental changes, as follows:

1. The engineer now has a clearer view of the track and signals because diesel or electric trains eliminated the boiler, firebox, and steam smoke.
2. Electric colored lights can be seen further than semaphore signals.
3. The trend toward "block" trains (trains handed to railroads by mines, factories, and so forth in completely marshalled form) removes need for further formation movements during which injury events may occur.
4. There is two-way radio communication between driver and conductor.
5. Improved emergency flares protect the rear of disabled trains.
6. All freight trains now have continuous automatic brakes that prevent the rear segment of a divided train from running back and hitting another train.
7. In 1936 only 1,000 miles of track were under Centralized Traffic Control, but by 1968 it was over 40,000 miles (one-fifth of total route mileage).

The Federal Railroad Administration publishes reports that of 215,000 crossings, 72 percent involved warnings of crossbuck type or less, 21 percent some form of lights or bells, and 8 percent gates.[14] The FRA also calculates crashes per crossing per year for each of these types of intersections. But without exposure data, these calculations are meaningless.

Berg and Oppenlander calculated the relative protection afforded by various devices to alert vehicles to a crossing or to an oncoming train.[15] Assuming that a painted crossbuck affords no protection, the relative protection of a reflectorized crossbuck is 0.021, a flashing light is 0.195, and a gate is 0.525. In other words, a flasher is over nine times as effective as a reflectorized crossbuck, and the gate is twenty-five times more effective than the reflector and 2.7 times more useful than a light.

Zalinger et al. note that in any one year a crash will occur at 2.5 percent of crossings, and over five years 10 percent of crossings will have one or more such events.[16] In Canada some communities have local ordinances prohibiting trains from blowing their whistles at crossings. The data below indicate relative increase or decrease in hazard if specific environmental features are present:

1. If the crossing is over mainline track the hazard increases 0.138 overall but only 0.037 in rural areas.
2. A flashing light and bell decreases the hazard by 0.070 to 0.073 in both areas, while a gate decreases the hazard by 0.306 in urban areas and 0.147 in rural areas.
3. An antiwhistling ordinance is found only in urban communities and increases the hazard index by 0.170.
4. An increase in road traffic from 100 to 1,000 vehicles per day adds 0.125 to the hazard at urban crossings and 0.099 at rural ones.
5. Doubling the number of trains from ten to twenty raises the urban and rural hazards respectively by 0.063 and 0.016.
6. Widening the road surfce at an urban crossing increases the hazard by 0.006 per foot, three times the increase experienced by widening rural roads.
7. An increase in sighting distance from 100 to 500 feet in rural areas reduces the hazard by only 0.009.
8. A change from 30 to 70 M.P.H. for cars in rural areas decreases the hazard by 0.035, while increases in train speed from 10 to 30 M.P.H. and 30 to 90 M.P.H. respectively increases the hazard by 0.118 and 0.038.
9. Factors that by themselves were found not to be significant overall were number or alignment of tracks, alignment of roadway, width of shoulder, grade of roadway, angle between roadway and track, and clearance between utility wires and roadway. Factors significant

only in rural areas were speed limit for trains or roads, sightlines, and road surface. Some of these variables—for example, number of tracks—are highly correlated with number of trains and track type but do not explain any variation in hazard not already covered by these other factors.

Many of the factors discussed here, including the existence of a right-of-way owned by the railroad, are to be found only in developed nations. A far different picture exists, for example, in Peru, where one-room houses open right onto the railroad tracks and young children can toddle or crawl onto them. Cummings and Molnar quote a study indicating that 14 percent of amputations in children in Chicago involved contact with 600-volt direct current in electrified third rails while playing around tracks.[17] Ideally, where railroad right-of-way exists there should be a fence to reduce the likelihood of trespassers in high-population areas, especially where high-speed trains are in use.

Particularly during rush-hour traffic, platform areas on rapid transit lines may become so loaded with would-be passengers that there is high risk of someone falling or getting pushed onto the tracks. The National Transportation Safety Board indicates that these falls are most frequent at car/floor height platforms[18] that lack barriers in order to enhance faster discharge and receipt of passengers. In urban areas, they note, there are few other places where the public is allowed to gather next to an unprotected opening that is four-feet deep and potentially lethal. For example, we do not expect elevator patrons to stand next to an open pit while waiting for an elevator.

That report also notes that third rails sometimes have no protective covering at all and that while satisfactory signal devices exist to separate trains, engineers are often permitted to ignore them, but with no clear instructions regarding when or how the message should be overruled.

In one study, a quarter of train/vehicle collisions involved the other vehicle crashing into the side of the train. Between the locomotive with its light and whistle and the caboose there are often up to a mile of freight cars without reflectors or other warning devices to alert a driver at night that the track is not clear. One solution is reflective devices on the sides of all rolling stock.

Collisions: Factors in the Injury and Post-Injury Phases

Early steam engines often had "cow catchers" in front that pushed animals off the track. Whether they worked or not, the goal clearly was to avoid injury to others. Modern rolling stock, however, lacks energy-moderating devices to reduce the effects of the overwhelming weight disparity between a train and almost any vehicle it hits.

Air-crash investigation techniques sometimes have been applied to train crashes.[19,20] According to one such report, most railroad passenger cars are designed first for longevity and easy servicing, second for passenger comfort, and hardly for passenger safety.[20]

One early train was the motor train, which had one to three cars. These vehicles carried mail and thirty to seventy-five passengers and were powered by an internal combustion engine in one of the cars. One reason why these vehicles fell out of favor is that they were ill designed to survive in collisions with much heavier locomotive-pulled trains with which they shared the rails and in collisions often caught fire because gasoline fuel leaked.[21]

Flammable and toxic materials carried by many freight trains have the capability of destroying large areas and substantial populations surrounding any collision. Factors that determine whether such a disaster occurs and what its extent will be are:

1. How much hazardous material is being carried?
2. Does a car with hazardous material derail and, if so, does it roll over?
3. The integrity of the containers. Are loading and discharge valves and coverings on tank cars leakproof?
4. Are several cars of hazardous materials grouped together so that a fire or explosion in one is likely to affect the others, or are they separated by other cars not carrying hazardous wares?
5. Have trains carrying hazardous materials been routed through areas with relatively low population density?
6. Are emergency services able to determine readily which cars carry hazardous contents, what the hazards are, and how to deal with them most effectively to avoid both short-term and long-term dangers (such as pollution of watersheds)?
7. Do emergency health services have appropriate disaster response plans that have been well rehearsed?

In collisions and derailments spillage of contents is most likely if cars uncouple (one couple would slide up vertically over the other) and then topple. The overriding coupler may strike the tank head, puncturing it. New regulations required couplers that cannot override each other. Tank cars are also required to have thermal protection or insulation to reduce the likelihood of presure buildup and explosion if they are exposed to an external heat source.

Shortly after these new regulations went into effect a freight train carrying both old and new type cars derailed in Texas.[22] No uncouplings, punctures, or dents attributable to override occurred in cars with protective couplers. In contrast, uncoupling occurred in 96 percent of the twenty-seven car ends connected with old-style couplers. None of the cars with protective couplers had head puncture attributable to coupler strike, but four head punctures and nine head dents were found in the twenty-seven ends without protective couplers.

Some cars were insulated against solar heating that can protect against a 2,200°F fire for twenty minutes. In contrast, a bare tank will survive this temperature for only four minutes. Three of the five thermally protected cars remained intact on exposure to fire, one was breached by fire but not explosively, and one ruptured violently. The single unprotected car also exploded. The investigators concluded that the evidence suggests thermal protection and insulation delayed violent ruptures.

Derailment

Derailments occur because of collision, failures in rolling stock, or more commonly, inadequacies of rails and rail bed. In nations such as France and Japan, where rail transportation is widely used for passenger travel, modern high-speed systems use continuous rail rather than old-style jointed rail. In most areas, however, jointed rails are used, resting on a subgrade, ballast, and nailed to wooden ties.

Based on numerous interviews with railroad officials, Tyworth and Reinschmidt describe a typical hypothetical medium-sized and financially weak class 1 railroad located in the northeastern region of the United States.[23] Main-line conditions are fair to poor, utilizing 1930s jointed rail with some rail-end batter, poor insulated joints, and inadequate surface grinding. Ties are in fair to poor condition, with last major renewals in the early 1950s, and have deteriorated because of derailments, single-shoulder plates, and missing spikes.

Surface and alignment problems result from these rail and tie conditions and poor drainage. During a recent season, 10.3 miles of the main line were under 5 M.P.H. slow orders, and there were numerous 10 M.P.H. slow orders on approaching bridges and at rail crossings. This track handles about 5,250 trains per year, with 3 locomotives and 70 cars per train. In another section of the main track there are 5.7 rail defects per mile per year and over 1,000 defective ties per mile.

The United States rail system has 8,000 derailments per annum in climate and terrain that are generally more amenable to rail transport than in many other areas of the world. In such other areas torrential rains, heavy snow accumulation, and rugged mountain terrain are constantly undermining the subgrade.

Tyworth and Reinschmidt indicate that one-half to two-thirds of expected savings achieved through track maintenance come from increased train speed with the other third to half coming from fewer derailment-related costs. Total costs of a derailment are about two or three times the direct costs. The average cost per derailment in 1977 was $16,000 in system costs plus $5,000 for wreck clearance.

They conclude that for most lines improved track maintenance will result in sufficient savings because of improved speed and fewer derailment costs to provide economic incentive for improvement, but track safety standards may not be worthwhile or necessary for low-density line segments, especially where hazardous materials are not involved. They urge emphasis on maintaining high-density segments where frequency and severity of derailments are greater.

Given limited resources, the necessity to make decisions such as these regarding the most appropriate allocation of resources cannot be denied. But a decision to downplay safety on low-density lines—as they suggest—should be permitted only where hazardous materials are not being carried; for where they are being carried the surrounding community is being asked—or forced—to share in a risk that may benefit only the railroad company.

Furthermore, under economic pressures, there is the ever-present urge to shave costs by exceeding low speed limit requirements on less adequate track segments. Tyworth's and Reinschmidt's assumption that posted speed limits will be followed needs to be validated before their conclusion can be accepted.

Failure of Rolling Stock Equipment

Equipment failures of rolling stock, such as brakes or couplings, "hot boxes" or failures of axle bearings, dragging equipment, and locomotive failures are of considerably more importance historically as causes of derailment and injury than they are at present. Sensing devices to alert crews to hot boxes or dragging equipment have reduced the frequency of serious results from these events although, even where such equipment is available, it is not always used.[18] Widespread conversion to diesel and electrical energy has largely done away with boiler explosions.

Injuries While Coupling or Braking or Stoking the Fire

Between 1897 and 1906 the two most dangerous occupations, based on mortality data, were brakeman and fireman on the railroad (with railroad engineers and conductors in the fourth and fifth positions behind electrical linesmen).[24] In fact, from 1902 to 1908 the Interstate Commerce Commission recorded 14,888 deaths and 218,082 injuries among trainmen! While railroading is still one of the more dangerous occupations, relatively speaking, it no longer plays as prominent a role, largely reflecting new technology, such as automatic coupling devices that do not require human contact, automatic braking systems for all cars that avoid having brakemen run along a moving train, and diesel or electrical engines that do not require exposure to open fire.

Such changes were often fought, however, by industry management. When federal regulations in 1893 required automatic couplings on all U.S. trains, industry spokesmen said the cost would put the railroad out of business.[25] They considered it less costly *to the railroad* to lose manpower through coupling-related injuries than to install the far safer automatic coupling devices. The cost to the employees, their families, and the public appears not to have been considered relevant.

Injuries to Passengers Who Fall from Equipment

In many developing nations overloading of trains as well as of trucks and buses is the rule and, as a consequence, passengers occasionally fall off. In the United States and Canada passengers who fall from trains are primarily individuals who have illicitly "hitched a ride," often in a dangerous location where they hope not to be discovered.

Countermeasures

As noted throughout this chapter, many of the relevant countermeasures have already been applied: for example, automatic couplers and braking systems and conversion to diesel or electric engines. Others already identified still need far wider application, in particular, separation of other traffic from approaching trains, better visibility for sides of trains, protection for elevated platforms and reduced access to electric rails, improved track, and the whole range of structural changes for both passenger and freight cars to improve crashworthiness. It is clear from the preceding discussion that most of these are feasible and that their effectiveness has been documented.

15

Water Transportation and Recreational Boating

The data on this subject are notoriously poor both within the United States and internationally. Where commercial vessels are involved, the reporting requirement for a "casualty" in the United States is any of the following:

1. physical damage to property in excess of $1,500;
2. damage affecting the seaworthiness or efficiency of a vessel;
3. stranding or grounding, whether or not damage occurs;
4. loss of life; and
5. injury resulting in incapacity lasting more than seventy-two hours (but not including injury to harbor workers unless 1–3 are also involved).

In the absence of a uniform international data collection and analysis system, casualty data collection procedures vary from one nation to another in their bases for calculation and in their standards for accuracy.[1] U.S. Coast Guard staff I have spoken with in Washington, D.C., feel reasonably comfortable with data for larger ships but were extremely skeptical about reporting of injuries for ships under 1,600 tons in size. Also, they noted, many fishing vessels leave the United States with limited crew and pick up foreign nationals once underway. Even deaths of such individuals, they believe, may not be reported.

Even if all injuries were reported, the seventy-two-hour disability criterion is not comparable with reporting criteria for National Safety Council, National Health Survey, Occupational Safety and Health Administration (OSHA), and other injury categories reported throughout this book. Because of international concern about inadequate health data on seafarers, the ILO and WHO have held meetings on this subject since 1949[2] and in 1973 WHO established a Pilot Health Center in Poland to obtain data on morbidity and injuries among seafarers.[2]

A reportable recreational boating event using U.S. Coast Guard criteria involves personal injury or property damage exceeding $100, but California requires reporting of all mishaps. A study of five state reporting systems indicates that the states themselves believe 90 to 100 percent of fatalities, but perhaps as few as half of property-damage-only events, are reported.[3] However, in 1974 California had reported events for 0.001 percent of all registered craft. At the same time, an insurance company had a 4 percent claim rate for its California craft.

It is estimated that at least 10,000 to 20,000 unreported reportable events occur each year among 500,000 registered boats in California. Furthermore, not all boats are registered. In 1976 only 7.7 million recreational boats in the nation were registered of an estimated 9.1 million in use.[4] It is also believed that in some cases casualties are being counted twice.[3]

Injury Experience

Keeping these limitations in mind, between 1970 and 1976 there were 320 to 477 fatalities annually on U.S. commercial vessels. A quarter to a third were on fishing vessels.[4] In 1976, for example, 52 of 477 deaths were to passengers, 16 to longshoremen or harbor workers (note that their deaths from shipping activities when not on board a vessel are not counted), 355 to crew members, and 54 to other individuals. Between 1970 and 1976 the mean number of seafaring jobs of U.S. ocean-going flag ships of 1,000 gross tons or over was 27,000, with mean annual deaths of 68, an annual death rate of 2.5 per 1,000 workers.

At the WHO Pilot Health Center injuries (both on and off duty) comprised 13.3 percent of all seafarer visits to outpatient clinics on shore and "unfit for work" certificates and 23 percent of all working days lost, and were the second most frequent cause for visits but the first cause of lost time.[2] Table 15–1 shows the distribution of all reported casualties in 1975 involving U.S. commercial vessels and of the 199 deaths and 104 injuries associated with them.[5] An additional 112 personnel deaths and 1,221 injuries on commercial vessels, but not considered vessel "casualties," are not included.

Between 1970 and 1976 there were a mean 1,480 deaths per year among about 8.3 million recreational boats (17.9 per 100,000 boats[4] and 0.5 per million occupant hours[5]). On average, 590 of these occurred during cruising or sailing, 290 while fishing, and 165 while drifting, these three activities comprising 70 percent of the total. The modal fatality configuration involved an operator age 20 to 28, on a summer weekend afternoon, with an open outboard motorboat or boat under 16 feet long with no motor (excluding sailboats), and with only two persons aboard. Capsizing or overturning was most common and was in nontidal calm water, with good weather and a light wind.[4]

Nonfatal recreational boating injuries in the United States are about

Table 15–1
Casualties and Related Deaths and Injuries, U.S. Commercial Vessels in 1975

Type of Event	*Casualties*	*Vessels Involved*	*Deaths*	*Injuries*
Collisions	1,213	2,708	34	48
Explosion/fire	183	198	19	26
Grounding	797	1,105	8	8
Founderings/capsizing	241	306	112	5
Heavy weather damage	86	105	0	0
Cargo damage	11	11	0	0
Failure of structure or equipment	756	820	11	13
Not classified	101	160	11	1

Source: *Annual Report to Congress, 1974* (Washington, D.C.: National Transportation Safety Board).

1,000 per year with about 5,000 reported boating mishaps annually.[6] There were 1,242 drownings and 225 other injury fatalities involving water transport (including recreational boating) in 1978 throughout the United States.[7] An additional 5,784 deaths from drowning did not involve water transportation.

Of 1,029 fatal drownings (suicides excluded) in the United Kingdom, 161 were boat related (58 motor boats, 38 rowboats, 28 canoes, and 5 sailboats).[8] Recreation accounted for 107, and in 82 of those the vessel capsized, the remaining 25 persons having fallen overboard. Forty-nine deaths were occupational. Boats were involved in 37 of 134 drownings in Geelong, Australia.[9]

During 1971 there were 4,963 drowning deaths in the United States, all except 952 of which were associated with recreation.[10] In this latter group, 343 involved a person fishing from a boat, 749 persons using powerboats, 113 rowboats, 48 canoes and 39 sailboats.

Human Factors in the Pre-Injury Phase

Recreational boaters commonly have neither interest nor time to learn rules of the water and how to operate a boat properly. Consequently, many mishaps, injuries, and deaths result from failure to observe basic safety principles about not venturing into waters that exceed limitations of the boat, ignoring weather warnings or overloading the boat.[11] These safety rules are not ignored. They are simply not known by the individuals involved.

With commercial vessels, safety and labor qualification standards differ between nations, and a ship's master is guided by the requirements of the nation of registration. However, under "open registry" a ship owned by American or other owners may be registered under the flag of a nation, such as Liberia or Panama, with less stringent requirements than the United States.[12] Ship's crews thus may be a polyglot combination of skilled and unskilled members who have limited ability to communicate with each other.

The most difficult part of vessel operation commonly occurs at the end of a voyage when crew members often are exhausted from standing long watches and other shipboard activities. In this condition they must venture into congested harbors for which no formal system of vessel traffic control exists.[13]

Alcohol is involved in both recreational and commercial boating disasters. A number of studies have reported on the high frequency of positive blood alcohol concentrations among adults who die of drowning or submersion.[9,14,15] Most of them, however, do not distinguish deaths involving boating from other water-related deaths.

Studies should be limited to individuals who have been submerged for six hours or less because with longer submersion fermentation may occur, resulting in endogenous alcohol. In one study alcohol was present in 29 percent of those with only brief submersion but more often among persons with prolonged submersion.[16]

Penttila et al. indicate that alcohol is involved in over half of all water traffic fatalities in Finland,[17] and others as well have reported alcohol in half of fatal submersions of Norwegian seamen and in half of their fatal injuries.[18] The epidemiologic question, if course, is whether alcohol is overrepresented among fatalities compared with uninjured persons at similar times and places.

Penttila et al. surveyed a representative sample of 424 drivers at two motorboat passages in Finland on summer weekend afternoons.[17] A surprising 30 percent had alcohol present, but all except 8 percent had BACs below 0.06 percent (4.0 percent, 3.1 percent, and 1.2 percent respectively had BACs of 0.06 to 0.10 percent, 0.11 to 0.15 percent, and over 0.15 percent).

Dietz and Baker reported alcohol in four of seven persons who drowned while boating.[19] Three had BACs of 0.15 percent or higher. Such deaths often occur when the individual falls overboard while standing up and urinating over the side of the boat. Also relevant is that the prevalence of alcoholism is substantially higher among seamen than among most other occupations.[20,21] Seven percent of seamen who have spent less than a year at sea are alcohol abusers, but this rises to 26 percent among those at sea over four years.[20]

Noted before, ships often leave home port with only a skeleton crew. This practice, calculated to save labor costs, sometimes results in a crew's having to cope with heavy weather or other emergency while shorthanded.[22] The task exceeds human performance in this case simply because a decision has been made to take certain risks.

But this is only one example of broader risk taking involving corporate policy abetted by national and international economic decisions. Because of the open registry system, a nation such as Liberia obtains 12 percent of its foreign exchange funds through registry fees.[12] Flags of Liberia, Panama, Singapore, and other open registry countries—which generally have more lenient safety requirements—fly over 28 percent of total tonnage. Three-quarters of these ships are owned by U.S., Japanese, Greek, or Hong Kong companies.[12] The apparent effects of this system are shown in table 15–2.[23] Clearly, tankers ten years of age or older have higher loss rates than do younger vessels. But at each age, vessels flying flags of nations with stricter safety codes have lower loss rates than do the open-registry vessels.

Older ships may be sold to someone willing to take on the headaches and risks. Often the new owner changes the name. For vessels with a name change during the previous year the loss rate is 1.4 percent. It then drops to 1.15 percent and 1.02 percent for the second and third years after the change, compared to the world average loss rate of 0.44 percent.[23]

About half of vessels in collisions and with cargo fires or explosions are ten years or older. The proportions rise to 73 and 79 percent for other fires or explosions and stranding or grounding and range from 89 to 100 percent for engine and engine room problems and structural failure. Carter says structural failure means than an "old rust bucket" broke up at sea and sank.[22]

Ship's masters sometimes decide to take shorter routes despite

Table 15–2
Total Losses of Tankers by Vessel Age and Country of Registry

	Vessel Age			
Registry	*0–9 Years*	*10–19 Years*	*> 20 Years*	*Total*
Japan	0.09%	0.44%	0.0%	0.18%
United States	0.00	0.22	0.26	0.19
Britain	0.10	0.26	0.44	0.19
Norway	0.29	0.52	0.00	0.37
Liberia	0.29	0.93	1.15	0.69
Panama	0.43	0.49	2.33	1.00
Greece	0.46	1.25	1.11	1.04
World average	0.21	0.59	0.67	0.44

Source: Adapted from A. McKenzie, "Tanker Losses," *Hazard Prevention* 15(3) (January/February, 1979):4–5.

threatening weather. Resulting tanker losses may involve not only a cost to a vessel's owners and insurance companies but also immense spillage and fouling of ocean and beach and disastrous effects on innocent human, animal, and plant inhabitants of these areas. Structural failures were involved in almost a third of all the oil spilled in oceans, and this exceeded losses from groundings and collisions.[22]

The last human factor applies to recreational boating alone. The casualty involvement for persons age 12 to 18 is 1.9 per thousand operators and then drops progressively to 1.6, 0.7, 0.5, 0.4, 0.3, and 0.2 respectively for persons age 19 to 25, 26 to 32, 33 to 39, 40 to 46, 47 to 60, and 61 or older.[24] Data not corrected for exposure wrongly suggest that middle aged adults have highest rates.

Environmental Factors in the Pre-Injury Phase

Size and characteristics of vessel is an issue involving both the largest of vessels—which are unable to maneuver rapidly when change of course is required—and smallest of recreational crafts—which may be of design and materials that permit easy tipping.[15] Dietz and Baker ask whether the least stable sailboats are being made primarily for the least experienced sailers.[19]

Weather conditions and floating or submerged debris are also problems for all water craft. In 1975 out of 3388 commercial casualties, the Coast Guard reported 19 collisions in fog, 292 episodes because of adverse weather, 74 events because of unusual currents, sheer, or suction, and 136 because of floating or submerged debris.[6] In 1972 weather or hazardous water conditions accounted for 7 percent of deaths in recreational boating.[25]

Even the ship *Titanic* was not immune, and this largest of many iceberg-related losses resulted in establishment in 1914 of the International Ice Patrol.[26] In the seventy years since, not a single life has been lost in a North Atlantic iceberg collision.

Besides equipment failures already discussed, hazardous cargo is another environmental preinjury factor in commercial shipping. Such cargo may catch fire or explode or toxic vapors may overcome crew members. Of 3,388 commercial casualty reports to the Coast Guard, fully 774 involved equipment failure, another 30 an unseaworthy vessel, and 13 explosion or fire in cargo.[6] The American experience is far better than that of the open-registry nations.

Engine fires because of flashback have been a problem in motorized recreational boating. This has been dealt with in the United States by requiring all such craft to have antiflashback devices.

Factors in the Injury and Post-Injury Phases

In writing about drowning, Dietz and Baker refer to the pre-immersion, immersion, and post-immersion phases rather than to the pre-injury, injury, and post-injury periods. In broader consideration of all water-related injuries, however, it is appropriate to use the latter terminology.

Severity in collisions or capsizing is determined both by the integrity of the vessel and its ability to remain afloat. In large tankers, use of "double bottoms," with segregated ballast tanks (SBT) located between the cargo and the hull, might prevent rupture of oil storage tanks in collision or grounding and give enough structural strength to avoid breakup.[22] The SBT also will prevent pollution of oceans during normal ballasting operations, which are the largest component of chronic pollution in shipping.

For a number of years the U.S. Coast Guard has required flotation devices in all recreational boats. While these devices keep a boat afloat, they have not necessarily kept it from capsizing or rolling about as people have tried to hang onto it.

The severity of fire is determined by amount and degree of flammable materials on board, presence of extinguishing devices, and ability of people to use them. Fires on both large and small vessels have not been uncommon, but the major approach to limiting their effects has been simply a requirement that fire extinguishers be available. There has been little attempt to limit flammability of cushions, curtains, and other components of the shipboard environment or to provide automatic extinguishment devices, such as inert gas, for holds that contain flammable materials.

Although fire extinguishers may be available, people commonly are not trained in their use, and coordination of fire management would be particularly difficult on ships where crew members speak different languages. Coast Guard staff have told me that loss of life in ship fires occurs primarily because seamen jump overboard without flotation equipment and drown.

Adding to the severity of submersion are the facts that many people are unable to swim, and they do not wear or have ready access to flotation devices. Dietz and Baker describe instances where the swimmers wore life vests while the nonswimmers had no life jackets and drowned.[19]

Consumer Reports points out, however, that most life jackets are incapable of keeping an unconscious person face-up in the water.[27] Those that can do so tend to be uncomfortable and, therefore, are not commercially popular. Recent labeling requirements in the United States now at least inform users about the capabilities or limitations of their equipment.

Blacks are reported to have drowning rates 2.6 times higher than those of whites, possibly because in the absence of bright clothing or swimwear they are harder to see in the water.[19] People who fall overboard at night may be impossible to find before they drown.

Temperature of the water also determines outcome. Many deaths alleged to be from drowning in fact are from hypothermia even in relatively warm water. Keating reports that almost all of the 124 deaths among persons who abandoned the liner *Lakonia* were from hypothermia.[28] Average age for survivors was 47 years and for fatalities 61 years. At an estimated temperature of 17°C (64°F), these people should have survived, he believes, were it not for the fact that old people have less ability than younger people to increase heat production, and to decrease heat loss in a cold environment. He also suggests that in cold water exercise accelerates heat loss, while conventional clothing retards it. Harnett and Bijlani conclude that 16 percent of deaths from recreational boating are from lethal effects of cold water.[29]

Providing adequate emergency and definitive care is a problem with smaller commercial vessels that do not have ship's doctors or anyone else trained in health care. Responsibility for care falls to a deck officer, who can get medical advice via radio but ultimately is limited by his understanding of that advice, the extent of his skills and those of other crew members, and the medicine chest and other equipment available.

Major ship disasters in the 1970s because of equipment failures have led to recommendations and proposed laws requiring all tankers to have backup radar, including a collision avoidance system and improved steering equipment.[22]

In 1966 only one tanker in the world was larger than 200,000 dwt.[22] Ten years later there were 583 of these "very large crude carriers" (VLCCs), or 9 percent of the world tanker population. Based on past experience with other tankers, the incidence of structural failure and catastrophic oil spills will rise dramatically in the 1980s when these ships are about fifteen years old.[22] In this case the stakes are so high regarding damage to a broad segment of innocent people, flora, and fauna that fail-safe mesures seem warranted not only to reduce but to virtually eliminate an unacceptable risk.

Regarding the injury and post-injury phases, double bottoms and segregated ballast systems are needed. Fires can be reduced by equipping tankers to inject inert gas (e.g., stack gas) into the cargo tanks as they are emptied, thus depleting oxygen so that an explosion is impossible.[22] Other forms of automatic sensing devices and/or extinguishing devices are also feasible.

For immersion, flotation devices need to be worn and, if possible, should be of design to support an unconscious person face up, especially if the person may be exposed to cold temperatures. Life jackets also should have a light source so that individuals can be seen after dark, and at least one item of clothing worn should be brightly colored. Neoprene survival suits now permit survival for several hours despite exposure to waters that under unprotected circumstances would kill in a matter of minutes.[33] Over 100 such prolonged survivals have been reported within the short time these suits have been sold in any quantity.

People also need to be taught at an early age how to swim or stay afloat, and those likely to have to ditch in cold water should be advised to wear clothing and to exert themselves as little as possible in order to limit exposure effects.

Lastly, better international standards for emergency care to people injured on shipboard are required, including periodic renewal of first aid certification for ship's officers, training for at least two crew members, and standardized medicine chests with at least annual inspection.

16
Air Transportation

From 1978 to 1980 the death rate per 100 million passenger miles in the United States was 0.04 for scheduled air transport versus 1.30 for automobiles and taxis and 0.15 for buses.[1] Comparable to the patterns with automobile fatality rates, there has been a progressive decline in both commercial and general aviation death rates over the years.[2]

As with water transportation this chapter will describe two different uses and groups of users: (1) commercial or "air carrier" transportation and (2) so-called general aviation, which consists of a combination of business-related enterprises such as aerial application of pesticides, air taxis, and use of aircraft for corporate and executive travel, as well as the use of aircraft purely for pleasure. As with water transport, these two groups share travel space and facilities, often with serious safety problems resulting.

Injury Experience

As of the late 1970s the number of aircraft in the U.S. air carrier fleet was about 3,500, or 10 percent of the worldwide scheduled and nonscheduled carrier fleet, which dealt with 40 percent of all passengers.[3] The U.S. general aviation fleet was approximately 200,000, or 69 percent of such planes worldwide.[3]

Not until 1975 did serious collection of international data on air fatalities begin through the International Civil Aviation Organization. ICAO receives no information from the USSR and probably gets only about half of reportable information from certain other areas of the world.[4]

According to these admitted underestimates, the annual average for commercial air crashes was 1,383 between 1975 and 1980 and 6,750 for general aviation. These resulted on average in 1,425 and 1,893 deaths annually for commercial and general aviation, respectively. Scheduled air services averaged 30 crashes per year in which passengers were killed for 0.36 fatal crashes per 100 million km (0.66 per 100 million miles) and

0.14 passenger fatalities per 100 million passenger km (0.23 per 100 million passenger miles).

U.S. data on air misadventures include some of the best statistics on injury. Reporting is virtually complete, and most events are investigated by the highly qualified multidisciplinary teams of the National Transportation Safety Board (NTSB). Data regarding numbers and rates for both fatal and nonfatal crashes in general and commercial aviation appear in table 16–1.[5,6] while tables 16–2 and 16–3, respectively, provide information on phases of operation in fatal and nonfatal events in both commercial and noncommercial mishaps.[5,6] Table 16–4 shows the causal factors involved.[5,6]

Briefly summarizing these last three tables, nonfatal air carrier events are most likely to occur in-flight, involving turbulent weather and personnel other than the pilot. Fatal events most often occur with collisions on landing, and pilot error and weather are common factors. In general aviation the modal pattern for nonfatal events is a bit less clear, involving problems either in-flight or on landing, with engine failure or malfunction or a loop-serve. Pilot error is involved in eight out of ten cases. Weather is less often a factor in these events. Fatal general aviation events involve pilot error even more often (84 percent), and weather quite often (41 percent). Usually these are in-flight happenings, most frequently with collisions but often with engine malfunction or stall/spin as relevant.

Human Factors in the Pre-Injury Phase

The public has always been anxious about air transportation, resulting perhaps in more official attention to safety than has existed for other modes of travel. Within the industry itself, however, schedules must be met in order to cut costs and fulfill public expectations, and employees feel pressures to cut corners. An NTSB study showed that the majority of in-flight injuries involving turbulence were associated with thunderstorms and could have been predicted,[7] but heavy flight-attendant workloads often compromised ability to monitor passenger seatbelt discipline.

Of even more serious concern, however, is the entire attitude regarding flight during hazardous weather. Lederer tells of a captain of a B-747 who was warned of hazardous icy conditions on the runway and strong crosswinds but who also got a message that unless he took off promptly, curfew regulations at his destination would prevent his landing.[8] Under this management pressure the plane started, slid off the runway, and had $20 million damage.

Testimony following a fatal crash of a commuter airline revealed that

Table 16–1
Event and Fatality Rates for U.S. Air Carriers, 1977–79, and Several Types of General Aviation, 1979

	Average All Carriers (1977–79)	*All General*	*Instruction*	*Pleasure*	*Business*	*Corporate*	*Aero Application*	*Taxi*
Events	27.3	4,023	515	2066	251	84	395	223
Fatal events	5.7	678	41	397	55	15	27	49
With serious injury	12.3	395	39	212	22	5	53	27
Fatalities	391	1,367	—	—	—	—	—	—
Injured (seriously)	?	700	—	—	—	—	—	—
Rate per 10^6 mi	0.0097	—	—	—	—	—	—	—
Rate per 10^5 hrs	.398	9.28	7.85	17.40	2.80	1.68	12.27	4.88
Fatality rate per 10^6 mi	0.0020	—	—	—	—	—	—	—
Fatality rate per 10^5 hrs	0.083	1.56	0.63	3.34	0.61	0.30	0.84	1.07

Source: Adapted from *Annual Review of Aircraft Accident Data: U.S. Air Carrier Operations 1979* (Washington D.C.: National Transportation Safety Board, Report NTSB-ARC-81-1, 1981); *Annual Review of Aircraft Accident Data: U.S. General Aviation, Calendar Year 1979* (Washington D.C.: National Transportation Safety Board, Report NTSB-ARG-81-1, 1981).

Table 16–2
Phases of Operation in All Events and Fatal Ones for Air Carriers, 1970–79, and General Aviation, 1974–78
(percentage)

	Air Carriers		*General*	
	Total	*Fatal*	*Total*	*Fatal*
Static	9.6	7.0	0.7	0.7
Taxi	9.9	7.0	3.7	0.4
Takeoff	11.3	14.0	19.5	12.6
In-flight	41.9	28.1	33.8	67.5
Landing	27.0	42.1	41.7	16.2
Unknown	0.3	1.8	0.6	2.6
Total	100.0	100.0	100.0	100.0

Source: Adapted from *Annual Review of Aircraft Accident Data: U.S. Air Carrier Operations 1979* (Washington, D.C.: National Transportation Safety Board, Report NTSB-ARC-81-1, 1981); *Annual Review of Aircraft Accident Data: U.S. General Aviation, Calendar Year 1979* (Washington, D.C.: National Transportation Safety Board, Report NTSB-ARG-81-1, 1981).

it was regular company practice to falsify fuel weights when carrying a maximum load of passengers and to fly the aircraft overweight if necessary. Following a crash in bad weather that killed 113 people near Kennedy Airport in 1975 the NTSB stated that in high-density terminal areas the air traffic system tends to resist changes.[9] Controllers and pilots try to keep traffic moving, particularly arriving traffic, because delays mean fuel consumption and late or missed connections with other flights. The system becomes even more inflexible as weather conditions worsen.[9]

Recreational pilots, just like recreational boaters, commonly get into trouble because they exceed their own capabilities and those of their crafts, especially in inclement weather. Wick observed that under Federal Aviation regulations a civilian student pilot flies with an instructor from fifteen to twenty-five hours.[10] He may never fly at night, has little instrument training, and only limited experience beyond his local area before being certified as a private pilot. Wick feels that the system to this point is a sound one. The problem is that no further training or refresher checks are required. The pilot literally is on his own.

Over 90 percent of all pilots in the United States are certified for single-engine land airplanes. A pilot who as a student may have flown only a Piper Cub is then permitted to buy and fly a complex, single-engine retractable-landing-geared airplane or a turboprop-powered short takeoff and landing aircraft. Because of limited training and experience, pilots fly into bad weather without checking weather conditions, do careless preflight inspection of the plane, fail to check fuel levels, or crash because the pilot is unfamiliar with the fuel system and doesn't know how to switch to a reserve tank.

Table 16–3
Most Prevalent Types of Events, for All Events and Fatal Ones Involving Air Carriers, 1970–79, and General Aviation, 1974–78
(percentage)

	Air Carriers		*General*	
	Total	*Fatal*	*Total*	*Fatal*
Turbulence	29.8	—	—	—
Miscellaneous/other	10.8	7.0	—	—
Collided with wires, trees, towers	8.3	14.0	7.9	14.1
Engine or propeller failure	8.3	10.6	23.8	12.4
Collision with ground/water	6.1	28.1	8.7	30.8
Gear collapsed	4.4	—	—	—
Fire/explosion on ground or in flight	6.3	3.5	—	—
Collision between aircraft on ground	3.3	—	—	—
Mid-air collision	—	7.0	—	5.1
Stall/spin/spiral	—	5.3	4.4	16.4
Ground/water loop-serve	2.8	—	12.2	—
Hard landing	2.2	—	6.5	—
Under or overshoot	4.2	7.0	4.4	—
Nose over/down	—	—	3.3	—
Air-frame failure in flight	—	—	—	6.3
Total of major causes	86.5	82.5	71.2	85.1

Source: Adapted from *Annual Review of Aircraft Accident Data: U.S. Air Carrier Operations 1979* (Washington, D.C.: National Transportation Safety Board, Report NTSB-ARC-81-1, 1981); *Annual Review of Aircraft Accident Data: U.S. General Aviation, Calendar Year 1979* (Washington, D.C.: National Transportation Safety Board, Report NTSB-ARG-81-1, 1981).

Parker points out that 38 percent of U.S. general aviation crashes in 1976 were weather related (31 percent in Canada) and that 39 percent of those involved flying with visual flight capability (VFR) and without a flight plan into weather requiring instrument flying.[11] The ten most common factors (each listed 150 times or more out of a total of 4,909 factors involving 4,023 crashes) in 1979 read like a litany of incompetence: continued VFR flight into adverse weather, failure to obtain or maintain flying speed, improper operation of brakes or flight controls, improper level off, inadequate preflight planning and/or inflight decisions, mismanagement of fuel, selection of unsuitable terrain, and failure to maintain directional control.[6]

This pattern for general aviation pilots contrasts sharply with both the training and the error patterns for air carriers, whose crews have far more extensive training, experience, and recertification requirements. Errors that occur among them more often involve role confusion among crew members or between crew and controller under demanding circum-

Table 16–4
Causes and Related Factors in All Events and Fatal Ones Involving Air Carriers, 1970–79, and General Aviation, 1979
(percentage)

	Air Carriers		*General*	
	Total	*Fatal*	*Total*	*Fatal*
Pilot	38.6	61.5	80.1	84.4
Personnel	50.0	48.1	9.1	12.4
Weather	46.5	46.2	21.9	40.7
Systems	6.7	7.7	1.6	1.5
Landing gear	10.2	7.7	3.5	—
Air frame	2.9	5.8	1.2	3.5
Power plant	9.1	5.8	14.8	8.4
Airport/airway/facility	8.5	5.8	8.1	1.5
Instruments/equipment	2.9	3.9	0.4	0.6
Terrain	1.8	—	22.4	13.9
Rotorcraft	0.3	1.9	1.1	1.6
Miscellaneous	6.4	7.7	3.7	3.2
Undetermined	1.0	3.9	2.5	8.4

Source: Adapted from *Annual Review of Aircraft Accident Data: U.S. Air Carrier Operations 1979* (Washington, D.C.: National Transportation Safety Board, Report NTSB-ARC-81-1, 1981); *Annual Review of Aircraft Accident Data: U.S. General Aviation, Calendar Year 1979* (Washington, D.C.: National Transportation Safety Board, Report NTSB-ARG-81-1, 1981).

stances. As one example, all may focus attention on a single problem instead of letting one deal with it while others continue to focus on their specific job areas.[12] Or, especially with pilot and air traffic controller, each may assume that the other has authority and responsibility to make a decision.

Alcohol is involved in at least a moderate proportion of fatal general aviation crashes, but rarely in air carrier mishaps. In 1964 Harper and Albers reported that alcohol was present in 35 percent of a series of 158 pilots killed in general aviation crashes.[13] Twenty-eight percent had BACs of 0.05 percent or higher.

Half of these individuals crashed within the first eighteen minutes of flight, and 18 percent did so in the first twelve minutes. Stall-spin crashes occurred in 33 percent of alcohol crashes but 13 percent of general aviation fatal crashes. Their sample, however, included tests on only 33 percent of pilot fatalities, thus introducing a question whether selection biases existed, a problem affecting other studies as well.[14] In a 72 percent sample involving 116 pilots, Ellis et al. found that 31 percent had BACs of 0.015 or higher.[15]

Because of delays in discovery, Dille says that, as with drowning, fermentation may create endogenous alcohol.[16] While 29 percent of 4,000 fatalities had alcohol, 55 percent of those involved samples that contained microorganisms capable of producing alcohol.

Extremely relevant is a study of 16 instrument-rated pilots at BACs of 0.00, 0.04, 0.08, and 0.12 percent.[17] Some were experienced, others inexperienced. At 0.04 percent, both groups showed significant increases in the number and potential seriousness of procedural errors, including ILS tracking errors in the inexperienced pilots.

At higher alcohol levels experienced pilots had minor errors, but less experienced pilots lost ability to track the vertical component of ILS. The number of major procedural errors rose almost linearly in both groups. At 0.12 percent BAC, catastrophic failures began to occur so that the safety pilot took control of the aircraft on sixteen of thirty flights. Two pilots became incapacitated with severe vertigo, nausea, and vomiting while flying by instrument. It is concluded that the *legal* BAC while flying should be no higher than 0.04 or 0.05 percent.

Regarding effects on inexperienced pilots, Harper and Albers noted overrepresentation of such pilots among their fatalities with alcohol, only three of fifty-six of whom held current instrument ratings.[13] Hricko reviewed driving records of forty-seven pilots in alcohol-related general aviation crashes and found that 30 percent had prior offenses involving alcohol, usually for DWI or public drunkenness.[18] The 30 percent figure, he said, is probably the tip of an iceberg involving alcohol problems.

Except for pesticide contamination in fatally injured crop dusters, examinations for other drugs generally have identified very small proportions of pilot fatalities with positive findings. Lacefield et al. found that over half of the agricultural pilots had below-normal cholinesterase levels, suggesting a continuing problem of acute and/or chronic pesticide toxicity.[19] Among aerial applicators, 6.9 percent had BACs of 0.05 percent or higher as compared to 8.7 percent of fatalities in other general aviation.

The subject of aging and physical or psychological impairment has been a source of much controversy among pilots and those who regulate their activities. Some aspects of the flying task can be quite demanding, and if failure occurs, the effects will be more serious than in typical automobile crashes.

Ebneter has categorized the flying task for jet transport aircraft into a series of pilot stress levels based on work load, skill demand, and anxiety involved.[20] Table 16–5 is an adaptation of his data and graphically demonstrates the effects of stress. This is one reason why there has been so much concern that the physical and psychological qualifications of air crews be sufficient to deal with extremely demanding situations.

Expansion of the air transport industry began after World War II utilizing healthy young pilots with military training and experience. Those commercial pilots and air crew have been aging and accumulating

Table 16–5
Relation between Flight Activities and Mishaps Involving Pilot Error in Jet Transport Aircraft, 1959–74

Stress Level	*Flight Hours*	*Pilot Error Mishaps*	*Mishaps Per 10^6 Hrs*
1	55×10^6	5	0.1
2	24×10^6	19	0.8
3	7.6×10^6	34	4.5
4	5.0×10^6	64	12.8
5	2.0×10^6	71	35.5
6	261,000	53	203
7	48,000	45	937
8	4,344	19	4,419
9	263 (levels 9–13)	13	104,000 (levels 9–13)
10		6	
11		4	
12		2	
13		2	

Source: Adapted from A. Ebneter, "Aircrew Error Rate Determination," *Hazard Prevention* B(3) (January/February 1977):17–19.

the medical conditions that accompany old age. In 1938, for example, United Airlines had one pilot age 50 to 59.[21] This rose to 1,650 in 1978. Between 1938 and 1966 the company's rate of medical groundings per 1,000 man years was 1.28 for pilots age 30 to 39, 4.13 for those in their 40s, and 10.01 for staff in their 50s. Almost half were for cardiovascular disease.

This disease group can precipitate sudden incapacity, especially under relative hypoxia, which is the environment in which flying occurs. The typical pressurized cabin simulates an altitude of 6,000 to 8,000 feet above sea level. If the plane is not pressurized, the oxygen deficit may be even greater. As a result all pilots, whether air carrier or general aviation, are required to have medical examination and certification every two years, and the air carrier pilots are retired at age 60.

Within this system few medically related crashes occur. In 1979, of 4,023 total mishaps and 678 fatal ones in U.S. general aviation, a total of 44 fatal crashes were reported to involve "incapacitation" or "physical impairment" and one involved a known "psychological condition."[6] In nonfatal events 11 were associated with incapacities or physical impairment.

Buley, Lane, and Chapman, among others, have tried to examine the frequency, causes, and effects of air crew incapacitation in air carrier operations.[22,23,24] Between 1962 and 1968 the 32 to 51 member airlines of the International Air Transport Association (IATA) reported 51 nonfatal incapacitations without warning in a total of 154,000 pilot years of exposure. The estimated annual incidence by age per 1,000 pilots of in-flight sudden complete incapacitation was as follows: under age 30—0.0002, age 30 to 34—0.0174, 35 to 39—0.0275, 40 to 44—0.0645, 45 to 49—0.1098, 50 to 54—0.1983, and 55 to 58—0.3615.

Chapman states that reaction and overreaction to pilot incapacitation, especially involving heart disease, has in part resulted from widely divergent definitions of the term.[24] In a fourteen-year period IATA reported 163 cases of acute in-flight illness, of which 17 were fatal. The majority involved gastroenteritis. Only thirteen (9 percent) of the non-fatal "incapacitations"—but all seventeen deaths—were cardiac in origin.

Of the thirty cardiac episodes, five (15 percent) are believed to have led to crashes. Such an incident rate applied to the U.K. pilot population would yield one fatal crash to a U.K. registered multi-crew public transport aircraft every thirteen years.

Using a different data base Lane calculates the probability of an incapacitating event causing a crash at 7 percent, rather than 15 percent.[23] But the probability can be reduced even further. Reflecting the widely divergent definitions of the term, a questionnaire survey of practicing pilots revealed 1951 episodes of in-flight incapacitation, 76 percent of which involved gastrointestinal symptoms, 14 percent earache or headache, 0.6 percent "faintness," and 0.3 percent vertigo or disorientation.

Regarding vision, one study suggests that pilots with monocular vision have no more difficulty in landing (although accomplishing the task differently) than do pilots with binocular vision,[25] while another study indicates reduced performance only for monocular pilots who were not permitted to adapt to their altered vision.[26] In a third study, monocular pilots had no more difficulty than matched controls in securing and retaining licenses or endorsements on different aircraft types or in accumulating flying hours, but the monocular pilots may have been involved in more hazardous mishaps and events than the controls.[27] Dille and Booze, however, reported crash rates of 21.1 per 100,000 recent flight hours for general aviation pilots versus 11.6 for the total active pilot population.[28] The rate for those with deficient color vision was 15.0 (not a significant difference, although there was a significant difference based on cumulative flight hours), while that for pilots with deficient distant vision was 11.0.

Despite the higher in-flight incapacitation rates for older pilots Booze found that after controlling for exposure young pilots with high exposure patterns had the highest crash rates (as did lawyers, physicians, and salesmen). What is not considered is whether these individuals were flying under different types of exposure than were persons with lower rates.[29]

Sanders and Hoffman report an ability to correctly classify 86 percent of aviators in pilot-error military events based on three personality variables.[30] Low-risk pilots are generally more self-sufficient, imaginative, and forthright. High-risk ones relied more on social approval and were more conventional, practical, worldly, socially aware, and willing to cut corners.

It is not possible to predict crash experience based either on recent life changes[31] or on biorhythms,[32,33] but Phillips found a significant increase in general aviation crashes killing both the pilot and one other person during the week after widely publicized murder-suicides.[34]

We turn finally to the role of the air traffic controller (ATC). Wiener documents the history of the field.[35] A system of "paper flight strips and mental arithmetic" was swamped by the volume and type of post–World War II air traffic. Using radar and then computers provided respite for additional years. But now the computers are overloaded.

As already noted, one of the major problem areas when a potentially hazardous situation becomes apparent involves uncertainty as to just who has the necessary authority and responsibility for what actions. Wiener suggests that one reason for this is a class difference between pilots and controllers, similar to that between doctors and nurses.[36]

Danaher believes that despite its limitations the ATC system basically functions well.[37] He says, however, that controllers sometimes cause or contribute to crashes and incidents through improper phrasing of communications, temporary lapses in attention, use of improper control procedures or techniques, and faulty judgment. In some pilot-caused crashes, controller action did not actually contribute, but a more alert controller might have averted the event. In other cases, however, pilots overlooked opportunities to avert controller-caused crashes.

Recently a system was established through NASA to permit air crews to report near midair collisions (NMACs) and related incidents in a nonpunitive environment.[38] The purpose of the Air Safety Reporting System is to identify potential hazards through study of near misses and thus avert some disasters. The rates of NMACs in air space with two methods of direct controller supervision were 14 and 18 per million operations per year, compared to 8 for airspace near terminals in which the controller has more of an advisory role. However, no one knows what biases of reporting might exist.

One thrust of Danaher's paper and that of other authors in a special issue of *Human Factors* is that controllers (and aircrews) can become overly reliant on automated equipment that was provided simply to complement standardized safety practices. As a result, they sometimes deviate from these practices, and collisions occur. Improved equipment, the authors point out, is no better than the attention that is paid to the interface between the equipment and its users.

Vehicular and Environmental Factors in the Pre-Injury Phase

The divergence in size and capabilities of airplanes is awesome, ranging from the tiny, slow Piper Cub to the jumbo jet or the Trident, and from the short take off and landing space for the helicopter and STOL to long runways for takeoff and landing needed for jets. All of these aircraft use the same terminal airspace and demand attention of the air traffic control system.

Even within categories important differences in capability are to be found. Crash rates for commercial craft per 100,000 aircraft hours flown show almost a tenfold variation from a low of 0.366 for the B-727 to a high of 3.401 for the L-188.[5] Fatal crash rates rise from none for two models (BAC 1-11 and Y.5-11), and 0.040 for the B-727, to 1.361 for the L-188.

Similar differences occur in the crash rates involving engine failure among single-engine and multiengine aircraft used in general aviation.[39] As described earlier, engine failure often occurs because a pilot mismanages his fuel or causes fuel starvation. Some makes and models of aircraft seem more prone to fuel mismanagement, suggesting that pilot error is something more (or less) than simple human mistake but involves some form of machine/user mismatch.[39]

A similar situation exists with the formation of carburetor ice, believed to be a cause or factor in 360 general aviation crashes during a recent five-year period.[40] Although an NTSB study says that these losses can be reduced by greater awareness and vigilance by pilots, the report also states that susceptibility to carburetor ice varies widely among the various aircraft models. An engine with a float-type carburetor is most susceptible to icing, while a direct-cylinder fuel-injection design is least. Theoretically, it is possible to design an engine not subject to icing, but this has not occurred in practice. Therefore, pilots still must remain alert and take preventive actions.

Frank mechanical failure because of design defects has also occurred; for example, cargo doors that depressurized and blew off in several DC 10s, flawed engine mounts in the same planes, and stabilizers in B 707s that developed metal fatigue at an accelerated rate. Philip Handler says in a report on FAA aircraft certifications that if evaluating the regulation of a different technology, aircraft safety could be considered a standard of excellence for comparison.[41]

Because of the large threat to life from even a single loss, however, a fail-safe philosophy with redundancy of safety precautions is required. For this reason the FAA certification process for aircraft design, production, and maintenance was found to be inadequate, despite the fact that only 16 of 216 fatal crashes of jet aircraft were primarily because of equipment failures. The regional structure of that agency was found in part responsible for fragmenting the work of engineering specialists among different functions, differing interpretations of regulations between regional offices, poor communication among personnel on issues of common interest and experience, and inability to maintain a cadre of highly qualified engineers.

Also recommended were earlier review of fundamental design concepts, the need to consider all possible failure modes of specific aircraft components despite a feeling that certain types of events just couldn't happen, unannounced spot checks by FAA of the manufacturing process, and manufacturer review of changes in airline maintenance procedures.

In 1979 a court awarded $3.5 million to widows of three pilots who were killed in a 1968 air crash.[42] The court found that a major manufacturer of aircraft instrumentation had poorly designed a flight director system so that because of its location the button was inadvertently activated while the plane was on its final instrument approach. This caused the plane to follow the wrong signal so that it stalled and crashed, killing twenty-eight. The decision reversed the findings of an NTSB investigation that had attributed the crash to "pilot error."

As long ago as 1947 researchers identified repeated pilot errors in reading and using aircraft instruments because of design features.[43] A conventional altimeter showed 15.9 percent errors, 11.7 percent errors of at least 1,000 feet, and an interpretation time of 7.1 seconds. In contrast, an experimental model yielded 3.5 percent errors, 0.7 percent errors of at least 1,000 feet, and an interpretation time of 1.7 seconds. "Confusion of controls" was reported to have caused fourteen crashes in 1948 and eighteen in 1949 and there were over 100 crashes those two years attributed to incorrect operation of landing gear. Between January 1943 and October 1944 there were 457 crashes because of confusion of landing gear and flap controls on military planes. Of these, 113 occurred on one model alone.

A quarter of a century later, Bullock described a whole series of cockpit design complaints by pilots relating to pilot accommodation and accessibility to controls.[44] Potential problems have also been described concerning effects of noise and vibration in helicopters[45] and distortion in windshields,[46] most of which already are so small that they offer a restricted view. For specific kinds of operations, such as aerial application of pesticides, some types of aircraft (high-wing monoplanes) appear to make for far more difficult maneuvering, and consequently more crashes, than do others.[47]

Despite this information, it is virtually impossible to identify definitively whether a pilot misread a display or activated a wrong control primarily because of its design features or for other reasons. It is simply possible to show statistically that certain design features are significantly overrepresented, and others significantly underrepresented, in certain types of crashes and to draw logical conclusions.

Instead of talking about the effect of environment on the flying task we will start by considering the effect of jet blasts on safety of the surrounding environment. A three-engine wide-body jet on starting to taxi may cause exhaust velocities of 75 M.P.H. for 200 feet behind the tail and 45 M.P.H. for 350 feet.[48] Personal injury and damage to other aircraft and property is widespread. One example was the demolishing of a small shack so that it in turn damaged eleven vehicles and injured a number of people.

Old runways that are too short for new aircraft types are an increasingly serious problem. In crowded urban areas, where larger craft and longer runways are most likely to be needed, land is scarce, and for political reasons the FAA has often backed off from requiring that runways be lengthened to serve the needs of large aircraft in wet or icy weather.[2] FAA tries to balance the cost of crashes and the cost of runway extensions or airline income and service reductions. In 1966, for example, there were several overshoot incidents, and in late 1967 one passenger was killed when a Boeing 707 ran off the runway during an aborted takeoff. The problem was simply that the runway was too short.

Because of land values, many airports are built on or near bodies of water and in some cases on filled land. This often places aircraft approach and departure paths in conflict with those of birds, and collisions inevitably occur. Jet engines, in particular, may suck in these creatures. Over a recent seven-year period the U.S. Air Force reported over 350 damaging collisions with birds annually.[49]

Visual miscues may occur when pilots make approaches over water at night, looking toward a brightly lit city. The runway appears larger, nearer, and lower than it does when viewed from the same flight path on a clear day, and on several occasions commercial planes have landed in the water short of the airport when approaching at night.[50] Pilots misjudge the height and "tilt" of the runway and consequently make low approaches under these conditions.

As we have already suggested in discussing the pilot/air traffic controller/ATC system triad, the nature of the traffic control system and the equipment available to maintain it are important factors in determining crash experience. Instrumented guidance systems and traffic control systems that give more information over large areas of air space, and that distinguish not only horizontal but also vertical proximity of aircraft, seem to offer best crash experience.[51,52,53] But such systems are of limited value unless they are well integrated with the behavioral patterns and physiological capabilities of the people who are using them.

Weather reports overall are accurate about three-quarters of the time.[54] They are correct a bit more often in identifying storm-associated turbulence but have been less able to warn of clear air turbulence (CAT), which accounts for about half of turbulence related mishaps.[55] CAT forecasting has recently improved,[56,57] but even with excellent equipment and efficient operators the equipment was always meant to be used for thunderstorm avoidance and never as an aid for thunderstorm penetration.[55]

Factors in the Crash and Post-Crash Phases

Despite public impressions that plane crashes are almost inevitably fatal, the data reveal that, as with automobiles, one's chances of survival in a plane crash are related to structural integrity of the craft, wearing of occupant restraints, avoidance of fire and toxic fumes, and adequacy of evacuation, rescue, and emergency care procedures.

Interestingly, the beginnings of crash injury research for motor vehicles began with Hugh DeHaven's survival in a plane in which his fellow occupant was killed.[58] He tentatively concluded that survival related directly to quality of occupant packaging and avoidance of ejection, but his recommendation of seat belts was met with ridicule among pilots. In 1942 he published his classic crash injury research paper in which he identified factors that led to survival in falls from 50 to 150 feet.[59]

Since all ticketed passengers in commercial aircraft are required to wear lapbelts, it is not possible to compare belted versus unbelted adult passengers in plane crashes. Children without tickets, however, often do not wear belts and have far higher death rates, even after correction for area of impact.[60]

Lapbelts have been required in general aviation aircraft since 1926, and their use has been required for takeoffs and landings since 1971. It was not until 1978, however, that the FAA required shoulder harnesses in *new* general aviation aircraft, with as yet no requirement for retrofitting of older planes, despite an estimate that as many as 60 to 70 percent of airplanes used in general aviation will be involved in a crash sometime during their approximately twenty years' use.[61]

Snyder cogently notes that for nearly thirty years general aviation occupants in low-energy crashes have received unnecessarily fatal injuries, although the cabin structure often remains essentially intact.[62] This occurs because in the absence of an upper torso restraint the forward seated occupant may strike sharp structures, in particular with head injury. These problems are easily correctible through engineering design changes. The fatality rate per 100 million general aviation passenger miles is at least seven times that for automotive transportation. Occupants of 1971 automobiles were far better protected against crashes than were occupants in 1971 general aviation aircraft, in which individuals capable of surviving 40g crashes were packaged into cabin-seat-restraint environments that often failed or disintegrated at 10g's.

In commercial crashes massive numbers of deaths have occurred because the upholstery and other cabin materials are not flame resistant and are capable of creating highly toxic fumes.[63] Consequently, passengers and crews have died in clearly survivable crashes. Nonetheless, FAA has been reluctant to deal with the problem, assuming instead that the major threat of fire and in fire involves the craft's fuel. Hazardous cargo has also been a problem that FAA has downplayed.[64]

Even if passengers survive the initial crash uninjured, there are repeated reports of injuries during emergency evacuation.[65,66] Often, these occur when people catch their legs in emergency slides or actually fall off the slide. Some passengers die of immersion and submersion in planes that crash into water. Some passengers pay little attention to crew briefings about safety and to written safety and evacuation materials at their seats because of the unattractive presentation style.[67] Assuming survival through each of these points we must then consider the availability of emergency care.

To the surprise and dismay of many people, airport emergency medical services were left pretty much catch-as-catch-can until the mid-1970s. Even major airports have often had inadequate or nonexistent emergency plans and communications with hospitals and ambulance facilities. It was not until 1976 that the FAA in the United States proposed a rule to upgrade medical preparedness.[68] Duffy emphasizes that such services should include attention to mental health needs of survivors, airline crew, ground personnel, and rescuers.[69] Lane and Brown estimate that in nineteen out of twenty cases the expected load of seriously but not fatally injured persons in a plane crash is unlikely to exceed 25 percent of the largest aircraft using an airport.[70]

Countermeasures

In terms of numbers of events and numbers of people killed, general aviation safety warrants higher priority than does commercial aviation.

Because of mixing of planes, an ill-equipped civilian pilot may put hundreds of commercial passengers at risk.

High priority would go to require that renewal certification for general aviation be linked to refresher training and that certification should more specifically be linked to type of plane being flown. Through simulation, both experience and judgment can be taught to some degree without the necessity of accumulating flight hours.[71,72,73,74] All airports and planes should have instrument capability, as should all pilots, no matter what their craft.

Regarding alcohol abuse and medical certification, despite its occasional lapses, the latter system appears to function reasonably well. Perhaps the major flaw in the system, as with medical examination of automobile drivers, is that it cannot now pick up people with diseases that generally come to medical attention only through history: for example, alcoholism and epilepsy. Closer linkage is necessary between automobile driving records and licensing to fly a plane.[18,75]

Especially in commercial operation I suspect there is an inescapable minimum of sudden incapacitation that must be accepted. Leighton-White and Chapman, however, have properly observed that air crews don't have to sit idly by, however, but can be trained to deal with such events as simply another form of manageable situation.[76,77]

To what extent is further instrumentation likely to be beneficial in air traffic control, especially around air terminals? In-board warning devices can be quite successful in preventing controlled flight into terrain and can do so with an acceptable—but not ideal—number of false alarms.[78]

It is not as clear to me that further instrumentation of air traffic control systems beyond the best currently available will necessarily have more than minimal benefit. Of higher priority, perhaps, is to bring more terminals up to the level of the best ones, to pay much more research and formal attention to how controllers interact with their equipment, with each other, and with pilots, and, at a few of the most crowded terminals, to take the politically volatile but necessary step of separating air carrier and general aviation traffic. Some success has been obtained in removing bird traffic by having falcons around.[49]

Desjardins has explicated eight successful principles for improving crash-worthiness of small aircraft,[79] while Peters provides evidence that in air carrier craft improved crashworthiness prevents injury.[80] The technology for flame retardance and for avoiding toxic fumes already is used elsewhere and needs to be transferred to aircraft. Finally, Abelson et al. point out that over the last decade crashes involving wide-bodied jets show approximately three times fewer fatalities per number of passengers than in piston aircraft.[81] A major reason, they believe, has been better mobilization of emergency services for larger disasters, including bringing hospital facilities to the disaster.

17
Injury in the Home Environment

No discussion of injury in the home environment is appropriate without some sobering comments about people and housing. There are 1.6 billion people under age 15 in the world today. An estimated 400 million of them have spent their entire lives in temporary shelter, and many of them may continue that way for their entire lives.[1]

Although most such individuals are in developing nations, about 25,000 people—mostly middle-aged and elderly—are homeless and shelterless in New York City. They may show up in injury data as persons found in public places with hypothermia or found in abandoned buildings or excavations where they have crawled and died after being injured in a fall, attacked by rodents or wild dogs, and so forth.

We have little information about the injury patterns of people living in temporary housing or, indeed, living totally without housing. Given their makeshift environment, it is reasonable to assume that their risks of injury are large, their likelihood of receiving care is small, and their residuum of unnecessary disability is substantial. But no one knows and few seem to care, either in the Third World or more affluent nations. The injuries of these individuals will not be discussed further, simply because no data exist, not because they are any less important than other people.

Injury Patterns

In the United States as of 1980 the home was the location of 22 percent of all 105,000 injury deaths but 39 percent of all 68 million nonfatal injuries.[2,3] The distribution of home injuries and fatalities appears in table 17–1.[2,4] Actually, the age standardized death rate from home injury in the United States has been declining consistently over the past several decades. In the early to mid-1930s, for example, the rate ranged from 23 to 29 per 100,000 population, whereas in 1980 it was 10.[2]

This reflects changes in death rates from falls, fires and burns, and drownings, a shift in ICD definition of injury deaths in 1948, and a

Table 17–1
Deaths and Injuries through Various Non–Motor Vehicle Modes in the United States and Their Frequency in and around the Home

	Fatalities 1980	*Number (%) in and around the Home*	*Persons Injured (in thousands) 1971–72*	*Number (%) in and around the Home*
All non–motor vehicle causes	52,400	23,000 (56)	54,775	24,012 (56)
Falls	12,300	6,700 (54)	13,611	7,183 (53)
Fires/burns	5,500	4,400 (80)	1,087	706 (65)
Poisons				
Solid/liquid	2,800	2,200 (79)	—[a]	—[a]
Gas/vapors	1,500	900 (60)	—[a]	—[a]
Suffocation				
Ingestion	3,100	1,800 (58)	1,465[b]	632 (43)[b]
Mechanical	—[a]	600	—[a]	—[a]
Firearms	1,800	1,100 (61)	155	97 (63)
Drowning	7,000	900 (13)	—[a]	—[a]
Other	18,400	4,400 (27)[c]	38,457	15,394 (40)

Source: Adapted from *Accident Facts, 1981 Edition* (Chicago, Ill.: National Safety Council); *Persons Injured and Disability Days by Detailed Type and Class of Accident, United States—1971–1972* (Rockville, Md.: Department of Health, Education and Welfare, Vital and Health Statistics Series 10 No. 105, 1976).

[a]Included in other, which includes exertion, bumps, twisting, struck by, cutting, piercing, crushing, pinching, and so forth.

[b]Foreign body in eye, windpipe, or other orifice.

[c]Percentage includes mechanical suffication.

probable shift in the definition of many infant deaths from mechanical suffocation to Sudden Infant Death Syndrome (SIDS) over the past ten to fifteen years. In 1960 there were 1,400 deaths under age 5 classified as mechanical suffocation; in 1980 there were 260.[2,5]

The number of persons injured in the home (requiring medical care or activity restricted) was 10.7 per 100 in 1959–61 and 12.2 per 100 in 1980.[3,6] The decrease in death rate, therefore, does not reflect a decrease in injury frequency but rather possibly a decrease in its inherent severity, an improvement in emergency and definitive care, or both. Nor does it reflect a shift in distribution of injury rates by age. The comparable injury rates per 100 persons by age in 1959–61 and 1980 are as follows: under age 6—21.0 versus 22.8; age 6 to 16—12.9 versus 14.8; age 17 to 44—5.7 (age 17 to 24) and 7.4 (age 25 to 44) versus 10.6; age 45 to 64—7.8 versus 9.9; and age 65 or older—11.1 versus 10.1.[3,6]

The injury rate in the home for women exceeds that for men once past the teen years, but the death rate for males at all ages to even age 75 or older exceeds that for women. However, the ratio of women to men is higher in older age, and therefore women comprise a larger *proportion* of persons injured and killed; but the sex-specific *rates* are greater for men. The death rates from home injury by age for 1980 are: age 0 to 4—15.5; age 5 to 14—2.5; age 15 to 24—5.4; age 25 to 44—5.3; age 45 to 64—8.2; age 65 to 74—19.7; age 75 and older—7.3.[2]

Home injury and fatality data from some nations are nonexistant or presented in incomparable ways. Table 17–2 shows relative proportions of all injury fatalities and of all nontransport injury fatalities that home injuries represent for several nations in a special study.[7]

The distribution of deaths according to age and sex is roughly similar for other nations and the United States. Reasons for death vary with environmental patterns, however. In the United States and Canada poisonings accounted for 8 to 9 percent of home deaths, whereas they were 22 percent in England and Wales and 30 percent in Scotland because of use of utility gas.[7] Burns from kerosene and paraffin lamps and cooking stoves in India, Ceylon, and Hong Kong are a problem,[7,8] as are falls in Hong Kong from high, overcrowded bunk beds,[8] ingestion of kerosene in India,[7] and electrocutions in England and Wales, where house current is 220 volts as opposed to 110V in the United States and Canada. In India a substantial proportion of fatal drownings are in domestic wells.[7]

In the United States unintentional injuries and deaths from firearms have been frequent and primarily in the home, a fact that has not deterred the National Rifle Association from placing its emphasis on

Table 17–2
Home Injuries as Proportions of All Unintentional Injury Deaths and of Nontransport Injury Deaths for Men and Women in Several Nations, 1960

	Percentage Home Deaths Are of All Injury Deaths		*Percentage Home Deaths Are of Nontransport Injury Deaths*	
	Males	*Females*	*Males*	*Females*
Canada	17.9	38.7	35.2	62.6
Finland	11.8	38.1	23.4	54.0
Hungary	17.8	49.3	30.5	62.3
Japan	11.3	32.3	21.8	53.6
Netherlands	18.7	56.4	48.1	86.8
New Zealand	18.3	43.1	34.0	60.2
Norway	23.4	69.3	42.3	84.7
England/Wales	21.2	51.4	44.7	70.3
Scotland	27.3	67.7	46.7	85.6
United States	19.2	39.7	39.3	64.5

Source: Adapted from "Accidents in the Home," *WHO Chronicle 20(1966):3–19.*

courses in hunting safety. In one year, there were 348 deaths among children under age 15 from this cause, and 250 were boys. In England and Wales, with a very rigid law limiting possession of firearms, only twenty-two unintentional deaths occurred in 1962.[7] The year 1980 saw 1,100 unintentional firearm deaths in U.S. homes as compared to 700 elsewhere.[2] This total, however, was outnumbered twentyfold by firearms-related homicides and suicides.

Causal Factors

There will be extensive discussion in the next several chapters of human and environmental factors in injury events within and around the home. At this time, however, I wish simply to provide an overview of the main themes that will run through these chapters.

The major human factors issues, again, are extreme youth and inexperience, abusive use of alcohol, and aging and medical impairment. Regarding the product and environmental contribution there is outright failure (such as building collapse or arcing in an electrical product), undue exposure to extreme hazard (unguarded blades, pinch points, or sharp parts), factors that increase error or have excessive task demand (such as poor lighting, slippery or uneven surfaces, or stoves with confusing knobs), components that increase severity (e.g., flammable fabrics or excessively hard or sharp surfaces) and factors that decrease likelihood of getting prompt care if injury results (hazardous chemicals that are not so labeled).

Young children are particularly vulnerable to injury because of their lack of experience, strength, and skill, which may result in touching hot surfaces, use of an open toy box that closes on the head of a child who has insufficient strength to remove itself, or knocking over a pot of boiling water. Their small size means that hot water, once spilled, may cover the entire body or that a small amount of ingested medicine may represent a fatal dose. In some cases, a head may be small enough to get caught between slats of a crib or play pen. Inadequate locomotion in a toddler results in frequent falls. Lack of experience and poor locomotion may mean inability to escape from a fire.

Many elderly persons have problems of locomotion, vision, and dizzy spells that may result in falls. They may also have decreased vision and altered heat sensation, which increase the likelihood of burns; confusion, which may contribute to several types of injuries; and disabilities associated with arthritis, stroke, or other health problems, which may result in dropping hot or heavy objects. In one study of home and other nonhighway injury fatalities age 15 or older, 10 percent died as a result of injuries incurred during an episode of altered consciousness and another 7 percent died of injuries attributable to other forms of medical impairment.[9] Such conditions probably also play a part in death from complications of moderate injury that a younger or healthier person often survives. Among persons who survived less than six hours after their nonhighway injuries, for example, 11 percent had medical impairment, whereas 23 percent had impairment among those who survived longer before death.[9]

A problem common to both young and old is the frequency of serious injury among persons with epilepsy or similar disorders of consciousness and, at least temporarily, of mobility. Such individuals are more likely to fall onto a hot or otherwise dangerous surface and once on it to be unable to remove themselves quickly. Consequently, injury is both more frequent and more severe than in less handicapped individuals.

In fatal injuries 54 percent of home fatalities age 15 or older who died within six hours had alcohol and 52 percent had BACs of 0.10 percent or higher. In contrast, 15 percent of adults who died suddenly in the home had alcohol, with 9 percent having BACs at or above 0.10 percent.[9] The vast majority of persons with alcohol had stigmata of alcoholism. Alcohol was found in 22.3 percent of nonfatally injured patients but 8.9 percent of patients treated for illness.[10] BACs of 0.05 percent or higher were registered by 11.3 percent and 2.6 percent respectively. Thirty-one percent of injured men and 15 percent of women had alcohol. Single, widowed, separated, and divorced persons and those in lower social classes had alcohol more often than did married or upper-class individuals.

Of forty-nine fatalities among children under age ten, thirty-five had no environmental contribution, ten product contribution to initiation of the event, and four contribution to its severity.[11] For sixty-two persons age 10 or older with neither alcohol nor impairment, 26 percent had environmental initiation, 6 percent environmental contribution to severity, and another 3 percent contribution to both initiation and severity of these sixty-two deaths.

Where alcohol was involved (forty-two cases), product or environment contributed to the injury phase 31 percent of the time, to pre-injury and injury phases 1 percent, was incidentally involved in 1 percent, but never contributed in the pre-injury phase. Thirty-five individuals had medical impairment as a pre-injury factor. In these cases there was environmental contribution to injury phase in 16 percent and incidental involvement in 3 percent.

Products or environmental components such as walls, stairs, floors, or windows were involved—not necessarily causally—in about 6.8 million injuries in the United States requiring medical attention.[12] About 4 million of these were products or environmental components in and around the house, and the rest recreational equipment. During that time about 10.8 million injuries in the home were medically attended,[2] thus indicating product or environmental involvement in 35 to 40 percent of all home injuries.

With this overview as background, we turn to an examination in the next five chapters of the home environment and injuries common to it. Drowning and firearms-related injuries will be considered under recreational injuries.

18
Issues in Building Design and Construction

While the discussion in this chapter deals with "typical" housing for developed nations, one must remain aware of the many people who have only temporary housing. In Cairo's severe housing shortage 100,000 people live in the local cemetery, while others are in decaying tenements, despite knowledge that annually 12,000 units are destroyed and about 100 people killed because buildings collapse.[1] Squatting in abandoned buildings, in fact, has become a way of life for many in developed nations as well.

Substantial portions of the Asian population live in houseboats or on piers above the water and are subject to the whim of the weather. So are many people living in mobile homes in the United States and elsewhere. If these structures are not properly tied down, they can be easily blown over in a severe storm.

Involvement of various building components in medically treated injuries in the United States appears in table 18–1.[2] Building materials have been included in this list, which totals about 1.8 million injuries per year. As noted in the previous chapter, an environmental component may contribute in the pre-injury phase, may determine injury severity, or may simply have incidental involvement. These estimates do not include injuries treated outside of the hospital emergency departments or not treated at all, two categories that overall comprise about 60 percent of product-related injuries.

Injury rates are higher for persons of lower socioeconomic status who live in delapidated housing,[3] but there is no way of determining whether the higher injury rates reflect effects of the housing, characteristics of residents, or a combination of both. Parents with young children, or older, impaired persons—two high-risk groups—may be less able to afford or obtain new housing than are young or middle-aged individuals without children. Delapidated housing is more likely to catch fire, from which the very young and the elderly are less able to escape. Rat bites clearly reflect housing quality. Where housing and food and garbage storage patterns attract rodents and permit them to nest, these animals

Table 18–1
Annual Emergency Department Visits in the United States Involving Architectural Components and Building Materials

Component	*Number of Injuries*	*Rate Per 100,000 Population*
Stairs	709,000	332.8
Nails, tacks, screws	226,000	106.2
Glass doors, windows, panels	193,000	90.8
Lumber (not part of structure)	129,000	60.8
Fences	95,000	44.9
Bathtubs and nonglass showers	73,000	34.4
Nonglass doors and panels	58,000	27.4
Porches, balconies, open side floors	55,000	26.0
Walls, interiors	51,000	23.9
Bricks, concrete blocks (not part of structure)	44,000	20.8
Pipes, heating and plumbing	33,000	15.9
Window and door sills and frames	31,000	15.0
Sinks and toilets	28,000	13.4
Handrails, railings, banisters	25,000	12.1
Roofs and roofing materials	25,000	12.0
Heating stoves and space heaters	25,000	12.0
Nonelectric wire	18,000	8.7
Cabinet or door hardware	15,000	7.0
Radiators, home	14,000	7.0
Chimneys and fireplaces	14,000	6.8

Source: Adapted from *NEISS Data Highlights. Hazard Identification and Analysis* 4(4) (October–December 1980) (Washington, D.C.: Consumer Product Safety Commission).

may bite sleeping occupants.[3] In Bombay, India, 20,000 cases of rat bite are treated in hospitals every year.

We will now examine specifically stairs, doors, windows, tubs and showers, electrical supply, and sources of heat.

Stairs

In many cases, part of the reason people fall is because they are very young, elderly, or impaired by alcohol. Whether these factors are involved or not, why do these individuals fall on stairs as opposed to elsewhere, and why on certain stairs but not on others? In an intriguing epidemiologic study, National Bureau of Standards (NBS) staff reviewed over 250 residences and then covertly videotaped stairways in public places to determine the frequency and circumstances of stumbles and falls.[4] They estimated that in the United States there were 1.95 billion stairway uses in 1975, leading to 264 million noticeable missteps (13.5 percent of uses!), 31 million mishaps (1.6 percent of uses), 2.66 million disabling injuries (0.14 percent of uses), 540,000 hospital treatments (0.028 percent of uses), and 3,800 deaths.

Particularly hazardous were uneven risers, riser height less than 6.25 inches, tread depth of 12 inches or less, low headroom, distractions on one side (such as pictures, glare, mottling effect from trees), frequent changes in direction of the stair on descent, polished terazzo steps, and tread edges that are poorly defined when viewed from the top either because one step seems to blend into another or because a highly decorated rug has a pattern that attracts more attention than the edges of the treads themselves. This visual confusion is particularly a problem for the elderly.

Presence of a banister decreased the severity, but not the frequency, of falls. While these issues are probably relevant throughout the world, ideal riser height and tread depth may differ in other nations where mean height and stride for both men and women are less than in the United States.

The major system for dealing with common problems and issues of design and construction is to establish and enforce standards by means of building codes, some of which date back to the Code of Hammurabi in 1700 B.C. Some insight into how effective such codes are concerning stairs comes from a study (subsequently referred to as the HUD report)[5] of 15,000 households in twelve U.S. cities.

The study pointed out that stair design and/or construction contributes to the incidence and severity of falls. Nonetheless, no codes dealt with prevention of slipping. Codes had conflicting and nonuniform requirements for stair slopes, riser heights, and tread width and reflect the fact that most designers and builders use values that have been developed entirely from instinct, logic, or arbitrary reasoning.

All codes studied required handrails, although some do not require them on the bottom few steps. However, many rails in the study had been removed or broken and not replaced. Load resistance requirements for hand rails varied from none to 20 and 50 lbs per lineal foot. Height of handrails was usually adequate, but many were of too large a diameter to be grasped in a hurry. Decorative wrought iron railings often have burrs that can catch on clothing and flesh. The physically handicapped or elderly user generally needs a handrail for even a few steps and may need rails on both sides of the stairway.

Most building codes do not deal with the placement of light switches, and consequently many basement stairways have switches only at the top of the stairs. Stairs should have no areas of either glare or shadow. The 95th percentile for vertical clearance on stairs in the U.S. is 73.1 inches, which should be considered in stairway design. Only two codes require solid risers on stairs, despite the fact that a small child can often crawl between steps that have open risers and then fall.

An exceedingly practical and well-designed summary of the NBS stairway and other research has been developed by the Buffalo Organization for Social and Technological Innovation (BOSTI) and will be referred to throughout this chapter concerning frequency of event and remedies that consider injury reduction, design process, initial costs, and lifetime costs.[6] Table 18–2 summarizes 68 percent of the injury events involving stairs and their remedies. One additional remedy is a barrel or basket at the head and foot of stairs to hold objects that otherwise would be placed temporarily and hazardously on the stairs as a reminder that they need to be carried to another level. Shelves placed clear of the path of travel will serve a similar function.

Doors

In the United States there are 835,000 injuries annually involving doors, most often injury to fingers, hands, arms, and heads.[6] Such injuries are most frequent among those age 2 to 4, followed by those under age 1 and those age 5 to 9. Over age 13 a steady decline in rate occurs, suggesting that learning occurs through experience. Injury rates are similar among males and females, and often occur during running, hurrying, or playing. Most result from acts of others or from performance errors by the person injured.

Most injuries (78 percent) occur inside the home, while a smaller—but still sizable number—occur in schools. In 24 percent door glazing is involved in the injury. According to BOSTI, there are over 785 million doors in extensive use in the United States, or an average of 11 per household. (Compare this with the single door to an entire dwelling that is the typical living arrangement in many Third World nations.)

BOSTI data[6] involving 70 percent of door injuries are summarized in table 18–3. The HUD report[5] deals more specifically with building code coverage to prevent injuries involving glass doors. All codes in the United States now pay attention to this issue, and, if enforced, all except the National Building Code ensure that safety glass is included in new construction. However, there is no easy and inexpensive retrofit for construction that predates the codes.

Three types of need are identified regarding glass doors:

1. Body contact must be avoided through increased visibility of the glass, proper handles on doors containing glass, and environmental design that prevents tripping near the glass.
2. The glass must safely resist shocks caused by unintentional contact or misuse.
3. The glass must be made of appropriate material so that injury is minimized even if the practical limits of its strength are exceeded.

The National Building Code fails to meet criteria 2 and 3 because it permits use of decals and muntins in place of safety glass. In fact, because decals often are not at eye level for children, the first criterion may not be met either. In a series of injuries with glass doors, 62 percent involved incorrect type of glass (nonshatterproof), 40 percent absence of markings on clear glass panels, and 15 percent incorrect glass thickness.[5]

One issue not considered in any of the codes is the proper method for installation. If glass breaks, the glazing should permit light pressure to push the glass out of the way but also retain pieces that might fall and cause further injury. Flexible adhesive glazing compound and rubber welt glazing meet this goal, but linseed-oil-based putty does not because it hardens over time. Nor are nonadhesive glazing methods useful for this purpose.

The HUD report notes almost a total lack of codes or specifications concerning doors in general, with attention directed mainly to the fire protection aspect of doors. In particular, it states that springs and cables on overhead garage doors need to be covered.

Windows

The estimated 266,000 injuries annually in the United States involving either residential window frames or glazing represent one injury for every 3,800 windows in use or one serious event for every 250 dwelling units.[6] Eight-one percent are amputations, fractures, or other injuries. Three-quarters are fingers, hands, or lower arms.

The typical injury involves a young male, and 37 percent are children under age 15. Where normal window use is involved, 60 percent of those injured are female. In 30 percent of cases people reported being angry, sick, hurried, drunk, or otherwise temporarily not following their normal behavior. One-quarter of events involved individuals on unstable footing, and in 43 percent the window involved was defective through poor maintenance, often with the defect (e.g., a stuck window) well known beforehand to the person injured. About 19 percent of windows in the Buffalo area had such defects, suggsting that windows should be selected

Table 18–2
Most Common Injury Events on Stairs and Their Remedies

Type of Event	*Number of Injuries (Percentage of Stair Injuries)*	*Remedies*
1. Elderly or impaired person misjudges tread length while descending and oversteps nosing.	505,000 (14.0)	a. Increase tread visibility by avoiding richly patterned surfaces. b. Illuminate flight with directional lighting from the lower landing. c. Use uniformly dimensional treads ⩾ 11 inches deep and riser 5 to 7 inches high. d. Install slightly rounded nosings.
2. Women carrying children or groceries down stairs have obstructed vision or can't turn on lights and overstep nosing. Severity increased by attempt to save child while falling.	290,000 (10.9)	a. If possible, don't place stairs where carrying is expected (such as from parking to kitchen or hamper to laundry room). Maintain flat floor surfaces here. b. Install light switches that can be activated by elbow or back of wrist or hand, as well as by fingers. c. Use uniformly dimensioned threads (see 1c). d. Install clearly visible handrails that break to horizontal in line with top nosing on lower landing and with top landing.
3. Women descending on high heels catch heels on nosing. Small children can't get foot high enough.	239,000 (9.0)	a. Use uniformly dimensioned treads (see 1c). b. Tightly affix tread coverings to avoid protruding edges. c. Use tread surfaces with uniform color and texture with rounded nosing. d. Use tread surface and handrails that stand out visually (use lighter value color).
4. Usually at night, person can't find light switch (or bulb burned out) and uses stairs in dark. Misjudges number of steps or size of tread.	173,000 (6.5)	a. Have two-way illuminated light switches at top and bottom of stairs. b. Increase tread visibility even in dim light (see 3d). c. Use permanent, unswitched low-voltage night light installed one riser height above nosing of second tread from top and at *every* landing. d. Use at least two bulbs for all stairs.

5. Foot too near nosing on descent creates slippage of tread covering material so that foot slides over edge of step.	162,000 (6.5)	a. Use uniformly dimensioned treads (see 1c). b. Affix all tread coverings tightly using durable bonding materials. c. Firmly anchor abrasive nosing strip to subflooring. d. Avoid tread or landing coverings of deep pile or shag carpet, linoleum, or abrasive mats.
6. Persons with crepe or rubber-soled shoes slip when descending wet or icy exterior stairs.	152,000 (5.7)	a. Paint exterior stairs with paint mixed with abrasive additives or use exposed aggregate concrete. b. Use tread materials that allow drainage and wear uniformly without dishing. c. Cover exterior stairs. d. Use heated treads and landings on exterior flights with ⅛-inch drainage pitch.
7. Person can't find or catch handrail on losing balance.	152,000 (5.7)	a. Use handrails on both sides, especially for stairs wider than 40 inches. b. Have adult handrail 2 inches in diameter 34 inches above nosing plus child rail 1½ inches in diameter 24 inches above nosing. c. Use handrail that stands out visually (lighter value and greater saturation than surrounding elements).
8. Person's attention is suddenly distracted by water from overhead gutter, stream of air from exhaust fan, and so forth.	133,000 (5.0)	a. Design stairs that either have no views of adjacent spaces or that have continuous view so no visual surprises occur. b. Design adjacent spaces to discourage placement of TV sets, mirrors, or art objects that can be seen while using stairs.

Source: Adapted from D. Alessi, M. Brill, C. Brady, K. Hammond, A. Schubert, and M. Wigglesworth, *Home Safety Guidelines for Architects and Builders* (Buffalo, N.Y.: Buffalo Organization for Social and Technological Innovation (BOSTI), Report NBS GCR 78-156, 1978).

Table 18–3
Most Common Injury Events Involving Doors and Their Remedies

Type of Event	*Number of Injuries (Percentage of Door Injuries)*	*Remedies*
1. Children or young adults in hurry push on glass to open door and break it or miss hardware and hit glass.	136,000 (16)	a. Install hardware easy to identify and grasp. b. Reduce size of glass and locate it at least 6 inches away from knobs, push plates, or panic bars. c. Use safety glazing (tempered, laminated, plastic). d. Use noninjurious barrier (such as grill) on both sides of glazing.
2. Person breaks glass by knocking on it to get attention or to gain access after locking themselves out, or in anger.	116,400 (16)	a. Alter size and position of necessary glazing to be unattractive for knocking or so inside handles are unreachable. b. Provide door knockers or bell. c. Use safety glazing. d. Use punch code numerical locks or combination locks that don't require keys.
3. Person (often child) on one side of door is struck by someone's opening door from other side who can't see them.	91,850 (11)	a. In building design place doors away from projected high-use areas. b. In room design use furniture to separate door areas from heavy-use areas in room. c. Place vision panels in and near doors to permit children to be seen. Use safety glazing for these. d. In design, selection, and installation of doors try to meet prior expectation of door users (which way door will swing, opens 90°, and so forth).
4. Fingers get caught between door and jamb.	66,800 (8)	a. Use door closing devices that control speed and rate of closure. b. Don't install unnecessary doors. c. Cushion or round door and/or jamb edges where they meet.
5. Children, usually playing with a friend, get fingers caught between door and hinge of jamb.	66,800 (8)	a. Set hinges in deeper or seal off hinge edges so fingers can't get in. b. Cushion or round door and jamb edges.

6. Person (usually age 5 to 25) slips near glass door and falls against glass.	66,800 (8)	a. Use slip-resistant floor surfaces on both sides of all doors. b. Install safety glazing. c. Alter size and position of glass to be away from falling children. d. In building design, position doors away from areas with slip hazard (such as sinks).
7. Person bumps into edge of door left partly open.	41,750 (5)	a. In building design, place doors near room corner so that when open 90° it rests against a wall. b. In room planning, place furniture far enough away so door can open 180° and lie against wall. c. Install door closing devices to ensure door is always either fully opened or fully closed. d. Pad or cushion door edges to reduce severity of injury if edges are bumped.

Source: Adapted from D. Alessi, M. Brill, C. Brady, K. Hammond, A. Schubert, and M. Wigglesworth, *Home Safety Guidelines for Architects and Builders* (Buffalo, N.Y.: Buffalo Organization for Social and Technological Innovation (BOSTI), Report NBS GCR 78-156, 1978).

which require little maintenance. Table 18–4 deals with the five most common injury event patterns responsible for 30 percent of window-related injuries.[6]

In the HUD report, 49 percent of the injuries involved windows that were hard to open, 16 percent each windows that were risky to clean or that were not secure when open and thus fell closed, 13 percent windows located in an awkward position, 11 percent non-safety glass, 9 percent low window sills, 7 percent absent or insecure screens, and 4 percent sharp edges on rollout windows[5] (total factors exceed 100 percent). The several building codes reviewed were virtually silent on design or construction issues dealing with all of these injury causes except for missing screens, the least common of the causal factors.

Tubs and Showers

Forty-five percent of the 152,000 tub and shower injuries each year in the United States are to children under age 10, who comprise 20 percent of the population. Three-quarters of such fatalities are in this age group. Slips and falls are the major type of event, with hot water burns less frequent but more severe. Elderly people are not overrepresented, apparently because they forgo baths and showers as too difficult to perform.

The BOSTI report says that bathtubs far exceed shower stalls both in absolute frequency and severity of injuries. The slipperiness of bathtub surfaces is the major pre-injury hazard, and the hardness is the chief cause of injury. The most frequent contact area in a fall is the tub edge. The hardness and slipperiness of all bathroom surfaces is a problem, coupled with the usual compactness of the bathroom.

Table 18–5 summarizes the seven modes that account for 98 percent of tub and shower injuries. The HUD report critically states that none of the codes are adequate to prevent bathroom injuries. The fact that only 6 percent of bathroom slips were due to wearing out of standing surfaces indicates that built-in slipperiness is a central issue, while service life is only a secondary concern. Nonslip tubs and showers must be required by codes.

Water controls are improperly placed, promoting loss of balance, handles come off easily, and faucet designs don't indicate the direction of movement required to adjust flow or temperature mix. The Federal Housing Administration code requires an electrical outlet near the bathroom mirror, which the report says should be prohibited because it is near water. Nor does the code deal with handholds. A towel rack is not a handhold because it can, and often does, pull out from the wall.

Protruding knobs and soap dishes and sharp edges increase the seriousness of slips in tubs and showers. No specification or code was found to reduce damages from these causes. Redesigned or recessed accessories and controls is one possible solution. Handholds need to protrude but can avoid pinch points, sharp corners, and edges and should be resilient to shock.

Electrical Supply

Relatively speaking, injuries in the home involving electricity are not very common or are not very serious.[5,7,8] One reason for this, at least in the United States and Canada, is that home current for most electrical outlets is 110 to 120 volts, as opposed to 240 volts in Europe and elsewhere.[9] In keeping with Haddon's energy aggregation model, larger currents mean more severe injury.[10] Of the approximately 1,000 electrical deaths in the United States annually, only about 20 percent are from home wiring and appliances,[11] and most burns from electrical currents are not very serious.[5] However, about 20 percent of serious home fires and 10 percent of minor ones appear to have begun in the electrical system.[12]

Electrical appliances are discussed in the next chapter. Here we will consider general issues of wiring and insulation. Four types of patterns are worthy of identification. The first is where an extension cord becomes worn or overloaded and shorts out or where a small child sticks the cord into its mouth.[13] With extension cords, the most *apparent* problem involving shorting is use of too old or too light a cord or intentional overloading, while the misguided action of a child seems to explain mouthing a cord. But the real problem often is that too few outlets and/or circuits have been installed, therefore requiring extension devices that are far easier for a child to mouth than is a wall socket.

For many years, standard fuses and circuit breakers have been far more successful than warning people not to overload circuits in preventing current overloads that can cause electrical fires. They function too slowly, however, to prevent electrical injury because a rather small current is enough to severely shock or even kill a person. The ground fault circuit interrupter (GFCI) is sensitive and responds quickly to these smaller currents and is now required by some codes for bathrooms, garages, outdoor receptacles, and near swimming pools.[14] Of course, installing closures on live receptacles is one way of keeping children away from them.

In recent years the electrical industry in the United States began using aluminum wiring, and at some junctions between aluminum wiring and terminal devices such as wall receptacles, hot spots and fires

Table 18–4
Most Common Injury Events Involving Windows and Their Remedies

Type of Event	*Number of Injuries (Percentage of Window Injuries)*	*Remedies*
1. People (often children) fall on or hit glass while playing, fighting, angry, or incapacitated.	88,200 (33.2)	a. Position windows in locations that discourage group gatherings but still permit access for operation and maintenance. b. Use safety glazing. c. Choose windows with large individual panes and with thicker glass. d. Cover window with nonbreakable, noninjurious barrier, easily removable for maintenance and emergency egress.
2. Arm slips and breaks glass while trying to operate stuck window.	44,200 (16.6)	a. Choose quality windows that are permanently painted, self-lubricating, with nonbinding frames, nondeteriorating sash weights, cords, and spring balances. b. Use safety glazing. c. Choose windows that prevent striking glass even if they are operated when defective (such as deeply recessed glass, bars over panes but not over frame, large easily grasped handles). d. Use nonoperable windows or combination crank operated louvers plus nonoperable glass panes.
3. Men and boys break uninstalled storm windows or glazing while working or playing nearby.	27,540 (10.4)	a. Select storm windows that needn't be stored in summer. b. Use safety glazing. c. Specify window sashes that allow easy removal and replacement of defective glass. d. Provide adequate secure storage for storm windows that must be removed.
4. Person struck while walking by a projecting awning or casement type window	15,970 (6)	a. Recess projecting type windows into wall. b. Don't place projecting type windows on ground floor or near walk areas. c. Select casement windows with an increased opening radius so they can open flat against exterior walls and be firmly held there against wind.

5. Persons with unstable body position who are fixing window or working near windows fall and strike window.	9,650 (3.6)	a. Don't place operable windows over fixed built-in equipment (such as washers, sinks, or bathtubs) or specify crank-operated louvers for such locations. b. Design areas near window to prevent unsafe positioning of people and with nonslip flooring. c. Select window types that can be easily cleaned from a stable position on interior floor. d. Use safety glazing.

Source: Adapted from D. Alessi, M. Brill, C. Brady, K. Hammond, A. Schubert, and M. Wigglesworth, *Home Safety Guidelines for Architects and Builders* (Buffalo, N.Y.: Buffalo Organization for Social and Technological Innovation (BOSTI), Report NBS GCR 78-156, 1978).

Table 18–5
Most Common Injury Events Involving Bathtubs and Showers and Their Remedies

Type of Event	*Number of Injuries (Percentage of Tub/Shower Injuries)*	*Remedies*
1. Children while bathing and adults while bathing or showering lose balance while changing body position, fall, and hit tub edge.	62,000 (40.8)	a. Use nonslip materials on tub and shower floors. b. Use seat and flexible shower hose in tub. c. Securely install grab bars that have rounded edges. d. Design or add on tub edges made with resilient material.
2. Child or adult slips and falls on entering or exiting wet tub.	32,300 (21.2)	a. Recommendations 1a, c, d above. b. Bathtub with slip-resistent edges whose width is suitable as handhold rather than as seat.
3. Person slips, falls, and hits faucets, soap dishes, towel racks, stall frames, and so forth.	15,000 (10.0)	a. See 1a above. b. Recess fittings where possible. c. Use rounded edges on fixtures that must protrude. d. Use enclosed stall door tracks rather than open-grooved types.
4. Person slips on wet bathroom floor and hits nearby fixtures.	14,000 (9.2)	a. Install slip-resistant flooring, such as textured impervious surface or wet-dry carpeting. b. Use tubs, toilets, and sinks with rounded edges and add on resilient materials. c. Install flooring that is resilient foam-backed carpeting or tile. d. Provide hazard-free area near door.
5. Person strikes and breaks glass tub or shower enclosure.	14,000 (9.2)	a. See 1a above. b. Use shower curtain or safety glazing. c. Provide adequate space outside tub/shower area for drying self away from glass.

6. Unattended child climbs into tub of hot water and is scalded.	7,900 (5.2)	a. Install automatic device limiting temperature to under 120°F. b. Install sliding tub enclosure panels with child-proof latches. c. Design layout so child can't reach tub by standing on toilet, shelves, and so forth. d. Use thermometer to warn if water is too hot.
7. Person grabs towel bar or soap dish for support and it breaks away.	4,300 (2.8)	a. Locate securely installed accessories where they can be used as hand holds. b. Install convenient auxiliary support devices. c. See 1d and 2b.

Source: Adapted from D. Alessi, M. Brill, C. Brady, K. Hammond, A. Schubert, and M. Wigglesworth, *Home Safety Guidelines for Architects and Builders* (Buffalo, N.Y.: Buffalo Organization for Social and Technological Innovation (BOSTI), Report NBS GCR 78-156, 1978).

developed because of different coefficient of expansion, oxidation, and corrosion.[15]

Also potentially of concern is the retrofitting of many homes with heavy layers of insulation, which often provide more buildup of heat around recessed lighting fixtures than was originally planned for. Use of only a moderately larger light bulb than recommended can result in very serious hot spots in such cases.[16,17] Furthermore, if fire results, some insulations release highly lethal gases.

When wiring is in walls, rats can gnaw insulation and initiate short circuits and fires. Old housing has more fires, but to identify the frequency of these from rat-caused short circuits would be impossible.

Home Heating Systems

Home heating varies from an open fire in the center of a hut through room stoves and space heaters to central heating. Local heating systems generally are hotter where people can contact them and thus have more injuries (discussed in chapter 20). Furthermore, injuries may occur from fuel preparation, such as logging and splitting of wood. With increasing fuel costs, many people have returned to wood stoves and space heaters. This is a technology that their ancestors knew how to handle, with many injuries but probably with fewer per unit of exposure than the neophytes are experiencing.

Developing Building Codes

What does it cost to include safety in the basic design and construction of a home? According to the HUD report, incorporating safety features in new housing should add less than 1 percent to the total building costs, while additional costs to include safety features in existing and rehabilitated housing will range between 1 and 2 percent of the value of the house.

These economic assumptions are based on reduction of a wide range of common injuries, usually involving kinetic energy. Another study examines specifically the cost per life saved of requiring ground-fault circuit interrupters throughout residential structures.[18] As already noted, electrical injuries in homes usually are minor and rarely fatal. The study estimated a cost of $4 million per life saved.

The HUD report states that building codes prescribe the standards for incorporating safety factors in construction and should be based on living habits and human behavior. If such codes are based on knowledge of these habits and behavior patterns, one would expect similarity between codes regarding important issues. What was actually found, however, were variations so great that they could not be based on scientific or objective criteria. Many code items were expressed in subjective language, based on subjective reasoning, and ignored requirements for family life. The codes were difficult to use, poorly organized, and subject to arbitrary interpretation by local building inspectors. Codes, they note, should cover the entire subject in one place, with clear, concise language expressing intent and purpose. Those same conclusions made in 1970 had, in fact, been identified by the U.S. Senate a half century earlier.

Ventre has examined the process by which technological innovations in the building industry are disseminated, including whether and how they are incorporated into building codes.[19] His observations make clear why it is so important to use a planning process for countermeasures, such as that reviewed in chapter 5.

Building technology, he notes, does advance, and building codes do get modernized, but only to the extent that a sufficient coalition of the building department's clientele concur. Local building departments must turn to their client groups to review potential code changes both because the clients may know about the technology under review and to maintain political legitimacy. The building department's clientele and the construction industry itself are so diverse that no group has the advantage of sole access to the staff during the decision on innovative technology. With potential influence fragmented among so many clients, decisions are influenced by ad hoc coalitions, and this accounts for the apparent irregularities in code development.

Ventre's study substantiates the widely made allegation that, overall, building trades unions vigorously resist building code accommodation to innovative technology. But equally important, such resistance varies between crafts and from one innovation to another and is influenced by occasional ad hoc coalitions of unions and building materials producers. Furthermore, even the most vociferous coalition in recent years has been unable to delay diffusion of those innovations that they have strenously opposed.

The fact is that so many countervailing forces exist within the building department's clientele that no single group of actors is sufficient to influence building code changes with any consistency. Therefore, there can be no predicting an innovation's fate because of the activities of any one part of the building department's constituency.

This generalization applies, however, only to conflicts surrounding local code change. Even the homeostatic properties of the building enterprise do respond to coordinated efforts of local groups, backed by technical support and advertising and lobbying assistance from outside. Industries can lobby as informed advocates of technological change but must do so with increased awareness and concern for the needs of the final users.

There remains a need for more consumer participation to represent the public interest. The diverse building department constituency considers, but does not give priority, to the public interest. Ventre says that only the low-paid and low-status local building official represents the public as a whole. Civic or voter groups only infrequently get involved in code changes and are accorded little standing when they do.

The National Commission on Product Safety repeatedly identified moral equivocation inherent in industrial self-regulation and provided several examples of failure of industrial consideration of public need in the built environment. In fairness, however, some of the standards-making bodies for the building industries have attempted to obtain direct consumer participation; but more public representation is needed if building regulations are to reflect public needs.

In stark confirmation of the need for such representation is the 1981 collapse in Kansas City, Missouri, of the suspended balcony of a new hotel, resulting in over 100 deaths and 200 injuries. The basic problem was that even if an adequate building code existed, it could not be enforced because the local regulatory agency was so understaffed and lacking in expertise that it did not routinely check on engineering calculations or pass on changes in building plans.[20]

Initially, plans for the balcony had provided, at best, a marginally safe structure that did not meet the existing building code. With unreviewed revision, the balcony became grossly unsafe and could scarcely support itself, much less several hundred people. If the building inspectors were too few and too hurried to inspect a major structure, one must ask how many other buildings of lesser community stature they were unable to inspect?

19
The Tools of Living: Furnishings and Appliances

Homes vary from the one-room woven hut in Papua New Guinea, housing the barest of clothing, carrying bags, axes and spears, an open fire, and a small supply of firewood and food, to such dwellings as Buckingham Palace with myriad and opulent contents. The relative frequencies of injuries involving four categories of home products in the United States are shown in table 19–1.[1] It is not appropriate to assume equal exposure to the products discussed in this table or this chapter.

Table 19–2 compares the priorities for products involving injury (including some discussed in later chapters) if one assumes that everyone has equal exposure or if one attempts to define a more appropriate denominator, namely the actual number of users.[2] Even this denominator is not fully adequate, however, because a television may be used on average several hours a day, a power lawnmower only once a week during summer months, and a power saw only a few times a year. Inadequate data are available, however, to compare injuries per unit exposure for very many products.

McAllister argues that none of the above assumptions are correct because many people discover the defects in their products—such as wearing out of a part—before serious trouble results and either correct the defect or discard the product.[3] I believe his assumption is limited, however, because he conceives of product-related problems as being defects, or equipment breakdowns. It is probably more common that a product functions as intended but does so in a manner that creates hazard by increasing task demand in subtle manner, not easily apparent to the user.

Why do people get into trouble involving various products? As a sociologist, David Klein's basic assumption is that what appear to be individual actions by individual people in fact to a substantial degree (but not entirely) are reflections of societal and subcultural structure and expectations.[4] And, he notes, these structures may have major effect—often negative—on our ability to educate and motivate people to achieve a safer environment.

To begin with, many lower-class families confront a higher-than-average number of environmental hazards, such as traffic congestion, dilapidated housing, unguarded railroad tracks, or faulty electrical wiring. One reason is that they are immune to middle-class modes of communication, such as pamphlets, community campaigns, group discussions, and school-oriented check lists, which have been conceived and developed by middle-class professionals who make ethnocentric assumptions about the information sources of people at other socioeconomic levels.

Even if they had read the pamphlets and attended the lectures, however, these families would have been financially unable to remove or

Table 19–1
Annual Emergency Department Visits in the United States for Injuries Involving Products in and around the Home

Product	*Injuries*	*Rate Per 100,000 Population*
Furnishings		
Chairs, sofas, sofa beds	212,000	99.9
Tables	207,000	97.3
Beds	177,000	83.3
Desks, cabinets, shelves, racks	118,000	55.5
Carpets, rugs	47,000	22.3
Electric fixtures, lamps	34,000	16.3
Furniture, not specified	25,000	12.1
Baby carriages, walkers, strollers	18,000	8.5
Mirrors	17,000	8.2
Benches	15,000	7.1
Cribs, playpens, baby gates	11,000	5.4
High chairs, youth chairs	8,000	3.8
Appliances		
Cooking ranges, ovens	38,000	18.1
Radios, stereos, and so forth	31,000	14.8
Television sets	22,000	10.6
Refrigerators and freezers	22,000	10.3
Electric fans	14,000	6.7
Irons, ironers	10,000	5.1
Housewares and containers		
Cutlery and knives	137,000	64.5
Glass bottles and jars	129,000	60.7
Drinking glasses	112,000	52.6
Cans and other containers	94,000	44.5
Tableware and flatware (except cutlery)	65,000	30.7
Cookware, pots and pans	27,000	13.5
Scissors	15,000	7.5
Skewers, ice and other picks	10,000	5.1
Small kitchen appliances except coffee and teapots	10,000	4.9

Table 19–1
Annual Emergency Department Visits in the United States for Injuries Involving Products in and around the Home

Product	*Injuries*	*Rate Per 100,000 Population*
Home repair and yard equipment		
Ladders and stools	92,000	43.2
Power home saws	71,000	33.6
Lawn mowers	64,000	30.1
Chain saws	63,000	29.7
Hammers	52,000	24.5
Manual workshop tools	42,000	19.7
Hatchets and axes	28,000	13.4
Hand garden tools	28,000	13.3
Other power home tools	24,000	11.3
Automotive tools, chemicals	22,000	10.4
Batteries	20,000	9.8
Wires/cords, not specified	20,000	9.4
Hoists, lifts, jacks	17,000	8.2
Screwdrivers	15,000	7.2
Garden hoses, sprinklers	12,000	5.8
Trimmers, other small garden tools	10,000	5.1

Sources: Adapted from *NEISS Data Highlights: Hazard Identification and Analysis* 4(4), (October–December 1980) (Washington, D.C.: Consumer Product Safety Commission.

get away from some of the hazards that these materials identified. Kerosene space heaters and floor heaters, for example, are extremely hazardous; but in many parts of the country they constitute the only source of heat available to low-income families, and the families themselves cannot replace them with something safer. Regulations have sometimes resulted in safer designs, but such regulations often contain a grandfather clause so that it could be decades before all the old-style products are eliminated.

Klein also observes important social-class differences in general styles of childrearing, with more fatalism among lower-class families, less supervision of children, a general style of household management that would appear to be irresponsible, unsystematic, or slovenly from a middle-class point of view. This disorderliness and lack of planning, he says, may be due to a lack of resources, or it may reflect a feeling of powerlessness to control life and hence an abdication of efforts to do so. It may be due to more stress, less ability to cope, or overload produced by too many children in inadequate quarters. It may also stem from a focus on the immediate present instead of the future. Under such conditions, child safety has low priority. This sense of fatalism is adhered to by some of the world's major religions.

Two observations from other sources suggest validation of Klein's

Table 19–2
Comparison of Priorities for Products Associated with Injury Based on Assumptions That All Persons in the United States Are Exposed or That There Are Fewer Users

Product	*Estimated Users*	*Estimated Injuries*	*Mean Severity*	*Frequency Severity Index (FSI)*	*Score (and Rank) Assuming Limited Exposure*	*Score (and Rank) Assuming Total Exposure*
Football	28,000,000	403,000	22	8.87	63.99 (1)	3.05 (4)
Bicycles	60,865,000	430,000	38	16.34	57.90 (2)	5.62 (2)
Baseball	41,102,000	401,000	21	8.42	41.20 (3)	2.90 (5)
Stairs	220,000,000	572,000	33	18.88	27.07 (4)	6.49 (1)
Lawn mowers	66,132,000	69,000	143	9.87	5.16 (5)	3.39 (3)
Power saws	31,870,000	68,000	56	3.81	4.08 (6)	1.31 (7)
Ladders	74,104,000	83,000	35	2.91	1.63 (7)	1.00 (8)
Floors	222,000,000	101,000	43	4.34	1.00 (8)	1.49 (6)

Source: F.P. Rivara and L.R. Berger, "Consumer Product Hazards: Setting Priorities for Research and Regulatory Action," *American Journal of Public Health* 70(1980):701–704. Reprinted with permission.

comments. Tokuhata et al. found that families reporting injury were more likely to purchase reconditioned products or appliances in a discount store and more likely to assemble parts or repair products themselves.[5] A survey from another source indicates that consumers believe that prices, but also quality, tend to be less in discount-type stores and that, for stores in general, about half of sales personnel are not very familiar with the products they are selling.[6]

A closely related issue is the frustration that both manufacturers and safety personnel often feel over the fact that people commonly innovate or use products in ways or for purposes not originally intended, to wit: the chair used as a step stool, the Coca Cola bottle that now holds kerosene or other poisonous material, or the cooking stove used to heat a house or apartment.

One reason for such behavior is the phenomenon of "satisficing": the choosing of an acceptable but less than ideal solution for an immediate problem, as described by economist, Herbert Simon.[7] It is reasonable to expect that those with the least resources available would be individuals most likely to satisfice by using their limited products for more than one purpose. Unfortunately, those products, because of low-cost design and workmanship, may be precisely the ones that are less amenable to safety despite innovative behavior.

Klein also points out that families introduce hazards into the environment because they serve as status symbols. Examples are snowmobiles, minibikes, high-horsepower boats, guns for hunting or for target shooting, high-powered woodworking and garden tools, which, he alleges, are more common in U.S. working-class than in middle-class households. One reason for introducing such hazards to children, he says, is that working-class parents regard their children's confrontation of physical risk as useful preparation for the realities of life, including ability to obtain personal distinction through competitive effort. This is a uniquely Western or frontier philosophy. In middle-class families, this competitive drive may be dealt with in ways that do not involve personal risk to the extent they do so in working-class families.

Turning to the role of the manufacturer, Clark points out that manufacturers usually measure the hazard of their products by looking only at the number of liability claims.[8] They are often incredulous on learning just how many medically treated injuries involving their products are not reported to them. In the absence of a liability claim, they assume that the "fault" for such injuries must lie entirely with the consumer.

Consequently, as documented by Bull et al. concerning fireplace guards, manufacturers and distributors may (1) not be aware of problems with their products, (2) either not know about or ignore standards or ideas available to avoid or correct hazards, (3) not provide adequate distribution of safer products, or (4) provide the safer product but in a way that makes retrofixing difficult.[9] Unsafe products whose sale is no longer permitted in the nation of origin may be "dumped" into a foreign market that lacks consumer safeguards.[10,11]

Manufacturers may not be aware of important human factors issues as new markets develop. More women, for example, are using tools at home and at work in the United States but are having problems with them because women have smaller hand size and less strength in upper limbs and shoulder girdle. Body size also varies between nations.

Advertising also may mislead the consumer. A panel of the National Advertising Review Board found no examples of blatant advertising of unsafe user behavior but did uncover examples of cues that could guide an unsophisticated person into using products inappropriately.[12]

Furnishings

Six types of contributory problems are identifiable regarding furnishings. We will begin with those that are most obvious and move then to the more subtle contributors.

1. *Furnishings that are of unstable design*. This category includes high chairs,[13] bar stools, and infant strollers[14] that have high centers of gravity and can easily tip with normal movement of the occupant. Some infant seats lose their wire bases and collapse or have tether straps that often are not used so that the child falls out.[15] Folding tables, chairs, beds, and related storable furniture may not lock in place and consequently can collapse.[16,17] Failure of high chair trays to stay locked in place has also been a reason for falls. Remedies for these problems are to provide a broader base or lower the center of gravity to reduce tipping and to design sturdy bases and passive restraint design for infant seats. More positive locking mechanisms are also possible, especially for folding furniture.

2. *Furnishings that have exposed pinch points that can grab, crush, and even strangle.*[16–20] Particularly hazardous are cribs or playpens with bars set just far enough apart so an infant or small child can get its head through but not back again. There are repeated reports of deaths from such strangulation. Collapsible furniture also has pinch points at the supports. Cabinet doors, as with larger doors, can pinch fingers if the hinges are not recessed or covered. Covering or rounding of most pinch points is quite feasible. The Consumer Product Safety Commission initiated an education program to get parents to cover the lower parts of crib bars and issued standards requiring that bars be placed so close

together that even the smallest head could not pass through. This has been associated with about a 40 percent decrease in injuries and deaths.[21]

3. *Furnishings that create an unmanageable task for a segment of the population.* The most obvious is the toy chest with a top lid too heavy for a small child.[22] The lid may fall on the child's head, causing death by asphyxiation. Lighter lids with balanced hinges permit a child to open the chest with little effort.

Innovative use of materials not designed as furnishing may also create hazard. Introduction of very thin sheet plastic for bags and covering for laundered clothing resulted in deaths to young children who suffocated while playing with plastic bags which they placed over their faces and to infants whose parents had used the plastic on crib mattresses in place of rubber sheeting. Educational efforts plus warning labels on the plastic have not reduced the number of fatalities, and it will probably be necessary to remove this plastic entirely from the marketplace if more deaths are to be prevented.

4. *Furnishings that place persons in unstable position.* In some cases this category overlaps the last one. One example is deep chairs, especially without arms, that pitch toward the back and make it difficult for elderly persons to stand up without losing balance.[24] Shelving that is both high and deep also may create an unmanageable task so that the person tips off balance to reach the back of the shelf.[17]

A well-known example is the throw rug that either slips underfoot or has a raised edge on which persons of unsure vision or footing can trip. Cribs and mesh playpens may permit young children to climb part way up, from where they then fall out onto the ground.[20] Bunk beds are predominantly a problem for older children and adults.[24] Falls from these beds occur to persons who roll out while sleeping, who are attempting to climb the ladder, or children who are jumping or playing in bed.

In Hong Kong the very crowded housing conditions require sleeping in tiers of bunks up to ten feet high. These bunks usually have no rails, and serious injuries are common. In one study there were eighteen head injuries, twelve lacerations, and fractures of skull, limb, and spine.[25] If elevated beds cannot be avoided, or their height cannot be limited because of shortage of space, sturdy guard rails are one preventive measure. Resilient flooring can also limit the effects of a fall.

Regarding chairs, Hiatt has suggested purchasing chairs for the elderly that have arms, are not exceptionally deep, and do not tip toward the back.[26] If faced with an existing chair that has too much tilt, it is sometimes possible to cut an inch or two off front legs, or to add slightly to back legs.

The usable depth of a shelf is a function of its height. For the woman

64 inches tall and a shelf 79 inches high only 6 inches of shelf depth is usable. A shelf 63 inches high could be 20 inches deep, and one at 48 inches could be 24 inches deep because the limiting factor is arm length rather than height.

Rugs can be stabilized through use of underpads that decrease the likelihood of slippage. Adhesive material that holds down rug edges reduces the risk of tripping.

5. *Furnishings that fail to provide adequate cues of their presence.* This is an extremely subtle contributor to injury events that is unlikely to arouse the attention of persons not specifically concerned with human factors research.

Zohar notes that unless they are in an unfamiliar environment, most people walk with their eyes tilted only slightly downward so that their "effective visual field"—the area they pay most attention to and in which they can readily identify objects—is above hip level.[27] They are thus far more likely to bump into objects, such as coffee tables or other low furniture or protrusions, that do not reach as high as the hips. One can increase effective visual field by use of contrasting colors or flicker or special lighting that calls attention to a protruding object below hip height. Drawing from the data concerning falls on stairs, I would also suggest that placing low objects in locations where people won't be distracted by interesting activities above hip level may also decrease frequency of striking low objects.

6. *Furnishings that increase the likelihood that injury will occur and that it will be severe.* Most household furnishings are either hard with sharp edges and corners or soft (as with upholstered furniture and carpeting) and highly flammable or capable of emitting toxic gases under extreme heat. (Flammability is discussed in chapter 20).

Furnishings with rounded edges and resilient surfaces are much less likely to cause serious injury. Where possible, breakable glass surfaces should be avoided in cabinets and coffee tables or should be thick or otherwise resistant to shattering. Designing for safety appears to have become a standard part of the curriculum in schools of architecture, but, to my knowledge, it is not a component of other educational programs teaching design concepts for industry. The costs of safer design in most cases are minimal.

Appliances

Again, we will move from those hazards that are most obvious to those that are least obvious but nonetheless harmful.

1. *Appliances that have obvious hazards that have been left readily*

accessible to the user or others. These include stoves and space heaters (in particular gas-fired ones), irons, fans, electric mixers, and washing machines with wringers. For some of these, such as space heaters and fans, better shielding is an appropriate preventive measure.[28,29]

Many injuries with electrical mixers occur because switches are placed where they can be inadvertently touched while a user is attempting to insert or remove blades.[30] Furthermore, some mixers have switches that turn the mixer completely on when the switch is moved only about one-eighth inch away from the "off" position. As a result, some users have found that the mixer is on when the switch appears to say "off." Better switch design and placement would avoid both injury modes.

For years, washing machine wringers have grabbed and mutilated hands and arms of children who are able to reach the switches, turn them on, and play with them.[31,32] Despite the advent of the spin drier, the wringer type remains available in the United States because families receiving welfare support are permitted to purchase a washing machine—but only if it is of the wringer type. Most wringer injuries, therefore, are in welfare families, and the medical costs of the injuries far exceed additional costs welfare departments would have to pay if they had authorized purchase of more expensive machines.

Ideally, these machines should be removed totally from the market. In lieu of this, starting devices should be made child-proof, a guard should be designed in front of the wringer, and a release mechanism should exist that is automatically activated if one attempts to pull back on an object entering the wringer.

Much rarer injuries involve children who have stuck arms into spin type dryers, with severe fractures or even avulsion resulting.[33] A spin drier should be designed either so that the door cannot open if the drum is in motion or so that the drum will stop almost instantly if the door is opened, instead of over a period of up to thirty seconds, as is now the case with many dryers.

2. *Appliances that explode or spontaneously catch fire.* Included in this group, which will be discussed in the next chapter, are gas stoves, kerosene space heaters, television sets, and electric blankets.

3. *Appliances that tip over easily, such as coffee and teapots, electric heaters, irons, and some humidifiers used to treat acute respiratory diseases in children.* Most of these appliances have long appliance cords. If the appliance is on an elevated surface, the cord may hang down and be pulled by a young child.[34,35,36] Retractable or spring type cords would be out of reach of small children.

Once pulled, these appliances tip over easily because of their narrow base and high center of gravity, both amenable to redesign. Finally, the contents commonly spill and cause extremely serious injury. Humidifiers have now been designed to disperse cool droplets rather than hot steam,[37] and electric space heaters currently on the market automatically stop if the heater tips over. Coffee makers and teapots that lose their covers on tipping immediately dump all of their boiling contents,[34] whereas those with retainable covers spill only a small amount at a time, resulting in less injury.

4. *Appliances that electrocute.* These are not common in the United States because many of the larger manufacturers have their products tested by Underwriters Laboratories. However, Christmas tree bulbs and various lamps and other small appliances periodically do reach the marketplace with errors of insulation design that under certain circumstances permit human contact with ungrounded electrical sources.[38,39,40]

5. *Applicances that release hazardous gases.* On the British Isles many heating appliances were operated with coal gas (with 10 to 20 percent carbon monoxide), with high loss of life until this was replaced with natural gas, which is virtually free of carbon monoxide.[41] Unvented or poorly vented space heaters, hot water heaters, and clothes dryers may also produce sufficient undispersed carbon monoxide to cause fatalities, especially if the appliance is not operating at maximum combustion efficiency.[42]

6. *Appliances that create an "attractive nuisance."* Children repeatedly crawl into abandoned refrigerators to hide and are then unable to escape because the doors are hard to open from the inside. In some cases children have crawled into clothes dryers, which have then been turned on by unsuspecting parents. Educating people to remove refrigerator doors when they throw them away has been partly successful. A better measure is to make refrigerators with doors that can be opened easily from the inside.

7. *Appliances that confuse.* The prime example is the four-burner stove. Turning on the wrong burner is common. But Chapanis and Lindenbaum showed that one arrangement of burners and their controls was associated with no errors even for neophyte users, whereas three other arrangements, even after extensive use, resulted in errors from 5 to 10 percent of the time.[43] Twenty years later Shinar and Acton attempted to learn whether stove manufacturers had used this information.[44] They found that the linkage designs most often sold not only ignored the earlier study but often ignored people's expectations of which knobs should control which burners.

Especially with electric stoves and those with ceramic tops, a person also may not realize which burner is hot because the burner may not turn red at low heat or may cease to glow once the coil has been turned off but while it is still hot enough to burn. The solution is to have an indicator light that not only indicates which coil has been activated[45] but that remains lit until the coil drops below a dangerous temperature. This would be especially useful for people with poor vision, such as the elderly.

Housewares and Containers

Probably little can be done to reduce either the number or severity of injuries involving sharp nonmechanized household equipment, such as knives.[46] But laceration from broken glassware, another common injury (table 19–1), may be amenable to prevention. Hard sinks, counters, or other working surfaces can be covered with resilient material (e.g., by a plastic tip on the end of a faucet or a rubber or plastic sink mat) so that bumping might result in fewer broken dishes and glasses and fewer lacerations. Reducing water temperature to below 120°F places less stress on weak glassware and on unsuspecting hands. Use of plastic utensils, of course, obviates the problem completely.

Another common source of laceration is from broken carbonated beverage and other bottles. This may occur as a result of dropping or otherwise striking the bottle, but since the advent of nonreturnable bottles there are annually about 32,000 injuries in the United States from explosion of thin-walled bottles housing carbonated soft drinks, despite little or no handling.[47] Plastic containers or stronger, thick-walled, returnable bottles avoid the problems. Where bottle return policies exist there is less litter and presumably fewer bottles around to get broken and to cause injury. Those bottles that do remain around are stronger and less easily damaged. Bottles can also be strengthened by applying a thin adherent outer layer of plastic, which softens the effects of bumps against the glass and also keeps pieces in place if the glass should fracture.

Mention should be again made of household containers that can be tipped easily, in this case the unpowered coffee or tea pot.[48] Around multiple dwellings, community refuse bins with uneven weight distribution have tipped over when small children have hung onto them.[49] More balanced design for the base and the lid reduces the hazard.

Equipment for Household Maintenance and Repair

Many of these appliances have exposed hazardous surfaces, such as blades in power mowers,[50–53] chain and power saws,[54–56] snowblowers,[57,58] or hedge trimmers.[59] Other equipment permits instability, such as ladders[60] and garden tractors.[61] In both cases the equipment usually is portable and must often be used on uneven surfaces, with unstable footing, in elevated position so that arms tire, or where tree limbs or other objects being worked upon require manipulation with one hand while the user tries to hold onto the equipment with the other hand. Less commonly, there may be fire from fuel leakage in gas-powered equipment, electrocution from defective or poorly grounded electrical equipment, and contact by lawnmower or other blades with stones or wire, which get thrown at high speed unless guarding mechanisms catch or deflect them.[53]

Collectively, injuries involving exposed blades are by far the most common. Especially on uneven ground feet can easily get under the housing of power mowers, resulting in amputation. Many people unsuspectingly stick their hands underneath clogged mowers or into snowblower shutes to clean the discharge area. In the latter case, they don't realize that the impellor blade has not yet stopped even though the auger is disengaged.[58] The result is a lacerated or amputated finger.

Chain saws or power saws, on the other hand, may bind while cutting wood and may kick back, lacerating the head or some other part of the body. With saws injuries also commonly occur because a hand or leg is in the way of the unguarded blade.

The most common approach has been to advise people to work in a clear area or on even surfaces, not to stick arms, hands, legs, or feet near the blade, or not to attempt to clear a piece of equipment that is still in motion. The reality, however, is that users often do not have the option to follow this advice, or they choose to ignore it.

A much more foolproof solution is the "deadman's switch," which stops blade motion within only one or two seconds if the hand is taken off a trigger that must be held to keep the blade engaged. Better guards can keep feet away from mower blades and hands or other parts of the body away from saw blades. Chain saws can also be designed with an antikickback device.[62]

Instability of ladders that occurs because the ground itself is uneven can be corrected with self-leveling mechanisms to lengthen one or more legs as necessary. Perhaps more common, the ladder may be placed at the wrong angle so that it slips when someone starts climbing. The Consumer Product Safety Commission now requires a label on the side of each ladder that describes and illustrates the correct angle for placement. Firmer traction on the feet of the ladder would also help to prevent slippage. Steps or rungs should also provide traction because some injuries occur when feet slip off the rungs.

Unbeknownst to most people, many ladders have been constructed so they break or bend under the weight of a person over about 200 lbs, despite the fact that most ladders are used by males and many males are over this weight. A weight standard is needed for ladder strength that will accommodate at least the 95th percentile male.

Finally, let us consider protection achievable through tempered, toughened, or impact-resistant eyeglasses while using other products. Before the U.S. Food and Drug Administration required such lenses in all eyeglasses in 1970, there were about 120,000 lens-related injuries each year in the home and school environment.[63] The cost of the stronger lenses at that time ranged from 50 cents to $3 per lens. Use of steel-tipped shoes and other protective devices is far less common for activities in the home environment but also has the potential for reducing frequency and severity of injury, such as amputation of toes by lawnmowers.

20

Thermal Extremes: Fire, Burns, Scalds, Hypothermia

An interesting dichotomy exists among professionals dealing with thermal extremes. Those concerned with the prevention and fighting of fires and their associated property damage have had little interest in thermal injury to people from contact with hot surfaces or liquids or from controlled sources of flame. On the other hand, health professionals concerned about thermal injury to people have cared little about fires and property damage issues.

Both areas are legitimate and important because fire without injury is a major cause of financial loss and hardship throughout the world, just as thermal injury without fire is a serious drain on health and social resources and a source of physical and psychological agony. The emphasis in this chapter, however, will be on the health aspects.

Frequency and Distribution

In 1980 a total of 5,500 fire-related deaths occurred in the United States, 4,400 of which were in the home.[1] Not included in these figures are those deaths from contact with hot or scalding materials or electrical current where fire was not involved. Table 20–1 shows the relative distribution of "burn" deaths when these other injury sources are added.[2] The mean death rate per 100,000 population in 1980 was 2.4 (not including hot surfaces, scalds, and electrical burns), compared to almost 9 in the years 1913–22. The crude death rates for other nations ranged from less than 1 per 100,000 to almost 10 for Egypt, with most nations recording rates between 1 and 2. This variation no doubt reflects differences in population distribution by age, reporting criteria and effectiveness, types of environmental hazards involving heating and cooking or types of clothing worn, and quality of medical care.

Deaths from burns occur predominantly among the very young and the elderly. In 1980 children under age 5 accounted for 700 of the 4,400 such deaths in U.S. homes, and an additional 1,300 deaths were to persons age 65 or older. The age-specific death rate is: age 0 to 4—4.3

Table 20–1
Distribution of Deaths Involving Fire or Hot Substances, United States, 1975

Heat Source	*Number*	*Percentage*
Conflagration		
Private dwelling	4,373	55.3
Other building/structure	199	2.5
Not building/structure	58	0.7
Ignition		
Clothing	429	5.4
Highly flammable material	147	1.9
Controlled Fire		
Private dwelling	54	0.7
Other building/structure	5	0.1
Not building/structure	18	0.2
Other specified fire or flame	364	4.6
Unspecified	432	5.5
Explosive material	393	5.0
Hot substances, corrosives, liquid steam	210	2.7
Electric current	1,225	15.5
Total	7,907	100.1

Source: Adapted from *Report on the Fire/Burn Problem in the United States, vol. 1, Analysis* (Virginia Beach, Va.: Systems Management Associates, Inc., Contract No. CPSC-C-76-0138, 1978).

per 100,000; age 5 to 14—1.0; age 15 to 24—0.9; age 25 to 44—1.2; age 45 to 64—2.0; age 65 to 74—3.8; and age 75 or older—7.2.

The overall death rate in the United States for blacks is twice that for whites, as is the rate for males compared to females. As Young and Baker point out, however, in 1959–61 the death rate for females age 3 to 14 exceeded that for males, presumably because of ignition of dresses.[3] The ratio shifted, they believe, because girls' clothing styles changed from dresses to less easily ignited pants. Death rates for young children have dropped markedly in recent years,[4] probably reflecting changes in clothing styles, some flame-retardant clothing for this age, and better emergency care.

Turning to nonfatal events, there are about 4.5 million residential fires in the United States each year, and fire departments are called for only 10 percent of them.[2] Even where the fire starts in furniture or wall and floor coverings, fire departments are called only 20 to 30 percent of the time.

Table 20–2 shows the distribution of nonfatal burns.[2] Note that major causes of nonfatal burns are only infrequent causes of fatal events

Table 20–2
Causes of Burn Injuries in and around the Home Based on 1974 National Household Fire Survey

Injury Cause	*Injuries*	*Percentage of Total*
Contact with hot objects	40,000	24
Scalds and burning grease	35,000	21
Explosions (including ovens/furnaces)	16,000	10
Fabric ignition only	21,000	12
Welding and soldering	7,000	4
Trying to extinguish fire in home	19,000	11
Electrical short circuits	2,000	1
Gasoline related	2,000	1
Motor vehicles	16,000	10
Other	12,000	7
Total	169,000	101[a]

Source: *Report on the Fire/Burn Problem in the United States, vol. 1, Analysis* (Virginia Beach, Va.: Systems Management Associates, Inc., Contract CPSC-C-76-0138, 1978).

and vice versa. About one in every twenty burns that are treated is serious enough to result in hospitalization. While this figure indicates about 170,000 injuries, a more accurate estimate might be 1.7 million.[2] With nonfatal fires women are involved three times more often than men.

Fatal burns are most likely to involve the very young and the elderly.[2] With less severe burns, however, children under age 11 comprise 20 percent of the U.S. population but 15 percent of persons burned. Persons age 11 to 20 are 19 percent of the population and 11 percent of those burned, while those age 21 to 45, 46 to 65, and 66 or older respectively are 31 percent, 22 percent, and 8 percent of the population but 53 percent, 8 percent, and 13 percent of those burned. Thus, only the age 21 to 45 and 66 or older groups are overrepresented in nonfatal burns.

Barancik and Shapiro, however, report a very different distribution of nonfatal injuries according to age, with overrepresentation of age groups 0 to 4, 15 to 19, and 20 to 24 and underrepresentation of persons age 5 through 14 and 45 and over.[5] In fact, persons age 65 years and older were burned only one-third as often as expected based on population. Similar underrepresentation of the elderly in both minor and serious residential fires is reported by Ducic and Ghezza in residential fires in Montreal.[6]

Data from other nations either are not forthcoming or are limited to hospitalized or other possibly nonrepresentative populations. Studies from the British Isles suggest that the relative distribution of injuries from scalds, hot substances, and open fires probably differs somewhat from the United States because of greater frequency of contact with open fires used for home heating.[7,8]

In Ceylon and India death from burns is far more common among women than among men, whereas in Japan males and females are almost equally affected.[9] Lockhart et al. report fewer burns by fire or hot substances than they anticipated in Hong Kong, given the crowded residential conditions and the use of unprotected charcoal and paraffin stoves.[10] However, their comparison with other nations is based upon burns as a proporation of all home injuries, which may be affected by the proportions of other injuries. They should have been comparing rates, rather than proportions.

In the absence of data I will suggest factors that could affect the rates of burn injuries in developing nations. Factors that would increase risk of injury would be crowded housing, often made of and containing highly flammable materials, with open fires, appliances not designed with safety in mind, and large numbers of children. Lack of sophisticated emergency, definitive, and rehabilitative care would increase the risks of death and of permanent disability.

On the other hand, a stove may have only a single burner so that people cannot reach over other burners that are lit. Absence in some cases of flammable (or any) clothing also reduces injury. If the stove and the food being cooked are close to the ground, it is also less possible for small children to pull scalding liquids on top of themselves but conversely easier to fall into them. In warmer countries people may spend less time in the home and thus are at less risk of injury. And it may be easier to escape injured but alive from a one-room, one-story structure with an unlocked door than it is from a typical house or multi-unit dwelling in the Western world. The net result, as suggested by the data in table 8–6, may be that the factors balance out so that the distributions of causes differ but the net rates remain roughly the same. In any event, the hypotheses, once stated, stand as a challenge for research to test them.

Severe burns, along with head injuries and spinal cord trauma may seriously affect quality of life among long-term survivors. Even a small annual incidence of such survivors may lead to a large prevalence. Individuals with severe head trauma seem to do poorly in social adjustments over the long-term.[11] Surprisingly, however, social integration, emotional adjustment, and self-esteem were generally good among eighty-nine young adults who were observed four to twenty-three years after burns that on average covered 27 percent of body surface.[12] Persons with burns literally are stigmatized, since the word *stigma* refers to a brand burned into the skin of a slave or criminal.

Human Factors in the Pre-Injury Phase

The predominant human factors in the initiation of burns appear to be associated, as in other injury events, with extreme youth, abuse of alcohol, and factors related to aging and medical impairment. The young child is at a disadvantage because of an innate curiosity associated with lack of experience, at least in initial encounters with hazard. Thus, the toddler who in normal developmental manner tests everything by mouthing it is at risk of being burned because it attempts to taste the end of an electric extension cord.

The onus for child management has often been shifted to the parents, who may have several children requiring simultaneous management, at a time in the parents' lives when they have not reached full economic growth and consequently must live in overcrowded and otherwise less-than-adequate housing. The combination of normative child development plus normative parental limitations of resources mitigates against total safety all of the time, especially since the child is in this environment for most of the day.

The young child is also particularly burn prone because of small size and coordination that is not yet well developed. A pot or electrical appliance dangling enticingly overhead can be easily pulled over so that it spills its liquid contents over a very large proportion of the body. A similar spill for an adult or a larger child would affect only a smaller body area and certainly not the head, neck, and shoulders, as with the younger child. Add to this the fact that the head represents a larger proportion of body surface in the child than in the adult.

Because of poor coordination a child who is attempting to deal with a hot substance may spill it, or he or she may drop a lighted match while learning how to strike matches (euphemistically known as "playing with matches") and not have the quick reflexes to put it out. Equally common is the toddler, just learning how to walk, who falls against a hot surface or the young child who bumps against such a surface while running because depth perception and attention span are not yet fully mature.

Finally, in a conflagration, the child may be trapped in a crib or playpen or be unable to run fast or negotiate windows or locked doors.

It is hardly surprising, therefore, that young children are overrepresented among fatalities in home fires.[13]

Serious scalds occur to infants and young children who are placed or fall into tubs of excessively hot tap water and are unable to remove themselves. Takafuji et al. found that the recommended temperature for water in living quarters at Ford Ord was 140°F and the mean temperature was actually measured at well over 130°F, both of which are clearly excessive from the safety viewpoint.[14]

We turn next to the role of alcohol. Heavy drinkers tend also to be heavy smokers. Levine and Radford reported that BACs were determined for thirty-four of fifty-five fire-related fatalities and that 20 percent of all fatalities, and 32 percent of those whose BACs were measured, had elevated BACs.[13] All, in fact, were over 0.15 percent. Waller found BACs of 0.10 percent or higher in 64 percent of twenty-two adult fire fatalities, all of whom had been tested for alcohol.[15] Most persons with alcohol had stigmata of alcoholism in the larger sample of nonhighway injury fatalities from which the fire-related deaths were drawn.

In 1969 Wechsler et al. reported that 18.2 percent had positive BACs among patients age 16 or older treated for nonfatal injuries involving home fire or explosion.[16] So did 16.1 percent of persons with burns. In contrast, 4.3 percent were positive among a control group of adult patients treated for illness.

Ducic and Ghezzo examined both alcohol use and smoking behavior in minor and serious home fires in Montreal.[6] They did not report on the severity of injuries involved, classifying the events according to property damage because, as Ducic observed in personal communication (May 13, 1982), the fire department reports were incomplete regarding injury.

These authors note that in the "serious" fires subgroup, the number of alcohol users per household was the single most important variable, and the number of alcohol users plus previous exposure to fire correctly identified 58 percent of households. Number of smokers per household was the most important variable for minor fires, and number of smokers plus crowding correctly found 61 percent of cases. Table 20–3 shows relationships between some of the human characteristics and fires in their study, including that of smoking in bed.

People are cautioned not to smoke in bed, with little awareness that those probably most likely to engage in such behavior are smoking while seriously impaired by alcohol. They are precisely the individuals who would be most resistant to behavioral modification through exhortation, most likely to fall asleep while smoking because of the depressant effect of alcohol, and least likely to be quickly aroused if fire breaks out. In fact, these individuals commonly die as a result of toxic gases during the

Table 20–3
Human Factors in Serious and Minor Residential Fires

	Serious Fires			Minor Fires		
	Case	*Control*	*Relative Odds*	*Case*	*Control*	*Relative Odds*
Age of occupants						
Under 15	31.1	26.8	1.16	31.3	28.6	1.06
16–60	60.8	60.8	1.0	61.8	60.0	1.0
⩾ 61	8.1	12.4	0.65	6.9	11.4	0.58
Sex						
Female	—[a]	—[a]	—[a]	46.0	52.0	1.0
Male	—[a]	—[a]	—[a]	54.0	48.0	1.28
Smoking in bed						
Never	68.7	79.5	1.0	70.1	82.2	1.0
Sometimes	31.3	20.5	1.8	29.9	17.8	1.97
Stay at home						
All day	63.1	65.8	1.0	—[a]	—[a]	—[a]
Not all day[b]	36.9	34.2	1.13	—[a]	—[a]	—[a]
Previously exposed to fire						
No	86.1	90.7	1.0	84.3	91.6	1.0
Yes	13.9	9.3	1.6	15.7	8.4	2.03

Source: S. Ducic and H.R. Ghezzo, "Epidemiology of Accidental Home Fires in Montreal," *Accident Analysis and Prevention* 12(1980):67–73. Reprinted with permission. Copyright 1980, Pergamon Press, Ltd.

[a]Not significant.

[b]These data differ from published paper and are based on personal communication with author, January 1984.

smoldering phase, rather than from burns per se. Heavy users of alcohol also are at risk of death from hypothermia. The "skid row bum" may have no indoor shelter or may sleep outdoors in a drunken stupor, with alcohol bringing about heat loss through dilatation of peripheral blood vessels.

One group at particular risk of serious injury from burns is individuals with seizures, cerebral palsy, or similar disorders of consciousness or coordination. Because of these problems, they are more likely to contact hot surfaces and more likely to be unable to remove themselves quickly, resulting in more severe injuries.[8] In Tempest's study, twelve of ninety-two burns to persons age 5 or older occurred as a result of a seizure, and another twelve as a result of a stroke.[7]

Besides more often having medical conditions that alter consciousness or attention, the elderly have other problems that may increase their risk of burns. As we have already observed, however, while there is no question about the higher mortality rate from burns for the elderly, it is not clear whether they are over or underrepresented in minor events.

1. Reduced or delayed peripheral sensation may result from aging per se or from diabetes. Twice as many burns among persons age 64 or older are full thickness compared to those of younger individuals.[5]
2. Reduced vision makes it more difficult for the elderly to pick out the proper control for a stove burner and to realize if a wrong burner has been activated.
3. Reduced mobility, both because of normal aging and because of conditions such as Parkinsonism, increases the likelihood of falling against hot surfaces and decreases the ability to escape in conflagrations.
4. The elderly spend more time in the home environment, which, because of limited finances, often is fire prone.
5. In the post-injury phase survival may be more tenuous because of complications from preexisting medical conditions but also because medical care for the elderly more often is of an expectant nature, rather than being aggressively therapeutic.[17]
6. The elderly also are at increased risk of hypothermia because they are uniquely sensitive to cooler environments. Because of poverty they may have less adequate housing or have to decide whether limited resources should be used for food or for heat. At least some apparently "natural" deaths of elderly persons in winter may be undiagnosed hypothermia. The risk of hypothermia from inadequate housing and nutrition poses an important problem as well in some developing nations.

Environmental Factors in the Pre-Injury Phase

We have already noted in the past two chapters some of the product-related contributors to the occurrence of burns. These can be classed as follows:

1. *Products that catch fire spontaneously or explode, such as electric blankets,*[18] *kerosene space heaters,*[19,20] *television sets,*[21] *ovens that lack pilot lights,*[22] *aluminum wiring,*[23] *heavily insulated recessed electric fixtures,*[24] *or woodstoves or other heating appliances that vent into soot-laden flues.*[25] Sometimes, as used in the real world, products can develop problems never anticipated by the manufacturer or even by a quality-control organization such as Underwriters Laboratory. A case in point is the kerosene-operated, cabinet-type space heater, malfunction of which caused at least 150 fires, 15 deaths, and 16 major burn injuries in Boston during six months between November 1959 and April 1960.[19] These heaters exploded because expansion of cold air in the fuel tank forced excess oil from the tank into the combustion chamber. This occurred only when the tank was partially filled with cold oil from a storage can kept outside. Development of an inexpensive device solved the problem by converting the heaters from barometric feed to gravity feed. But there were still 40,000 old-style heaters in use in Boston alone. An educational program to inform people to fill the fuel tank to capacity if cold oil was used was carried out by radio, TV, newspapers, pamphlets delivered through schools, neighborhood councils, fuel oil dealers and door-to-door peddlers of kerosene. As of mid-March 1961, only six additional fires with injuries had been recorded. Nonetheless, some fifteen years later some explosions of kerosene heaters were still being reported.[20]

2. *Hot appliances that can be tipped over easily, such as electric irons, kerosene lamps, teapots, coffee makers, vaporizers, or pots with long handles.*[7,26] In Ceylon, soda bottles are filled with kerosene and a cotton wick and used as "bottle lamps."[9] They are easily knocked over, with over 400 deaths per year as a result.

3. *Hot appliances such as stoves, radiators, open fires, and other heating devices whose hot surfaces have not been guarded and thus can burn people or ignite clothing, draperies, or other nearby materials.*[7,8,26,27] Bull et al. have described some of the political and economic issues that keep people from having adequate guards on fireplaces and gas or electric space heaters.[8] A similar pattern has existed in the United States regarding floor furnaces, gas-fueled heaters that are located just below the floor with a grate placed in the floor. In 1961 I reported on burns to children who fell against or touched the floor furnace grate and shortly after showed that in temperate climate these heaters were the most

frequent single cause of burns to children under age 5.[27] The industry responded by trying to get permission to use floor furnaces in mobile homes, where it would be literally impossible for a resident to walk (or to crawl, if an infant) from one room to another without contacting the grate.[28] Second, they testified that the industry-developed standard for such furnaces was quite adequate for safety, even though it permitted the surface of the grate to reach a temperature of 350°F above room temperature—or about 425°F. At that temperature the cooking of human flesh is instantaneous.[28] Several technically and economically feasible countermeasures have been proposed.

4. *Stoves that have confusing display-control arrangements.*[29] This problem was described earlier in the book. To these we will add some more general environmental factors as observed in the Montreal study of residential fires.[6] These are shown in table 20–4. Clearly, some of these factors represent an interaction between the human and the environment. Boarding houses, for example, are probably more likely than single-family homes to house the elderly, poor, and those addicted to alcohol. The authors state that the single most important variable for serious fires was type of building, followed by the number of stories. Number of stories, number of rooms, and building use for nonresidential purposes correctly labeled 61 percent of fire households. In minor fires type of building was the most important variable, and type of building, its conditions, and the presence of fire-fighting equipment correctly identified 67 percent of the fire locations.

Throughout this and the preceding chapters there has been emphasis on different experiences associated with different technologies and life styles. This is nowhere more obvious than with fire. Automobile radiators and electric cords can hardly be a problem in populations that have neither automobiles nor electricity. Where there is central heating—as in the United States and Canada—burns from space heaters for individual rooms are few, while nations such as the British Isles report many serious injuries of this type. Countries with 220 volts have more injuries from electricity than do those with 110 volt outlets.[9]

Especially in the United States prices of fuel began rising in 1973, and many homes have switched to wood stoves to supplement or supplant central heating. This return to a previous technology immediately brought a rash of burns and residential fires such as had been seen decades earlier, as well as lacerations, amputations, and other injuries to people carrying out logging and log-splitting activities. Between 1975 and 1978 about 12,000 home fires related to wood-burning appliances were reported from only twenty-one states. The most important problems identified were ignition of adjacent combustibles by heat from wood-burning equipment, chimney fires resulting from improper, defective, or poorly maintained chimneys, and ignition of building exteriors by sparks from chimneys.[25] Because of inadequate clearance, walls and especially floors near stoves often become dangerously hot in the absence of protective shielding. Chimney fires are a centuries old problem. In 1647 the Dutch governor of New Amsterdam (later New York City) established a Fire Commission, which recommended outlawing wooden chimneys.[30]

Factors That Increase Energy Load and/or Promote Transfer to People

In this section we will examine matches, materials that spill or spread highly flammable gases or liquids, clothing and fabrics, and toxic gases. On first thought it would hardly seem appropriate to consider matches here instead of in the pre-injury phase. In the Montreal study, 9 percent of both minor and serious fires were reported to have been started by children playing with matches,[6] while in a Baltimore study 54 percent of residential fires were stated to be caused by "careless smoking or children playing with matches."[11]

But not all matches are the same. Some book matches have the strike bar on the front, permitting ignition of the entire book, while others, more appropriately, have the strike bar on the back. More important, some matches have been designed so that they burn at a relatively slow rate (i.e., less thermal energy) and extinguish themselves before the entire match is used up. Such a match, if dropped, is far less likely to ignite other materials. In similar fashion, some ash tray designs do not permit a lighted cigarette to fall out and may even extinguish it. While all matches are capable of causing burns, the design of the individual match and of the matchbook can determine whether that burn is likely to be insignificant or more serious.

If a utensil or appliance with hot contents is uncovered or has a cover that falls off, the high-energy contents are dumped in their entirety.[26] For a small child, this may mean a serious or even fatal scald. If a bottle lamp is involved, a conflagration may result. In areas of Peru, where houses are close together on hillsides, the spilled contents of an overturned paraffin stove are likely to run downhill, igniting all of the houses that are in their path. Besides providing a broader base or lower center of gravity for such containers, or having a tight-fitting cover that prevents contents from spilling, it is also possible where fuels are involved to use gels or semisolid materials that spread only with difficulty. At the same

Table 20–4
Building Characteristics in Serious and Minor Residential Fires

	Serious Fires			*Minor Fires*		
	Case	*Control*	*Relative Odds*	*Case*	*Control*	*Relative Odds*
Type of construction						
Single	4.1	9.5	1.0	5.2	9.9	1.0
Duplex	12.0	15.1	1.83	9.0	16.3	1.02
Apartment house	75.0	71.6	2.42	73.9	69.2	2.06
Boarding house	8.9	3.8	5.35	11.9	4.1	5.58
Number of stories						
1	1.6	4.4	1.0	2.1	5.4	1.0
2	31.0	48.6	1.75	32.6	46.9	1.78
3	54.2	40.1	3.71	49.9	38.1	3.36
4	9.1	4.4	5.68	10.8	6.3	4.41
5	0.3	0.9	(0.83)	0.5	—	—
⩾ 6	3.8	1.6	6.53	4.1	3.3	3.19
Number of rooms						
⩾ 5	45.9	59.8	1.0	46.5	62.9	1.0
2–4	48.2	38.6	1.62	46.2	33.5	1.86
1	5.9	1.6	4.79	6.3	3.6	2.36
Condition of building						
New/good/fair	77.9	88.6	1.0	87.2	91.5	1.0
Poor/dilapidated	22.1	11.4	2.20	12.8	8.5	1.58
Ownership						
Self	14.6	22.7	1.0	12.0	25.1	1.0
Owner in building	21.2	24.9	1.33	21.2	23.2	1.89
Owner not in building	64.2	52.4	1.91	66.8	51.6	2.69
Use of building						
Dwelling only	85.9	94.2	1.0	82.9	94.5	1.0
Other use	14.1	3.6	4.17	17.1	5.5	3.53

Previous fire in building						
None	78.5	87.1	1.0	74.9	91.3	1.0
⩾ 1	21.5	12.9	1.85	25.1	8.7	3.52
Duration of occupancy						
⩾ 3 yrs	46.9	68.1	1.0	48.6	70.4	1.0
1–3 yrs	17.0	16.4	1.50	26.1	14.4	2.62
1–12 mo	33.0	14.2	3.36	23.1	22.1	1.50
< 1 mo	3.1	1.3	3.45	2.1	1.1	2.90
Fire fighting equipment						
No	67.8	76.7	1.0	67.8	77.8	1.0
Yes	32.2	23.3	1.57	32.2	22.2	1.67

Source: S. Ducic and H.R. Ghezzo, "Epidemiology of Accidental Home Fires in Montreal," *Accident Analysis and Prevention* 12(1980):67–73. Reprinted with permission. Copyright 1980, Pergamon Press, Ltd.

time, however, it is necessary to avoid materials that stick to the skin as they burn.

Fire may become widespread because the material involved is both highly flammable and easily dispersed. Tile and linoleum cements sometimes use an easily vaporized solvent with a very low flash point. The vapor may travel along the floor until it contacts a spark from a refrigerator or other motor and flashes back to set the can on fire. Quite often, it is possible to substitute a solvent with a higher flash point, lower vapor pressure, or both.

A major source of serious burns is clothing, curtains, bedding, and upholstery that catches fire easily and burns at a high temperature or that forms a molten mass that sticks to skin. Colebrook et al. pointed out that such burns were not always a problem.[26]

In the nineteenth century in England, and presumably even today in some nations, woolen and silk garments, which are less flammable, were in common use. In the 1940s and 1950s they were replaced by highly flammable cotton, rayons, cellulose nitrate lacquers, nylon (some types of which become molten on contact with heat) and loosely woven or brushed materials, all reflecting changes in clothing technology. In the thirty years after the introduction of cotton flannelette to England, burns to children increased by 62 percent.[26] By the 1940s and 1950s four out of every five deaths from burns resulted from injury inflicted by burning clothing.

Barancik and Shapiro reported that full-depth (third-degree) burns were 26 percent of clothing cases but 6 percent of other cases.[5] Hospitalization was required for 33 percent versus 10 percent, and the average length of hospital stay was thirty-one days, as compared to eleven days for other burns. Fourteen percent died among persons hospitalized with clothing burns, whereas 4 percent died among patients hospitalized with other burns. This 14 percent added to an additional excess of clothing burn victims who died before arrival at the hospital.

During the mid-1940s deaths in the United States from ignition of brushed rayon "torch" sweaters and long rayon pile cowboy chaps for children[26,31] led to protective legislation in 1953, as did the death of a physician's wife in New Zealand when her lacquered net dress caught fire.[26] White notes, however, that this legislation, developed by an industry committee, allowed 99 percent of all fabrics involved in serious burns to pass[31] and excluded from the market primarily explosively flammable brushed rayon imports. Enforcement proceedings were rarely used and ineffective. The 1953 act was amended in 1967, but White notes that at the time of his paper the only new standards proposed were for children's sleepwear, carpets, and rugs. Less than a month after the rug standard was published, a nylon carpet with foam rubber backing that met that standard caught fire and killed thirty-two residents of a nursing home. Since 1970 standards have also been passed to cover mattresses and upholstered furniture.

Several potential problems need to be considered in making fabrics and clothing flame retardant or nonflammable. First, in an international market with low profit margins and high marketing risks, there must be minimal addition to cost. A 5 to 10 percent increase in cost of manufacture can have economic repercussions that most people not in retail or wholesale business are hardly aware of. An item that goes through several intermediaries between manufacture and sale to the public may have as much as a fivefold markup because each intermediary requires a 100 percent markup to meet overhead costs. Thus, a 10 percent increase in cost to manufacturer could possibly mean a 50 percent increase in ultimate price. Unless all manufacturers are required to meet the same standards, severe economic disadvantage will occur to some that is sufficient to negate the safety requirement.

The issue is not just that all manufacturers selling in the United States must meet a standard. The U.S. manufacturers who are trying to sell to international markets as well as the U.S. market have already tooled up for the safety requirement and thus may not be in a position to make a safe product for the U.S. market and an unsafe one for other markets. Nor should they be permitted to do so. If it is unsafe in one country, it is probably a hazard elsewhere as well. This is why international standards and agreements are needed.

Second, the flame-retardant process must not degrade other qualities of the product, such as softness, color, or strength. Some of the processes in current use do make fabric stiffer and decrease its life span. Third, the retardant material must not be harmful to the user, such as causing allergies or being carcinogenic, as was found with TRIS treated sleepwear,[32] nor must the retardant create toxic fumes when it comes into contact with heat.

Last, the fabric must remain flame retardant during its entire usable life, after many washings, after dry cleaning, but also despite the fact that the fabric may be used in a variety of ways. A flame-retardant fabric does not necessarily produce a flame-retardant garment. It may pass a vertical flame test due to shrinking or melting but may still burn vigorously if supported by a structure or "scaffolding."[33]

Despite these problems, the industry has shown an ability to develop treatments that have considerable potential for flame retardance. Also useful is the avoidance of open weaves and clothing designs that promote fire. At least one large store in England no longer carries nightgowns because they more easily catch fire than do pajamas. Large flowing sleeves and bell-bottom trousers have similar propensity for brushing against hot surfaces and igniting.

The last type of problem in the energy transfer phase is the development of toxic gases. In home fires the majority of deaths are caused by carbon monoxide and possibly other toxic gas poisoning, not by burns or oxygen depletion per se. Many of the newer synthetic fibers used for rugs and drapes, plastics, and fire-retarded polyurethane foam produce other poison gases that have been implicated in deaths. To what extent they actually contribute to such deaths is the subject of intense argument, some study, but no definitive conclusions.[34]

Toxic fumes are often generated during smoldering, preceding open conflagration. Recent work with the National Bureau of Standards indicates that dyed upholstery fabric containing the sodium salt mordant emits more toxic gases than does fabric that has gone through a rinse to remove the salt. Some individuals have opposed dissemination of this information for fear that requiring a low-salt final product for upholstery fabric would be economically disadvantageous to the American textile industry.

Substantial benefit can be gained from the installation in all homes and other buildings of smoke and fire alarms that are sensitive to excessive but survivable levels of carbon monoxide or of heat. This is one area where there is also excellent evidence that public education can be successful. Where pediatricians have recommended the installation of such devices in homes, almost half of parents complied, and a third installed the device correctly.[35] No parents in a control group took similar action.

Pezoldt and Van Cott have pointed out, however, that an alarm that is capable of effectively arousing a young person cannot be assumed to have comparable effect on the elderly,[36] and Rohles has documented the problems of persons with hearing deficits in responding to such alarms.[37] But once aroused, people often lose valuable time in actual fire situations by attempting to seek further information or consulting with others rather than taking prompt appropriate actions.[38] Smoke alarms, therefore, are an aid, but not *the* solution to escape in a fire.

Another area where public education appears to have had some success concerns the emergency treatment of burns. In previous years the use of butter, grease, or other home remedies to cover localized burns was common. Since the advent of cold water application as the method of choice, the public appears to be both aware of the method (which reverses the direction of heat flow) and willing to apply it.

Countermeasures

Several countermeasures have already been noted, including broad bases and lower centers of gravity for many utensils, covers that don't fall off, chemicals with higher flash points that do not spread as easily, pilot lights for stoves and ovens, better shielding for floors and walls near wood stoves, guards for hot surfaces or controlled flames that can be easily touched, stove displays and controls that avoid confusion, periodic cleaning of flues and chimneys, safer matches and ash trays, flame-retardant design and materials for fabrics, and smoke alarms.

We will close the chapter with consideration of two final issues: the value of evaluation systems to determine whether a house or other building is at substantial risk of fire and the effectiveness of broad community education for fire safety.

The general assumption that underlies fire safety codes and inspections is that it is possible to examine an environment and its occupants, to assess factors that increase or decrease the risk of fire or fire-related injury, and to formulate a summary "Fire Safety Effectiveness Statement." There are many schemes for carrying out such inspections and for formulating such statements. Watts has examined fourteen typical systematic methods for grading fire safety, with three questions in mind:[39]

1. Do they have internal validity? Are their basic assumptions explicitly identified and do they have logical and scientific derivation?
2. Do they have external validity? Do their methods collaborate existing knowledge of fire safety and have wide applicability?
3. Do they have utility? Are they relatively easy to use, requiring minimal level of judgmental fire skills and analytical skills, utilizing data readily available, and being insensitive to vagaries of data but yet accurate enough to permit sound decisions?

The fourteen methods divided into two different approaches for grading fire safety. Eight were theoretical methods, using probability theory, simulation, network analysis, and calculus. They tend to have both internal and external validity but little utility, usually requiring at least extensive analytical skills.

The remaining six methods were schedules or checklist types of approaches. They are simple to use but seldom justified in their selection of items or in the assumptions regarding these items. In general, they require a fair degree of judgmental skill in assessing fire-related situations. While three of the fourteen schemes appear to have more potential than the rest, Watts concludes that at present no method meets all three criteria—and all three are needed, he feels, to serve the needs of fire prevention and life safety.

We turn to the issue of community education as a method of promoting fire prevention and life safety. During the years 1954–63 the average annual death rate from fire was 4.3 per 100,000 for the United States, 4.8 for the state of Missouri, but 10.5 to 20.9 for six counties in the southeastern corner of that state.[40] After analysis of the pattern of fires and deaths, a three-year project was established in 1966 to provide community education through the schools, letters from the health department to the homes of 140,000 residents in the area, and through demonstration talks to community groups about the causes and prevention of the types of fires that were common to the area.

The report on this project states that there was a 43 percent reduction in death rates for the three years of the project, from 12.9 to 7.4, and that on multiple choice questions concerning this subject junior high school students averaged 75 percent on a pretest and 91 percent after the demonstration talk, with 46 percent getting scores of 100 percent.[40]

I met the former director of this project and asked the inevitable epidemiologist's question. Had he compared the rates with those of other counties not exposed to the project? Such analysis had in fact been done and showed only slight decrease in the nonproject area. Furthermore, as of 1972–77 the six-county area still had 50 percent fewer fire deaths than before the project began.[41] He further wrote that the project cost 17 cents per capita per year, or 50 cents per capita over the three years.

Why did this project succeed, and why did its success appear to continue for so long? I suspect there are several reasons. First, the project was based on careful in-depth investigation of over 1,000 fires and burns in the area and was modified from time to time to include new information identified as a result of these investigations.

Second, the project focused on a single type of event, rather than on all injuries. Third, the effort was not a safety week or safety month but an extensive and intensive activity over a full three years. Fourth, the project sought to involve all of the residents through contact with *all* students, establishment of community councils, and letters from the health department to *all* homes. It is relevant, for example, that nonwhites, who comprised 16 percent of the area population, were 39 percent of the burn population. For any effort to succeed, it was essential to reach this segment of the community.

Fifth, the project staff spent considerable time in developing educational materials that are not only educational but highly entertaining. I have seen the demonstration unit, which is used to show how fires occur and how they can be avoided, and it literally rivets one's attention. Finally, and of substantial importance, the project aimed at behavioral and environmental changes that, once understood, are relatively easy to accomplish without serious effect on ego structure. Improving the fire resistance of insulation around a chimney is nowhere near as threatening as trying to change drinking behavior.

All of these, but probably especially the last, help explain the continuing effect of the project. Environmental changes to a home, for example, are likely to remain for a number of years, long after students had grown up and left the area.

Also important is the fact that this project was developed because of long-term trends and not in response to brief changes in rates that might merely be random deviation from the mean, and the evaluation was designed to observe who was being reached and how. In short, the project appears to have succeeded because it is one of those all-too-rare efforts that was really designed so it would have a chance to succeed.

21
Falls

As a cause of death from unintentional injury throughout the world, falls are exceeded only by highway injury. And none of the types of injury events exceed falls in the range of death rates among the various nations. As shown in Table 8–6, the crude death rate goes all the way from no reported deaths in Syria to 26 per 100,000 population for France and Austria. Among the developed nations death rates are usually 15 or higher, while they tend to be below 7 for most of the developing countries listed in the table. At least some of the reasons for this diversity are differences in age distribution among nations and different reporting criteria and completeness.

The death rate in the United States as of 1980 was 5.4, having ranged from 13 to 17 between 1913 and 1952.[1] Beginning in the 1950s it began to decline, with a 35 percent decrease between 1970 and 1980 alone. At least in part, this may reflect improvements in treatment for hip fractures and for complications associated with aging. Hip nailing and related procedures that permit early ambulation of patients, for example, became popular in the United States by the late 1950s. It may also reflect the fact that many delayed deaths from falls in the United States are probably attributed to cardiovascular or other chronic disease.[2]

The U.S. death rate in 1980 translates into 12,300 deaths, 6,700 of which occurred in the home and 8,500 of which occurred to persons age 65 or older (5,200 of whom died of falls in the home). The death rate from falls in the home environment is: age 0 to 4—0.9; 5 to 14 and 15 to 24—0.2; age 25 to 44—0.5; age 45 to 64—2.0; age 65 to 74—7.0; and age 75 or older—42.3. Overall, the rate for males slightly exceeds that for females.

Around 1971 there were estimated to be 4.4 million falls per annum in the United States from stairs or other heights and 9.2 million falls on level surfaces, for an overall rate of 67.0 per 1,000 population, again with about equal rates for both sexes.[3] Rates for children under age 6 were 106, age 6 to 16 were 91, and for age 15 to 24, 25 to 44, and 45 to 64, respectively, were 54, 41, and 47. Among older persons they rose again to 84.

The nonfatal injury rate (treated injuries and those affecting usual activities for a day or longer) for falls is higher than for any other single type of injury.[3] About a third involve fall from a height, such as on stairs. Gordon et al., reporting on injury in four rural villages in Punjab, India, where stairs do not exist, noted that falls comprised only 9 percent of fifty injuries and were exceeded by several other types of injuries: cutting and piercing instruments (21 percent), cutting and piercing objects (17 percent), injury by animal (13 percent), striking against or by blunt objects (11 percent), and contact with hot or corrosive substances (9 percent).[4]

Iskrant and Joliet state that under age 5 both sexes have about 4,000 to 5,000 nonfatal falls per fatal event.[5] This ratio increases for age 5 to 14 to 24,000 to 1 for girls and about 12,000 to 1 for boys. It decreases rapidly over the next decade and more slowly thereafter, until by age 65 or older the ratio is equal for both sexes with about 1 death for less than every 1,000 injuries. For all age groups except age 5 to 24, the nonfatal injury rate for females exceeds that for males. Men are somewhat more likely to fall from heights and to be injured in the occupational environment. There have been suggestions from limited data that blacks have lower rates of hip fractures than do whites.[6]

One measure of the societal impact of falls is in their contribution to head and spinal cord injury. According to the National Head and Spinal Cord Injury Survey falls were the initiating event in 515,000 of the 2.02 million head injuries in the U.S. over a five-year period and in 10,000 of the 54,000 spinal cord injuries during those years.[7] (About half the head injuries and 16,000 spinal cord injuries were from highway crashes, and 27,000 spinal cord injuries were from other causes, predominantly recreational activity in teenage and young adult males, which will be discussed later).

The direct care and indirect economic costs during 1974 for all persons with head injury that year or still alive after injuries in 1970 to 1973 was $2.384 billion, of which falls contributed $316 million and motor vehicle injury $1.64 billion. Serious head injury in falls tends to involve subdural hematoma, whereas motor vehicle injuries tend to involve concussion with brain contusion or laceration.

Overall costs of spinal cord injury during these years was $234 million, with cost by cause not specified. I suspect, however, that the contribution of falls to this exceeds the 20 percent that one might ordinarily extrapolate based on its proportion of all spinal cord injuries because survival after six years is achieved by 70 percent of persons with spinal injuries from falls versus 95 percent for recreational injuries, but 50 percent to less than 60 percent for motor vehicles, firearms, and all other causes.[8] Thus, costs for long-term care would be greater for injuries from sports and falls.

Human Factors in the Pre-Injury Phase

Extreme youth, alcohol, aging, and medical impairment, again, are important factors. Toddlers and slightly older children have poorly developed locomotive skills, inordinate curiosity, and limited strength and coordination. They often climb into untenable positions, lose their balance, and fall.

Gibson and Walk tested the hypothesis that some falls occur because children develop ability to locomote at a faster rate than they develop depth perception.[9] Infants capable of crawling were coaxed to crawl toward their mothers from a clearly solid surface across a heavy sheet of glass that appeared to be either a shallow or deep dropoff into open space. While most children were unwilling to crawl out—indicating well-developed depth perception—some were willing to crawl out. Had the glass not been there, they would have fallen.

On average, center of gravity is higher for younger children than for older ones, promoting ease of toppling.[10] While the mean center of gravity decreases only slightly for a standing child between birth and age 13, that of the 95th percentile child drops more markedly from about 65 percent of standing height around age 25 to 36 months to about 59 to 60 percent in children age 10 or older. The mean center of gravity while seated decreases progressively from about 57 percent of seated height under age 4 months to about 32 percent in children age 13.

Turning to the subject of alcohol, there has been a general misperception that "drunks never get hurt when they fall because they are so relaxed." Trained acrobats seldom injure themselves in falls because they know how to spread the energy loading over a large body surface. But this does not mean that anyone can avoid injury, no matter how clumsily they fall, if only they are relaxed.

In my own study of nonhighway injury fatalities only 30 percent of persons age 15 or older who died within six hours after a fall had no alcohol in their blood, 10 percent had BACs of .01 to .09 percent, and 60 percent had BACs of .10 percent or higher.[11] Wechsler et al. reported positive BACs in 22.8 percent of persons treated for fall related injuries, whereas 2.6 percent of persons treated for illness had positive BACs.[12] There have also been anecdotal reports, but little documentation, of individuals who have fallen from windows while "high" on drugs such as LSD.

In mostly nonfatal falls among the elderly, 13 percent admitted to alcohol consumption before the fall, and in 8 percent the drug was felt to have contributed to the event. Among those who had consumed alcohol, 47 percent were either daily medium (three to four drinks/sitting) or daily heavy (five or more drinks/sitting) drinkers, whereas only

3 percent of those who had not consumed alcohol were daily medium drinkers and none were heavy drinkers. An additional 18 percent of the alcohol group and 2 percent of the no alcohol group were weekly medium or heavy drinkers.

Honkanen et al. have examined alcohol in nonfatal falls in public places of persons age 15 or older who were compared with uninjured persons at the same location and time of day.[13] Most of the falls involved slipping on ice in winter or stumbling in summer. In winter 73 percent of males and 16 percent of females had BACs above .05 percent, and in summer the comparable figures were 83 percent and 24 percent. The relative risk (RR) of falling compared to the control was 0.5 at .03 to .05 percent, 1.8 at .06 to .10 percent, and, respectively, 6.5, 13, and 29 in BAC ranges .11 to .15 percent, .16 to .20 percent and .21 percent or higher.

In another study of nonfatal falls positive BACs were as follows: falls while going to or from work—28 percent (11 percent were .15 percent or higher); falls at work—28 percent (8 percent); falls at home—37 percent (20 percent); falls during other free-time activity—45 percent (22 percent in the very high range).[14]

Mention was also made in the last chapter about persons with seizures, cerebrovascular disease, or other chronic conditions who have suffered severe burns. Commonly, these occur when the person falls, strikes a hostile surface, and is unable to remove him or herself.[15,16]

The elderly are by far the largest single group to die as a result of falls. In my own study of persons age 60 or older treated for falls and matched with the nearest neighbor of similar age and sex, 40 percent of injured population and 32 percent of comparison sample reported one or more fall during the previous year.[2] But 22 percent of persons with falls for medical reasons, compared to 7 percent and 3 percent of persons with other falls or no falls, had had three or more previous episodes (usually not medically attended) during that time, clearly identifying falling as a repetitive problem for those with medical impairment.

An acute or chronic health problem (excluding alcohol) contributed to the fall in 34 percent of events, health or alcohol was definitely not a factor in 50 percent, and its role could not be determined in 8 percent. These health problems included dizzy spells, insecure footing because a leg buckled or because of arthritis, general debilitation or multiple sclerosis, stroke or similar disorder of mobility, or confusion related to poor eyesight or senile dementia. As noted before, an additional 8 percent were attributable to acute impairment from alcohol.

Important differences were apparent at time of interview between those whose fall was precipitated by a health problem, those who fell for other reasons, and the comparison group of age/sex matched neighbors.

Only 35 percent of the first group were lucid and had no reported limitations of mobility, vision or stamina, and 27 percent were clearly not lucid. In the second group 75 percent had no physical limitations and only 5 percent were not lucid, while in the comparison group 49 percent had no physical limitations and 4 percent appeared confused. Most persons lacking lucidity had physical limitations as well.

Sheldon identifies several reasons why the elderly more often fall.[17] In drop attacks the person may suddely collapse with loss of muscle power in legs and trunk, sometimes lasting for several hours. This loss of postural control is similar to what is seen in decerebrate animals.

Second, he identified falls from true vertigo, often associated with defective hearing. Next are falls due to disease of the central nervous system, such as a cerebral or carotid artery thrombosis, preexisting hemiplegia, or paralysis agitans. Other or related factors identified were falls due to kinking of the vertebral artery on throwing the head back, postural hypotension when standing up or getting out of bed suddenly, loss of vibratory sense in the legs, and severe deterioration of gait with consequent postural instability, actual mechanical weakness in a leg, and mental confusion. These factors have been implicated by others as well.[18–24]

Of particular importance in the elderly is a shift forward in center of gravity. Perhaps this is one reason why, as Sheldon observes, older people are unable to regain their balance once they begin to fall, as they did when they were younger.

Other reasons for falls are cardiac arrhythmias,[25] severe arthritis, and disorders of vision (many of which are normative with aging) such as increased sensitivity to glare, yellowing of the cornea with loss of ability to distinguish visual cues on the ground by difference in color, decreased dark adaptation, and cataracts or glaucoma. The elderly are especially sensitive to highly polished floors (found in many nursing homes or public buildings), patterned stairs, or places where lighting is either excessively bright or only modestly dark, or where the level of light changes suddenly. Because of problems in gait and postural control elderly persons may become especially dependent on vision to help locomotion.[26]

It is sometimes suggested that some elderly persons break a hip (or a vertebra) because of osteoporosis or osteopenia and then fall. While this hypothesis is enticing—and while weakness of bone undoubtedly contributes to severity of fracture once the fall is initiated—I have not seen any data with definitive "proof."[2,27,28]

The elderly also have decreasing muscle mass to maintain position over the range of environmental obstacles. Data do suggest that the frequency of falls in this population is correlated with the amount of muscle mass,[29] and it has been suggested without documentation that older black women in the United States may have lower hip fracture rates than white women because on average they may have larger muscle mass.[29,30]

Although judging from prescription patterns many physicians are not aware of it, a medication dose half that given to a younger person may be adequate for the elderly. When tranquilizers and similar medications have been reduced in nursing homes, there is less confusion and fewer falls.[30]

Haddon et al. make the important observation that insights in Sheldon's research came primarily from an adequate knowledge of medicine, human pathology, and physiology.[31] As their comments are meant to suggest, the sorts of research into causal factors identified here for children, the elderly, and persons with other forms of impairment are a far cry from simply urging people to avoid throw rugs and rickety stairs or to watch their step, as safety practitioners are so prone to do based on superficial analysis and minimal understanding.

Environmental Factors in the Pre-Injury Phase

Previous chapters have already considered many of the major environmental factors in the initiation of falls. We will review them briefly. Where a building is more than one story high or has a basement, there is the possibility of falling from a high window or down stairs. In New York City in 1966, for example, 20 percent of injury deaths to children were from falls, and 97 percent of those were from a height in a multiple-level dwelling, such as from a roof top, window, or fire escape.[32] A number of these children had previous history of major falls, mental retardation, or seizures.

The typical tenement in some New York neighborhoods has a prominent fire escape, which is frequently used as a play area by children. Since air conditioning is not available in these apartments, people often sleep on fire escapes or roofs on hot nights, a pattern that is common in many cities where multilevel tenements exist.

Chapter 18 has dealt at some length with factors that increase the hazard of stairs: visual confusion because of sudden distraction, poor lighting or patterned covering for steps, banisters that do not delineate beginnings, endings, and landings on stairs, inappropriate step dimensions, rugs that are capable of slipping forward as one walks down the stairs, and number of landings. Regarding ladders, we have spoken about slippage because the user has no information about the proper angle for placement and because of actual breaking of ladders that are inadequately constructed.

Other lesser heights that have been discussed are bunk beds without side rails, especially in Hong Kong, and high chairs or baby carriages that have narrow bases and hence can tip over easily if the child moves about and thus shifts the center of gravity. Regarding falls on nonelevated levels, mention was made again of effects of poor lighting or surfaces that are highly reflective. Because of sensitivity to glare, an elderly person can be confused by a waxed linoleum or marble floor that appears to be wet. This causes a sudden change in gait, which increases the likelihood of falls.

Older people who shuffle along without raising their feet completely are also likely to trip on edges of rugs, to cause motion or slippage in rugs that do not have good traction with the floor, or to trip on uneven surfaces. The hazards of wet and slippery surfaces in bathrooms, often associated with absence of grab rails, have also been indentified. Surprisingly, slipping on icy surfaces does not appear to be associated with impairment in the elderly.[2] Table 21–1 shows environmental factors according to presence or absence of precipitating health problems.[2]

When flared or "bell bottom" trousers were popular, falls increased because people tripped on them, as they did when clogs and platform shoes became popular as footware.[33] Sheldon identifies another hazard when talking about the pleasures that the elderly can derive from having pets.[34] He warns that cats take perverse delight in tangling themselves

Table 21–1
Environmental Factors in Initiation of Falls among Elderly According to Presence of Precipitating Health Problem in Fall

Environmental Factor	*Precipitating Health Problem*	*No Health Problem*	*Total*[a]
Slippery ground	3	41	22
Rough ground	11	13	12
Ladder/chair	2	11	6
Walker/wheelchair	13	3	7
Rug	9	1	5
Other	19	16	17
None	43	7	24
Unknown, possible	0	8	7
Total			
%	100	100	100
(N)	(63)	(75)	(150)

Source: J. Waller, "Falls among the Elderly: Human and Environmental Factors," *Accident Analysis and Prevention* 10(1978):21–33. Reprinted with permission. Copyright 1978, Pergamon Press, Ltd.

[a]12 persons included with falls in which role of health problems is unknown.

around people's legs, especially in the dark. As a result, he says, he has treated fractures in elderly women who have tripped over the family cat.

Factors in the Injury and Post-Injury Phases

The three major human factors that contribute to severity of injury—and that have already been noted—are alcohol and its effects on sensitivity of nervous system to trauma, increased bone fragility in the elderly, and medical impairment that prevents people who fall from removing themselves from hot or other dangerous surfaces. The fact that unguarded hot surfaces, easily breakable glass, or hard sharp corners on furniture are available for contact also markedly increases severity. Banisters on stairs, if properly designed and installed, give people cues regarding the length and configuration of stairs, and they also help to break the force of those falls that do occur. Resilient floor covering spreads kinetic forces so that injury may be less severe.

If the injured person is unable to move and is living alone, as the elderly and the alcoholic often are, considerable delay may occur before discovery and treatment. Delay may also occur because of procrastination. Among a group of patients with fracture of back or leg bones, only 57 percent sought care within the first hour after injury, and 26 percent waited six hours or longer.[2] Only head injury brought prompt request for treatment (75 percent in less than an hour), probably because of the extensive display of blood.

Once in the emergency department one is not necessarily ensured of prompt and compassionate treatment. For a given severity of injury those arriving by ambulance are likely to be examined more quickly than those who arrive by other transportation.[2] In addition, evidence exists that the elderly and those impaired by alcohol at least on occasion receive less enthusiastic or, in some cases, more hostile treatment than do other patients.[35,36]

Countermeasures

Before discussing new countermeasures it is worthwhile to briefly highlight those already discussed in previous chapters. These include in the pre-injury phase the range of design and construction issues concerning stairs and bathrooms described in chapter 18 and use of bars or grillwork on upper-story windows. These must be capable of being removed quickly in an emergency, since, as we have already observed, fire is particularly a threat to life for persons living on upper floors. Furthermore, where laws requiring such installation exist, as in New York City, their effectiveness is no greater than the degree to which they are enforced.[37,38] Bunk beds with side rails, furniture with more stable base for children, and chairs that are easier for the elderly to get out of have also been mentioned in the pre-injury phase, as have adequate, nonglare lighting and nonglare, skid-resistant surfaces without excessive patterns on floors for the elderly.

Many elderly persons, at least in the United States, are overdosed with medications. For persons who appear to be falling excessively, medication regimens need to be reconsidered.[21,22,23] Abuse of alcohol must also be kept in mind as a possibility requiring therapeutic intervention.

Studies have suggested that in some cases fluoride and calcium or estrogen therapy may strengthen bone and either reduce the frequency of falls or the severity of their results.[27,28] Both regimens, however, carry risks of side effects that must be considered.[27,39] Exercise for the elderly is another useful option, both to increase muscle tone and to give better balance and confidence.[18,29] For elderly persons who have compromised vertebral artery circulation it is helpful to rearrange storage so that most commonly used items are on lower shelves. Such individuals should also be advised to try to arrange their activities so they do not raise their arms above their heads.[34]

Some communities have laws or regulations requiring cleaning of walks within a limited time after snowfalls, and at least one report from Chicago indicates that peer pressure by neighbors can increase the proportion of people who shovel their walks.[40]

Countermeasures already identified in the injury phase are rounded, resilient corners and surfaces in bathrooms and on furniture, resilient flooring, glass that doesn't break easily, banisters on stairs, grab rails in bathrooms, and guarding around hot surfaces or open flame. In the post-injury phase some communities have established programs to identify elderly persons who should be looked in on regularly, thus potentially identifying more quickly if help is needed.

22
Poisoning

Unintentional poisoning is a difficult phenomenon to determine both regarding fatal and nonfatal events. Mention was made in chapter 6 about the possibility that many deaths from suicide are listed instead as unintentional poisoning. Barraclough points out that if poisoning deaths are truly unintentional, they should involve a distribution of lethal preparations similar to that found in the home and not favor the less unpleasant toxic substances available (such as psychotropic drugs), which would be a more common choice in suicide.[1] But while only 28 percent of a random sample of homes contained sedatives, sleeping tablets, or tranquilizers, 80 percent of poisonings classified as nonsuicide are caused by these drugs and at least that proportion are from mixtures of psychotropic drugs that have been ingested in large quantity.

The evidence, he suggests, supports the view that most deaths from poisoning are suicides that are not classified as such by the coroner. Even if all poisoning deaths classified as unintentional or unknown were really suicides, underestimation of the suicide rate itself would be less than 23 percent, in contrast to some statements that the true suicide rate is two or three times the official one.

Injury Patterns

Given this warning, let us examine some of the official data on death from unintentional poisoning. These data internationally appear in table 8–6. The crude death rates per 100,000 population range from a low of 0.2 for Chile to a high of 5.8 for Czechoslovakia. There are relatively few outliers, however, and over half of the rates range from about 0.7 to 1.4.

The death rate in the United States declined from 3.3 in 1913 to an all time low of 0.8 in 1957, then rose steadily to 2.2 in 1975 and decreased again to 1.2 in 1980.[2] Most of the changes since 1957 reflect increases in deaths among persons age 15 to 44 to a peak in 1975 and a decline in this age group since then. Table 22–1 shows the distribution of deaths according to age, sex, and type of poison involved.[2] Forty

Table 22–1
Deaths from Poisoning by Type, Age, and Sex, United States, 1978

	Both Sexes			
Type of Poisoning	*Number*	*Rate Per 1,000,000*	*Males Number*	*Females Number*
A. *Solids/liquids* (includes B and C, below)	3,035	1.4	1,800	1,235
Under age 5	81	0.5	45	36
5–14	37	0.1	25	12
15–24	577	1.4	405	172
25–44	1,210	2.1	811	399
45–64	725	1.7	334	391
65 and older	405	1.7	180	225
B. *Drugs/medications*[a]	1,906		1,036	870
Under age 5	48		24	24
5–14	25		14	11
15–24	400		274	126
25–44	798		495	303
45–64	336		117	219
65 and older	299		112	187
C. *Other solids/liquids*[a]	1,129		764	365
Under age 5	33		21	12
5–14	12		11	1
15–24	177		131	46
25–44	412		316	96
45–64	389		217	172
65 and older	106		68	38
D. *Gases/vapors*[a]	1,737	0.8	1,260	477
Under age 5	51	0.3	26	25
5–14	76	0.2	45	31
15–24	525	1.3	362	163
25–44	492	0.8	404	88
45–64	356	0.8	268	88
65 and older	237	1.0	155	82

Source: Adapted from *Accident Facts, 1981 Edition* (Chicago, Ill.: National Safety Council, 1981).

[a]Major contributors in drugs were analgesics (including aspirin) 452, other sedatives 231, tranquilizers 168, cardiovascular 172; in other solids and liquids—alcohol 363; in gases and vapors—motor vehicle exhaust 863, carbon monoxide from incomplete combustion 172, other carbon monoxide 194.

percent of the deaths were from drugs and medications, and males exceeded females at almost all ages and in deaths from each major class of substance. The age group at highest risk is persons age 25 to 44. In 1980, 3,100 of a total of 4,300 poisoning deaths occurred in the home.

The numbers and types of fatal poisonings clearly reflect the environment and technology in any area and at any moment in time. In the United States, with a largely urban population, deaths from snake bites and insect venom are rare. Between 1950 and 1954, for example, there were 215 deaths from venomous animal stings or bites, 71 from reptiles, 86 from bees and wasps, and 39 from spiders.[3] The annual death rate from snake venom is 0.09 per million population. Throughout the rest of the world, however, there are 300,000 poisonous bites annually from snakes alone resulting in 30,000 to 40,000 deaths.[4] About 25,000 of these occur in Southeast Asia, and 3,000 to 4,000 in South America, especially Brazil.

In years past, when strychnine, arsenic, caustics, and kerosene lamps were in common use in the United States, deaths from these causes were more common. In Ceylon, with use of kerosene bottle lamps, ingestion of kerosene by children is still a major problem.[5] For reasons to be discussed later, overdoses of aspirin were a more frequent cause of injury and death in the United States in years past than they are now, while deaths from utility gas were a major problem in the British Isles. And with the widespread use of illicit drugs in the 1960s and 1970s, deaths from these recreational chemicals have been increasing.

We turn now to the vexing problem of nonfatal poisonings. Where toxicology laboratories exist and are used, the fact of death from poisoning is less difficult to identify than is the intent of ingestion. With nonfatal ingestion, however, it is hard to tell whether there has been true poisoning (cellular damage) or simply seeking of health care because of a known or suspected ingestion that doesn't involve true poisoning. These false alarms would be countable as injury under the National Health Survey definition. On average, poisonings in the United States result in only one day of reduced activity for those who report ingestions, by far the shortest period of altered activity for any category of injury.[6]

The first formal poison information center was established in Chicago in 1953.[7] Within ten to fifteen years there were several hundred of these centers located throughout the United States and Europe. In the United States, all except the centers in California accept calls directly from the public, and these calls form the basis of estimates of poisonings in the nation. Such estimates range from 500,000 to 2 million per year,[7] but no one knows how many are "real" poisonings and how many are known or suspected ingestions that are nontoxic.

Since likelihood of injury usually is a function of dose, some authors have examined the accuracy of patient and physician estimates of quantity ingested. These authors report a tendency at least initially to overestimate the amount ingested.[8] If this is true, calls to poison information centers—which are usually the first contact with the health system—would probably have greatest susceptibility to overestimation.

Other researchers have pointed out that there often is little correlation between serum level of a chemical and the clinical picture.[9] They suggest that a better measure of toxicity might be the proportion of persons with ingestion who are hospitalized.[10] Using this as a measure it might be possible to adjust the number of *ingestions* reported by poison information centers to provide an estimate of the number of *poisonings*, thus reducing the effect on statistics of specific nonharmful chemicals that are ingested frequently simply because they are very common in the environment or are attractive to young children.

According to the National Clearinghouse for Poison Control Centers, fifteen products (acetyl salicylic acid, kerosene, and ammonia each count as a single product) account for 1 percent of all products but 69 percent of reported ingestions. The thirty-one products named 100 times or more are 2 percent of all identified products but 76 percent of ingestions.[11] The remaining 98 percent of products represented only 24 percent of cases. Table 22–2 shows what would happen if the incidence of poisoning ingestion involving these substances were adjusted to reflect the proportions hospitalized, thus giving an estimate of actual poisoning.

In marked contrast to the distribution of fatal injuries involving solids and liquids, about 90 percent of reported nonfatal ingestions involve children under age 5. Stallones and Corsa report that 8 percent of injuries to children under age 15 are poisonings, and they comprise 15 percent to children under age 5.[12]

Manheimer et al. report an annual rate of 6.2 poison ingestions per 1,000 children under age 16, equivalent to that for contact with hot objects or substances, motor vehicle injuries, and suffocation.[13] Unlike most other injuries, ingestions were considerably less severe: 0.5 severe injuries per 1,000 population, 7.3 percent severe, and an average of 1.1 physicians' visits per injury. For ages 0 to 3 the rate per 1,000 is 16.7 for both sexes, 20.0 for boys, and 12.9 for girls. From there it drops markedly to 1.6 (1.7 for males and 1.5 for females) at ages 4 to 7, 0.8 (1.0 and 0.5) for ages 8 to 11; and 0.3 for both sexes and each sex for age 12 to 15.

In 1968 Verhulst and Crotty found a quarter of ingestions by children involved aspirin, almost all of which was child size (0.08 gm or 1¼-grain) tablets and equal to ingestion of all other internal medicines.[7] Cleaning and polishing agents comprised 15 percent, with pesticides, turpentine products, petroleum products, and cosmetics comprising 5 to 6 percent each.

If tables 22–1 and 22–2 are compared, it is clear that aspirin is a problem in both nonfatal and fatal ingestions, and other medications are important as causes of death but not as substances nonfatally ingested. Alcohol, which isn't even noted among the top thirty-one products, is a major cause of death among the nonmedicinal liquids and solids.

Table 22–2
Thirty-one Products Most Often Involved in 34,653 Reported Nonfatal Poisonings, United States, July 1959–December 1961

Product	A *Number of Cases*	B *Number of All Cases*	C *Percentage Hospitalized*	D *Column A × Column C*	E *Rank Based on Column A*	F *Rank Based on Column D*
Aspirin	15,546	44.9	13.9	2,161	1	1
Clorox	1,855	5.3	14.3	265	4	4
Kerosene	1,656	4.8	39.5	654	3	2
Ex-Lax	1,021	2.9	6.0	61	4	12
Drano	989	2.9	50.9	503	5	3
Ammonia	420	1.2	40.8	171	6	5
Pride furniture polish	360	1.0	32.6	117	7	8
Lysol	356	1.0	29.0	103	8	9
Old English polishes	303	0.9	50.3	152	9	6
Gator Roach Hives	275	0.8	21.3	59	10	13
Lestoil	262	0.8	27.9	73	11	10
Lye	245	0.7	55.1	135	12	7
Purex	240	0.7	13.0	31	13	18
Pine-Sol disinfectant	212	0.6	31.5	67	14	11
Black Flag	200	0.6	25.5	51	15	14
Real-Kill	194	0.6	26.3	51	16	14
Raid	192	0.5	22.7	44	17	15
Windex	173	0.5	3.1	5	18	27
Comet	169	0.5	0.0	0	19	28
Harris Famous roach tablets	168	0.5	5.6	9	20	25
6–12 insect repellent	168	0.5	8.5	14	21	22
Poly-Vi-Sol	166	0.5	0.0	0	22	28
Mr. Clean	162	0.5	13.8	22	23	20
Sani-Flush	161	0.5	22.5	36	24	16
Carters Little Pills	161	0.5	7.5	12	25	23
Roman cleanser bleach	158	0.5	6.5	10	26	23
Joy	145	0.4	5.7	8	27	26
Chocks vitamins	127	0.4	0.0	0	28	28
Ajax	121	0.3	13.6	16	29	21
Lilly's ant cup	119	0.3	27.3	32	30	17
Easy Off oven cleaner	101	0.3	29.8	30	31	19

Source: *Survey of the Most-Frequent Accidently Ingested Products* (Washington, D.C.: National Clearinghouse for Poison Control Centers, Department of Health, Education and Welfare, 1963).

Human Factors in Pre-Injury Phase

Although other human factors issues are relevant, especially where fatalities are concerned, the major issue for discussion involving nonfatal poisonings is that of early child development. Corsa and Stallones found that, compared to a cohort of neighbors with children under age 5, those who had been poisoned were more often age 18 to 35 months (60 percent versus 44 percent among neighbors).[14]

These are months when the child is increasingly able to climb and to reach new things but is without experience about what is to be avoided. It is also the time when assertive behavior is at its peak and when mouthing has not yet decreased. Sense of taste develops at this time, and Stallones and Corsa believe that unpleasant experiences of touch, taste, and perhaps odor help to develop avoidance reactions and decrease the likelihood of injury.[12]

It is generally suggested that young children are not deterred by substances that to adults do not have acceptable taste. Temple and Stremming indicate that taste can be a deterrent in nursery school age children, but unfortunately, no data are provided on actual age of these children, and it is likely that many, if not most, were above the peak months for ingestion.[15]

Most studies comparing behavioral characteristics of ingesters or repeat ingesters and noningesters are hampered by possible biases of selective memory by parents of the ingesters. In addition, the samples studied often are quite small. Sibert and Newcombe found that ingesters were more anxious and active than controls, cause more worry, and more often put things other than food in their mouths.[16] Following the line of hyperactivity, Stewart et al. conclude that one out of every three or four boys brought to hospital for poisoning is a hyperactive child, whereas in that age group they would predict this behavior problem by chance in one boy out of seventeen.[17]

Margolis reevaluated poison repeaters, single ingesters and noningesters five years after an initial study and found that poison repeaters continued to have behavior problems more often than did noningesters, including hyperactivity, destructiveness, uncooperativeness, stubbornness, fighting, and temper tantrums.[18] These characteristics were more common among repeaters than among single ingesters, and repeaters were more often labeled "aggressive-impulsive" and "passive-anxious." In fact, the entire families of the ingesters, and especially the repeaters, had more ongoing stress from marital conflict, mental and physical illness, separation and loss of family members, and so forth than did control families.

Sibert reports similar results.[19] Thirty of 100 families with ingestions, but 4 of 100 comparison families reported one or more of five major stress factors (serious family illness, pregnancy, recent family moves, one parent away from home, anxiety or depression in one or both parents).

Sobel asserts that the poisoning episodes seem to be related to a power struggle with the child because of inept role performance by the mother.[20] Depending upon the situation, he believes that the poisoning can be seen as an act of defiance, a bid for attention, an attempt to achieve dependency through coercion, or an expression of anger against the mother deflected onto oneself.

One problem with studies of this type is that authors or readers are tempted to conclude that they have identified a sine qua non, rather than simply one factor among several that predispose to injury. To place this issue in better perspective, note that Sibert's study found stress factors in 30 percent of ingestion families but no stress factors in 70 percent.

Corsa and Stallones also found that "slightly more" ingesters were considered to be independent, active, contrary or stubborn, restless, disobedient, and difficult at bedtime, and slightly fewer were thought to want support and comfort to an unusual degree or were considered to be too shy.[14] They note that this difference is too small to be of any value for prediction. This statement is especially important given their observation that families with one poison case were more likely to have had similar events in the previous twelve months. Concordant with Sobel's comments about mothering, they found that parents of the poisoned children were three to five years younger than either of the comparison groups, and they asked whether lesser maturation of these parents is a significant factor in increasing the risk of poisoning in their children.

Other factors that may be working simultaneously to increase the risk of ingestion are hunger and thirst on the part of the child and task demands on parents that may draw their attention away from the child at crucial moments. Carithers suggests that children may drink kerosene in summer because of thirst,[21] while Meyer notes that 57 percent of ingestions of aspirin occurred less than an hour before the child's mealtime, when the mother was especially busy with meal preparations and related household activities, and that a third of these children were just recovering from illnesses and just beginning to get back their appetites.[22]

Both he and Corsa and Stallones also found a high proportion of mothers who were working outside the home, and for the poisoned group not only were three times as many mothers (15 percent) working as for the comparison group, but these working mothers also tended to be younger than comparison mothers.[14]

De Castro and Kocur comment about children who are early risers and get into trouble presumably while parents are asleep[23] (and conceivably because the child has gotten hungry and sought something to eat). Echoing Sibert's finding of families with recent moves, Maragos et al. have described paint ingestions occurring in families that have just moved and where access to both usual and unusual substances (such as paint) is altered from that of the previous household pattern.[24] Again, this is a time when parents are likely to be faced with greater task demands that affect their ability to monitor children's needs and to cope with them.

Moving to the subject of human factors in poisonings of adults—which tend to be true poisonings rather than harmless ingestions—conscious risk taking by persons who use drugs for recreation or who are actually addicted is an important contributor to the problem. Abusive alcohol consumption is also a major issue. In Krakow, Poland 63 percent of fatal, unintentional poisonings involved this drug,[25] and in North Carolina about half of poisoning deaths in 1973 resulted from rapid ingestion of quantities equivalent to 500 to 1,000 ml of 50 percent ethanol.[26] These quantities (BACs of .30 percent or higher) are usually associated with identifiable alcoholism.[27] Alcoholics have higher death rates from barbituates and other sedatives as well.[28]

Although death from poisoning in the elderly is not overly common, clinical signs and symptoms from unintentional overdose—and falls or other injuries as a complication—are more frequent.[29] Elderly persons often are taking a number of medications and because of renal or hepatic degeneration may have lesser ability to detoxify drugs, and because of failing memory, poor eyesight or other reasons may overdose themselves. In fact, medication errors have been observed among a majority of ambulatory patients age 60 and older.[30]

Environmental Factors in the Pre-Injury Phase

Regarding solids and liquids, the major environmental factor appears to be the extent to which access is possible because of location and ease of opening the container. Cann et al. point out that products were not in their original containers for 51 percent of ingestions by children younger than one year, 40 percent of one-year-olds, and 26 to 28 percent of two-, three-, and four-year-olds.[31] These data certainly suggest that, at least for children under age 2, between a quarter and a half of ingestions might not have occurred if original containers were involved and that the preventive suggestions to leave drugs and chemicals in original containers appear to reflect common sense.

On the other hand, data such as these are based on cases only and ignore the basic epidemiologic question whether substances in homes with ingestions are in their proper places and containers any less often than in homes without ingestions. This question has been examined by Corsa and Stallones, who report no difference in basic safety practices, except that families with poisoning *less often* had items accessible to small children.[14]

With aspirin, for example, the drug was accessible in 27 percent of ingestion homes but 36 to 37 percent of comparison residences. It is not clear whether the difference reflects "closing the barn door after the horse has escaped" or a true difference. Given the fact that there is a tendency in some families for repeated ingestions, one must suspect that factors other than accessibility per se are at work.

The other component of access is ability to open a container. It has become quite clear that this is of utmost importance, and this has resulted in laws and regulations in the United States to make "child-proof" containers for all medications and for household substances such as pesticides, caustics, and sprays.

Once the container is opened, Jolly and Forrest have shown that magenta, pink, blue, orange and brown pills are mouthed more often than are yellow, white, green, black and wine ones.[32] Among the preferred tablets—which were mouthed despite a disagreeable taste—all except brown were bright colors. It is hypothesized that brown, however, already has association with chocolate among children age 1 to 8 in this study. Age apparently made no difference in the color selection.

The selection of brown tablets assumes particular importance because of the unfortunate practice by drug companies of making candy coated children's aspirin. This practice can do nothing but add to the problem many children have in distinguishing medicine from candy. Time of year also is important in considering access. In summer time pesticides and paints are more likely to be ingested, while medicines are more common in winter.[31]

Given its large contribution to fatalities there are, relatively speaking, few recognized nonfatal poisonings from carbon monoxide in the United States. The annual incidence is believed to be about 10,000 known cases, although undoubtedly more exist that are not identified.[33] Exposure to 100 parts per million of the gas results in appreciable clinical effects in only two hours. The problem occurs in several ways.

In a few cases, as with a baseboard gas-fired heater produced and distributed by a major retailer, there may be a product defect so that a large proportion of the devices do not function properly.[34] More commonly, however, gas appliances are "out of tune," or their vents are clogged. In a survey of homes in Memphis, Tennessee, 24 percent of homes with gas appliances were found to have at least one that was emitting CO in the range of 200 ppm or greater, in some cases reaching as high as 2,500 ppm![34]

Perhaps even more common, however, appliances that should be vented or used only outside are used indoors and are unvented. Examples are automobiles left with the motor running to warm up in a closed garage or charcoal burners that are used indoors. Also a problem are various solvents and cleaning compounds that are meant to be used with active localized ventilation but where the instructions about the meaning of "adequate" ventilation are vague.[35] To most people, the term means that a window should be opened, which usually is inadequate compared to active localized ventilation that draws out the hazardous vapors with a fan in such a way that the gases do not travel past the nose.[36,37]

It has been known for some time that mobile homes present a unique problem with respect to pollution by CO and other gases because the small space permits high levels to gather rapidly. With the increasing insulation of many residences since 1973 in order to conserve fuel, the spare capacity that many larger homes have had to disperse excessive amounts of CO or other gases is being severely compromised. It is quite likely, therefore, that better insulation to improve fuel efficiency will also mean more deaths from carbon monoxide poisoning.

Baker et al. identified that some recent model automobiles operated outdoors were implicated in CO poisonings because they had been designed with a tail pipe that does not extend beyond the rear bumper.[36] If the vehicle is not in motion for even a relatively short period of time, and if the underside of the vehicle is in any way compromised, enough exhaust can accumulate to cause serious symptoms and even death.

Turning last to the subject of poisonous snakes, access in southeast Asia and some other locations may occur during flooding, when both animals and humans are driven from their usual habitats. Occupational activities in and around trees also promote contact. In southwestern United States encroaching suburbs have put more people into contact with poisonous snakes, with summer being the time when both snakes and humans are likely to be out and active.

Injury and Post-Injury Phases

The most important determinant of severity of injury with poisons is the toxicity of the substance involved. This is nowhere more apparent than with the change in suicidal and unintentional deaths in England when utility gas rich in carbon monoxide was replaced with a product that was almost free of CO.[39]

Dose, too, is important. A quantity of baby aspirin ingested will be less harmful to a child than will the same quantity of adult aspirin. With snake bites the amount of venom potentially available is related to the size of the animal, although many bites result in little injury because for some reason no venom is injected. Body weight is also an important factor, since dose plus body weight determines serum level of the substance. Because of this, it has been assumed for years that poisonous snake bites to children have more severe outcome than do those to adults. Sadan and Soroker, however, have shown just the opposite to be the case.[38]

In the post-injury phase an important issue is early identification that poisoning has occurred. One of the obstacles to such identification has been that what are labeled as "inert ingredients" in pesticides often are petroleum distillates that may be inert as insect killers but are hardly so as child killers.[39] Delay may also occur because physicians are unable to get accurate information about product ingredients, their toxicity, and treatment. The poison information center network was specifically established to deal with this problem.

Countermeasures

Nine potential types of countermeasures have been used or warrant application regarding poisoning of single individuals. First, and perhaps most important, is the substitution of less toxic substances for more toxic ones. Examples include removal of carbon tetrachloride from the market, replacement of arsenic, strychnine, and more hazardous pesticides by less harmful substances that serve the same purpose, use of lead-free paints, and removal of carbon monoxide from utility gas in the United Kingdom. In the latter case, unintentional deaths from gas and vapors declined from 3.9 for males and 5.1 for females in 1926–63 to 1.5 and 1.2 for each of the sexes in 1970–71.[37]

The second most important countermeasure has been to reduce access. The major example of this is the child-proof cap for medicines and particularly harmful household chemicals. These were tried successfully as long ago as 1959,[40,41] and initial community trials resulted in a 91 percent decrease in poisoning rates where these containers were used for aspirin and prescription medications.[42]

Nonetheless, it was not until 1972 that the Poison Prevention Packaging Act was passed in the United States. Survey results indicate that about 85 percent of the population approves of this countermeasure, although 14 percent of adults under age 30 and 33 percent of those age 60 or older report having trouble opening these containers.[43] When this has happened, most people have left the top off or loose or have switched to another container.[43] Most ingestions from child-proof containers have been where the tops were not closed properly or contents were transferred,[44] although a few children seem able to open even properly closed safety packaging.[44] Such packaging has been associated with a 76 percent drop in aspirin-related deaths among young children, a 65 percent decrease in poisonings from automotive windshield cleaning compounds, turpentine and related paint thinners, and 51 percent and 58 percent declines respectively in poisonings.[45]

However, probably not all of the effectiveness can be attributed to better closures alone. At the same time that the program was underway to create child-resistant closures, a third type of countermeasure aimed at the injury phase was also being applied, namely a nationwide effort to limit the number of baby aspirin tablets per container. This would reduce total dose for a child who did attempt to ingest the entire contents of a bottle.[46] (Similar efforts have been undertaken to reduce the quantity of lead in household paints but, unfortunately, not to limit the size of packages of Lomotil or certain particularly toxic drugs.[47]) The net result is that aspirin ingestions declined both in absolute numbers and from 26 percent of all ingestions in 1965 to 7 percent in 1973.[46]

Child-resistant cabinets have also been designed, although as yet they do not show the acceptance that has accompanied the child-proof medicine packages.[49] The fourth type of countermeasure is the avoidance of packaging that permits confusion of toxic substances for harmless ones, such as use of candy-coated infant aspirin.

Fifth is community and family education. Evaluations of these programs have in general been poorly designed or totally absent. All of the programs discussed below lack truly adequate outcome evaluation. Goals of such programs have been:

1. To help young children identify directly what substances might be poisonous or to identify a standard surrogate label, such as the "Mr. Yuk" label that has replaced the traditional skull and crossbones;
2. To promote behavioral change in these children by helping them to understand the serious consequences of poison ingestion; and
3. To help parents understand which household materials present a hazard and to promote safer storage of these materials.

The best effort described is a three-year project in Monroe County, New York,[48] which sought to alter knowledge and behavior through five approaches:

1. community outreach seminars for firemen, visiting nurses, social workers, and so forth;
2. school curriculum;
3. efforts to get retailers to put toxic products on higher shelves in

their stores, to post signs near these products indicating how they should be stored at home, and to encourage sale of safety latches;
4. distribution of poison information leaflets to all mothers of newborn infants; and
5. mass media efforts on radio and TV and in newspapers.[50]

Samples of homes with young children and of retail stores were surveyed pre- and post-intervention. In post-intervention homes 36 percent, 32 percent, and 27 percent fewer homes, respectively, had accessible aspirin, drain cleaners, and furniture polishes. Substances not in their original labeled containers decreased from 13 percent to 2 percent. The number of households where people knew or had posted the poison center number increased from 20 percent to 78 percent, and safety latches in homes increased from 4 percent to 15 percent.

Twenty-two percent reported getting their information about poisons from a Blue Cross Immunization Record booklet given in hospitals at time of birth or from physicians or neighborhood health center, 12 percent through the health department mailing to new mothers, 11 percent from older children who brought the information home from school, 10 percent from shelf signs in retail stores, and 18 percent from media. (No information was provided on the remaining 27 percent.) Forty-five percent of the stores displayed information placards and the proportion of stores selling safety latches jumped from none in the pre-intervention period to 30 percent, often with advertising displays and discount coupons.

The ultimate outcome was evaluated by comparing the trend of poison ingestions reported through neighboring NEISS-affiliated hospitals with that of such hospitals nationally. There was a continuous decline in reported treatments and hospitalization throughout the program area, totalling over 60 percent by the end of the project compared to the baseline years, and 71 percent in the NEISS hospitals. In comparison hospitals there was a 15 percent decline. The project was believed to have a crude benefit of $25 for each $1 spent.

Another project attempted to help nursery school children distinguish poisonous from nonpoisonous products through education and through the use of a brightly colored poison logo with a serpent named, "No! Siop!" (*poison* spelled backwards).[49] Those children who had both verbal and visual cues for discrimination were more able to identify poisonous substances than those who had to rely on either cue alone. In a similar program using the "Mr. Yuk" logo, recognition of the meaning of the symbol by children at day care centers increased from 41 percent pre-intervention to 99.5 percent post-intervention.[50] Unfortunately, unlike the Monroe County effort, these two programs were aimed at children age 30 months or older, which is past the peak for childhood ingestions.

The last program to be described for preventing ingestion by children involves an effort to reduce pica—the eating of plaster, paint, and dirt—by small children in dilapidated neighborhoods where chronic lead poisoning from such behavior was common.[51] Although it deals with chronic rather than acute poisoning, the study presents several interesting components.

First, 41 percent of children in old housing, compared to 18 percent in new housing, had evidence of lead in their urine, although a negative history of pica from the mother showed little correlation with presence of lead. Second, mothers far more often reported pica if the questions were quite specific and if they understood the implications of pica. Third, 90 percent or more of mothers who learned about hazards of pica from their physician, formal teaching, or news media attempted to change their children's habits, compared to 63 percent and 25 percent among mothers who learned through unknown sources or by word of mouth.

Four out of every ten mothers learned through their physicians, 23 percent by word of mouth, and 18 percent through news media. This clearly emphasizes the value of health providers in imparting knowledge and changing behavior. Lastly, children age 3 to 4 stopped the habit easily, whereas younger children were far harder to change. However, with young children, simply moving furniture in front of areas with worst peeling was enough to slow up or stop ingestion in some cases.

Two types of education regarding adults should be mentioned. One is the need for active, local ventilation by artists, craftspeople, hobbyists, and others who are exposed to solvents, heavy metals, photographic developers, and various other toxic chemicals. Widespread education for this group began in the mid-1970s, but there is little information about the extent to which the target audience is responding.

Physicians must be alerted to the fact that elderly patients frequently get into trouble if given medication dosage that is appropriate for younger adults. Patients who are receiving drugs that are detoxified or excreted through liver or kidneys often need to start on lower doses and to be monitored carefully.

The sixth of the nine countermeasures is proper installation and periodic checking of gas-operated appliances to determine that there is no buildup of carbon monoxide. In some communities health departments have played this role,[34] but it can be done as well, or perhaps better, by the companies supplying utility gas and who deliver their product directly to the home or check flow meters periodically. A seventh approach is the installation of CO sensors that either alert people or automatically shut off an appliance that is spewing out 100 ppm or more of CO.

The eighth category of countermeasure is early case finding and prompt and appropriate treatment for those who have had potentially toxic exposures. One method is observation by alert physicians and laboratory technicians of the color of venous blood when samples are taken for laboratory tests. The telltale "cherry red" has on occasion suggested CO poisoning as the true reason for unexplained nausea, headaches, and inability to pay attention.[52]

Once diagnosis of ingestion or of contact with a product has been made or suspected, information is needed about product contents, toxicity, and treatment. Poison centers can help physicians to obtain answers quickly. Initially, there were many small centers, and few of them were able to keep up with the extensive task of research and filing as new product formulations came onto the market and old ones were discarded. This problem has been dealt with through the establishment of a national clearinghouse in the United States that can be reached easily by the local centers.

The last type of countermeasure is intervention for families where there have already been ingestions in order to avoid repeat performances. As Sobel and others have suggested, ingestion often is a red flag warning the alert health professional of intrafamilial stresses that may require outside help to promote resolution.[20] But while urging physicians to be alert to such needs and opportunities, Sobel also wisely observes that environmental countermeasures may be more effective than education.

23
Schools, Playgrounds, Camps, and Parks

These four locations of injury events have been grouped into a single chapter because all are public places, are heavily frequented by children or teenagers who are either unsupervised or under nonparental supervision, and often are the locus of special equipment. They also, unfortunately, share a sparcity of data about both the numbers, rates, and types of injury and about the extent of exposure. Excluded from this discussion are school recreational injuries not involving playground equipment, which are in the chapter on recreational injury.

Injuries Involving Schools

The school environment in Western society, with separate buildings, is different from that in some developing countries, where training for tribal children may occur in a tent or outdoors. Furthermore, unacceptably large segments of the world's population receive little or no formal education and thus are not "at risk."

In the United States, 22,000 school jurisdictions reported about 62,000 school-related injuries among almost 1.7 million children of elementary and high school ages for the 1977–78 school year.[1] These data are summarized by sex and activity or location in table 23–1.[1] The injury rates for males by grade are respectively 6.3, 5.8, 9.0, 12.1, and 12.3 per 100,000 student days for kindergarten, grades 1 to 3, 4 to 6, 7 to 9, and 10 to 12.[1] For girls the comparable rates are 4.0, 4.2, 6.0, 7.9, and 4.7.

Typically, about a day of activity is lost per injury. Trauma involving unorganized activities on school property is highest among children of both sexes in kindergarten and the first six grades and then declines markedly. Those injuries involving physical education and sports activities begin to increase with fourth to sixth grades, and are highest among boys in grades 10 to 12 and among girls in grades 7 to 9. In fact, the major difference between males and females in total injury rate is

Table 23–1
Injury Rates Per 100,000 Student Days Related to School Activities by Sex and Location or Activity

	Males	*Females*
Shops and labs	0.64	0.14
Building, general	1.86	1.23
Grounds, unorganized activities	1.94	1.19
Grounds, other	0.37	0.22
Physical education	2.92	2.14
Intramural sports	0.12	0.04
Interscholastic sports	1.15	0.23
Special activities	0.05	0.05
Going to/from school (motor vehicle)	0.18	0.16
Going to/from school (other)	0.16	0.08
Total		
%	9.39	5.48
(N)	(39,000)	(23,000)

Source: Adapted from *Accident Facts, 1981 Edition* (Chicago, Ill.: National Safety Council, 1981).

attributable to the substantially higher rates among males involving physical education and interscholastic sports. Males also have higher rates than females in injuries incurred in shops and laboratories almost entirely related to their exposures to vocational and industrial arts activities.

The many articles about injury in the elementary and high school environment are almost invariably inadequate regarding epidemiology, or safety program design and evaluation. The reports do suggest that the teaching of safety practice and use of safety equipment is often neglected in chemistry laboratories and in vocational and industrial arts programs.

One publication produced by an insurance company in 1962 does offer a guide to safety program development for education in agriculture, home economics, science, and technical and industrial arts, but it provides no information whether such programs appear to work or not.[2] As this publication suggests, however, safety training in the schools can have at least theoretical potential, not only for reducing injuries in the school setting but also for imparting appropriate knowledge, skills, and habits for the future. This is applicable as well to the use of passenger restraints and to education about alcohol and other drugs.

Somewhat more information is available about injury in the college and university setting. Leard reports that 48 percent of 10,700 students (3,500 in dormitories) annually sought care from the Student Health Service, with a total of 23,325 first visits over a five-year period.[3] Of these, 25 percent were for injury, equivalent to the number of first visits for the common cold.

Table 23–2 shows data from thirty-six institutions in the United States[4] and one in Uganda.[5] The U.S. data provide much more detail about type of activity or location of event. But since we are given information only about the total population at risk it is not possible to identify an injury rate for specific activities. The overall annual on-campus rate is 82 per 1,000 students, with a disabling injury rate of 6 per 1,000. Trying to extrapolate to all U.S. college campuses, the author estimates 100 medically treated on-campus injuries per 1,000 students per academic year, 115 to 120 per 1,000 for males and 75 to 80 for females.

The Uganda study reports that 9.7 percent of students overall were injured, with 10.6 percent for males and 5.6 percent among females. The on-campus rate is 60 per 1,000 students among 2,035 students living on or off campus. Among approximately 55 students who owned scooters, motorcycles, or automobiles, 32 (mainly scooters) were injured in a single year, with one death and one disabled for almost a year.

The importance of alcohol in injuries on U.S. campuses is not well documented, but shortly after the beginning of the 1982–83 academic year the University of Vermont was severely shaken by serious injury or death among eight students in one month because of falls from roofs or porches of fraternity and sorority houses and elsewhere, in several cases directly associated with use of alcohol.

A majority of injuries involve recreational activities and are discussed in another chapter. Laboratory injuries are of concern because most, if not all, should be preventable through training of students, faculty, and staff in handling procedures, through both passive environmental protection such as automatic pipettes, self-activating hoods, and proper storage devices and through active protective devices, such as gloves, aprons, or shatterproof glasses.

Larger institutions have a greater proportion of their injuries in this setting because of more graduate-level and research laboratory activities, sometimes including radioactive materials.[6] Injuries in academic activities ranged from 8 to 9 percent for institutions with fewer than 10,000 enrollment to 11 percent for those with 10,000 to 20,000 students and 15 percent for larger campuses.

Some appropriate countermeasures are considered in chapters on highway, home, and recreational safety. Because of the diversity of special occupational and environmental problems that affect universities—including the storage, use, and disposal of dangerous chemicals—each campus should have an equally diverse, well-trained safety committee with authority to require incident reports and environmental and other safety procedures.

At many schools students living both on and off campus now

Table 23–2
Injury in College and University Activities by Location/Activity, Sex, and Severity
(percentage)

	United States						*Uganda*
	Disabling[a]			*All*			*All*
	Males	*Females*	*Both Sexes*	*Males*	*Females*	*Both Sexes*	*Both Sexes*
Academic							
Academic Buildings (excluding lab/shops)	1.9	6.0		3.8	8.3		
Laboratory	1.5	.7		5.3	5.0		
Shop	.8	1.5		.9	.8		
Public assembly	.3	.7		1.0	1.6		
Total academic	2.7	8.9	4.9	11.0	15.7	11.6	19.5
Associated campus							
Residence halls	8.9	22.4		13.8	29.4		
Service buildings	1.1	1.8		1.8	2.6		
Pedestrian	6.4	13.8		7.6	15.1		
Vehicle use	1.6	3.8		2.9	4.1		
Total associated	18.0	41.8	24.7	26.1	51.2	34.9	37.4
Sports/recreation							
Varsity	26.8	1.0		13.9	0.3		
Intramural	19.2	4.3		17.1	3.2		
Physical education	13.8	34.9		12.7	19.2		
Recreation	15.8	6.8		16.9	7.7		
Other	1.8	2.3		2.2	2.4		
Total recreation	77.4	49.3	68.5	62.8	32.8	51.4	43.1
Total							
%	99.9	99.9	98.1[b]	99.9	99.7	97.9[b]	100.0
(N)	(1,220)	(398)	(1,618)	(16,214)	(6,657)	(22,871)	(197)

Source: Adapted from G. Scheffler, "Student Accidental Injury Experience," *Journal of the American College Health Association* 16(1967):85–90; A.P. Arya and C.B. Bosa, "Injury in the University Environment," *East African Medical Journal* 48(1971):420–426.

[a]Death, permanent disability, or loss of activity for one day or longer.

[b]These summary figures quoted from the study do not add to 100 percent, even assuming small variation because of rounding of decimal places. The reason for the discrepancy is not obvious.

commonly engage in drinking and other activities limited only (but not entirely) by what is legal in the community rather than by what the institutional administrators believe is behavior that a parent would wish to see. The rules of yesteryear were often unduly arbitrary, but the complete laissez faire approach is also inappropriate. Specific rules for students regarding alcohol use and education about patterns and effects of abusive behavior are needed, as are alcohol and drug counseling services for all members of the campus community.

Students must cope with learning curves involving alcohol use, first emancipation from the home environment, and extraordinary peer pressures for risk-taking behavior unguided by parental advice and caution. Any program, therefore, to alter behavior should be based, not so much on preaching what is "right" or "wrong" or "safe" or "unsafe" but rather on helping students to develop inner strength and to find group support among those who have misgivings about some of their activities.

While this suggestion may seem to emphasize those who already are less likely to engage in serious risk-taking behavior, it is based on an awareness that even this group often engages in substantial and potentially harmful experimentation, especially involving use of alcohol.[7] Other approaches perhaps are needed to reach that segment more willing to take risks.[7,8] A plea must again be made, however, for adequate evaluation of the effects of any behavior modification schemes.

Playground Equipment

Before discussing the details of injury involving playground equipment, mention should be made of its safety advantages. Children in preschool and elementary school years are more likely to be struck by motor vehicles if they live in communities without backyard play space[9] or public off-street play areas.[10] But while such facilities can provide safety for children, they can also present unnecessary safety problems.

Several studies of injuries involving playground equipment have been carried out by or for the U.S. Consumer Product Safety Commission. There were about 177,000 medically treated playground equipment-related injuries in the United States in 1981, for an overall rate of 83 per 100,000 population.[11] These occurred overwhelmingly among children under age 15, with rates of 327 and 302, respectively, for age 0 to 4 and 5 to 14 and with a decline to 15 for persons age 15 to 24, and 5 or less for older persons. Males had 93 injuries per 100,000 and females 74.

Another study suggests even higher medically treated injury rates for children under age 13, with 6.4 injuries per 1,000 boys, 4.4 per 1,000 for girls, and 5.2 to 5.7 for both sexes combined in age ranges 2 to 4, 5 to 9, and 10 to 11.[12] Half the injuries occurred on public playground equipment, and half involved private equipment, while national data indicate that injuries on public equipment may slightly exceed those occurring elsewhere.[13]

Table 23–3 shows this national distribution and the types of equipment involved in both home and public environments.[13] Probably reflecting a greater availability of swings among playground equipment around the home and a greater availability of climbing apparatus in public places, the data show that these two types of equipment, respectively, were the types most often involved in these different environments. A survey of public playground equipment does not suggest overrepresentation of any particular type of equipment when compared to frequency of its presence in that location.[13] No information is provided, however, regarding relative frequency of use.

Almost three out of every four injuries involved falls from equipment: 59 percent falls to the ground and 12 percent falls with striking of some equipment. Another 7 percent resulted from impact with moving equipment, 5 percent contact with protrusions, pinch points, or sharp edges or points, 8 percent a fall against, onto, or into equipment by a child not on the equipment, and 8 percent unknown. Only 7 percent of injuries resulted in hospitalization. The most common injury (59 percent) was a laceration, contusion, abrasion, or avulsion, followed by fracture, dislocation, sprain, or strain (35 percent) with concussion or internal injuries 6 percent of the time.

The overriding human factor in playground injuries is the fact that children lack skills, strength, and judgment, although older children

Table 23–3
Distribution of Playground Equipment Injuries in Home and Public Places According to Equipment Type, U.S. 1977 Modified Estimate
(percentage)

	Location of Equipment			
Type Equipment	*Home*	*Public*	*Other/Unknown*	*Total*
Swings	68.6	23.0	72.5	43.3
Slides	13.9	16.3	5.9	14.9
Seesaws	5.7	4.7	0	5.0
Climbing apparatus	7.2	41.8	21.7	27.0
All other	4.5	14.3	0	9.8
Total				
% down	99.9	100.1	100.1	100.0
% across	40.6	55.7	3.7	100.0
(N)	(67,521)	(92,560)	(6,217)	(166,312)

Source: *Public Playground Equipment: HIA Hazard Analysis Report* (Washington, D.C.: Consumer Product Safety Commission, 1979).

more often use climbing equipment that requires skill and strength, while younger children are more often on a less demanding swing or slide. In one Vermont study, 33 percent and 50 percent, respectively, of injury events involved poor judgment or lack of skill or strength in the injured child and 13 percent in another child. Crowding was the primary factor in 8 percent, equipment failure 13 percent, other environmental factors 3 percent, and a combination of factors 24 percent of the time.[11] Even excluding several children who were injured the first time they used a particular piece of equipment, injured children averaged fewer previous exposures to the equipment on which they were hurt than did uninjured children of similar age and sex.

Equipment factors have already been noted; episodes of equipment failure, often involving homemade playground equipment, and contact with protrusions, pinch points, and sharp surfaces. Public equipment appears to be built more strongly than that for private use, although there is no evidence that this difference is associated with any difference in injury frequency or patterns. In one study, 60 percent of private equipment and 90 percent of public equipment had been dug into the earth, but, again, there is no evidence that movement of equipment played a significant role in the occurrence of injury events.

As noted earlier, fully 86 percent of injuries involved a fall from, against, onto, or into equipment or being struck by moving equipment. For this reason, despite the fact that 76 percent of falls from known height were five feet or less, [13] the nature of the object or surface struck in the injury phase is important. Of fifty-eight fall injuries, 46 percent resulted in fractures or concussions, compared to 5 percent for other playground events.[12] The proportions of injuries designated as severe were 42 percent, 53 percent, and 31 percent, respectively, for contacts with paved surfaces (asphalt, macadam, and concrete), natural surfaces (grass, bare earth, and rocky earth), and protective surfaces (sand, gravel, rubber matting, or wood chips).

A laboratory analysis of peak accelerations at impact showed that asphalt, synthetic turf, and pea gravel do not attenuate impact very well, with asphalt producing an average peak acceleration of 400g's at a drop height of approximately 0.4 feet.[14] Soils produced lower peak accelerations, and loose surfacing materials (6 inches in depth) lower yet.

Another report includes the following illustrative peak accelerations.[15] At a drop height of one foot it reports: concrete—475 to 525g's; asphalt 140 to 160g's; two-inch gym mat 1 to 2g's; rubber mat (1 ⅛inch thick) 3 to 5g's; double rubber mat—1g. At a drop height of 8 feet they record: double rubber mat—50 to 58g's; sand (10 in. deep)—10 to 13g's; pea gravel 1 (8 in. deep)—15 to 40g's; pea gravel 5 (8 in. deep)—15 to 30g's; wood chips (12 in. deep)—30 to 35g's.

Regarding injuries from being struck by moving equipment, such as a swing seat, fewer injuries involve swings with canvas seats than might be anticipated when exposures of uninjured children are compared with those of injured ones.[12] Werner and the Consumer Product Safety Commission have developed guidelines for playground equipment, many of which follow from the above data.[16,17] Some of these are listed below, with modifications or comments where appropriate:

1. Equipment should avoid sharp edges and protruding parts. Cover exposed screws and bolts, and check regularly to ensure that the covering hasn't fallen off because of weather.
2. Use absorptive surfaces beneath and around equipment to keep peak accelerations below 40 to 50g's. Sand, wood chips, pea gravel, shredded tires, and so forth are recommended surface materials.
3. For stability, anchor equipment in concrete placed below ground level and covered with absorptive material.
4. Avoid open-ended S hooks because they catch clothing and skin.
5. If possible, cover moving parts, such as on gliders and seesaws, which can pinch or crush fingers.
6. Swing seats should be of lightweight, absorptive materials. Store indoors in winter to prevent weather damage. If used, metal seats should have rounded edges.
7. Climbing equipment should have steps no greater than the knee height of those who will use the equipment.
8. Spaces between bars of horizontal climbing equipment should not exceed 14 inches.
9. Rails on equipment should be cylindrical and about 1 inch in diameter.
10. Equipment should never extend more than 6 feet from the ground.
11. Slides should be wide enough to permit more than one child at a time.
12. Avoid radical angles for sliding or climbing equipment.
13. Standing surfaces need protective rails that children can reach.
14. Crawl spaces should be large enough to permit access by adults.
15. Equipment should be designed to preclude entrapment or strangulation. Avoid swinging exercise rings.
16. Equipment with inertial effects or rotary motion should not cause dizziness or spatial disorientation.
17. Use nontoxic preservatives for wood materials.
18. Drill drainage holes in the bottom of all tires.
19. Metal equipment should be in the shade or facing a north/south direction.
20. Locate moving equipment (such as swings and merry-go-rounds)

toward the edge or corner of a play area to avoid hitting children who run from one apparatus to another. Swings should be at least 6 feet away from fences, walls, walkways, or other play equipment.

21. Arrange equipment so that children playing on one piece will not interfere with those playing on, or running to another piece of equipment.

A state health department project provided thirty standardized, forty-minute workshops for 1,500 professional leaders involved in the purchase, installation, maintenance, and supervision of public playgrounds.[18] Facilities in the areas of the program were surveyed at the beginning of the effort and a year later, at which time the average number of hazards per playground site had declined from 8.85 to 5.11 (42 percent reduction). In one county, hard surfaces declined from 72 percent to 26 percent of playgrounds. At the same time the two largest hospitals in the area reported a 22 percent decrease in injuries involving playground equipment. Unfortunately, comparison data were not collected for an area in which the effort was not being carried out.

Camps

Estimates range from 8,000 to 11,000 resident or day camps in the United States serving between 7.5 and 11 million children.[19,20] Camps vary widely in size, facilities, type of camper and program, qualifications and training for counselors and supervisory personnel, preparedness for health and safety, and state or local regulations to which they may be subject.

Most camps have traditional or multidirected programs for a general camper population, but some cater specifically to tennis or horse enthusiasts or to special health problems (such as obesity, diabetes, or cerebral palsy). Fewer than 40 percent of camps require counselors to be age 18 or older, a third some college education, and 15 percent certification in first aid.[19] Only one in every six give counselors one week or more of precamp training, even though less than a third require staff to have previous counselor or camping experience. Although several accrediting organizations exist, at least two-thirds of camps are not accredited.

The same data source also reported five to six injuries per 1,000 days of camper exposure but noted that a number of the reporting camps apparently provided information only about more serious events, rather than about all injuries, as instructed.[19] Probably for this reason, other studies have indicated much higher rates, in one case calculated at over 40 per 1,000 camper days.

The earliest of four noteworthy studies on this subject was by Meyer et al. in 1962.[21] They found 296 injuries among 1,192 campers and staff at three camps over an eight-week period, for a rate of "12.4 injuries per 100 campers per month" or, as I have calculated it, 44 per 1,000 camper and staff days. Of interest, they found that the incidence of injury was inversely proportional to the supervisory ratio. A Scout camp with the lowest injury rate had one supervisor for every 18 campers while, at the other extreme, a guidance camp had one supervisor to 2.3 campers. With the exception of the guidance camp, staff experienced higher injury rates than did campers. Overall 12.3 percent of the injuries were "disabling," that is, resulted in exclusion from usual camp activities for a period of time. This proportion ranged from 22.8 percent for the Scout camp to 6.7 percent and 0.7 percent for a private camp and guidance camp, respectively. Scout camp injuries usually got first aid at the place of injury and were less often reported to medical personnel, whereas guidance camp injuries often involved the campers' concern about themselves, and medical visits were encouraged. Clearly, the nature of the reporting mechanism has markedly affected conclusions about absolute injury rates or about relationships between such rates and supervision.

Almost all injuries required treatment by the medical staff, but only two needed medical or surgical care beyond routine first aid procedures. According to the authors' classification scheme, 42 percent of injuries resulted from impact, with 23 percent and 22 percent, respectively, from falls and cuts and 7 percent and 6 percent burns and other injuries. A subsequent report found 16.5 injuries and 8 treated illnesses per 100 campers per week (23.6 and 11.4 per 1,000 camper days).[22]

Cosand reported that 47 percent of 34,000 complaints at sixty-eight California camps over two years were for injury.[23] In this latter study 56 percent of injuries occurred during unscheduled activity, 17 percent while hiking, and about 10 percent each during swimming, camp duties, or athletics. While exposure data are not provided, I would suspect that considerably less than 17 percent of camper activity is spent in hiking, thus suggesting overrepresentation of injury risk. Contact with sharp or rough objects accounted for 40 percent of injuries, falls 20 percent, rubbing (such as blisters) 16 percent, collision with person or object 7 percent, and other or unknown 16 percent.

No relationship was reported in the Meyer et al. study between injury rate or pattern and weather, hour, day, camper age, or living arrangements. At the Scout camp, only those with previous camping experience had higher injury rates. On the other hand, young campers without previous camping experience had significantly more injuries than did young campers with experience. "Well-coordinated" campers tended to have fewer injuries.

Campers who had two or more injuries within the study period tended to be healthier, more aggressive, more impulsive, and more hyperactive than other campers. But campers with an illness some time during the study period also were more likely to have repeated injury than were those without illness. At the guidance camp, those with higher intelligence were more likely to have two or more injuries. Overall, 13 percent of all injuries were repeats.

Finally, Barrett provides a comparison not only with the Meyer et al. data but also with injury rates for boys not camping.[24] Boys age 10 to 14 living at home had a higher frequency of injuries than did boys at camp. Furthermore, the injury rate for boys under supervision at home (playgrounds and so forth) was less than that for boys not under supervision. He concluded that supervision improves safety but noted that Meyer and others had come up with a different assessment (the reason for which we have already noted). Whereas Meyer et al. reported 41.2 injuries to 1,000 camper days, Barrett found a rate of 25 based on eight years of data. He concludes that supervision is only one determining factor and that the programming of camping may have considerable influence on the rate. Boy Scout and Girl Scout camps averaged 15 per 1,000 camper days for aquatic camps, while the regular Boy Scout camping experience ranged from 20 to about 25.

Barrett also notes that the injury rate for counselors was about 20, or slightly less than for the average camper. This may reflect effects of a staff training week conducted before the camping season opened. Bites by animals are rare, but Barrett points to the potential for rabies or bites by poisonous animals. Less uncommon, but equally serious, are allergic reactions to insect stings. He estimates 4 to 6 per 1,000 days of exposure, compared to 0.1 per 1,000 each for snake bites, other animal bites, fractures, and hospital admissions.

Although such injuries require prompt and knowledgeable treatment, a fifth of ninety-two camps in Vermont had no qualified person responsible for first aid, half had a nurse, and one-sixth had a resident physician.[21] The majority (eighty-four) reported having physician service available, usually "on call," but one-third of these physicians were engaged in busy practices ten miles or more away.

A survey of 95 Connecticut camps in 1967 showed ninety-two with a licensed registered nurse in camp and eighty-nine with a physician on call.[24] However, only fifty-five had standing orders available for the nurse. In a 1974 national survey, 56 percent of camps had a registered nurse in residence, 80 percent an M.D. on call, and 5 percent an M.D. in residence.[19] The median time for ambulance or rescue squad to get to the camp was 15 minutes and to get to the nearest hospital about 20 minutes. Furthermore, rural ambulance and hospital staffs often have difficulty in keeping skills and capabilities continuously honed.[25] Thus, even if emergency care were immediately available, its quality would not necessarily always be adequate to the need.

We turn last to the issue of safety programming for camps. Appropriate suggestions exist and can be expanded upon, but I can find no instance of actual program evaluation for such suggestions. In my opinion, five types of program efforts are warranted to promote camper and staff safety. These are:

1. Minimum qualifications should be required and training provided for all staff. Counselors should be at least 18 years of age, with at least basic first aid training, and at least one week of preseason training *at the camp* to familiarize them with the environment and expected activites, potential hazards, and how to deal with emergencies. An adequate number of personnel should have advanced training in water safety, with the number specifically a function of the minimum number of children expected to be in the water at any time. At least 20 percent of staff members should have advanced first aid or greater training (such as an EMT course). Where special camper activities are to be carried out staff should have specific training and *experience* in these areas.
2. A specific individual or group of individuals should have responsibility for reviewing each aspect of camping environment and activities based on a comprehensive checklist and to make recommendations, where appropriate. This should be done at least twice per season. State or local health departments can often assist.
3. A record system should exist with information about previous health status for campers and staff, including required tetanus immunization. Where special health problems exist, environment and activities should be checked with these conditions specifically in mind. An adequate record in a form that permits statistical analysis and review should be kept of all injury and illness problems referred to health staff. Such data should guide staff training and environmental and activity evaluations noted above.
4. Equipment for water safety in all except pools should always include a boat specifically available for rescue purposes. While boating, all campers should be required to wear flotation vests capable of keeping an unconscious person face up in the water.
5. In most cases, given the ratio of persons with advanced training in emergency care suggested above, it is sufficient simply to have a nurse in residence and a physician on call, provided the nurse has specific training in first aid, such as that offered by the Emergency Department Nurses Association[26] or similar training[27] *and* specific

written standing orders jointly developed by the nurse and physican to cover possible emergency situations. The local health department should have an active program for both prehospital and in-hospital emergency services in the community.

Parks

In an increasingly urban society millions of people seek out regional or national parks, wilderness areas, or other rural locations for exploration and camping. Commonly, they are inexperienced with this environment and unprepared from the viewpoint of safety. Unfortunately, park personnel may be equally unprepared to help because park service rangers are often individuals who grew up in the outdoors and do not realize that some natural aspects of the parks can present dangers to urban residents.

In 1969 the 280 parks in the U.S. national system had 1.11 deaths for every million visits.[28] The next year a nine-year-old boy visiting Yellowstone National Park fell from a walkway without a guardrail into a thermal pool and was scalded to death. The boy's father initiated a one-man campaign to evaluate and improve safety in the system.

In response, the number of full-time safety officers increased from seven in 1969 to twenty-four in 1976, with a budget in 1970 of $115,000 and in 1976 of $450,000. Information about injuries was methodically collected and environmental assessments made so that patrolling could be directed to more hazardous areas. Also, written and verbal information provided to visitors now specifically makes reference to aspects of safety, and warning signs have been reworded to offer more specific advice.

By 1976 the death rate had been cut to 0.57 per million visits, and this was attributed specifically to efforts growing out of the initial tragedy. Not noted was the improvement of emergency medical services occurring at the same time throughout the United States, with particular attention to many of the rural areas in which these parks are located.

One rather special problem in parks and other wilderness areas is that of exposure to wild animals that may attack humans. Between 1900 and 1949 usually only one or two people per decade were injured by grizzly bears in North American national parks.[29] In the next decade this rose to thirteen, and in 1960–69 to over fifty. Herrera reports that only five of seventy-seven such events resulted from active provocation of the bear, twenty-four while hiking in back country areas, and forty-seven while camping, usually in developed areas.

Overwhelmingly the attacks during hiking occurred when hikers, walking quietly, inadvertently came upon a sow with cub. Since the bear can run at speeds of up to 30 M.P.H. and when standing can reach to a height of ten to twelve feet, the only protection is for a person to promptly clamber higher than this distance up the nearest tree. Running is not effective. Traveling noisily in groups or by horse has been beneficial in warning sow bears that humans are approaching and gives them time to remove their cubs from perceived harm.

Injuries in developed areas generally have not involved sows with cubs but rather animals that have learned to forage for human garbage. Programs to limit the amount of garbage, to warn people not to camp where bears have been seen looking for garbage, and to trap and remove bears that continue to be a problem appear to have some value, although evaluation of these activities is still under way.

Finally, camping areas tend to be placed near especially scenic or interesting locations such as lakes created by dams, volcanoes, or similar sites that may be subject to disaster. This is considered in the chapter on disasters.

24
Recreational Activities

In previous chapters we have touched upon several activities that sometimes are recreational, including use of motorcycles, minibikes, bicycles, boats and planes, camps, and playgrounds. In this chapter we will review a generous sampling of other forms of recreation, starting with discussion of some general principles involving recreation and recreational safety. This will be followed by several subchapters covering specific activities, including toys, water recreation, body-contact team and martial sports, winter sports, noncontact competition, firearms and firecrackers, and outdoor competition with nature. Countermeasures will be dealt with generically at the beginning of the chapter but will also be identified where relevant within the subchapters.

Overview

Judging from the behavior of both humans and other mammals, recreation is an integral part of preferred life style, ranging at one extreme from killing or maiming of fellow humans or other animals through hunting, gladiatoral, and jousting contests to, at the other extreme, reading, watching movies or TV, listening to or making music, painting, or playing sedentary games.

Estimates in the mid-1960s were that 100 million people in the United States were involved in water sports (including 39 million boating, 34 million fishing, 9 million waterskiing), 57 million in riding bicycles, 40 million in volley ball, 25 million in softball, 20 million each in ice skating, table tennis, shooting activities, and 6 to 9 million each in skiing, tennis, horseshoes, archery, golf, and handball.[1,2]

Lehr places the annual loss of life from these activities at 5,000 to 6,000.[2] They also result in at least 2.5 million medically treated injuries annually in the United States, 250,000 involving skates and skateboards and 50,000 involving toys.[3]

One study of all treated injuries to school-age children showed that recreational injuries were sustained by 3 percent of all elementary school students, 7 percent of those in junior high school, and 11 percent in high school grades.[4] Nonorganized sports and physical education classes each produced nearly twice as many injuries as organized sports. One in every five injuries was considered serious. As others have pointed out, however, injuries do not become more severe until the mid-teens. Especially serious is football played by those who have left school and who are in their formative years at work, marriage, and home building. Injuries for such individuals may impose a severe financial burden.[5]

Recreational activities contribute to 7 percent of all spinal cord injuries in the United States[6] and about 3 percent of serious head injury,[7,8] but far more to long-term disability. Whereas survival six years or longer is achieved by only half of persons with spinal cord injury from motor vehicle crashes or firearms, 70 percent from falls, and 60 percent from all other causes, about 95 percent of those with recreational injuries are long-term survivors.[9]

Especially with organized sports, it is often possible to measure injury experience per unit of exposure. Although this is helpful, it does not deal with other relevant issues involving comparative risk. Various recreational activities differ not only in the risks that participants are willing to take but also in the ages of the individuals involved. And as Burdge has shown, there are distinct social class differences in preferred recreation.[10]

Waller and Klein have hypothesized that lower-class individuals bound to repetitive, boring employment, seek excitement and high risk through recreational endeavors that give immediate satisfaction.[11] They are likely to choose high-energy equipment (such as motorboats, motorcycles, and snowmobiles), which, they believe, does not require long training for proficiency. Persons of higher socioeconomic level, they suggest, more often choose activities, such as sailboating, which demand training and a longer apprenticeship to assure competence.

Huberman explores several other hypotheses, including the question whether people who engage in high-risk sports do so to overcome phobias about danger that they had as children.[12] He concludes that many people take risks simply because they like to test their capabilities and because from an early age they are taught a positive attitude toward risk taking by people they love and respect. This explanation is offered by Orlick as well.[13]

One explanation why people engage in aggressive sports is that aggression is a basic human trait, that we need to "work off" competitive energies, and that body contact sports provide a constructive outlet for aggression. Others, however, hold that such activities teach and positively reinforce aggression.

These hypotheses were tested in a study of outwardly and inwardly directed aggression by basketball players and wrestlers who had just won their competition versus those who had lost.[14] Overall, both groups showed a drop from the normal level of outwardly directed aggression following competition, with the sharpest decline among winning basketball players. Losers, particularly wrestlers, however, actually showed an increase in aggression. And while competitors generally became less ego defensive after winning, losers tended to become more defensive. Competitors in individual sports, it is suggested, suffer a loss more keenly than do team players, apparently because there is no one else with whom to share blame for a defeat.

Within the context of these limitations of ability to compare type of exposure, data from several studies are presented in table 24–1 on relative injury rates.[15–21] A study of rugby football showed 198 injuries per 10,000 player hours,[22] and one of equestrian activities had 23 per 10,000 rider hours.[16]

Comparison of data in column 1 of this table, which were collected in the 1930s, with those of subsequent columns, collected in the 1970s, suggests that football has become a safer sport over time. Unfortunately, the bases for defining which injuries are to be included and which excluded in these studies are not always clear. The apparent trend, therefore, cannot be verified.

Body-contact sports, whether of an individual or team nature, tend to be associated with higher injury rates than do other sports, and recreational activities such as sky diving, SCUBA, hang gliding, mountain climbing, and similar efforts that are generally seen as feats of daring have far higher fatality rates than does football, which is seen by the public as one of the more hazardous of the popular sports.

According to one study, the injury rate for contact sports is 13.9 per 100 males per year and 9.6 females. It is 4.5 for males in noncontact sports, but 8.9 for females in such sports.[23] Another study, however, which dealt only with injuries to female participants, showed different results. In that report, the injury rate (defined as more than one day of sport disability) was 8.9 in high school contact sports and 4.9 in noncontact sports. In college athletics the rate was 28.1 for contact sports and 17.1 for noncontact sports.[17] Major injuries, defined as more than three weeks of sports disability, were twice as common in high school and collegiate contact sports (1.3 and 3.5 per 100 participant years) as in noncontact sports (0.7 and 1.7). Between 34 and 45 percent of major injuries in high school but about 15 percent of those in college occurred without a health care person available.

Four basic ingredients underlie the injury experience associated with specific recreations. The first is the degree of sanction to take personal risks or to injure an opponent. This is determined both by the basic rules of the sport and its application by coaches, umpires, and other team officials and by the attitudes and behaviors of spectators. Soccer

Table 24–1
Injuries and Deaths Per Unit Exposure for Various Forms of Recreation

	Injuries Per 1,000 Exposures		*Injuries Per 1,000 Participant Years*			*Deaths Per 1,000[f] Person Years*
	Study A[a]	*Study B*[b]	*Study C*[c]	*Study D*[d]	*Study E*[e]	
Football	87.9	3.0–6.3(M)*	46.9	16.1	—	0.008
Rugby	1.0	—	23.0	—	14.7	—
Soccer	6.1	2.3(M)	7.9	1.2	7.9	—
Basketball	2.5	2.1(M) 2.5(W)	3.6	6.5	11.3	—
Ice hockey	2.5	2.5(M)	6.4	—	5.3	—
Lacrosse	9.3	2.5(M)	5.6	—	—	—
Boxing	4.6	—	20.3	—	—	0.45 (professional)
Wrestling	10.7	4.2(M)	41.2	4.7	—	—
Judo	—	—	25.9	—	—	—
Skiing	—	—	23.9	—	—	0.02 (racing)
Cricket	—	—	—	—	6.6	—
Track	0.7–1.0	1.9(M)	1.2–2.6	1.4–1.8	—	—
Gymnastics	0.1–2.1	1.5(M)	14.1	2.1	15.5	—
Baseball/soft	1.5	1.3(M) 1.8(W)	—	1.3–1.5	7.1	—
Badminton	—	—	2.6	—	1.5	—
Tennis	0.1	0.6(W)	0.3	0.3	1.8	—
Squash	—	—	1.5	—	1.7	—
Volleyball	0.2	2.1(W)	0.6	0.7	3.0	—
Fencing	1.3	—	1.7	—	—	—
Equestrian	2.0[g]	—	—	—	—	1.4 (racing)
Horse polo	11.2	—	—	—	—	—
Swimming	—	0.6(M) 0.2(W)	1.4	2.1	—	—
Sky diving	—	—	—	—	—	1.6
Gliders	—	—	—	—	—	0.39
Hang gliding	—	—	—	—	—	0.3–0.94

Mountain climbing	—	—	—	—	—	0.57
Spelunking	—	—	—	—	—	0.04
SCUBA	—	—	—	—	—	0.42
Power boat racing	—	—	—	—	—	0.8

Source: Adapted from (a) F.R. Eastwood, "Hazards to Health: Athletic Injuries," *New England Journal of Medicine* 271(1964):411–413; (b) K.S. Clarke and W.E. Buckley, "Women's Injuries in Collegiate Sports," *American Journal of Sports Medicine* 8(1980):187–191; (c) D.L. MacIntosh, T. Skrien, and R.J. Shephard, "Physical Activity and Injury," *Journal of Sports Medicine* 12(1972):224–237; (d) W.A. Grana, "Summary of 1978–79 Injury Registry for Oklahoma Secondary Schools," *Oklahoma State Medical Association Journal* 72(1979):369–372; (e) R.N. Marshall and H. Sandes, "Dunedin Sports Injuries 1974–1976," *New Zealand Medical Journal* 86(1977):423–427; (f) "Sports Hazards" *Statistical Bulletin* 60(3) (July–September 1979):2–5 (New York: Metropolitan Life Insurance Co.); (g) G.R. McLatchie, "Equestrian Injuries: A One Year Prospective Study," *British Journal of Sports Medicine* 13(1979):29–32.

*M = Men; W = Women.

and rugby matches in Europe and South America may generate more mayhem among spectators than among players.

Generally, in this century—but not in the past—actions associated excessively with serious injury are declared illegal: for example, spearing in football or hard checking of an opponent in hockey with use of the stick. But players quickly learn how much the officials are willing to look aside without applying penalties. And, of course, many athletic activities are informal "pick up" games that have no officiating.

Within this context of what is permissible, the physical condition of the player is the next ingredient to be considered. The more developed and conditioned are the muscle masses that are used for a specific sport, the less likely is there to be an injury from overexertion of those muscles or from equivalent forces by an opponent. This requires initial training, maintenance of tone, adequate warmup, and sufficient rest periods during the activity to prevent excessive stress. Maintaining condition is especially a problem for the weekend athlete.

Such muscle conditioning is no guarantee, however, against injury from a larger opponent—as sometimes happens in teen and preteen body-contact sports, where players may vary widely in physical maturity. Nor is it protection against external forces that can impart high energy load because of their size and shape or against acute loss of coordination and judgment because of alcohol.

Third is the nature of the equipment. Certain protective equipment, such as helmets, face masks and mouth guards, shin guards, or boxing gloves afford distinct protection in the injury phase. What has attracted less attention is the extent to which equipment can also injure: that is, ski tows that break down, golf balls and other small hard spheres, the outsides of football helmets, which can wreak havoc both on an opposing team and on one's own teammate during scrimmage, and bicycle parts, such as spokes. Much more concern has been aroused over "new" recreational activities, such as use of skateboards or trampolines.

Fourth is the nature of the recreational environment. Terrain, weather, and environment are obvious issues in skiing, mountain climbing, spelunking, SCUBA or skin diving, hang gliding or skydiving. Far more common hazards are pot holes and trash on playing fields, generation of heat on artificial turf, or collision into benches, posts, or other impedimenta placed close to the edges of fields or courts. Cleared space and "forgiving" quality for obstacles that must remain (such as padding of posts in boxing rings) are as applicable to the playing environment as they are to avoidance of injury on the highway.

The basic principles of injury avoidance and amelioration therefore are:

1. For more hazardous sports, the injury experience should be reviewed periodically to identify which actions are associated with the most

serious injuries and to alter those activities through rules and officiating or to limit their effects through changes in training, equipment, or environment.

2. Standards for health status and training and conditioning of participants often exist but are not always followed by teachers and coaches, especially at the elementary or high school level. Participants need to be medically screened, to receive appropriate training for muscle development and to perform procedures properly, to be given necessary conditioning and warm-up periods, to be matched with opponents of equivalent size, skill and maturity, and to be given sufficient rest periods, especially early in the season and in warm weather. Hogue describes two horror stories in which these rules were not followed.[24] One involved a frightened thirteen-year-old who was forced by the instructor to do a gymnastic maneuver without either demonstration or instructions and had a severe head injury. The other case involved a 128-lb fourteen-year-old who, a few minutes after being stunned, had to tackle a seventeen-year-old weighing 205 lbs. The result was a C5 quadraplegia. The coach had left the boy in the game because he wanted him to "toughen up." Furthermore, the boy was handled improperly after he was injured.
3. Use of safety equipment of proper design and construction must receive high priority for all sports. Equipment for playing and for protection of participants often seems to receive less attention than do uniforms meant to impress the public and to massage the egos of coaches, players, and parents. Especially in lower grades and for intramural play, participants may have to choose from a pool of equipment that fits poorly or is badly worn out and, therefore, is unable to serve the function for which it was designed. Or participants may be given no protective equipment at all. Hogue describes brain injuries in nine- and ten-year-olds playing softball and football at school without protective headgear.[24]

   Much of the equipment on the market was never designed for adequate energy attenuation, a fact of which physical education teachers may be quite unaware. One study showed high correlation between differences in injury rates among high school football teams and make and model of equipment being used.[25] Despite documented head injuries involving inadequate football helmets, representatives of the helmet manufacturers stated in testimony that they had never looked at the excellent energy attenuation standards for motorcycle helmets because they assumed they were irrelevant to football. As Dr. George Snively cogently pointed out, the head cannot tell whether it is being traumatized by hitting a tree at 25 M.P.H. or by contacting someone's knee at the same speed.[26]

   Equipment standards based on biophysical data are needed for each skill/stress level of recreation and should be distributed widely throughout the schools and official community recreational programs. In order to meet state and regional certification, each school or program should be required to demonstrate that it is adhering to these safety standards for all participants in intra- and interscholastic sports.

4. Similar standards are needed for public recreational spaces: that is, playing fields owned by schools and municipalities, ski slopes and similar recreation areas offered to the public for a fee, and bodies of water used for public recreation despite known submerged hazards. Attention needs to be paid to removal of potholes, uneven surfaces and trash on playing fields, or moguls on ski slopes and to obstacles on the sidelines against which participants may be propelled.
5. Many injuries become unduly serious because teachers, coaches, and officials are not alert to early signs and symptoms of head or other injury and do not take necessary and timely therapeutic steps. This occurs because of competitive pressures and inadequate training in health status evaluation and emergency care. Also for these reasons, players may be permitted back into activity before they are physically ready to return.

   Higher injury rates exist for high school football teams with young coaches who have only limited experience, limited help, and limited training in first aid.[25] Faculty, coaches, trainers, and officials need specific training—with periodic refresher courses—in identifying and dealing with injuries, and all public spectator sports should have at least one independent person on hand who is trained in health care and whose job it is to guide evaluation and treatment. Medical clearance should be obtained before injured players return to sports activities.

Toys

Toys provide the equipment for socialization of the young child into recreational activities. Parents and other relatives guide the timing and selection of toys and to some extent the training in their use. With few exceptions, a child gets only what the parents permit, when they permit it, and may use the toy only in the ways they permit.

In the United States, the year 1981 saw 18,000 injuries involving projectile or flying toys, 11,000 from children's tricycles, 24,000 from wagons and ride-on toys, 235,000 involving skates (including ice skates), and 24,000 with skateboards.[3] Since many toys have an element of fad in them, however, these figures are relevant only to a specific time and place. During the 1970s, for example, skateboards were more of a problem than were skates. But, after a decline in use in recent decades, skates have had increasing popularity in the late 1970s.

The types of problems most often encountered with toys are the following:

1. *Difficulty in control of direction.* This is defined as a problem only in that it is the basic mechanism of initiation of the pre-injury phase. But this difficulty of control is precisely what makes the toy so exciting. Examples are skates and skateboards. Using either requires skill, and the fact that people are going to fall off seems to be a foregone and often even an accepted conclusion.

   Skateboards became popular in California during the early 1960s. From there they spread rapidly across the United States[27,28] and to Great Britain about ten years later,[29] bringing with them an epidemic of fractures, which comprise about one-third of the treated trauma.[30] Serious head injuries and deaths have occurred as well because of attainable speeds of over 50 M.P.H. on a "vehicle" that cannot be easily directed and that provides no protection either for the user or for anyone he contacts.[30] Injuries appear excessively to involve new and unskilled users who strike discontinuities on the street surface.[30]

   Because of the hazards, several cities have banned their use on city streets and have established skateboard parks with smooth riding surfaces and where users must wear protective helmets and knee and elbow pads.[31] Morgan et al. contend, however, that the pads are largely cosmetic, protecting against contusion and laceration but not against fractures.[32] Between 1977 and 1978 the number of injuries treated in hospital emergency departments declined from 140,000 to 87,000, probably in part because the skate fad replaced the skateboard "rage."[33] Skating injuries are now rapidly increasing, again with many fractures and probably overrepresentation of less experienced and unskilled users. But unlike the skateboard, more women are being injured on skates.[34,35]

   Loss of control in skateboards occurs because of lack of inherent guidance mechanism. But some tricycles, wagons, or other riding toys fall over on turns because their centers of gravity are too high. This problem is readily correctable by widening the base and lowering the center of gravity.
2. *Toys that have pinch points.* Some toys are designed so that it is easy for a small hand or head to get caught and damaged.[36] We have already noted this problem with toy boxes and some play pens.[37]
3. *Toys that permit ingestion or inhalation of small parts.*[38] Examples include rattles that break open, dolls with removable eyes[39] (espe-

cially if the attachment point is sharp), and balloons that can get sucked into the trachea or larynx.[40]

4. *Toys meant to be moved or propelled that, because of their design, transmit an excessive loading of kinetic energy.*[41] Examples include darts, arrows with sharp points and air guns. Sometimes, however, a toy that was quite satisfactory in one culture becomes dangerous when its concept is translated in another culture but employs a different technology. Such was the case with the infamous clacker balls introduced into the United States around 1970. Both the Eskimos of Canada and the Maoris of New Zealand have toys consisting of two soft balls, each attached to the opposite end of a long string. A skillful participant can manipulate these balls so that they twirl gracefully or strike against each other and reverse direction. While one is learning this skill, however, he or she may strike an arm, face, or other parts of the body. If balls are made of heavy plastic, as happened in the United States, the energy involved can be sufficient to break an arm or a facial bone. In addition, pieces of plastic spalled off and caused serious eye injuries when the balls clacked together.
5. *Toys with easily reached sharp edges or burrs.* This is avoided by paying closer attention to design and quality control in the manufacturing process. One interesting example of this type of problem is that penetrating injuries of the skull have occurred when small children have fallen head first on toy trucks or cars made out of soft plastic but with metal axles.[42] As the head hits the toy, the soft plastic is compressed, leaving the stiff axle to penetrate to brain tissue. Use of soft plastic instead of metal axles obviates the problem.
6. *Toys that carry thermal or electrical load.* Sesser noted in 1969 that parents often assume their children's toys are protected by some sort of safety code. But a toy stove, for example, may reach temperatures of 200°F on the sides, 300° on the top, and 660° inside the oven.[43] A hard-to-read cautionary label appears only on the underside of the stove. Such toys should be removed entirely from the market.
7. *Now much less common, toys that contain toxic pigments, or caustic materials, such as grout in tile sets.* In most cases a nontoxic material could be easily substituted.

Water Activities

Besides immersion and drowning, four other types of injury are also associated with water activities. These are cervical cord and other injuries associated with diving; similar injuries (plus trauma from blades on motor boats) to persons who are water skiing, surfing, or skin or SCUBA diving; attack by sharks or contact with poisonous water animals; and decompression injuries to SCUBA divers.

Immersion and drowning involve people swimming in pools or natural bodies of water, children who fall into pools, bathtubs, ponds, wells, or even buckets of water, individuals standing or walking on the steep banks of lakes or rivers or who get caught in flood waters, and persons who incidentally have seizures, heart attacks, or other health problems while bathing, swimming, or standing near water.

The availability and nature of bodies of water is closely related to the frequency and mode of drowning. India—with open wells and major periodic flooding—sees many deaths from drowning, as do such nations in close proximity with water as Japan, Mexico, the Netherlands, and France.[44] In Tehran drowning is the most important cause of nontransport injury fatalities and is responsible for 65 percent of injury deaths in children.[44]

By definition, all drownings are fatal. Near drowning or immersion are the terms used for nonfatal events. Of 134 drownings in Geelong, Australia, 28 percent involved boating, 26 percent swimming or diving, and 24 percent slipping or falling into the water from the shore or pier.[45]

Dietz and Baker reported that 29 percent of 117 deaths in Maryland were associated with boating, 34 percent swimming, 19 percent adults and 9 percent children who fell or stepped into deep water, and 9 percent who died during other activities.[46] Sixteen persons were drowned in a tropical storm, in several cases when their cars were swamped, while 3 of the 117 deaths occurred in bathtubs, and none in swimming pools.

Press et al. studied 1,201 deaths in five large states across the United States.[47] Of these, 6 percent involved swimming pools and 5 percent bathtubs. Relevant activities were 20 percent boating, 24 percent swimming, 16 percent playing or wading, 2 percent skin or SCUBA diving or surfing, 6 percent other water activity, 11 percent nonwater activity, and 21 percent activity unknown. Eighty-five percent were males, 10 percent under age 5, 8 percent age 5 to 9, 24 percent age 10 to 19, and respectively 12, 7, 10, 13, and 8 percent age 20 to 29, 30 to 39, 40 to 49, 50 to 64 and 65 or older. Age was unknown for 6 percent. Overall, in the United States there were about 7,000 drownings in 1980, of which 1,100 were associated with boating, 900 in the home environment (pools and bathtubs), and the remainder elsewhere.[48] This total figure has been fairly stable over the past several decades. If a person survives immersion even after being comatose, the chances for permanent neurological deficit are minimal.[49,50,51,52]

Schuman et al. examine the question of "near-misses."[53] They note that to the health profession the term *near-drowning* means a serious hypoxic episode during submersion with circulatory arrest. To the general public, however, it means a serious risk of drowning not necessarily resulting in submersion, aspiration, or severe hypoxia.

In South Carolina during a recent year, 182 persons drowned, and 13 of 100 consecutive persons hospitalized for near-drowning (medical definition) subsequently died after surviving for twenty-four hours or longer. The death rate was 12.6 per 100,000 for persons age 25 to 64 and 2.8 for older persons, 9.7 for white males, 25.7 for black males, 1.7 for white females, and 2.7 for black females. In their survey of school children, 15 percent reported at least one episode of near-drowning (public definition) during the previous year. The authors estimate that over 350,000 South Carolina residents had had a near-drowning episode during that year and that the 182 deaths were drawn from this population at risk.

Throughout the world, extreme youth contributes to drownings involving wandering into a dangerous environment, such as near a well, pool, or river edge, being unsteady on the feet, and unable to escape once immersed.[50] Bathtub drownings occur when a child under age 1 year is being bathed or watched by other siblings who themselves are little more than toddlers.[54] Pearn and Nixon also identify "parental vulnerability"—that is, distraction because of ill health, argument, unexpected visitors, and so forth—in 44 percent of pediatric drownings, and poorly defined monitoring assignments—where each of two persons thought the other was assigned the task of watching a child—in 20 percent.[55] This problem has been noted as well by Thorson et al.[56] Several small children have drowned in pails of water.[57]

Dietz and Baker found alcohol in eleven of fourteen persons who drowned while swimming and in three of eleven who fell or stepped into deep water.[46] Twelve of the fourteen persons with alcohol had BACs of .10 percent or higher, and eight had BACs over 0.19 percent! These authors also describe seven drownings in which preexisting medical conditions may have played a part, involving seizures, severe mental retardation, organic brain syndrome, and myocardial infarction. Others have also noted these conditions as risks for drowning.[45,47,56,58,59]

Lack of ability to swim or to remain afloat with face up has been emphasized repeatedly as a factor in drownings, although no real epidemiological analysis has been undertaken. It is possible, for example, to identify what proportion of drowned persons are excellent, good, fair, or poor swimmers.[47] But it is also likely that the excellent and good swimmers take risks that less competent swimmers would never think of assuming. Unless one could compare abilities of swimmers who drown with those of uninjured persons exposed to similar circumstances, it would not be possible to determine the safety benefits of swimming ability per se.

Illustrating the complexity of such study, drownings in Huntington Gorge, Vermont, usually involve reasonably good swimmers in good health, who lack familiarity with the Gorge and its idiosyncrasies. They get into trouble while swimming within a day after a heavy rain, when the water level has risen about a foot and the water flow is much faster than usual in an area with smooth walls that offer no surfaces to catch and avoid being swept under. Many of the fatalities also have BACs between 0.05 and 0.09 percent, although usually not higher. According to Pearn and Nixon only 14 percent of child drownings involve just a single factor, with pool drownings averaging four simultaneous factors and other drownings two factors.[56]

Schuman et al. point out that black youths, who have higher drowning rates than whites, tend to be poorer swimmers and to overestimate their swimming ability more than do white youths.[53] They also offer evidence that swimming ability alone does not determine drowning rate because black males, who often can't swim, have higher drowning rates than white females, who usually can swim, or black females, who are even poorer swimmers than black males. One reason suggested for higher drowning rates for black children is that in addition to having less access to organized training in swimming, they also are more likely to have recreational access only to unguarded swimming areas such as rivers, canals, and ponds rather than pools.[60]

Be that as it may, it intuitively makes sense to teach people how to handle themselves in deep water. Schuman et al. observed that ancient Hebrew scholars said that parents have three teaching responsibilities toward children: to teach them an occupation, to follow the Torah (Bible), and to swim.[53]

The "rule of thumb" has been not to swim for at least one hour after eating, to avoid abdominal cramps that may interfere with ability to swim. At least one study, however, suggests that swimming shortly after eating is not associated with abdominal cramps.[61]

Water speed and depth are relevant environmental issues in drowning, as is a means of escape. A small child who falls into a pool is likely to find that the water level is about a foot below the edge of the pool, too great a distance for it to pull itself up. The hard vertical sides of a deep well are even more difficult.

According to Pearn and Nixon, the ideal fence to keep children under age 4 away from an unsupervised pool is 1.2 meters high with a high, hidden, self-closing, and self-locking latch.[56] One proposal in Australia to require fencing of swimming pools resulted in 44 letters to the editor, 7 in favor, 2 neutral, and 35 against fencing. Those in opposition were against bureaucratic control, thought it was the parents' responsibility to watch their children, or thought that the fences would be costly and ruin the landscape and property values.[62] Above-ground swimming pools seem to have fewer drownings than do ground-level pools, perhaps because they are harder for a young child to reach and are of smaller dimensions than ground-level pools.[63]

Many of the flotation devices sold for children and adults are quite inadequate for the alleged task.[64] Pearn and Nixon identified failure of these devices as a factor in only 5 percent of child immersions.[56] But false sense of security by parents or others, who thought the devices reduced the requirement for their own vigilance, was a factor in almost one out of every five immersions.

In the injury and post-injury phases rescue may be delayed because, especially with black swimmers, dark skin color and dark swimming clothes make discovery more difficult.[46] Also, flotation equipment may not be immediately at hand or, if it is, isn't used. Equally dangerous, however, are rescue attempts by nonswimmers who jump into the water to help and themselves are drowned.

Once rescued, victims must be followed for at least several hours for signs and symptoms of respiratory distress. Aggressive treatment of hyperhydration, hyperventilation, hyperpyrexia, and hyperexcitability even in severely comatose patients can markedly improve survival and decrease long-term morbidity.[52]

About 71,000 persons are treated annually in U.S. emergency departments for impact injuries associated with in-ground swimming pools.[65] Three-quarters are contusions and lacerations from "rough housing," slipping on the pool apron or ladder, or using a sliding board. Twenty percent involve fractures, sprains, and strains. Injuries from ladders are common with above-ground pools.[66]

Only 7 percent of spinal cord lesions in the United States occur during recreation, but three-quarters of those involve swimmers, usually young males who become quadraplegic. Kewalramani and Kraus report that 45 percent of these result from diving into a river or a stream, 27 percent into swimming pools, and 28 percent into lakes, reservoirs, or the ocean.[67] Usually there is a wedge fracture despite no objective evidence that the diver struck bottom or a hard object. This suggests hyperventroflexion as a common mechanism for injury.

But a study of seventy-two serious injuries in pools reports that thirty-six of fifty-seven quadraplegic cases resulted from plunges into four feet of water or less, that forty-six of the pools had no depth markings, and that striking the head on the bottom was common.[68] Few of these individuals received proper first aid. Another study reveals that it is possible for a diver to strike with some force the bottom of the deep end of most pools as they are currently designed.[69] Burke's study in Australia[70] and Mennon's in South Africa also implicate striking bottom upon diving into shallow water, often after consuming alcohol.[71]

Impact injuries also occur with surfboarding, although with the recent development of lighter boards they have become less serious. The injury occurs when the person falls off the board, which then strikes him about the head, arms, or shoulders. Cervical fractures also occur from cervical compression if the head strikes the sand while in flexion. However, surfing injuries are reported to be quite uncommon.[72,73]

In water skiing impacts, the person operating the boat usually has guided the skier too quickly and at the wrong angle into the shore.[74] When a third person is not available in the boat to keep an eye on the skier, boats have even run over the skier or someone else in the water, usually with extremely serious outcome.[75]

SCUBA (Self-Contained Underwater Breathing Apparatus) diving has become increasingly popular in temperate climates since World War II. Caisson's disease, or decompression sickness, is relatively uncommon,[76,77,78] but lacerations from underwater objects are frequent, and there are occasional drownings from exhaustion because relatively weak swimmers outdistance their abilities, since underwater things look 25 percent closer than they really are. In some cases nitrogen narcosis may contribute to poor judgement that leads to overexertion. Exhaustion of air supply because of failure to check tanks, and barotrauma to ears, sinuses, or lungs also are common, the latter occurring because people attempt to dive with head colds or to ascend while holding their breath. Diving after ingestion of alcohol has also been implicated in some of the deaths.

Most decompression illness comes from failure to follow standard decompression tables. Those tables, however, had been developed for U.S. Navy divers, who are carefully selected and then kept at ideal body weight and in good training. In the general population, some people, especially obese ones, are particularly sensitive to decompression effects. Such individuals, who would usually be culled from the navy diving squad, may remain as recreational divers and may get into trouble even if they follow the navy tables precisely. For this reason, some diving organizations now recommend tables that are more conservative.[79]

Problems also occur because some individuals dive without use of a buddy system (where two persons dive together and are responsible for each other), have no plans worked out for getting help, and do not know where recompression facilities are located. For this reason, SCUBA activities should be carried out through organized clubs, after completion of a formal course and formal certification in diving, and in accordance with club rules as to who is skilled and experienced enough to dive to deeper levels.[80] Sources of air supply also need to be checked to avoid carbon monoxide contamination. Such programs have also been developed by some college athletic departments as well.[81]

Despite widespread fears of shark attack, injury by stinging jellyfish, sea anemones, gastropods, anelid worms, and sea urchins probably is far more common, especially in tropical areas. Poisonous snakes and fish also may cause excruciatingly painful and sometimes dangerous injury, but the frequency of these events usually is not known.[82] Russell estimates, however, that sting rays cause about 750 injuries annually in the United States.[83]

In contrast, since 1600 about 1,000 shark attacks have been recorded throughout the world, about 800 unprovoked, and all attributable to only 20 of the 350 different species of shark.[84] The case fatality rate is about 50 percent. No foolproof system for avoiding these animals has yet been found. In high attack areas, such as Australia and South Africa, extensive and costly systems of sea nets have been built to keep sharks separated from bathers. These, and heavy fishing for sharks in high-risk areas, have been of some value in reducing the population of this predator near swimmers.[84] Worldwide, the shark population may be increasing because sharks no longer have commercial value for their livers (a source of vitamin D) or their skin (used for sandpaper).

Sharks seem most likely to attack in warm, turbid, partly fresh water that is relatively shallow but near a deep channel and to go after a person whose skin or clothing contrasts sharply with the surroundings.[84] The single most useful lesson learned so far is how to bring emergency care to the scene to help a severely shocked and agitated individual who usually has had to struggle through strong surf while hampered by a useless limb. Having reached shore, the victim is usually handled by untrained people with inadequate first aid facilities.

In order to counter these deficits, an emergency care system was established along a heavily shark-infested area of the Natal coast.[84] This system includes plasma deposits at thirty locations along eighty miles of beach, stationing of lifesavers expert in the emergency measures for beach treatment and able to reconstitute plasma, and excellent organization of local and vacationing physicians to ensure that a physician will be on the scene within minutes after an attack.

The injured person is kept at the site, given plasma, and not moved until his condition has stabilized. Then, and only then, is he moved slowly by ambulance to a hospital prepared to receive him. Using this approach, the medical community in the Natal has almost routinely achieved survival of severely mauled individuals who almost as routinely have been dying elsewhere in the world.

One of the undocumented types of injury along beaches and waterfronts is laceration of feet from broken beer and soda bottles. In recent years, several states in the United States have reinstituted a small deposit charge for such bottles, which can then be returned for cash instead of being thrown away. The net result is that people litter less, since bottles are worth money. No data exist, however, about the possible effects of this change in behavior on fewer broken bottles at beaches, fewer lacerated feet, and reduced need for surgical care. Such data may provide economic and injury prevention incentives for bottle-return laws.

Body-Contact Team Sports

We begin this section with discussion of soccer, which probably attracts more adherents worldwide than any other sport. Nilsson and Roaas report injury rates ranging from a low of 3.6 per 1,000 hours of adult play and 14 per 1,000 hours of professional play to 13 and 32 per 1,000 hours for adolescent boys and girls, if abrasions and blisters are excluded.[85] They attribute the higher rate in girls to less experience and skill with this sport. Qualifying rounds in league play saw fewer injuries than did final rounds. Overall, 39 percent of 858 injuries during games were abrasions and blisters, 36 percent contusions, 20 percent sprains and strains, 3.5 percent fractures, and 1.5 percent other injuries. Sixty-eight percent of the injuries were to lower extremities.

In one season of play, according to Lingard et al., there was 1 treated injury per 1,000 players per week among boys under age 18 and 6 among those over age 18 in New Zealand soccer.[86] According to McMaster and Walter, while both soccer and American football are contact sports, the purpose of contact in football is to neutralize an opponent, whereas that in soccer is to control the ball.[87] Attempting to neutralize the opposing player in soccer carries a penalty, which, they suggest, is invoked without hesitation and consequently keeps down unwarranted aggression. Some unavoidable injuries do occur in soccer as a result of unintentional contact between players, who may wear no protection except for a thin shin guard in some instances.

Because agility and maneuverability are essential, soccer players tolerate only a minimum of taping or protective equipment. Anything more, they feel, would interfere with the game. Avoidable chuck holes and other objects on the playing field pose a serious threat and can cause foot, ankle, and knee injuries.

Looking at insurance costs for medical care to soccer players,

Pritchard concludes that soccer has only one-fifth the frequency of injury and 16 percent the medical expenses per unit players as does football.[88] The most costly type of injury is internal derangement of the knee.

Rugby football, like its American sibling, is far more hazardous than soccer. In contrast to the low injury rates in soccer, Lingard et al. noted 30 treated injuries per 1,000 players per week in rugby play among seniors, 12 in open grade play, and 6 to 7 in secondary school play.[86]

At the Rugby School in England, the injury rate is a phenomenal 198 per 10,000 player hours, compared to 103 for basketball, 27 for field hockey, and 3 to 37 for a range of other sports involving the same students.[22] If one assumes that students at this school are individuals who like to work out their aggressions through sports, it would also be necessary to conclude that rugby affords a far more hazardous way of doing so than do any of the other sports.

Rates at other schools were also high (almost all over 100 per 10,000 player hours), although not as high as at Rugby School. The differences may possibly reflect age, other player characteristics, officiating, playing surface, or criteria for counting injuries. Overall, about 40 percent of injuries are to lower limbs, 25 to 30 percent to upper limbs, 20 percent to head and neck, and 10 percent to trunk.[22]

The types of injuries noted in rugby are lacerations 35 percent, fractures 27 percent, soft tissue injury 24 percent, dislocations 8 percent, and concussion 6 percent.[89] The highest injury rate per player involved is incurred by the fullback. Forwards receive more cuts, bruises, and hematomas and fewer joint injuries than do backs,[90] while highest tooth injury is among the front five, next the back row, and least at three-quarter, halfback, and fullback positions.[91] In fact, 42 percent of players who broke or lost teeth did so during play in the front five positions. It is not known, however, what proportion of player time was spent in those or any other positions, therefore limiting any conclusion that might be reached.

While 45 percent of players had lost or fractured teeth, none had done so while wearing mouthguards. One in every four players reported currently wearing a mouthguard regularly, with half of these starting to do so only after injuring a tooth. Another 22 percent had worn a guard in the past but had ceased to do so, usually because it was uncomfortable, interfered with breathing, or was loose. Only half of those currently wearing a guard had had it provided by a dentist. Two out of every three players said they would be willing to wear a guard if it was provided.

Among 221 students in New Zealand who were fitted with mouth-guards by local dentists, 135 wore them regularly during rugby and 86 did not.[92] During the next season, 15.6 percent of wearers had mouth injuries, usually soft tissue laceration. Only 4.4 percent had tooth fractures, but even less—0.7 percent—were above minor Class I injuries. Among the nonwearers, 17.4 percent had oral injuries but 16.1 percent had tooth fractures, and 3.5 percent had Class II or more serious damage. The risk of tooth fracture was almost four times greater without mouthguards, while the risk of serious damage was five times greater.

This obviously preventable injury should be subject to compulsory equipment standards. These standards for equipment design, construction, and use should apply not only to mouthguards but as well to other protection for head and other parts of the body. Such equipment is especially important, since rugby injuries are particularly likely to involve injuries of the central nervous system and other complicated injuries requiring special services.[86]

Davies and Bigson note that almost half of injuries in rugby occur during the last quarter of play and that foul play might have caused as many as 31 percent of all injuries in their series.[93] There is ample room here for more sensible rules and rigorous officiating, especially during the latter half of games. Each sport seems to have its own signature in the medical literature. That of football, for example, is a deep concern about methods to prevent head, lower limb, and heat-stress injuries. The literature on rugby simply documents the high frequency of injuries but then rarely suggests prevention. This apparent absence of preventive concern given the extent of injury is both surprising and disturbing.

In contrast to rugby, concern about prevention of injuries is almost as old as American-type football itself. Rugby is played without protective equipment, but photographs of early football players show helmets and padded equipment, and currently protection is provided for head, shoulders, thighs, and lower trunk.[94]

Nonetheless, the injury rate remains high but not as high as for rugby. CPSC reports that there are about five injuries per game and the high school seasonal rate is about 0.5 per player season, with many of these injuries occurring during practice.[94] There are currently about 18 deaths per year in the United States directly related to football (under 3 per 100,000 participants) and at least 300,000 injuries treated in emergency departments.[94] Another 10 deaths occur from heat stroke or heart failure and are listed as "indirect deaths."

The best overall study is an epidemiological analysis of high school football injuries in North Carolina between 1968 and 1972.[25] All forty-three randomly chosen schools with over 8,700 players in this study used similar injury definitions, and data collection was obtained by interview, with data on uninjured as well as injured players. The major conclusions of the North Carolina study were as follows:

1. The injury rate per player per season was 0.488, including all injuries

whether treated or not. Those injuries comprising 5 percent or more of the total were sprain 20.4 percent, contusion 17.7 percent, fracture 10.6 percent, pulled muscle 8.8 percent, strain 7.4 percent, laceration 5.8 percent, concussion 5.4 percent, and torn ligament 5.1 percent. Nineteen percent were to the knee, followed by 15 percent to ankle, 7 percent to shoulder, 6 percent head, and 5 percent each upper leg and back. Overall, 46 percent of injuries were to lower extremity, 24 percent upper extremity, 13 percent each trunk and head/neck, and 3 percent other.

2. Over 95 percent of injuries resulted in loss of participation for one day or more, and 35 percent for seven days or longer. A quarter of those injured received no medical treatment, while a third were seen by a physician the same day. Fifteen percent were treated only after a delay of two days or longer.
3. Injury rate was 0.529 for schools with less than 500 pupils, decreasing to 0.470 for those over 1,000 in size. Over half of injuries occurred during practice, especially during tackling drills. Based on time in game, rates rose to a peak with 11 to 15 minutes' participation and then fell, with lowest injury rates for those who played 26 to 45 minutes. Boys playing more than 45 minutes again had somewhat higher injury rates.
4. Injury rates rose from 0.250 and 0.278 for those age 13 and 14 to 0.621 and 0.680 for those age 17 and 18 and then fell to 0.353 for those age 19. Taller and heavier boys had higher injury rates. The 28 percent of players previously injured averaged 0.624 injuries versus 0.437 for those not previously injured. Based on exposure, the most hazardous position was fullback, followed by quarterback, defensive tackle, offensive halfback, and tight end.
5. The most frequent cause of injury was a blow from an object (31 percent)—usually a helmet (with spearing) or a shoe—followed by collision with another person (20 percent), torsion or twisting (11 percent), and collision with an object (8.6 percent). Also noted were illegal acts (3.7 percent), improper technique (1.9 percent), heat stress (0.8 percent), ill fitting, broken, or defective equipment (1.7 percent), contact with hard or sharp object, such as fence post, bench, glass, or rock (4.1 percent), or stepping on or in a hole, uneven surface, rock, or equipment (2.7 percent).
6. Injury rate was a direct function of age of coach (0.623 for those under age 30, decreasing to 0.422 for age 45 or older), of coaching experience (lower for more experience), and education (lower for those with a master's degree). The more assistant coaches available, the lower the injury rate (from a high of 0.719 for one assistant, down to 0.385 for seven assistants).

7. The concussion rate ranged from 0.009 for one helmet make and model up to 0.125 for another, with a mean of 0.25 ($p < 0.01$). No significant difference was noted according to type of suspension, helmet fit, or condition of helmet. In similar fashion, shoulder injury rates varied significantly with type of shoulder pad, from a low of 0.019 to a high of 0.167, but no difference was found according to fit or condition. The biggest reductions in knee and ankle injuries were associated with resurfaced fields and use of soccer shoes.
8. A significant reduction of injuries came from adopting training programs that limited player contact. Not only was the injury rate less but the percentage of games won was greater. The authors note that this refutes the theory that it is necessary to have hard contact in practice in order to have a successful team.

Work by Kraus and colleagues at two universities provides the best information about intramural touch football.[95] Both schools had crude injury rates of about 8.5 per 100 players. The serious injury rate was 4.7 percent at one and 2.2 percent at the other, a difference thought to be associated with hard, grassless fields at the former school. Women had more injuries (33 per 1,000 participations versus 20), but men had twice as many serious injuries. Eighty percent of championship games and 39 percent of all games ended with at least one injury, and half of championship games, but 12 percent overall, had a serious injury. This study indicated higher injury rates during the second half of games, a conclusion not reached in the North Carolina report. Another Kraus et al. study showed no relationship between injury rate and training or experience of officials in touch football.[96]

No mention is made of the use of alcohol, known to be an important social lubricant for many intramural games. In fact, the rugby club at the University of Vermont advertises for players with the motto, "Blood, Sweat and Beers." Scandals have occurred involving the use of amphetamines by professional football players,[97] and alcoholism treatment programs have been established for professional players. But to date there are no data concerning either the frequency of alcohol or other drug use in this sport or the results of such use with respect to injury.

Face guards and the mouth protectors are now routinely used in football. But in years past oral injuries were 50 percent of all football injuries, and each player had a 10 percent chance of such an injury during any playing season.[98] Face guards eliminate about half of oral injuries, and mouth protectors prevent most of the remainder. Together they may prevent more than 100,000 oral injuries annually among over 1 million players.

Regarding quality of the playing field, Garrick et al. reported that 95 percent of the time when football players run out of bounds they stop within eighteen feet, and that on average there are forty-two such excursions per game (ranging from thirty-six for professional games to fifty-six for college).[99] Clearing this area, they suggest, would reduce 7 percent of offensive player injuries requiring hospitalization and an estimated 2 percent of injuries overall.

Higher ambient temperatures exist with synthetic turf than with natural turf, thereby possibly increasing the likelihood of heat stress.[100] This has been an often fatal type of injury, and its likelihood is exacerbated by making players do too much work too soon early in the season, especially with inadequate salt and water replacement and while wearing heavy clothing that limits evaporation.[101]

Some have questioned whether artificial turf also results in more injuries to knees and ankles. Grass absorbs more energy than does either uncovered ground or ground covered with certain forms of synthetic turf.[102] No really definitive data are yet available, however, because studies of such injuries have failed to control simultaneously for type of turf, type of preseason conditioning of players, type of footwear, and wetness of playing surface, all of which undoubtedly interact.[103–108]

As autumn turns to winter, so attention shifts from football to basketball and then hockey. The most interesting thing about the medical literature on basketball injuries is its relative absence.[108] We have already noted a high injury rate with basketball at the Rugby School (103 per 10,000 player hours), but no other information is provided in that study. Zariczny et al. indicate 0.30 injuries per 1,000 participating hours, which is less than for football, baseball, wrestling, gymnastics, and track and field but more than for volleyball, swimming, field hockey, golf, tennis, cross country, or badminton.[4] A Canadian study reports that 58 percent of injuries are sprains and strains, 14 percent contusions, and 5 percent each fractures and abrasions or laceration.[18] Thirty-two percent of injuries involve the ankles, 20 percent the hands, 11 percent knees, 7 percent head and face, and 4 percent elbows and shoulders. For a contact sport without protective clothing, the injuries are relatively modest. As with soccer, the emphasis is on agility and control of the ball more than on neutralizing an opponent, and there are penalties for unnecessary body contact.

This brings us to hockey, where, despite primary emphasis on control of the puck, attempts to "neutralize" opposing players is common. According to one study, so-called competence players play for the joy of it and are not influenced by movies showing aggressive hockey, but so-called noncompetence players are interested primarily in winning and show significant increase in aggressive behavior during their next game after seeing an aggressive movie.[109]

A Czechoslovakian study identifies 30 injuries per 1,000 hockey players per annum, 45 percent occurring in training and 82 percent resulting from physical contact with another player, 9 percent from defects in rink, uniform, or equipment, 7 percent from improper warmup or action, and 2 percent for other reasons.[110] The actual cause of 54 percent of injuries was being struck by an object, with another 17 percent from impact against the boards, 16 percent body contact between athletes, 11 percent falls on ice, and 2 percent other reasons. Over 70 percent of injuries were evenly divided between head and lower limbs.

In 1972–73 and 1974–75, respectively, Canadian ophthalmologists reported 287 and 258 injuries to eyes of hockey players, the vast majority occurring as a result of "high sticking": that is, checking an opposing player with the stick held above shoulder level.[111] During the 1975–76 season, this practice was declared illegal, and simultaneously use of face masks was heavily promoted. The next year, masks were made compulsory for younger players but still were not being used by many of the older players, for whom they were not compulsory.

The results are clear. Between the 1976–77 season and the 1979–80 season, total reported eye injuries ranged from 43 to 90. Furthermore, most of these injuries were now in older players. Between 1972 and 1975, about 25 percent of eye injuries were to players over age 21. From 1976 to 1980, about 75 percent were in that age group.

Given the fairly large proportion of injuries from contact with the boards, it is surprising that no real attempt has been made to pad the boards. In hockey, with an audience that appears to play an important role in maintaining aggressivity, it appears that achieving a game that is fast but safe will be a long, slow task.

Individual Body-Contact Sports

The goal of boxing is to injure one's opponent, predominantly through concussion but short of permanent damage.[112] In wrestling, the goal is not to injure but to prevail over one's opponent. Karate's goal is to sufficiently impair an opponent so that he is unable to rise within five seconds.

Between 1946 and 1952, boxing saw eighty-eight deaths (usually from head injury) in more than 200,000 bouts, for a death rate of "only" 0.04 percent compared to most other sports where no deaths are tolerated.[112] But while the immediate goal of a single bout is to end up short of permanent damage, the long-term effect is a person who has mental and other neurological deficits, often of profound and progressive nature.[112,113]

The most common apparent injuries in boxing are facial contusions and lacerations, with fractures or other injuries being rather uncommon.[113,114] However, "minor" repetitive scarring of brain tissue is probably equally common. A study of 224 boxers, age 50 or older, showed that of those who had boxed ten years or more, over half had some brain damage, with less damage for those who had boxed fewer than ten years.[113]

Among amateur boxers at an air force base, over a four-year period, 4 per 1,000 had injuries that kept them from their work for forty-eight hours or longer and there were two deaths and one permanent invalid.[113] The six-year record (1952–57) for 9,871 professional boxers in New York State was 259 knockouts, 502 technical knockouts (TKOs) for injury, and 216 TKOs for inability to defend oneself, 9 serious head injuries requiring hospitalization, 16 eye injuries, 29 fractures (mostly metacarpal and nasal), 4 shoulder dislocations, and 138 boxers who retired or were denied license.[115]

Given the inherent blood-letting intent of this sport, what can be done to limit the most harmful effects? Some recommendations that have been made are:

1. Each boxer should have a precareer examination, including chest X ray, EEG, EKG, complete blood count, and urinalysis.[116]
2. Before each bout, boxers should also have complete examinations in private.[116] As Elia notes with a whole litany of horror stories, severely ill or damaged boxers have repeatedly been permitted to fight because their obvious problems have either been overlooked or ignored.[113]
3. Officials should undergo annual reexaminations to ensure that they are in good health and competent to promote the safety of boxers.[115]
4. Gloves that do not retain moisture should be used, since those that do not meet this criterion can add a pound of weight to the hands in the course of a fight.[113] Ideally, a body-weight-glove-weight formula should be used to overcome weight disparities between boxers and the glove should imprison the thumb so that it can't be applied as a weapon.[113] Except for championship fights, an 8-oz rather than a 6-oz glove should be used.[115]
5. The target area should be discussed with both boxers before each fight and rabbit punches should be heavily penalized.[113]
6. During the bout itself, there should be much more leeway to delay or stop the fight than now exists or is applied.[113,115,116] The referee should stop the fight if one boxer seems excessively tired, and the ring physician should be authorized to call "time" anytime he feels it necessary to examine a contestant and to stop the fight if he feels

it is appropriate. If a fighter is on the ropes, the referee should begin his count at that point, and if a fighter is knocked down, the count should continue even though the bell has rung. After a knockdown, a boxer should be questioned concerning his awareness of time and place to ensure that "he has his wits about him."[112]

7. New type plastic ensolite fiber board ring padding should replace old style felt padding.[115] All boxers should have properly fitting mouth pieces.[115]
8. No fight should be held in a community that does not have neurosurgical capability immediately available,[113] and a portable resuscitator with oxygen equipment should be available at all rings.[115]
9. Any person who sustains a knockout, technical knockout, or other serious injury should have an automatic suspension of thirty days or longer.[115,117]

Injury patterns in wrestling contrast substantially with those of boxing. Most result from impact with the floor or from twisting of muscles rather than from impact by another human being. Snook reports a very high injury rate because of inadequate floor mats.[118] Overall, including both practice and meets, U.S. college wrestlers in 1979 had a 9.2 reportable injuries per 1,000 athlete exposures, 3.8 "significant" injuries, and 0.6 major ones.[119] The rates for game-related exposures were considerably higher, being, respectively, 28.1, 12.7 and 6.2 per 1,000 exposures for reportable, significant, and major injury.

The 1979 experience, incidentally, involved 550 participants in 22 teams who over a season had 56,000 exposures, 10 percent of which were game related, and who had 363 injuries, 153 of which were game related in this time. Between 1975 and 1979, there were a total of 2,129 injuries, 895 of which were significant. By far, the most frequent location of these significant injuries was the knee (308 injuries), followed by the shoulder and arm (116), ankle and foot (97), torso (93), and forearm and hand (81). The remaining 201 injuries involved mostly head and spine, and face and scalp, with smaller numbers to hip and leg and "miscellaneous."

During US Olympic trials—where participants were not required to wear head protection—81 (26 percent) of 313 participants in 1,141 bouts had 83 injuries, or one injury per 14 bouts.[120] Almost one in five injuries was an exacerbation of a preexisting injury. In this environment, without head protection, about 30 percent of injuries were to face, head, and neck, 16 percent to shoulder, and 14 percent to chest. Free-style wrestling produced far more knee injuries than did Greco-Roman wrestling. No trend in injury rate was found according to weight of wrestler. Only 10 percent of Greco-Roman wrestlers, but 27 percent of free-style ones, had injury requiring treatment. The authors urge use of head protection for all wrestling, including the Olympics.

Karate contests last only two minutes but seem aimed at maximum mayhem. McLatchie reports on 295 contests fought over three days in which 25 percent resulted in injury, and in 10 percent the injury was severe enough to cause withdrawal of the participant. Injuries included 7 concussions, 2 blows to the trachea, 18 blows in solar plexus, 4 to testes, 4 dislocations of fingers or toes, and 3 nerve injuries.[121]

He reports without supporting data that injuries were more common in the first hour of the contest and to persons below brown belt capability. Nor is a subsequent paper by him very encouraging regarding injury to brown and black belt contestants.[122] In that report, 37 of the 70 contestants sustained injury, 15 of which were potentially serious. Again, concussions, blows to solar plexes and testes, and dislocations occurred, as well as rib trauma, a corneal laceration, and several severe hematomas to arms and legs.

Contestants were required to break two one-inch boards with their hands or arms. This spectacular activity resulted in frequent and substantial injury to hands. Groin guards being used were considered inadequate, and protective padding was recommended for fists, forearms, shins, feet, and mouth. Also recommended was mandatory presence of a physician at all such contests to do prematch examinations and provide emergency care.

During 1974 and 1975 there was an average of one injury for every five contests in the Scottish games.[123] Shortly after, the use of protective padding was strongly encouraged by the Karate Board of Control in Scotland and was used by 75 percent of competitors in the area. During 1976 the injury rate dropped to one per twenty-two contests. However, in this year a new and more dangerous sport—"full contact" karate—became popular, with bouts lasting three to five rounds of three minutes each. This is a more dangerous sport than traditional "no contact" karate, but apparently is also made less dangerous through use of protective padding.

Another interesting paper points out that Caucasians who practice the Oriental martial arts of Kung Fu, Karate, Judo, and Aikido often have knee injuries, whereas the incidence of this type of injury is relatively rare among Asian competitors.[124] The author suggests that the difference is because the Japanese have wide, strong popliteal tendons, rare transverse ligament, and wide range of mobility of the medial meniscus. In contrast, Europeans have small popliteal tendons, commonly have a transverse ligament, and have very small range of motion in the medial meniscus. He suggests that Caucasian participants be taught to limit maneuvers that require deep-knee flexion.

Winter Sports

In addition to ice hockey, the most popular outdoor winter sports are probably skiing, snowmobiling, and sledding. The literature on skiing is, relatively speaking, gargantuan. Fewer physicians have dealt with snowmobile injuries, and virtually none have written about sledding.

Skiing in the United States sees about 55,000 product-related injuries per year treated in emergency departments, snowmobiling almost 20,000, sleds 30,000, toboggans 9,000, and snow disks 1,000 injuries.[125] These figures are probably a substantial underestimate.

Garrick and his associates suggest that only about half of skiing injuries are reported to ski patrol or area physicians.[126,127] Reporting to ski patrol ranged from a low of 24 to 37 percent of injuries incurred for skiers age 40 or older to a high of 73 to 79 percent for children under age 16. As skiing ability improves, there is a progressive decrease in the proportion of injuries incurred that are reported to the patrol, from 72 percent for persons who can snowplow to 38 percent for those who can do the Wedeln. Women who are injured are more likely to come to the attention of ski patrol than are men. Because of the nonuniform nature of underreporting to the ski patrol, studies using only these injuries are likely to suggest lower injury rates for males, older persons, and experienced skiers than actually exist.

Based on reporting both to ski patrol and physicians, Garrick and Kurland have estimated 4.3 and 4.5 injuries per 1,000 skier days, respectively, for males and females.[127] Children under age 10 had 23 injuries per 1,000 skier days, with the rates for other ages ranging from 3.1 to 6.8 but with no specific trend apparent. Skiers who could do only a snowplow or snowplow turn and traverse averaged 10 injuries, while intermediate skiers averaged 3.4, and advanced skiers 5.0 injuries per 1,000 activity days. (More recent training techniques using short skis permit beginners and novices to carry out maneuvers that used to be limited to more advanced skiers. Therefore, some researchers now ask respondents whether they classify themselves as beginner, novice, intermediate, or advanced, rather than whether they can perform certain maneuvers.)

Eriksson and Johnson conclude that reported rates internationally range from 2 to 7 per 1,000 days but possibly would be as high as 1 percent if unreported injuries were also included.[128] The rate appears to be declining somewhat in recent years. They also estimated that there are about a million ski injuries annually worldwide, of which one-quarter to 60 percent occur among the 14 million downhill skiers in the United States. Fatalities are rare, especially considering that many ski areas are also potential avalanche areas.[129]

There is an absolute dearth of formal information about the role of alcohol in ski injuries. Anecdotal information suggests that alcohol is a factor in at least some skiing injuries. A study currently being completed, however, revealed only a handful of persons with positive BACs among injured adults consecutively tested for this drug.[130]

The literature on ski injuries deals predominantly with leg injuries. Downhill or alpine skiing became more popular during the 1950s as lighter skis were developed and boots and bindings changed from the earlier leather straps and thongs. New, tight metal bindings without releases, however, were associated with frequent and serious tibial fractures.[128]

Early attempts in the search to balance safety, maneuverability, and inadvertent binding releases perhaps even increased the incidence of fractures.[128] Johnson et al. believe that 80 percent of lower-extremity injuries are equipment-related.[131] No one knows what the frequency of injury would be if the old type of equipment were still in use because new equipment simultaneously improved maneuverability, probably reducing the frequency of falls, but also increased the severity of falls that did occur. The current approach seeks the best of both worlds.

Eriksson and Johnson note that in recent years the fracture strength of the tibial shaft has been the criterion for design and settings of bindings.[128] The ski binding should release before the threshold of injury to the tibia is reached. This is quite difficult, however, because a binding that will release in any direction the skier can fall also is likely to have an excessively large number of "unnecessary" releases during normal skiing maneuvers. Consequently, most binding manufacturers have chosen to produce bindings that have a side-to-side (twist) release capability at the heel (that is, a two-mode release system).

But if the skier falls directly backward, the tibia may still be fractured by the boot top. Binding function is determined by binding settings, maintenance and lubrication, and antifriction devices (sole pads), as well as by the basic binding design.

During the mid-1970s, the most common injury in downhill skiing was knee sprains (22 percent), followed by thumb injuries (9 percent), leg contusions and sundry lacerations (8 percent each), and ankle sprains (7 percent).[128] Tibial fractures were only 6 percent, and ankle fractures 3 percent. All other injuries comprised less than 5 percent of the total. Table 24–2 shows comparative injury patterns for cross-country and downhill skiing and ski jumping.[132,133]

The last of these is by far the most hazardous, with high injury rates and high proportion of head injuries. The frequency and severity of these injuries can be reduced through use of properly designed helmets. Cross-country skiing has the lowest injury rate, with a greater tendency toward

Table 24–2
Injury Patterns in Different Types of Competitive (C) and Noncompetitive (NC) Skiing

	Downhill		*Cross-Country*		*Long-Distance*	*Ski-Jump*
	C	*NC*	*C*	*NC*	*NC*	*C*
Percentage injured in 3 years	18		3		—	47
Fracture rate per 1,000 athletes over 3 yrs	4.8		0.7		—	13.3
Area Injured						
Head	19	3	9	5	7	33
Trunk	7	2	12	9	2	13
Upper limb	19	10	35	25	29	25
Lower limb	56	84	44	61	62	30

Source: Adapted from N.E. Westlin, "Injuries in Long Distance, Cross Country, and Downhill Skiing," *Orthopedic Clinics of North America* 7(1976):55–58; J. Sandelin, O. Kiviluoto, and S. Santavirta, "Injuries of Competitive Skiers in Finland: A Three Year Survey," *Annals Chirurgiae Et Gynaecologia* (Helsinki) 69(1980):97–101.

trauma to the upper extremity. Performing of tricks while skiing—or "hot-dogging"—is reported to increase the risk of spinal cord injury.[134]

Although always a potential problem, hypothermia has received little attention in the literature on ski injury, and I can report nothing on its relative frequency. Nor is there much information about the relative frequency of injuries involving ski tows. Beginning about twenty years ago, virtually all lifts have been required to pass periodic government inspections.[135] Nonetheless, occasional failures occur, sometimes of a spectacular nature with injury and even loss of life. Anecdotal reports, however, also suggest that an unknown number of people are being injured in the process of getting on or off chair lifts.[136]

Improvements in the grooming of ski slopes to remove "moguls" and provide a smoother surface and availability of snowmaking equipment to provide a thicker blanket of snow have been suggested as possible reasons for the reduction in downhill ski injuries in recent years.[131] There is no documentation, however, of the relative contribution of slope quality to either the initiation or the severity of falls.

In the post-injury phase, one of the most sensible and positive programs in the field of sports medicine has been the development of the ski patrol, a corps of well trained and equipped rescue personnel who patrol the slopes and can deal not only with sprains, strains, lacerations, and fractures but also the prevention of hypothermia and, if necessary, search procedures for lost individuals.

During summer months, some ski slopes made of solid cement bases are now being used as slides for snowless "sledding."[137] One sled type is placed on a track and the riders are strapped in. They can control the speed of the vehicle but not its direction. If one sledder slows down suddenly, others may crash into him, with resultant injuries that in some cases have been rather severe.

Other slides use free-riding sleds. While collisions between sleds are not common, riders sometimes fall off, getting abrasions of arms or legs as they scrape along the slide. Unfortunately, during pollen season the slide surface may have large amounts of pollen, which gets "injected" into the abraded skin, and anaphylaxis has resulted in several instances.

Snowmobiling developed during the 1930s to 1950s following Bombardier's 1923 invention of a motor vehicle capable of skimming the deep snowy surface.[138] By the late 1960s numerous reports of injuries began to appear in the medical literature. In the winter of 1970–71, for example, 118 fatalities occurred in Canada, and 102 in the United States.[139] This concern, however, was not merely about the injuries, but also represented a cultural clash between people who like a quiet, pristine environment and those who want to explore rapidly, albeit noisily, sometimes cruising from one tavern to another.[140]

Dewar reviewed eighteen of these papers in 1973 and concluded that most of the data were meaningless because of unreliable methods of data collection and absence of baseline data on snowmobile use and user characteristics.[139] These problems have largely been dealt with in studies by Waller and Lamborn.[141,142] A random 10 percent sample of licensed snowmobiles in Chittenden County, Vermont, showed an average seasonal use of 470 miles for males and 260 for females, and 650 for males under age 29 versus 300 for males age 40 or older. Very few persons (13 percent) reported that they *did not* go snowmobiling at night, while 59 percent averaged half or more of their use after dark.

Overall, there was one property-damage event reported per 7,000 miles of riding and one injury event per 16,700 miles. The loss rate varied widely according to make of machine—from 0.69 per 10,000 miles to 5.41—with the most popular machines having by far the lowest loss rates. There were nonsignificant differences ($p > 0.25$) in loss rates among owners who had highway crashes and citations (47 percent) versus those who had clear motor vehicle records (35 percent).

The second study involved 133 injured persons who were treated at a hospital that provided about 80 percent of trauma care for the county. Forty of those injured were passengers. Overall, 26 percent of injuries involved collision with an obstacle, 19 percent hitting a bump, or hard landing after jumping, 10 percent each collision with another vehicle or snagging on a wire or other object, 6 to 7 percent each snagging on equipment or vehicle overturning on a slope, and 21 percent miscellaneous other reasons (often involving product failure). Contusions and lacerations were most common (38 percent), followed by fractures (30 percent), sprains (22 percent), concussions (3 percent), and miscellaneous other injuries (6 percent).

Forty percent of injured adults, but 22 percent of comparison snowmobilers, reporting consuming alcoholic beverages on their most recent excursion, but the two groups did not differ in their usual drinking patterns. Injury events involving alcohol occurred at higher speeds than did those not involving this drug. Generally, the injured population expressed frustration or violent response to frustration more often than did the comparison group. Almost half the injured drivers, versus a quarter of uninjured ones, reported at least one fight in which they hit another adult.

Injured snowmobilers averaged 3.4 crashes and 2.7 citations per 100,000 highway miles versus 1.6 crashes and 1.3 citations for the comparison. Many of the injured group had accumulated high mileage through driving pickup trucks or motorcycles in addition to automobiles, results largely consistent with those reported by Carlson and Klein.[143] Eleven percent of drivers with current injuries, but 4 percent of comparison drivers, reported a snowmobile injury during the previous year among those who were at risk the previous season.[142] Injured drivers tended to drive their snowmobiles at higher speeds than uninjured ones and either to have much less exposure or much more exposure than the uninjured snowmobilers.

Environmental factors—usually rough terrain or slick ice—were involved in almost 40 percent of all injury events, and snowmobile factors contributed 33 percent of the time. These included inadequate lights, running board too narrow, skis or track exposed or hazardous, throttle stuck in open position, exploding clutch, and inadequate guards or bumper. Poor stability and handling, inadequate windshields and lights, and inadequate padding and guards were the major vehicle design problems reported by both injured and comparison snowmobilers. The overall interaction of human, vehicular, and environmental factors in initiation of these injury events is shown in table 24–3.

With respect to vehicular inadequacy, Waller and Lamborn noted the following areas of suboptimal function that warrant standards for improvement:

1. inadequate suspension systems;
2. high center of gravity and narrow track;
3. inadequate front and rear lights;
4. poor traction on ice;
5. windshield too small to give protection;

Table 24–3
Interaction of Factors in the Initiation of Snowmobile Injuries

	Injured Person							
	Driver under Age 18		*Driver Age 18 or older*		*Passenger*		*Total*	
	No.	%	*No.*	%	*No.*	%	*No.*	%
Human	4	24	8	12	8	26	20	17
Environmental	1	6	14	20	6	19	21	18
Machine	1	6	3	3	0	0	3	3
Human and environmental	6	35	28	41	9	29	43	37
Human and machine	1	6	5	7	2	6	8	7
Environmental and machine	3	18	6	9	3	10	12	10
All three	1	6	6	9	3	10	10	9
Unknown	1	—	5	—	7	—	13	—
Total	18	101	74	101	38	100	130	101

Source: J.A. Waller and K.R. Lamborn, "Snowmobiling: Characteristics of Owners, Patterns of Use and Injuries," *Accident Analysis and Prevention* 7(1975):213–223. Reprinted with permission. Copyright 1975, Pergamon Press, Ltd.

6. narrow running boards and other features that make it difficult for passengers to avoid being tossed about;
7. exposed track and other moving parts that catch riders; and
8. handlebars, seats, and so forth with poor energy-attenuating ability.

These design problems were thought to contribute to occurrence, severity, or both in at least half the injuries. Considerable redesign and improvement by manufacturers has occurred in these areas since the original observations were made.[144,145]

Others have also noted that long scarves on snowmobilers get snagged easily.[146] Hypothermia is a potential risk if people are not well insulated and get stuck or injured some distance from help or if their vehicles go through soft ice on a lake or river. The possibility of avalanche is also an issue for snowmobilers who travel in groups.

Fatalities have often occurred when snowmobiles cross roads designed for automobiles at night, with a poorly lit snowmobile suddenly coming up over a snowbank and onto the road.[147] Snowbanks should be kept low for at least 500 feet around crossing points.[148] Another unexpected hazard is that some injured snowmobilers who seek treatment meet with open hostility and "lecturing" by hospital staff who don't like snowmobiles or snowmobilers. Literally, in these cases, insult is added to injury.

Sleds, toboggans, and snow disks account for about 40,000 injuries per year treated in U.S. emergency departments.[125] The major injuries appear to be lacerations, and contusions/abrasions (almost 30 percent each), followed closely by fractures and sprains/strains (20 to 25 percent each).[149] A third of sled and snow disk injuries, but 18 percent for toboggans, are to head, face, and neck. Injuries to lower limbs predominate (33 percent) with toboggans. Between 80 and 90 percent of patients are under age 20, with the biggest single age group (about 40 percent) age 10 to 14.

All three "vehicles" contribute to the initiation of the event because they are so difficult to steer and control, especially the snow disk.[125] And the environment is likely to be a bare spot that produces a sudden and unexpected stop, a parked or moving automobile, or a curb struck in an attempt to avoid going into traffic.[125] Flimsy materials that break or splinter during use are also noted as a contributing factor.

Miscellaneous Other Sports and Recreation

This section considers several sports that are competitive but do not involve body contact—racket sports, track and field, gymnastics, and baseball—as well as "toys" for adults—amusement parks and mechanical bulls. Equestrian injuries will also be examined, as will bites from pets and other animals.

The epidemiologic quality of "research" concerning the racket sports is quite poor, and the data below are presented simply because they are all that is available. Hensley and Paup report that 82 percent of 231 players indicate that they have had at least one injury over ten to fourteen years, for rates of 0.09 and 0.14 injuries per person per year for male and female badminton players.[150] Forty-four percent reported sprains or ligament injuries, 39 percent blisters, 28 percent strains or tears, 21 percent each muscle cramps or tendon injuries, 7 percent each eye injuries and bursitis, and 3 percent fractures.

Most of the injuries resulted from intrinsic stress on muscles or ligaments, but 19 percent were from collisions between humans, 6 to 7 percent each from contact with racket or shuttle, and 3 percent from collisions with environment. Over these several years of exposure medical care was sought by 78 of the 231 players, and 13 were hospitalized.

To the extent that they are comparable, the reports on acute injuries in squash and tennis also suggest that many involve intrinsic injuries to muscles, tendons, and ligaments, with few fractures.[151,152] Several papers emphasize the number of injuries to face and eyes from balls or rackets and the fact that these are largely preventable with use of protective face shields or goggles.[152–155] Failure to warm up properly is also an important and preventable reason for injuries.

Such training and warm-up inadequacies are also commonly pointed out as causal factors in the frequent musculoskeletal injuries among runners.[156–159] Poor shoe design is another factor, as is running only on hard surfaces. I can find no data on either the absolute frequency or the rate of injury to runners (overall rates of track injury appear in table 24–1). With the increasing popularity of jogging—from 2 million residents of the United States and Canada in 1972 to 30 million in 1979[158]—collisons between joggers and automobiles have also become a problem.[160] Usually they occur after dark, with a young male jogger being struck from behind by a vehicle traveling in the same direction. One study reports 60 collisions throughout the United States in a one-year period resulting in thirty deaths and thirty-five nonfatal injuries. Potential solutions are not to run on roads after dark, to run single file and against traffic, and to wear light-colored clothing and reflective materials.

Another problem becoming common among joggers and long-distance runners is heat stroke, especially among novices who attempt to run long races without adequate acclimatization.[161,162] In such individuals, injury may occur despite consumption of fluids before and during the race. One 10 km race saw 15 people (1.2 percent) hospitalized among 1,250 participants. In another race, there were 11 hospital admissions (0.7 percent) among 1,658 racers.[161]

There is relatively little information on injuries in field events, as opposed to track overall. Serious facial injuries to persons who are near hurlers have been reported, usually from contact with the hurley, and helmets have been recommended.[163] There is a report of quadriplegia in a pole vaulting champion, but this occurred while warming up on a trampoline rather than while vaulting.[164]

Garrick and Requa describe a rate of 40 lost-time injuries per 100 participant seasons in 17 women's teams.[165] Thirteen percent were to spine and trunk, with 52 percent and 31 percent, respectively, to legs and arms and 4 percent to head. Most injuries (68 percent) were sprains and strains, 10 percent fractures, 5 percent contusions, and 17 percent other. They suggest without documentation that use of trampoline is overrepresented among the injuries.

Among 198 persons with 201 trampoline injuries, 49 had permanent residua, such as permanent back pain or painful joint instability.[166] Many of these injuries occurred while doing simple exercises under careful supervision. The mid-1970s saw about 19,000 trampoline injuries annually in the United States, with 50 serious spinal cord injuries, while in Germany there were 7,000 injuries annually among school children.[166] Even the best safety mattresses appear not to offer adequate protection.[166]

We turn next to baseball, one of the favorite sports of Americans and Japanese but not the subject of much medical literature,[108] except for concern about chronic stress to elbows of young pitchers.[167,168,169] Among professional and college players sprains and strains comprised 46 percent of all injuries, contusions 17 percent, pulled muscles 11 percent, and fractures 8 percent (from sliding or being struck by a pitched ball. Skull fractures and contusions are largely preventable through use of helmets.). Among pre–high school players, an annual injury rate of 2 percent requiring treatment is reported among 750,000 boys age 8 to 12 in Little League play.[170] Fractures were 19 percent and concussions 3 percent. Ten percent of injuries were from sliding.

Data are also sparse concerning the remaining forms of recreation to be discussed in this section. An estimated 6,000 to 8,000 nonfatal injuries and 10 deaths occur annually involving carnival amusements in the United States.[171] Many of these events involve simultaneous injury to many individuals when gondolas fall, doors fly open, or aerial cars collide. While some states require inspection of such equipment before operation begins, many do not, and because traveling carnivals move from one jurisdiction to another, it has been difficult to determine whether repetitive problems are occurring. CPSC tries to serve as a clearinghouse.

In Britain injuries, especially to the perineum, have been reported from the use of go-karts on tracks at amusement parks.[172,173] These small carts offer very little protection for the operator, and when vehicles collide in the limited space—as they often do—face, perineal area, and limbs may be thrown against the steering wheel or caught between cars or parts of a single car. Again, inspection of the track and equipment usually is not required.

At one track, the injury rate was reduced from 1 per 12,000 laps to 1 per 20,000 by increasing the length and breadth of the track to reduce the severity of bends and prevent pile-ups, providing crash barriers that offer more energy attenuation, providing a protective barrier so carts enter the pit area more slowly, and reducing the number of vehicles on the track at any one time, especially in wet weather.[172] Padding has been placed around the steering wheel, and helmets and seatbelts have been promoted. These latter two have not been at all popular, however.

Riding the bucking mechanical bull has become a new fad in the United States.[174] Those who use these "toys," which often are placed in taverns, commonly have no riding experience, have been drinking heavily, and may be "egged on" by spectators. In one series of twenty persons with injuries, all had been drinking. Injuries resulted from being thrown to the ground, from striking part of the bull itself, or from concussive effect of the "animal," which is capable of moving in three directions.

Sprains predominate, but vertebral and other fractures are not uncommon.

Reports of injury rates for equestrian activity range from 0.7 to 2.0 injuries per 1,000 rides.[16,175–177] Fewer than one rider in every five uses a protective helmet, and head injuries appear to be both frequent and serious, especially from falls.[175,178]

Among 622 patients, falls accounted for 44 percent of injuries, including 34 of 38 brain injuries, 33 of 50 injuries to back and spine, and 54 of 69 injuries to shoulder and clavicle.[178] Next were kicks (24 percent), over a third of which were to the head. Being stepped on or crushed (where the animal fell or rolled over) each were 6 to 7 percent of injuries, usually to the ankle or foot. Remaining injury causes were bites (3 percent), caught in rein (3 percent), struck an upright object (2 percent) or the horse's head (2 percent), and miscellaneous other (8 percent).

Almost half of households in the United States have dogs, and from 13 to 34 percent have cats.[179] More than a million dog bites occur each year, and they probably represent only 25 to 50 percent of the total bites, which cost municipal governments about $50 million per year, exclusive of medical treatment.[180] Fewer than 5 percent of bites are serious. In some areas only a third of dogs have rabies vaccination, making many more bites potentially serious.

In an excellent study at two air force bases, males and females, respectively, under age 19 had 2,419 and 1,883 bites per 100,000 population per year, while those over age 18 had 830 and 488 bites per annum.[179] The crude attack rate was 7.4 bites per 100 animals, with significantly higher rates for collies (20.0), German shepherds (17.4) and cocker spaniels (13.7) and highest rates for sporting and working breeds. Male dogs under age 5 have highest attack rates, with older male dogs, female dogs of all ages, and cats having lower rates. In this study—as in several others[180,181]—most bites involve a person actively interacting with an animal that is not a stray and that is on its owner's property, perhaps trying to protect the owner.

Letter carriers are bitten about fourteen times more often than the general population.[182] In such cases, they usually either have not had a chance to use a chemical repellent, or the repellent has not worked. Carriers who own dogs are more likely to be bitten than those who do not.

Bites, of course, occur from other animals as well, especially from rats in dilapidated housing. A study in New York City described 892 human bites in one year, for a rate of 11.3 per 100,000 population but ranging from 0.9 in one neighborhood to as high as 60.9 in another.[183]

Three-quarters of these bites were associated with fighting or other aggression, with most occurring between the ages of 10 and 40.

Guns and Fireworks

In countries such as the United States and Afghanistan, the right to have guns is prized, while in nations such as Britain ownership is relatively rare. In the United States 90 million firearms are owned by one-half of the population.[184] Of these, about 27 million are handguns, usually purchased for protection against intruders.

In 1980 the number of unintentional firearm deaths was 1,800, of which 1,100 occurred in the home.[48] The total number of unintentional firearm deaths has decreased, however. Each year, about 100,000 nonfatal injuries, unintentionally incurred, result from firearms, usually handguns.[185] But such unintentional deaths represent only about 7 percent of all firearm deaths in the United States, the remainder being almost equally divided between homicides and suicides. Thus, firearms are the second leading cause of injury deaths in the United States,[182] in marked contrast to other nations where such deaths are few.

Since the mid-1960s ownership of guns has increased markedly in the United States, in part as reaction to riots at that time.[181–186] Homicides have increased in proportion to the number of weapons owned, as have the number and rate of unintentional firearm deaths in some metropolitan areas. The total number of unintentional firearm deaths, however, has decreased progressively from a peak of 3,000 between 1923 and 1932. (How many of those were really covert suicides during the depression?)

In Cleveland, Ohio, the unintentional death rate for white males increased from 0.3 per 100,000 for 1958–62 to 0.6 for 1963–67 and 1.4 for 1968–73.[186] Among black males, the rate rose from 1.5 to 1.7 to 5.6 during comparable time periods. In the suburban areas, the rate among white males increased from 0.2 to 0.3 to 0.6. The highest rates were 14 and 4, respectively among nonwhite and white males age 25 to 34.

At the same time, a hospital in Detroit, Michigan saw an increase in unintentional gunshot wounds to children from about two per year between 1962 and 1965 to over thirty per year in 1969–71.[184] Half of these involved handguns, usually obtained illegally for protection, owned by a parent of the victim, and kept easily accessible on a bedroom table or under a bed. Sixty percent were kept loaded at all times without any safety precaution, and only 13 percent were under lock and key. When these families were interviewed months to several years after the event, the same conditions prevailed.

The usual sequence is that a child—almost always a boy—was playing with the gun, and the bullet hit a bystander, although in eighteen of sixty cases the child who was struck was actually aimed at. Thirteen percent were fatally wounded, 59 percent recovered completely, and 29 percent had a disability that usually lasted for months or years.

Klein et al. stated that in Michigan between 1970 and 1975 handguns were reported in 30 percent of urban child fatalities but no rural ones.[187] Between 33 percent and 58 percent of the time, however, no information was available about type of gun involved. Death rates for black children were higher than for whites, and handguns were more often involved with deaths to blacks. The authors present data, however, to suggest that poverty is the strongest predictor of gunshot death in children, rather than racial factors or population density. Furthermore, urban residents, regardless of race or socioeconomic status, are more likely than rural ones to get a handgun that they keep for self-protection.

A study by Waller and Whorton of sixty-four unintentional shootings in Vermont in 1967 found handguns involved in one-third.[188] Half of the shooters were age 10 to 19, 30 percent age 20 to 29, and 19 percent age 30 or older. However, among persons shot, 7 percent were under age 10, 33 percent age 10 to 19, 39 percent age 20 to 29, and 30 percent age 30 or older. Ninety-seven percent of the shooters and 80 percent of those shot were males. Vermont is a predominantly rural state in which hunting is an important recreational activity, both for residents and nonresidents. Yet only 37 percent of the injuries occurred during hunting, 31 percent during target practice (especially Western style "quick draw"), 8 percent while the gun was being cleaned, and 24 percent during other activities, such as transporting the gun or showing it to someone. Four out of every five injuries were minor, while 6 percent resulted in death.

This study examined personal characteristics of the shooters, those whom they hit, and an age/sex matched comparison group, most of whom also own guns but who had not gotten into trouble with them. In several cases, the shooter struck himself (especially while playing "quick draw"). Persons shot by someone else turned out to be similar in characteristics to the comparison group. Not so, however, for the shooters.

Forty-one percent of the shooters but 14 percent of the comparison group were already known to the police for nonhighway offenses. Among shooters, 32 percent, 21 percent, and 50 percent, respectively, had previous contacts for deliberate violence, misuse of alcohol, and highway crashes in the previous three years. Comparable figures for the comparison were 5 percent, 5 percent, and 29 percent. Nineteen percent of shooters, but 1 percent of comparison drivers, had previous suspension or revocation of driver's license.

Persons who shot themselves or others while hunting were similar to the comparison group, whereas those with incidents during target practice or other nonhunting activity frequently had previous arrests. Only one out of eight hunters, but six of fourteen persons in shootings during target practice, had previous arrests, and all six had previous arrests for violence. Heins et al. comment that boys learn about violence through television and toy guns, which are models of tools used by adults.[184] As the Vermont data suggest, at least some males carry their play as gunslingers into their adult lives, reflecting arrested development in several areas of social interaction.

The subject of countermeasures to gun injuries, at least in the United States, is emotionally charged. Registration of handguns is vehemently opposed by the National Rifle Association, which instead promotes gun safety programs predominantly aimed at hunters, although even in rural areas only a minority of the shootings involve hunting.

Klein et al. maintain that handgun control legislation is not likely to be very effective. First, more than half the deaths are caused by long guns. Second, handgun owners probably believe that compliance with a gun control law would remove their only protection against what they see as a real threat. Nor are they likely to follow advice against keeping a loaded gun in the house because the fact that it is loaded is seen as protection against intruders. In the long run, there must be enough police protection available so that the poor no longer perceive the need for guns as a means of self-protection.

Baker and Dietz, however, suggest other options, such as using less hazardous ammunition, for example, that already developed for police use in crowd control.[185] Unpublished data from the Vermont study suggests that in several cases unintentional discharge occurred because the weapon had a "hair trigger." Also in the Vermont study, at least one death probably occurred because of inadequate emergency care. In hunting, the use of blaze orange has been found to offer greater conspicuity for wearers than does red, yellow, or fire orange.

Regarding a requirement that potential buyers of handguns be screened to make sure that they do not have criminal records, Baker and Dietz point out that under such a policy most murderers would have qualified for ownership. Most murders involve acts of passion among people who already know each other, and often one or both is under the influence of alcohol.

One final remark by Klein et al. is cogent not only to gun injuries but to most research involving recreational injury. The need, they note, is not for more research but rather for better data on which to base such research.

Unlike guns, fireworks and firecrackers almost invariably are used for recreation. In China and other Asian nations this occurs to a far greater degree than in the United States and has religious overtones. While U.S. data are available, they may not be comparable to those from elsewhere because the size of powder charges and types of fireworks vary from one nation to another.

In the United States, for example, beginning in 1966 explosive charges larger than 2 grains (130 mg) were prohibited.[189] (This is equivalent to a device 1½ inches long and ¼ inch diameter and removes cherry bombs from the marketplace.) As of late 1976, the permissible amount decreased to 0.77 grains (50 mg).[190] Several states, however, prohibit private use of fireworks and firecrackers entirely. Other nations permit larger firecrackers or have no regulations at all.

The new U.S. regulations appear not to be very effective, both because of smuggling of illegal devices from Canada and Mexico and some degree of illegal manufacture.[190] In addition, the 2-grain firecrackers still are capable of producing injury, and it appears the smaller ones may be also.[189] As of 1980 there were about 9,000 treated injuries, although the rate per exposure is not known.[190] A report from New Zealand suggests that the injury rate is about one per 10,000 persons exposed during the week or two before Guy Fawke's Day.[191]

A CPSC study in 1973 indicated that 30 percent of injuries occur among boys between age 10 to 14 and after age 25 the number of injuries was negligible.[189] About half of injuries were burns, usually of an arm or hand, but one in every five involved the eye, sometimes with blindness resulting. In that study, only 5 percent of injuries resulted in hospitalization, but a 1979 report had a much higher proportion (16 percent).[192] Homemade explosive devices almost invariably resulted in hospitalization and accounted for most of the very rare fatalities. Some types of banned explosives—in particular, bottle rockets—had high injury rates, usually from improper use. These devices seem especially likely to cause eye injury.[193]

The vast majority of injuries involving oversize fireworks resulted from improper use, while half of the injuries from permissible displays resulted from apparent malfunction.[189] In 1978, however, illegal fireworks distributed in two states resulted in more than 150 injuries within a matter of days.[194] These defective devices exploded immediately when lighted, instead of providing the usual delay from the fuse, and at one hospital alone, twelve young users were seen, seven of whom each lost one or more fingers.

Challenging the Great Outdoors

There are about 60,000 mountain climbers in the United States, between 2,000 and 10,000 of whom are "serious climbers."[21] According to official records—which are known to be an underestimate—the number of deaths among these was 308 between 1970 and 1978.[21] Falls and slips are the most common cause, with exposure, exhaustion, and physical illness next in importance.[195] Attempts to perform beyond one's abilities, climbing unroped, and using inadequate equipment were often implicated. The European Alps saw 268 deaths during 1961 alone.[196]

For club-sponsored climbs Ferris reports 6.88 injuries per 1,000 man-mountain days for persons age 10 to 14, 3.20 for age 15 to 20, and decreasing to 0.80 for those age 36 to 55.[196] The overall injury rate was 2.31, and the mortality rate was 0.65. Again, the highest rates were among the young (1.14 and 1.24 for age 10 to 14 and 15 to 20) and the lowest among the oldest (0.21 for age 36 to 55). His data on frequency and case fatality rates for the most common causes of death in U.S. climbing appear in table 24–4.

Ferris warns of hazards of high-altitude pulmonary edema at heights above 12,000 feet and of the possibilities of freezing to death even at temperatures of 40 to 45°F.[197] Yet it is not uncommon to find individuals attempting casual hikes in dangerous territory while scantily clad, with inadequate shoes, and not even a map.[198]

Burns from portable cooking, lighting, and heating equipment used in camping have been a problem. Often these occur as flashbacks when

Table 24–4
Ten Most Frequent Apparent Causes of Mountaineering Injuries in the United States, 1951–60

Cause	*Number of Cases*	*Case Fatality Ratio (percentage)*
Slip on rocks	156	41
Slip on snow or ice	72	21
Falling rock or object	45	20
Avalanche	45	18
Failure in rappel	23	22
Loss of control in glissade	20	5
Exposure or exhaustion	18	50
Miscellaneous	17	12
Lightning	11	46
Fall in cravasse	10	40

Source: Adapted from B.G. Ferris, "Hazards to Health: Mountain-Climbing Accidents in the United States," reprinted by permission of the *New England Journal of Medicine* 268(1963):430–431.

campers spill fuel on their clothing.[199] In the United States, tents for campers are now required to be flame resistant.

Less information is available about spelunking or exploring of caves. There may be 10,000 participants in the United States, and deaths are rare.[21] Flash flooding and other water exposure is a problem here, and falls, exhaustion, and exposure to cold also appear to be important, again, sometimes involving casual explorers.

The modern sport of hang gliding began around 1971,[200] and now has 20,000 to 60,000 participants in the United States alone.[21] Yuill estimates that about 1.8 percent of participants are injured annually,[201] while Tongue reports 2.7 fatalities per 1,000 participants annually, compared to 1.85 for sky divers and 0.6 for persons using sail planes.[202] Frequencies of exposure are quite unknown and the data, therefore, may or may not be comparable.

Tongue's study covers 144 injuries and 37 deaths. Nonfatal injuries were upper extremity 31 percent, lower extremity 23 percent, spine 17 percent, head 16 percent, and other 13 percent. Included were five paraplegias and one quadriplegia. Most deaths involved massive head and chest trauma. Two deaths were by electrocution. A small number of deaths involving less serious circumstances—including falls of less than 30 feet—were to individuals who did not wear helmets, which are highly recommended and widely used. Of 37 autopsies, 24 included tests for alcohol. Four of these (17 percent) had BACs of .02 to .05 percent.

Tongue also provides an analysis—unfortunately unimodal—of causal factors in 104 of the nonfatal events and all 37 of the fatal ones. He attributes 35 of the nonfatal events to poor preflight judgment and 43 to poor inflight judgment. In 26 he could not determine cause. Most of the preflight errors were attributed to inadequate education, while most of the inflight errors were attributed to inexperience.

The 37 fatal events involved improper inflight maneuvers for 16, equipment problems for 12, and peer pressure in 9 cases. Less than 10 percent of fatal injuries, but about 40 percent of nonfatal ones, involved persons with 1 to 13 previous flights. About 60 percent of fatalities but 20 percent of nonfatal ones were to persons with 200 or more flights.[202] Krissoff identifies vagaries of terrain and wind, as well as personality, experience, and equipment as contributory factors. In particular, he suggests that certain glider designs may be more difficult to control under certain conditions than are others.[203]

Krissoff and Eiseman recommend the following safety practices:[204] (1) approved schools with minimum hours of instruction before allowing independent flights; (2) licensing of flyers; (3) licensing and certification of airworthiness of equipment; (4) improved equipment, and considera- tion of using nonconductive tubing, perhaps fiberglass; (5) safety clothing, including a helmet, gloves, shin pads, long-sleeved shirts and pants, and sturdy ankle-top boots; (6) approved areas for flying, with no obstructions or equipment hazards; and (7) airspeed indicator or variometer to aid in speed and height judgment. To this Tongue adds an energy-absorbing seat for seated harness or inflatable vest for prone harness.[202]

Tongue's study also includes a comparison with injuries among sky divers, of which there may be 20,000 participants in the United States with 37 deaths per year.[202] Among 135 nonfatal injuries, 71 percent involved a lower extremity, 17 percent an upper extremity, 9 percent the spine, 2 percent head, and 1 percent other.

Whereas, as we already noted, fatal hang gliding episodes most often involve experienced participants, the sky divers show a U-shaped curve with highest proportions among the novices (1 to 24 jumps) and the most experienced groups (200+ jumps). Without knowing about the population at risk, however, it is not possible to reach any substantial conclusions about his data. He does appropriately note, however, that the "panic, no rip cord" reaction of novice parachutists is more hazardous than the "panic, stall" response by persons learning to hang glide.

Hallel and Naggar's study of 84,000 jumps by Israeli Armed Forces indicates 6.26 injuries per 1,000 jumps overall, 4.62 in daytime jumps, and 11.25 at night.[205] Nine percent of the 723 injuries were serious (fracture of long bone, spine, ankle, or tear of knee ligament), 26 percent moderate, and 65 percent minor.

Rates of 3.37 per 1,000 jumps overall and 1.87 among students (less than 15 prior jumps) are noted by Ryan and Thomas,[206] while Istel reports having reduced the injury rate from 1 per 300 jumps to 1 per 1,000 by giving students radio receivers so they could be guided by the instructor to a soft target area.[207] The fatality rate dropped from 1 per 3,300 jumps in 1958 to 1 per 17,000 in 1963.[208] Of 100 fatalities studied, 34 involved not pulling the rip cord or doing so too late, 16 malfunctions of main chute and nondeployment of reserve, and 19 water landings.

One study found that many female parachutists could not exert the maximum force permitted under specifications to release the rip cord and urges design of parachutes for the weakest individuals likely to use them.[209] However, Istel's data indicates that women made between 15 and 20 percent of the jumps but had 13 percent of injuries.[207] He also notes that half of 125 fatalities could have been prevented by having a reliable device to activate the reserve parachute. Use of flotation devices would have prevented the 20 percent of deaths that resulted from drowning.

Injuries in hot air ballooning are not common among the small number of enthusiasts and tend to be similar to those among sky divers.[210] Often the chase crew will be dragged and injured as they attempt to bring the vehicle and its occupants under control.[210] The United States saw 16 deaths from 1960–74 as the number of certificated pilots increased from 25 to 700.[211]

The fatality rate for gliders is 5.0 per 100,000 aircraft hours.[211] As of 1973 there were 13,000 certificated pilots and 2,000 active gliders in the United States, totaling 197,000 hours of flight. The year saw six deaths.

Some Additional Observations

My review of the literature on recreational injury has impressed me in that it is as spotty as it is massive. Most physicians who write on this subject tend to chose a sport—and an aspect of that sport—that interests them, often because they themselves are, or have been, participants. Consequently, some forms of recreation—such as skiing—are vastly oversubscribed, while others are scarcely touched upon. The net result is that even where much is written, little appears that truly represents an adequate understanding of the epidemiology of the activity and of its associated injuries. Recommendations for prevention often reflect this limited viewpoint.

As Haddon has commented as well, the epidemiology of recreational injury has barely been touched.[212] Exceptions are a handful of studies of drownings and recreational injuries involving spinal cord, football, skiing, and snowmobiling. At present, in the absence of good and comparable data about exposure, there is little or no way to assess the relative risk of one type of recreation—or one type of activity within a specific recreational form—versus another. Clearly, there is wide room—and a desperate need—for someone who has a broad view of the field and who knows what he or she is about. The recent establishment of a national registry of athletic injuries gives hope that a few such individuals may be starting to bestir themselves.[119]

25
Hospitals and Nursing Homes

The hospital and nursing home differ from every other situation in this book because the people involved are not in charge of their own destinies and may even be subject to invasive procedures, albeit with an expectation or hope for personal gain in the form of renewed or maintained health. Furthermore, personal integrity is surrendered under conditions of considerable stress, both for the patient and often for the staff. This surrender occurs under circumstances that are usually pressed and rushed in even the best equipped and staffed facility and that in many parts of the world—both "developed" and "developing"—fall far short of the best.

For this reason the subject of iatrogenic or treatment-caused injury is regularly discussed in medical publications with considerable anxiety about both ethical and legal issues. Concern by a hospital about a perceived excess of medication errors represented my own entry into the field of designing injury research. And their even greater concern that the results of such research might have legal ramifications made them decide not to do the study. Knowledge can be a two-edged sword.

In some hospitals "incident" or "episode" rates may be high but with relatively fewer injuries in those events than in other hospitals where the mishap rate is lower. In the former case all known mishaps are reported for legal protection of the hospital against possible patient suits. In the latter case, only those mishaps with likelihood of injury may be reported.

In illustration, the east south central states of the United States reported a rate of 3.5 hospital employee injuries per million person-hours worked but a high severity in average days of work lost.[1] Pacific states, on the other hand, had a very high rate of 14.0 but low average severity, suggesting differences in reporting, rather than in occurrence. Few authors describe the de facto reporting policies in their institutions, making it impossible to know whether apparent differences between institutions are real or artifact.

The description that follows is of hospitals and nursing homes on the North American and European continents, where patients are usually isolated from their families, placed in beds—often very high ones, and fed from a central dietary facility run by the hospital. In many non-Western hospitals patients may sleep on the ground and be surrounded by their families, who live at the hospital with them and bring and prepare meals for the patient. I have found no data concerning in-hospital injuries under such arrangements.

Also noteworthy is that nursing homes are a Western phenomenon. They do not exist—and don't need to exist—in rural agrarian societies, where disoriented or otherwise disabled family members can be kept in the home and protected by an extended family.

This chapter and chapter 23 represent a transition, in that both deal with two different groups of individuals, campers and patients on the one hand and staff on the other. We will begin first with patient injuries and then turn to those of staff.

Patient Injuries

According to a study of six hospitals in England (one geriatric and one a large mental facility), 71 percent of 3,100 incidents were to patients, 28 percent to staff and 0.6 percent to visitors.[2] This is equivalent to 0.39 incidents per bed per year for patients, and 0.53 if all events are counted, or 9.6 patient episodes and 14.5 total episodes per 10,000 patient days of exposure. One U.S. hospital reported data equivalent to 36.1 injuries per 10,000 days, of which 26.5 were falls,[3] and another hospital, describing falls only, indicated 17.2 reported events per 10,000 exposure days.[4] The annual toll of in-hospital mishaps to patients in the United States is 550,000.[5]

Several studies permit calculation only of rates per 1,000 hospital admissions, with all of them showing about 20 to 25 events per 1,000 admissions.[6,7,8] This base, however, is inappropriate for comparing the experience of groups that have widely divergent durations of hospital stay.

Fagan and Vita note, for example, that the rate for males is 23.4 while that for females is 14.9.[8] They attribute the difference to the fact that men are intolerant of enforced passivity. An equally logical explanation, however, is that young pregnant women, who comprised almost a quarter of admissions, had short hospital stays compared to the men and the older women. Weil et al., however, also reported that males had twice as many mishaps as females (45.6 per 1,000 patients versus 18.0), which could not be accounted for by differences in length of exposure.[8]

Table 25–1 shows rates per 1,000 admissions from Fagin-Vita study (column 1) compared with those per 1,000 admissions and per 10,000 exposure days from the Weil and Parrish study.[9] Weil and Parrish note

Table 25–1
Reported Patient Incidents by Age Per 1,000 Admissions and Per 10,000 Patient Days

	Events Per 1,000 Admissions[a]	*Events Per 1,000 Admissions*[b]	*Events Per 10,000 Patient Days*[b]
Newborn*	0.36	} 23.40	} 34.41
1 wk–1 yr	5.49		
1–10 yrs	12.1		
11–20	11.9	12.82	11.99
21–30	4.99	25.78	28.02
31–40	7.95	13.94	14.37
41–50	12.1	22.57	22.57
51–60	21.8	37.61	26.67
61–70	39.6	46.02	32.64
71–80	62.0	37.34	24.40
Total	20.0	28.47	25.00

Source: Adapted from (a) I.D. Fagin and M. Vita, "Who? Where? When? How? An Analysis of 868 Inpatient Accidents," *Hospitals: Journal of the American Hospital Association* 39 (16 August 1965):60–65; (b) T.P. Weil and H.M. Parrish, "How Did It Happen? An Analysis of the Causes of 2,036 Patient Accidents at New York's Mt. Sinai Hospital," *Hospitals: Journal of the American Hospital Association* 32 (1 September 1958):43–48.

*Ages for column 1 are as noted. Those for columns 2 and 3 are 0–9, 10–19, 20–29, ≥ 80.

that while the very young and old had the most injuries, the differences in rates, when corrected for 10,000 days of patient exposure, are considerably less than reported by other investigators.

Overwhelmingly, falls are the most common of the episodes reported. Snell notes, for example, that 91.3 percent of 653 incidents were of this type, with the remainder being burns 2.6 percent, bumping against objects 2.5 percent, and other 3.7 percent.[7] No medication errors were mentioned. In Fagin and Vita's study, falls comprised 68 percent, as shown in table 25–2, with medication errors and bumps against objects as next most common events.[8] Falls were 83 percent of events at Mt. Sinai Hospital.[5] One study from Israel among 3,000 nursing home residents[10] reported 5.1 mishaps per 100 residents per year, or 1.4 per 10,000 patient days. Falls were 95 percent of these episodes.

In the Mt. Sinai study, 59.9 percent of reported events were not associated with injury, 30.1 percent with minor injury only, 7.6 percent with moderate injury, 1.9 percent severe injury, and 0.5 percent death.[5] Snell reports no injury for 53 percent of incidents.[7] Grubel's data provided the highest estimates of episodes among those quoted: 36.1 and 26.5, respectively, per 10,000 patient days for all incidents and for falls.[4] However, 83 percent of the falls and half of other episodes were without injury. For injuries only, the rates are 4.5 per 10,000 patient days for falls, 4.7 for other injuries, and 9.2 overall.

Table 25–2
Types of Mishaps in Hospital

	Percentage	
Falls	68.3	
From bed		28.3
Elsewhere		39.9
Medication or treatment error	6.9	
Hit or bumped object	6.9	
Injured by hospital equipment/furniture	6.8	
Burned, liquid, chemicals	2.9	
Damaged teeth during anesthesia	2.3	
Cut by broken glass/sharp object	1.9	
Self-inflicted	1.4	
Injury to dentures	1.1	
Injured by other person	0.9	
Other	0.6	

Source: Adapted from I.D. Fagin and M. Vita, "Who? Where? When? How? An Analysis of 868 Inpatient Accidents," *Hospitals: Journal of the American Hospital Association* 39 (16 August 1965):60–65.

Discussions of proportions of events that involve falling out of bed with and without siderails, and percentages of events that occur in bed, near bed, in bathrooms, in corridors, at specific times of day, on certain services, and so forth will not be quoted because almost without exception there is no information about exposure to risk. The fact that a certain percentage of falls occur between the hours of 8 and 9 A.M., or to patients without siderails, has little administrative value unless it can also be demonstrated that such episodes are overrepresented with respect to specific activity exposure or with respect to the proportion of beds that do have siderails.

A bare handful of papers involving long-term care facilities do offer scientifically more acceptable information. I can find no definitive risk-related studies in acute care facilities.

Ballinger and Ramsay note in a psychiatric hospital that 75 percent of patients with mishaps (mostly falls) had received a psychotropic drug on the day of the event, as compared to 61 percent of matched patients without mishaps.[11] Excluding episodes involving aggression or intentional self-injury, 75 percent of the injured patients had received such a drug, compared to 58 percent of the controls ($p < 0.001$), suggesting postural hypotension or neurological side effects as causal factors.

Foerster points out that in attempting to relate drug use to falls the researcher needs to be extremely careful.[12] On the one hand, medications such as for Parkinsonism might prevent some falls, whereas diuretics may contribute to falling by increasing the need to void. Research should examine specific medications and dosages between fallers and nonfallers.

Her comment about diuretics suggests that if an association were found between this drug group and falls, it may simply reflect greater *exposure* to risk through increased walking, rather than increased risk per se. In her nursing home study, no difference was found between fallers or nonfallers in number of medications taken daily.

The Foerster work considers age, sex, medication, functional status, and use of walking aids. The population under study consists of twenty-one men and forty-five women residents in a health-related facility, all being able to walk unassisted by nursing personnel, and thirty-four men and fifty-eight women with a range of walking capabilities who were residents in a skilled nursing facility. All were age 60 or older, and 86 percent were 70 or older. No association was found between sex and falls or age and falls. Corless points out, however, that by analyzing fall relationships and sex separately for the two different facilities, instead of for both facilities combined, possible associations may have been overlooked.[13]

In another nursing home study, Margulee et al. report fracture rates in falls of 1.5 and 3.1 per 100 residents, respectively, for males and females.[10] That study, however, reports that 80 percent of falls resulted in fractures, compared to Foerster's comment that 39 percent of falls resulted in minor injuries and that "no major injuries occurred." The two studies, therefore, may not have used comparable methods of data collection.

One might anticipate greater correlation between functional ability or "functional age" and falls than between chronological age and falls. Table 25–3 shows this to be the case.

Two other studies with larger populations of "young" elderly do show relationships between falls and age.[10,14] Table 25–4 shows bone fracture rates by age and sex in the Margulee et al. report, while table 25–5 shows fall relationships with age, functional status, and involvement of host and environmental factors in that study. Clearly, as age increases and/or functional ability decreases, internal factors assume a more important role and external factors seem to become less important in fall initiation.

Several reports mention the frequency of falls at night among hospital and nursing home residents who need to use toilet facilities. Hiatt has suggested that the elderly are particularly hampered both by low levels of illumination and by glare, such as one gets from highly polished floors in nursing homes and hospitals and from tile floors and walls in bathrooms.[15] The possible contribution of these visual factors is not likely to be identified in any of the studies described.

Hiatt has also pointed to the inadequacies of the so-called geriatric wheelchair and to the fact that it promotes poor posture, poor function,

Table 25–3
Relationships between Falls in Nursing Homes, Walking Ability, and Use of Walking Aid

	Nonfallers	*Fallers*	*Fell 1–2 Times*		*Fell ≥ 3 Times*	
			Weak	*Strong*	*Weak*	*Strong*
Uses aid						
N	48	19	6	7	6	0
(%)	(41)	(48)	(21)[a]	(24)	(55)[a]	(0)
Walks Alone						
N	70	21	5	11	3	2
(%)	(59)	(52)	(17)	(38)	(27)	(18)
Total						
N	118	40	11	18	9	2
(%)	(100)	(100)	(38)	(62)	(82)	(18)

Source: Adapted from J. Foerster, "A Study of Falls: The Elderly Nursing Home Resident," *Journal of the New York State Nurses Association* 12(2) (June 1981):9–17.
[a]Percentage of all who fell 1 to 2 times or all who fell ≥ 3 times.

Table 25–4
Fall-Related Bone Fracture Rates Per 100 Persons by Age and Sex

	Age					
Sex	*< 75*	*75–79*	*80–84*	*85–89*	*≥ 90*	*Total*
Males	0.7	1.8	1.3	1.5	3.3	1.5
Females	2.3	2.8	3.2	4.3	6.7	3.1
Total	1.9	2.5	2.6	3.2	5.3	2.6

Source: I. Margulee, G. Librach, and M. Schadel, "Epidemiological Study of Accidents among Residents of Homes for the Aged," reprinted by permission of *Journal of Gerontology* 25 (1970):342–346.

and likelihood of falls.[16] In her opinion, such chairs are an abomination and should not be used.

One small ten-week study of thirty-seven beds with rails and of thirty-eight with rails only if the physician ordered them suggested no substantial difference in the rate of falls.[4] The sample size and time, however, were unacceptably small for reaching adequate conclusions. Certainly, from the safety viewpoint there do seem to be major advantages to using hi-low beds, which in the low position both approximates the height of beds found at home and decreases the impact distance if a fall should occur.[4] In nations where patients lie on the ground such problems do not exist.

We turn next to three types of in-hospital problems that are reported infrequently, namely medication errors, injury from electrical diagnostic

Table 25–5
Fall Rates Per 100 Persons According to Age, Prior Functional Status re Activities of Daily Living (ADL), and Contributing Factors

Functional Status re ADL	*All Falls*	*Host Factors*			*Environmental Factors*		
		Total	*<75 y.o.*	*≥75 y.o.*	*Total*	*<75 y.o.*	*≥75 y.o.*
Independent	7.9	5.3	1.2	6.3	2.6	2.9	2.6
Partially or totally dependent	13.1	10.1	3.9	12.9	2.0	3.9	1.2
Total	9.7	7.3	2.8	8.8	2.4	3.4	2.0

Source: I. Margulee, G. Librach, and M. Schadel, "Epidemiological Study of Accidents among Residents of Homes for the Aged," reprinted by permission of *Journal of Gerontology* 25 (1970):342–346.

therapeutic equipment, and fire. In their classic 1962 study Barker and McConnell classified seven different types of medication errors: omissions, wrong dosage (more than 5 percent off), extra dose given, unordered drug given, wrong dosage form, wrong time (thirty minutes or more before or after ordered), and wrong route of administration.[17]

Their study included not only use of official signed mishap reports but also anonymous error-in-medication reports and actual covert observation of the preparation and administration of 572 medications by nine registered nurses, each of whom was observed for two consecutive eight-hour shifts. A total of 365 errors were officially reported over 59,470 patient days of exposure, or 0.6 per 10,000 patient days. Based on disguised observation, however, the extrapolated number of errors was 56,000 or 9,429 per 10,000 patient days.[a] The observed error rate, in fact, was one error for every six medications prepared and administered. These data are shown in table 25–6.

These authors observe that while 75 percent of nurses stated that all errors should be reported, only 48 percent included omissions, and only 21 percent included early or late doses in their personal definition of errors. Furthermore, nurses often exhibited a divergence between what they said should be reported and the fact that they didn't report 36 percent of such reportable errors known to them. Nurses were markedly influenced by physician's attitudes. Only 36 percent of the nurses said they would submit an incident report if the physican disagreed, and 21 percent felt the physician's opinion would be the decisive factor in reporting.

---

[a]The actual paper refers to 51,200 extrapolated errors by multiplying each observed error by 603. In doing so, however, the authors neglected to extrapolate correctly on the number of "wrong time" errors, thus listing 600 such events when the correct figure was 5,400.

Table 25–6
Officially Reported and Covertly Observed Medication Errors Per 10,000 Patient Days by Type of Error

	Officially Reported over 59,470 Patient Days		*Observed (Extrapolated) to 59,470 Patient Days*	
Type of Error	*Rate*	%	*Rate*	%
Omission	0.20	33	3565	37.7
Underdose	0.01	3	1211	12.9
Overdose	0.13	22	706	7.5
Extra dose	0.05	8	908	9.6
Unordered drug	0.18	31	1732	18.4
Wrong dose form	0	0	404	4.3
Wrong time (late or early)	0.02	3	913	9.6
Total				
%	0.61	100	9429	100.0
(N)	(36)		(56,000)	

Source: Adapted from K.N. Barker and W.E. McConnell, "How to Detect Medication Errors in Hospitals," *Modern Hospital* 99 (July 1962):95–106.

Several other authors before Barker and McConnell have studied reported medication errors.[18–22] These studies are noted here for historical completeness. But in light of both the extent and biased nature of underreporting as described in the Barker-McConnell study, it is not appropriate to give credence to either the frequency or the distribution of events noted in these other papers.

Even the Barker and McConnell study may contain an underestimate of misdosage. Whitcomb has compared actual doses of liquid medications given, as measured with calibrated pharmaceutical glassware, compared to what appeared to be given using a marked paper cup or glass cup of the types commonly used at nursing stations.[23] In illustration, an apparent "2 cc" dose of paregoric in a paper cup was actually 5 cc; "5 cc" of cough syrup was really 7 cc; "5 cc" of gelusil was 8 cc; and "10 cc" of distilled water was 13 cc. Using glass cups, "5 cc" of distilled water really measured 4.5 to 5.75 cc and "10 cc" measured 8.5 to 10.5 cc. Clearly, product control in manufacturing is inadequate to the purpose for which the cups are being used.

The environment for dispensing medicines also plays a major role in determining the types and frequency of errors. Hartley, for example, describes the "combination" system, in which some medication orders are filled from the pharmacy and others are dispensed by nursing staff from open stock on the wards, and he identifies at least forty opportunities for error in every dose given the patient under this system.[24] Errors occur in transcription, in misfiling, mislaying or misreading medication cards, in pouring wrong medicines, or in identifying the wrong patient.

The probability of error increases, he states, with increases in the number of people involved, the number of transcriptions, the amount of confusion and number of interruptions at the nursing station, and the work load on the floor. Better personnel qualifications decrease the risk. Perhaps because of such stresses, one study reports higher error rates for those student nurses who have had more life changes and adjustment demands during the previous two years.[25]

What actually happens is discussed in a study by Safren and Chapanis of 187 medication errors and near errors.[26] Ninety percent of the events could be classified into five categories as follows: failure to follow required checking procedures 36.4 percent, misreading or misunderstanding written communication 21.9 percent, transcription errors 18.2 percent, medicine ticket misfiled in ticket box 8.0 percent, and calculational errors 5.9 percent. Repeatedly, mention is made in studies of the poor quality of physicians' handwriting, misreading decimal places or abbreviations, continual interruptions, and lack of qualifications of many personnel for the jobs they are expected to perform.

Hartley observes that although the hospital pharmacist is by far the best trained and qualified person to handle and control medications, he or she is usually assigned to repackaging drugs into more convenient containers.[24] Tasks of interpreting and transcribing physician's orders and selecting, pouring, and measuring medications are done by nurses, who lack training and adequate inservice education for this purpose.

MacRostie's 1958 survey of 100 nurses acting as night supervisors also is illuminating.[27] Seventy of them substituted as pharmacists, with 30 percent doing so several times nightly, and 60 percent going for everything except narcotics. Ten of the supervisors sent floor nurses or aides to the pharmacy. Only a quarter of trips to the pharmacy were for real emergencies.

As countermeasures to a clearly archaic system of preparing and administering medications Hartley has recommended: (1) reducing or eliminating open floor stocks, (2) eliminating transcription of drug orders at the nursing station, instead having medication cards typed in the pharmacy, and (3) using unit-of-use packaged medications, which would be transported in small mobile medication carts that contain drawers for individual patients in which all medications for twenty-four hours or longer can be placed.[24] These carts would be filled in the pharmacy, thus providing a centralized unit dose system, as developed and described by Barker and his colleagues.[28,29,30]

In 1969 Barker reported on an observation study comparing error rates utilizing the traditional system for administering medicines with the centralized unit dose system.[29] In the former case the error rate was 25.9 percent, including 12.9 percent involving wrong time of administration, a type of error that one would not expect to change with the new system. With initiation of the centralized unit dose system the error rate was 12.0 percent, including 10.1 percent wrong time. If wrong time errors are excluded, the error rates are 13.0 percent for the traditional system and 1.9 percent for the new one. Furthermore, the new system costs less to operate.[30] Other more recent studies validate these results.[31] Nonetheless, a substantial proportion of hospitals in the United States still use the traditional approach.

Substantial underreporting is alleged also for injuries from electrical current coming from diagnostic and therapeutic equipment. In 1969 Ralph Nader asserted that there were 1,200 patient deaths a year from this cause.[32] One reason this occurs, he said, is because as much as 40 percent of new equipment at some medical centers arrives in defective condition.

One report noted leakage of small amounts of current in a variety of equipment in a newborn nursery and stated that this was a more subtle hazard than grossly faulty equipment.[33] In another study, however, involving fifty-five incidents in an 1,100 bed hospital over forty-two months, Bruner et al. argued that the failures they saw were rarely subtle and that microshock was not a large problem.[34] Grossly inadequate cords and connectors and ungrounded equipment were much more important.

These 55 episodes resulted in 3 fibrillations, 22 shocks, 14 skin burns, 10 electric arcs and fires, and 6 instrument and component failures. Twelve each were in electrically operated beds and high-frequency electrosurgical instruments, 10 in monitors, 6 in cords and connectors, 3 each in defibrillators, and pacemakers, 2 in immersion heaters, and 7 miscellaneous (TV sets, thermal blankets, lamps, and so forth). Almost half (23) of the episodes occurred in the operating room, with another 19 in recovery room or intensive or coronary care units. Ten were in patient bedrooms. These locations probably reflect where most of the heavy use of electrical equipment is occurring.

Both Bruner et al. and Stanley point out that plugs molded onto the cord seem especially prone to develop failure of the ground connection in the third prong.[35,36] Stanley offers the following recommendations for hospitals to reduce electrical hazards:

1. All personnel using electrically operated equipment should have safety training, including courses in electrical technology.
2. All equipment connected to one patient should go through a single positive earth ground.
3. If possible, isolated and monitored ungrounded power should be used for hospital rooms, particularly those with patient monitors or cardiac catheterization. Less costly are portable units, which can

detect leakage currents of 200 microamperes and interrupt the circuit if such leakage exists.

4. Trained personnel should be employed to guide purchase of electric equipment and to provide preventive maintenance.
5. All areas where electric instruments are used should be regarded as hazardous for the patient.

Representatives of three hospitals have described what appear to be effective and not especially costly programs to check electrical equipment in their facilities.[36,37,38] Authors of one of these papers note an 80 percent reduction in both major and minor electrical incidents,[36] while another paper states that the costs of the preventive program are partially offset by a substantial reduction in equipment repair costs.[37]

The last issue is fire safety. In 1973 the United States experienced an estimated 10,700 fires in hospitals and 6,400 fires in homes for the aged.[39] Between 1951 and 1970, 486 patients in long-term care facilities in the United States died as a result of multiple death (that is, three or more) fires in long-term care facilities, and an additional 500 or more patients a year died in single-fatality fires in health-care institutions.[40] However, the annual death rate from fires in health-care institutions was 0.0248 per thousand as compared to 0.06 per thousand overall for the nation.

This difference is due at least in part to the development and revision every three years of a model institutional life safety code by the National Fire Protection Association (NFPA). A model code standard is not synonymous with a compulsory requirement or building code, but pressure to comply exists through the Joint Commission on Accreditation of Hospitals.[41] Hospitals and nursing homes at any moment have far more impaired individuals than do other structures, individuals who are less able to escape a fire and more sensitive to injury from smoke inhalation. At the same time, however, such individuals also have much closer supervision twenty-four hours a day than exists in homes and elsewhere.

NFPA codes deal with use of fire-rated materials in construction as related to number of floors and presence of automatic extinguishing systems, adequacy of egress, use of smokestop partitions, sensing and warning devices for smoke and fire, and flammability and smoke requirements for gowns, bedding, curtains, wall finishes, and furnishings.[40] Single-fatality fires have also been reduced by supplying flame-resistant pajamas to all patients.[40] Complete compliance with life safety code standards is quite expensive.[42] The National Bureau of Standards, therefore, has developed a Fire Safety Evaluation System (FSES) to integrate multiple factors in assessing what changes are needed for maximum safety at minimum cost.[43]

Fineberg et al. argue that with the development of acceptable nonflammable anesthetics there is no longer any reason to use flammable ones.[44] Even though only 15 percent of American hospitals still use flammable anesthetics, this use adds approximately $9.4 million annually to the cost of surgical care in the United States.

Well-designed training programs and plans are needed to help hospital employees cope quickly and competently with fire and with the need for evacuation.[45] These should be based on actual observations about how people behave in fire situations. In four separate fires, eighty out of eighty-five people did not use the fire escapes, and seventy-four people did not even try to do so. Only one of sixty-one people with a workable fire extinguisher available managed to get the first extinguisher to work, while two succeeded with a second extinguisher. Four were unable to operate an extinguisher at all, nine fought the fire in some other way, and forty-five made no attempt to fight the fire. People misinterpret the warning signals, such as odd noises and odors, and thus do not detect fires early enough.

This paper noted that only 6 percent of hospital fires in the United Kingdom required patient evacuation, but when this was necessary, numbers of evacuees were large. The size and the design of hospital exits make evacuation difficult, especially if two rescuers carrying a person must move side by side down a stairway. Canadian research has shown that the speed with which people can be evacuated from a building can be overestimated by 50 to 100 percent. In planning fire and evacuation procedures for nonhospital situations, the emphasis must be on evacuating the building within three minutes. In hospitals, however, evacuation of patients to outside the building should be an absolute last resort. Patients should be removed, however, from danger at the point of the fire.

Employee Injuries

The employee injury rate for hospitals is higher than that for industry in general.[46] The reported rate for 326 hospitals was 7.34 per million hours worked; that for all industry was 6.04. Schauer's analysis from 5,004 hospitals with 1.3 million employees identified 31,000 disabling injuries annually.[1] As observed before regarding patient injuries, some studies have only limited value because numerator data only are presented. Table 25–7, however, shows injury rates for various staff and their monetary costs in relation to actual staff distribution.[46]

Table 25–7
Injuries and Their Cost among Different Categories of Hospital Employees According to Their Proportions of Hospital Work Force
(percentage)

Staff Category	*Total Employment*	*Total Injuries*	*Total Cost*
General nursing	33.6	39.6	48.0
Dietary	8.2	18.0	11.2
Housekeeping	5.8	10.7	8.0
Maintenance and engineering	2.4	7.0	6.8
Laboratory, X-ray, EKG, EEG	5.4	3.9	5.4
Laundry	1.5	3.0	3.7
Pharmacy	0.8	0.3	0.1
Outpatient department	0.9	0.8	2.0
Business, medical, clerical	13.5	6.3	7.5
Student nurses	1.7	0.9	0.6
Surgery, obstetrics, central supply	9.9	9.0	6.3
Volunteers	16.3	0.5	0.4

Source: Adapted from T.H. Rockwell, D. Nameche, and W.E. Tarrants, *Work Injuries and Accident Causes in Hospitals* (Washington, D.C.: U.S. Department of Labor, BLS Report 341, 1968).

Table 25–8
Injury Rates Per Million Hours Worked According to Hospital Type and Employee Category

	Hospital Type			
Employee Category	*General*	*Psychiatric*	*Specialty*	*All Hospitals*
Professional care	5.9	12.4	16.1	7.3[a]
Plant operation/maintenance	11.7	15.5	21.8	12.9
Administration	2.1	2.0	3.5	2.2
Total	6.9	12.6	16.7	8.3

Source: Adapted from L.R. Schauer, *Work Injuries and Work Injury Rates in Hospitals* (Washington, D.C.: U.S. Department of Labor, BLS Report 340, 1968).

[a]Attendants 17.9, orderlies 11.7, nurses's aides 9.7, practical nurses 9.5, registered nurses 4.8, student nurses 2.2.

Table 25–8 shows injury rates per million worker hours according to both employment category and hospital type.[1] Higher rates in psychiatric and special hospitals reflect injuries from trying to lift patients, often without adequate assistance. In psychiatric or pediatric hospitals, some injuries are from attacks by patients. Reflecting these differences in population, the rate for long-term care facilities is 13.5, while that in short-term facilities in 6.9. Also reflecting differences in care activities are far higher injury rates among attendants, orderlies, nurse's aides, and practical nurses, who may do much of the lifting, and lower rates among RNs involved in charting, preparing medicines, and similar physically less strenuous activities.

Schauer notes marked differences in injury rates according to hospital size (table 25–9) and observes that in industrial operations large plants (over 500 employees) have low rates because of organized safety programs. Small ones (under 100) have low rates because of closer supervision. Middle-size operations are often too large for effective supervision but too small to warrant elaborate safety programs and thus have higher rates.

That this typical occupational pattern is not found in the hospital situation he attributes to the fact that, in contrast to industry, many large hospitals do not have safety programs. More logical in my opinion are two other possibilities. First, the low injury rates in smaller hospitals are accompanied by higher average disability days per injury, while the opposite pattern exists for the larger hospitals. This suggests, among other things, differences in reporting practices, with possible underreporting of minor injuries in the smaller facilities. Another possibility is that the larger hospitals more often are psychiatric and other long-term care facilities with larger proportions of attendants, nursing aides, and other high-risk personnel engaged in dealing with a different type of patient population.

A comparison report to Schauer's written by Rockwell and associates, deals with types and reasons for hospital work injuries.[46] Falls and overexertion were the two most common mechanisms (28 percent and 24 percent, respectively), followed by "struck by" 15 percent, "struck against" 3 percent, caught in, between, or under 5 percent, contact with noxious substance 6 percent, temperature extreme 4 percent, and other 7 percent. Sprains and strains represent 40 percent of the injuries, and contusions and lacerations another 34 percent.

Of particular note, and reflected in the above data, is the large proportion of injuries to patient care personnel from lifting, pulling, or occasionally restraining patients without adequate help or proper footing. For food service workers, falls on wet surfaces are a common event. One study indicates that nurses who are working rotating shifts have significantly higher injury rates (23.3 per 100 person years) than do those on straight night shift (18.0), day shift (16.8), or afternoon (15.7).[47] One possible reason for this is less adequate sleep and fatigue recovery pattern. Injury rate in this group was not associated with age, length of employment, or marital status.

At least in theory, overexertion injuries involving movement of patients can be reduced by not attempting to do such activities alone if they are to be done manually, by use of mechanical lifting aids to assist

Table 25–9
Employee Injury Rates Per Million Hours Worked and Average Disability Days Per Injury by Hospital Size

	Hospital Size (Number of Beds)							
	<20	*20–49*	*50–99*	*100–249*	*250–499*	*500–999*	*1000–2499*	*≥2500*
Rate	6.2	6.6	6.7	6.7	7.5	9.2	8.4	14.5
Disability days	51	56	79	44	38	35	34	18
Disability days, fatalities excluded	51	56	53	36	36	29	29	18

Source: Adapted from L.R. Schauer, *Work Injuries and Work Injury Rates in Hospitals* (Washington, D.C.: U.S. Department of Labor, BLS Report 340, 1968).

in patient transfers, and by initial training and periodic retraining of personnel in lifting procedures. In actual practice, however, many, if not most, hospitals and long-term care facilities have such serious problems of personnel shortage and frequent personnel turnover that reducing this type of injury requires constant *and formal* dedication beginning at top management levels. The basic methods of safety management and programming for hospitals are the same as in other occupational settings and will be discussed in the chapter on occupational injuries.

The two major types of exposure for hospital personnel not found in most other work environments are contacts with laboratory chemicals, radiation, needles and glassware, and with infectious agents. Arbitrarily, infections are considered as diseases, rather than trauma and are not considered here. However, illnesses comprise only 5 percent of occupational mishaps in the hospital setting.[1]

Table 25–10 shows the distribution of injuries among laboratory personnel in one study of two hospitals.[48] One of these, a university hospital, had 8.3 mishaps per 100,000 laboratory worker hours, while the other, a private hospital, had a rate of 23.5. This and other reports contain extensive lists of potential hazards and safety procedures for hospital laboratories, which will not be reviewed here.[48,49,50]

Table 25–10
Vehicles, Mechanisms, or Types of Injuries Reported for Two Hospital Laboratories
(percentage)

Vehicle, Mechanism, or Type of Injury	*Occurrence*
Glass	36.7
Acid or alkali	13.3
Serum/spinal fluid over pipetting	7.5
Blades	9.2
Microtome	13.3
Scissors/paper	3.3
Formaldehyde	0.8
Needles	2.5
Bruise	8.3
Burn	5.0
Total (N = 120)	99.9

Source: Adapted from G.M. Ederer and B. Tucker, "Accident Surveys and Safety Programs in Two Hospital Clinical Laboratories," *American Journal of Medical Technology* 26 (1960):219–227.

26
Occupational Injury

In many areas of the world, unemployment is the chronic status for a relatively large segment of the able bodied community. For such individuals any job, no matter how risky, is often perceived as a godsend. Any consideration of occupational injury and of our ability to institute appropriate safety measures must be grounded on this sobering reality as a serious but not invincible countervailing force.

A number of books have already been written about occupational health and safety in developed nations,[1] although I am not aware that this subject has been considered for hunter-gatherer or other less technologically advanced societies, except for discussion of bites and stings from poisonous animals among agricultural workers in those areas of the world. This chapter, therefore, will make no serious effort to be truly comprehensive in the international sense of considering many of the idiosyncracies of work throughout all cultures. Nor will it attempt to discuss all Western occupations in depth.

For one thing, organized concern with occupational safety has been overwhelmingly with industry: that is, with those places of business that employ large numbers of persons. Even within those industries, there have been strong biases as to where attention has been directed. Baker et al. state that occupational safety literature, regulations, and training programs emphasize injuries in manufacturing, although only 14 percent of all work deaths occur there, and virtually ignore transportation vehicles, which are involved in about 40 percent of all work injury deaths.[2] Even in manufacturing, more employees are killed by vehicles than by fixed machinery. The self-employed and the businesses that employ only a handful of workers have been largely excluded from this concern and from the various studies. In Allegheny County, Pennsylvania, 69 percent of places of employment have less than eight workers, while only 2 percent have 100 or more.[3] In Hong Kong 57 percent have fewer than ten employees and 5 percent have 100 or more.[4]

This chapter, then, will include an examination of costs and comparative injury rates and countermeasures for a variety of occupations in more developed nations, plus what comparative data I have been able to find for other areas of the world. Some categories of occupational risk have already been considered elsewhere in this book in chapters on trucks, air, rail, and water transportation and hospitals and nursing homes.

Injury Patterns

In the late 1950s, when the rate of work-related injury and deaths in the United States had already dropped to about two-thirds of what it had been only a quarter of a century before,[5] U.S. Secretary of Labor, James Mitchell, pointed out that one out of every 100 teenagers entering the labor force would die as a result of work injury, six would incur a permanent impairment, and seventy would have one or more disabling work injuries before reaching retirement.[6] Since organized safety programming and the occupational activities in many of the developing nations appear to be comparable now to what they were in the United States around the turn of the century or earlier, it seems likely that Mitchell's statement represents a very conservative estimate for the United States in previous years and for many of the less developed nations at present.

In 1980, according to the National Safety Council, there were 13,000 deaths and 2.2 million disabling injuries at work in the United States, yielding death and injury rates, respectively, of 0.07 and 11.4 per million hours of exposure.[5] The estimated costs of these was $30 billion, an average cost of $310 per worker. National Health Survey data (for 1977–79), however, suggest as many as 11.3 million work-related injuries annually.[5] Of these, 2.6 million result in confinement to bed, and 4.1 million are associated with activity restriction.

As we noted before, these discrepancies are hardly unusual. Baker et al. state that work-related injuries are rarely subjected to sound epidemiologic investigations because often there is no single source of data.[2] Among 161 occupational injury deaths in Wisconsin, only 76 percent could be identified from death certificates alone, 57 percent from Workers' Compensation records, and only 35 percent were reported to OSHA (Occupational Safety and Health Administration).

In 1933 the death rate from injury per 100,000 workers was estimated to be 37, and it was probably higher around the turn of the century or earlier, although data are scarce.[7,8] By 1980 the figure had dropped to 13 (13,000 deaths in 97 million workers). Some of the earliest U.S. data for injury by specific occupation were calculated in 1913 based on estimates of numbers of workers and numbers of fatalities.[8] These rates per 1,000 workers are shown in table 26–1.

Note that the death rate for employed males in 1913 was ten times

Table 26–1
Estimated Fatal Injury Rates for Males Per 1,000 Employees by Industry, United States, 1913

Industry	*Rate*
Metal mining	4.20
Coal mining	3.50
Fisheries	3.00
Navigation	3.00
Railroad employees	2.40
Electricians (light and power)	2.25
U.S. Navy and Marine Corps	1.85
Quarrying	1.70
Lumber industry	1.50
U.S. Army	1.49
Building and construction	1.25
Draymen, teamsters	1.00
Street railway employees	1.00
Watchmen, police, firemen	0.75
Telephone, telegraph (including linesmen)	0.50
Agriculture	0.35
Manufacturing (general)	0.23
All other occupied males	0.75
All occupied males	0.75
All occupied females	0.075

Source: Adapted from "Golden Anniversary," *National Safety News* (May 1963):33–92 (Chicago, Ill.: National Safety Council).

higher than for employed females. These data in themselves mean very little, however. While women at that time were often engaged in activities that were hazardous because of unguarded equipment, the men were—and still are—engaged to a far greater extent in more hazardous occupations.

Pochin summarized U.S. occupational fatalities from 1955–75 per million hours worked as follows: trade 83, manufacturing 103, service and government 131, transport and public utilities 373, agriculture 613, construction 717, mining and quarrying 994, for an overall rate of 200.[9] Because they vary in the number of employees at risk, the actual *number* of injuries and illnesses in U.S. industry may differ from the *rates*. Thus, almost 2.6 million of 5.8 million private sector injuries and illnesses in 1978 involved manufacturing, with another 1.25 million in wholesale and retail trade, 676,000 in services, 577,000 in construction, and 463,000 in transportation and public utilities.[10] Mining, agriculture, forestry, fishing, and finance/insurance industries combined contributed fewer than 300,000 injuries.

More recent data available by industry are incidence rates of occupational injury *and illness* per 100 full-time employees (or 200,000 employee hours, based on OSHA definitions of these events). Table 26–2 shows cases involving death or lost work days per 100 full-time employees for each major occupational category and for each industry within the category that exceeds the category mean.[5] One reason why some industries have higher injury and fatality rates than others may be

Table 26–2
Injuries Per 100 Full-Time Employees (200,000 Hours) Involving Death or Days away from Work by Industry Category and All Industries Exceeding Mean for Their Category

	Category Mean	*Exceeds Category Mean*
All industries	2.79	
Mining	2.13	
Metal		2.41
Coal		2.81
Nonmetal minerals		3.89
Construction	4.29	
Manufacturing	2.32	
Food		4.19
Meat products		8.47
Paper		3.52
Printing and publication		4.41
Rubber and plastics		2.66
Leather		2.72
Lumber, wood products (excludes furniture)		6.06
Stone, clay, glass		4.94
Cement		2.77
Iron and steel foundries		4.83
Nonferrous rolling, drawing		2.54
Fabricated metal		2.97
Machinery except electrical		2.71
Ship building, and repair		5.40
Railroad equipment		7.67
Transportation and public utilities	2.72	
Railroad		6.50
Local and suburban transit		4.45
Trucking		17.65
Air		7.09
Gas production and distribution		2.85
Wholesale and retail trade	2.82	
Services	3.78	
General government		7.20

Source: Adapted from *Accident Facts, 1981 Edition* (Chicago, Ill.: National Safety Council, 1981).

that a single event is more likely to involve two or more workers. This is especially true in occupations such as mining and construction, for example.

The OSHA definition counts only injury events that result in loss of at least a full day of work activity. A person with a walking cast, for example, may be able to continue to work at substitute activities in one industry and thus not be counted as injured, but have no substitute activities available in another industry, and thus be counted with substantial lost time. The OSHA data, therefore, may not be comparable between industries.[11]

Furthermore, differences may exist between and within industries for other reasons that also do not reflect severity of injury per se. Stable regional differences exist in average days lost per injury in coal mining and other industries in England, perhaps, according to Harper et al, reflecting regional social norms.[12] They noted an inverse relationship between the number of injuries per annum at each colliery and the number of days away from work per injury.

In the United States, National Health Survey data indicate that work related injuries comprise 35 percent of all injuries, 16 percent of those with activity restriction, and 15 percent of those with bed disability.[6] Occupational deaths were 12.4 percent of all U.S. injury deaths in 1980.[5] In a rural population in Punjab, India (with transportation only by boat or domestic animal), Gordon et al. found that 24 percent of all injuries and 22 percent of the twenty-three deaths were of occupational origin.[13] No deaths resulted from transportation mishaps, in stark contrast to the United States.

That study involved collection of data by home health visitors who asked about injuries, whether medically treated or not. More recently, Datta and Verma carried out a study in ten rural villages in southern India.[14] They included only injuries resulting in treatment at the rural health center. The overall injury rate in a population of 8,728 was 51.9 per 1,000 population, with rates of 76.2 for males and 28.6 for females. Work-related injuries (usually from agriculture) accounted for 79 percent of all injuries, 85 percent of those for males and 63 percent of those for females. Again, transportation injuries were virtually absent.

Causal Factors: An Overview

We will examine first overall factors associated with places of employment that have high injury rates versus those with low rates and then turn to an examination of individual factors, such as age, sex, experience, alcohol, fatigue, personality, and characteristics of equipment used.

A study by Saari and Lahtela is based on information flow theory: namely, that an injury event occurs if the worker's information processing is disturbed by the characteristics of the job, existing hazards, or his own incapacities. Thus, hazards must be present, but the event itself is triggered by a malfunction in worker's information processing.[15] General demands of a job can contribute to malfunction, or the worker's perceptions of the hazards may be poor. Thus, if the complexity or speed of stimuli exceed man's ability to assimilate them, an injury event may occur.

They compared work and environment characteristics in four light metal working factories with very low injury experience in Helsinki, Finland, and in five plants in the same industry with above-average injury experience. The latter plants more often had either fixed or mobile machines with unguarded parts, large objects capable of falling, materials on the floor on which one might stumble, and oil or rubbish on the floor, supporting the portion of the theory stating that hazard must exist. Regarding the job characteristics, workers in high-injury plants had to perform more demanding tasks, often having to rely on senses other than vision and more often using manually controlled machines that require high precision and exact timing.

Furthermore, even for very large jobs, they more often had to plan their own work, the order of tasks and subtasks being less often predetermined. In illustration, where a run of 1,000 pieces or more was being produced, about 90 percent of the workers in high-injury plants, but half of those in the safer plants, had to plan their own tasks. The high-experience factories more often used universal or multipurpose machines and tools, while the safer locations more often had production machinery originally designed for a specific product. High-experience plants also were ones in which the location of work was more varied, so that workers found it necessary to walk around more often.

On its surface a somewhat similar study by Simonds and Shafai-Sahrai examined very different factors.[16] They compared eleven pairs of industrial firms matched for state, type of industry and size, but differing in frequency of work injury. Those plants with low frequency showed the following characteristics:

1. top management involvement in safety;
2. better injury recordkeeping systems;
3. use of injury cost analysis;
4. smaller span of control at foreman level;
5. recreational programs for employees;

6. higher average age of employees;
7. higher percentage of married workers;
8. longer average length of employment with the company;
9. roomy and clean shop environment; and
10. more and better safety devices on machinery.

Unrelated to injury frequency were safety programs for workers' families and quality of safety rules.

A third study examining severity, rather than frequency, of injury in Maine sawmills found that youngest and oldest workers had most serious injuries and that greater severity was associated with temporary job assignments, suggesting that lack of familiarity with the job increases exposure to more serious injury.[17] Also, hardwood sawmills had more serious injuries than did softwood mills, presumably because the raw material is harder, heavier, and contains more defects, in essence making the sawing job much more demanding.

Despite differences in focus, these studies appear to identify three common threads to high injury frequency/severity: (1) laxness of the management process, (2) presence of hazardous environment, and (3) factors associated with inexperience, such as youthful employees, lesser time on job, and job situations that result in frequent changes in task requirements.

Human Factors in the Pre-Injury Phase

A number of human factors have been considered in an excellent and comprehensive review of the literature carried out in 1974 by Sleight, Cook et al. for NIOSH.[18] For ease of access to this extensive subject area (a total of over 1,300 references were considered) this single summary source is used unless another reference number appears.

Table 26–3 shows rates of disability injury according to age.[19] Overall the nonfatal injury rate is highest among workers in their late teens and twenties, then decreasing progressively. Just the opposite pattern, however, occurs for fatalities, with a progressive increase with increasing age, from a low of 0.089 per 1,000 male employees ages 20 to 24 (the youngest group reported), to a high of 0.210 for workers age 65 to 69 (the oldest group reported).

The following questions, however, have been examined in very few of the many studies that consider age as a risk variable:

1. Are younger and newer employees placed in more hazardous activities

Table 26–3
Disabling Work Injury Rates Per 1,000 Employed Males in California According to Age (Mean of Years 1960, 1965, and 1968)
(occurrence per thousand)

Age	*Rate of Occurrence*
14–15	5.26
16–17	19.26
18–19	45.49
20–24	46.33
25–29	44.22
30–34	34.74
35–39	31.67
40–44	29.64
45–49	28.38
50–54	27.73
55–59	27.05
60–64	24.61
65–69	17.53
70 and over	9.36
Total	32.41

Source: Adapted from A. Akman, M. Brooks, and J. Gordon, "Use of Work Injury Rate Tables in Estimating Disabling Work Injuries," *American Journal of Public Health* 62 (1972):917–923.

because they lack seniority and also because they have greater strength and speed for certain jobs that require these attributes?

2. To what extent is injury risk and age a function of general experience with the type of work and/or specific experience with the particular job? Since, in general, younger employees are more likely to have several job changes, to what extent is higher injury frequency in the young really a measure of greater job mobility and less experience?
3. Are younger employees less cautious because they usually are unmarried and lack family responsibilities?
4. Are older employees protected from injury by being placed in safer, less demanding jobs, by the early retirement of less capable older employees, or both?
5. Is injury more severe in older employees because they are less able to respond quickly to impending hazard, because of greater tissue sensitivity to damage, or both? Some studies suggest that young employees also may have greater severity of injury.[17] Is this because they are in more hazardous types of jobs that are associated not only with greater frequency but also greater severity of injury?

The data permit one only to hypothesize on some of these issues but do provide firm evidence regarding others. The placement of young employees in more hazardous activity, less caution by younger unmarried employees, and greater severity in older employees because of slower responses do not have firm documentation, although they remain, to my mind at least, reasonable explanations.

Several studies have shown that injury rate goes down as experience increases, but there are some variations in the results. The relationship between age, experience, and injury rate varies with individual plant factors, and Thorndike hypothesized that the most important variable may be the nature of work performed by different age groups and their levels of experience.

Burov and Bizyayev found that the lowest injury group was workers age 26 with one to two years of experience.[20] The results of this study appear in figure 26–1. Among new employees both youngest and oldest workers have highest injury rates, with the "safest" new employee age being 22. Especially for the young, however, injuries decrease as experience increases.

This study also noted that workers who constantly change places of

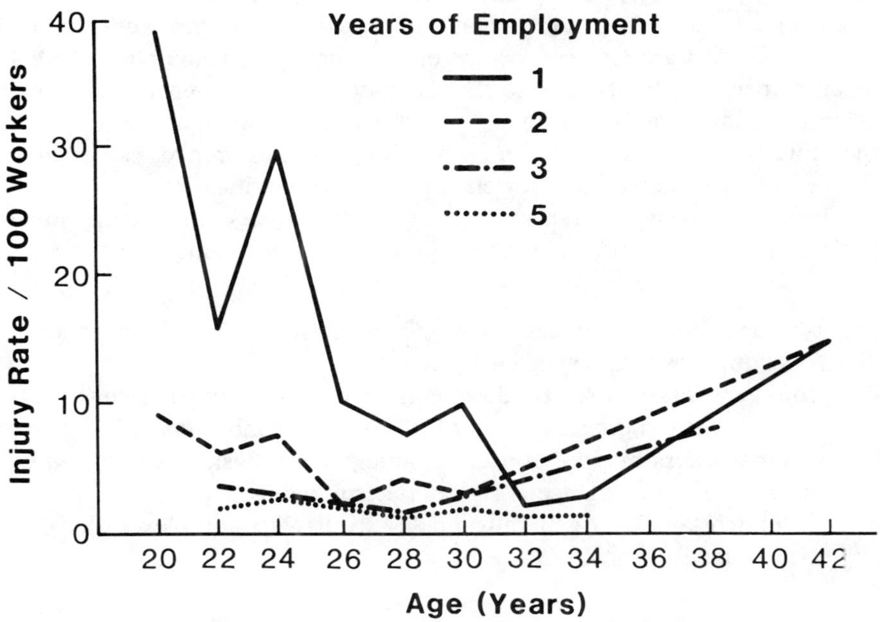

Source: Adapted from N.F. Burov and V.P. Bizyayev, "The Effect of Workers' Age and Length of Employment on Industrial Injuries," *Bezopasnost Truda v Promyshlennosti* (May 1967):11–13, as quoted by C. Fried, V.M. Forbes, K.P. Giles, S.J. Mumford, et al., *The Miner, His Job and His Environment: A Review and Bibliography of Selected Recent Research on Human Performance* (Washington, D.C.: National Bureau of Standards, Department of Commerce, NBS Report 10868 for Bureau of Mines, Department of Interior, Working Fund Agreement HO-122019, April 1972).

Figure 26–1. Injury Rates of Underground Miners According to Age and Years of Employment.

work and occupation were more likely to be injured. Other studies as well document that inexperience with the specific task rather than general level of experience may be the major factor in mining mishaps. Older workers may have problems because technology for a job may change. Thus, they may lack experience for the specific job despite long general experience.

Older employees do have alterations in hand/eye coordination, reaction time, various aspects of vision, and stamina. Whereas about 80 percent of watch and clock makers are physically able to continue work after age 65, this drops to 70 percent for carpenters and bricklayers, 60 percent for mine surface workers, plumbers, and plasterers, 50 percent for riveters, cabinet makers, and underground miners not at coal face, 40 percent for foundrymen and papermakers, 30 percent for construction engineers, and 10 percent for coal-face workers. Older workers employed in jobs usually occupied by younger workers (electrician, miller, grinder) tend to have more injuries than expected, perhaps reflecting greater difficulty in meeting the demands of certain types of work.

It may also be, however, that those older employees who change jobs often, or who remain in jobs usually occupied by younger workers, are individuals who are less competent or who have problems with alcohol or other personal limitations so that they do not "move up the ladder," as do most individuals their age. The association between age and injury, therefore, may in this case reflect other factors not examined, rather than age per se. Well-designed research is needed for clarification.

In summarizing the various studies relevant to age and occupational injury, Sleight, Cook et al. reach the following conclusions:

1. Workers from about age 25 or 30 to 55 generally appear to have fewer injuries than expected by chance.
2. Younger workers are at a disadvantage in tasks requiring considerable judgment and anticipation of unexpected conditions.
3. Older workers may be at a disadvantage if the task is structured or the pace of performance is rigidly determined.
4. Older workers also generally do less well with complex tasks that require fast response.

Reference has already been made to differences in work fatality rates for males and females and the fact that these differences may not reflect gender per se. Beginning with World War II, women have been an increasing proportion of the work force in the United States, including occupations traditionally filled by men. In some European nations this male/female distinction has never been very strong in recent years, whereas in some other societies it is even more rigidly applied than in the United States.

Some of the issues either associated with or confounding sex as a variable are the following:

1. Women *on average* are smaller and may have lesser musculature for specific occupations, such as those requiring heavy lifting. On the other hand, studies of differences in muscle strength have rarely considered the fact that men may be using certain muscle groups to a greater extent than women and, therefore, that at least part of the difference may be a function of training rather than inherent muscle strength.
2. Women often have more extensive work loads at home in addition to their out-of-home jobs than do men, thus raising the greater possibility of fatigue because of an average sixteen- to eighteen-hour day.
3. Variations associated with menstrual cycle and in some cases with premenstrual tension (PMT) syndrome may be a potential factor in variability in work performance, as may pregnancy and post-delivery condition.
4. Furthermore, since child-raising responsibilities usually are assigned to women, whether employed or not, rather than to men, the female employee often may have to be concerned simultaneously with that job as well as with the job that is offering monetary remuneration. Thus, the female employee may have a split task requirement more often than may the male counterpart.
5. Tools, machinery, and safety equipment may be designed only with male employees in mind, thus putting the average woman at a distinct disadvantage.

Furthermore, various legal and social restrictions may affect the types of jobs available to women or the number of hours or time of day they may work. Thus, there may be limited ability to make adequate epidemiologic comparison between work-related injury rates of men and women.

Overall, women employees not only have lower fatality rates than men but lower injury rates as well. This may vary widely. One study found that women had higher rates than men in ordnance and food industries, equal rates in the apparel industry, and lower rates in printing, publishing, chemical, and leather industries. According to Mohn, the mean annual injury rate for males was one in 85 workers and in females one in 205. But the rates for females showed the following range: chain groceries 22, drug stores 26, slaughtering and meat packing 67, stamped and pressed metal products 76, fabricated metal products 55, and textiles and cotton yarns 186. Mohr further notes that when rates are comparable for men and women, the hazard exposure is also similar in the industrial environment.

Vernon found that the hourly rate for minor injuries in a fuse factory was 2.7 times greater during a twelve-hour day than during a ten-hour one, with a greater increase noted for women than for men, perhaps because women were more often fatigued as well by preshift and postshift work at home. Other studies, however, have not found an association between hours worked and female injuries, and Baetjer states that lengthening of hours does not result in disproportionate increase in work injuries if a good safety program exists.

Dalton and others have documented that injuries of women tend to cluster during premenstrual and early menstrual days. While these studies compare the timing of injuries in women, they do not deal with the relative injury rates of men and women or whether women with PMT have higher rates than do women of comparable age and occupation without PMT. Distinct problems have been identified in the design of tools and equipment within the work environment that are particularly relevant to women.

Back pain, presumably at least in part from overexertion, has been one of the most frequent and disabling problems in employed populations. In 1967 there were at least 400,000 disabling back injuries per year in the United States that were work related. Some places of employment screen all new employees with spinal X rays, which certainly increases exposure to radiation but probably is useless for prevention.

Studies suggest the following associations:

1. The incidence of back injury peaks in the age group 31 to 40. However, in a study of a single industry (food chain distribution) the average number of days lost per year increased progressively from fifteen for workers under age 20, to thirty for those 51 to 60, and then dropped sharply to five for those over age 60. Neither of these studies considered whether people were performing similar tasks.
2. According to one study, younger persons with back pain were most likely to be in jobs that required either prolonged sitting or hard physical work. The hypothesis, therefore, would be that lack of physical exercise increases risk of injury, as does assignment to tasks that make physical demands. But it is not clear if a greater frequency of back pain with hard physical work occurs even if one is in a good physical condition.
3. Other studies also suggest that emphasis on physical fitness is

associated with lower back injury rates and that obese persons have higher injury rates.

4. One recent study shows an association between cigarette smoking and back pain.[21] Do smokers cough more, have less physical fitness, engage in different work activities, or a combination of these factors? The study controlled for age but not for these other variables.

In recent years there has been increasing attention to biologic rhythms and the possibility of their effects on productivity, successful endeavor, and injury. Some of these have been founded on sound biological theory and knowledge, such as the menstrual cycle. Indeed, as already noted, variations in timing of injury experience have been shown with this particular cycle. However, the assumption that, if one knows the date and time of day of a person's birth, it is then possible to predict exact rhythmical patterns over many years, has no scientific basis, and there is no association between such alleged rhythms and occupational injury.[21]

Fairly strong evidence exists that efficiency is lower at night,[23,24] that workers with alternating shifts experience reduced capacity, probably because of cumulative fatigue from altered sleep patterns,[23,24] and that such alterations are associated with increased risk of injury.[23] Of equal importance, however, is that there are marked variations in individual sensitivity to Circadian shifts and to sleep deprivation.[23,25,26] Some individuals, therefore, suffer severe decrement in capacity and increase in injury risk under such circumstances, while others show little or no effect.

The issue of alcohol abuse and inadequate employee behavior is an exceedingly important one, causing extensive work-related problems throughout the world and resulting—and rightly so—in alcoholism treatment programs in some of the more enlightened places of employment. It is not my purpose here, however, to deal with the larger issue of lost time, production errors, and other worker inefficiencies but rather to focus on occupational injury involving this or other drugs.

In surprising contrast to the situation involving alcohol and home or highway injuries, no consistent pattern shows up regarding alcohol and work injuries. Shain states that there is vast underestimation of the role of alcohol in occupational injury, and he presents some interesting and frightening data on the frequency of alcohol use and impairment in some railroads.[27] Some of the European data that he offers, however, suggesting that as much as a third of work injury fatalities have alcohol are based on sampling of fewer than half of eligible subjects.

Honkanen has reviewed a number of studies involving both fatalities and nonfatal injuries in the United States and Europe, including several where most or all of the eligibles were tested.[28] The following are the proportions with alcohol for fatalities in the more adequate studies: Wilentz (USA)—7 percent, Hansen (DDR)—10 percent, Waller (USA)—0 percent (18 cases), Alha (Finland)—9 percent, Naeve (Germany)—7 percent. The one nonfatal injury study with adequate sampling (80 percent tested) was by Verhaege in France and reported 36 percent with alcohol. Baker et al.[2] found 11 percent with alcohol in a complete sampling of occupational fatalities around Baltimore, Maryland.

Three important studies of nonfatal work injuries in Boston,[29] Helsinki,[30] and a rural Finnish hospital[31] are presented in table 26–4. They again highlight the wide range in observed results. What these and other studies lack are comparison data on BACs in persons with similar work exposures who are not injured. Were these available, I would anticipate (based on experience with home and highway injury) no excess among the injured of persons with BACs below 0.05 percent and that the contributory role of alcohol to injury probably is only at BACs of 0.05 percent or higher.

Some possible explanation for these inconsistencies comes from the work of Observer and Maxwell[32] and from Roman and Trice.[33] The

Table 26–4
Distribution of Blood Alcohol Concentrations in Nonfatal Occupational Injuries in Boston, Helsinki, and Rural Finland

	B.A.C. (Percentage by Weight)				
	0	*0.01–0.05*	*0.06–0.15*	*≥0.16*	*Total % (N)*
Boston[a]	84.4	10.6	4.9		99.9(969)
Helsinki[b]					
Traffic to/from work	94	3	3	0	100(36)
Fall to/from work	72	11	6	11	100(46)
Fall at work	72	10	10	8	100(63)
Machine	89	5	5	0	100(62)
Other work-related	83	9	9	4	100(46)
Rural Finland[c]	91	2	2	3	100(69)

Source: Adapted from (a) H. Wechsler, E.H. Kasey, H.W. Demone, and D. Thum, *Alcohol Level and Some Home Injuries: Final Report to U.S. Public Health Service on Grant 5 ROI UI-00022* (Boston, Mass.: The Medical Foundation, 1969); (b) R. Honkanen and T. Visuri, "Blood Alcohol Levels in a Series of Injured Patients with Special Reference to Accident and Type of Injury," *Annales Chirurgiae et Gynaecologia (Helsinki)* 65 (1976):287–294; (c) R. Honkanen and J. Ottelin, "Blood Alcohol Levels in Injury Victims at the Emergency Station of a Rural Central Hospital," *Annales Chirurgiae et Gynaecologia (Helsinki)* 65 (1976):282–287.

former conclude that problem drinkers have an excess of on-the-job injuries only during the early stages of their abusive drinking but that as their problem becomes "full-blown" they learn how to be more cautious in the work environment. In their study, the problem drinking employees had many off-the-job mishaps, while the normal controls had none.

Trice's interviews with members of Alcoholics Anonymous supports these conclusions. He and Roman quote work indicating that alcoholics are two times as likely to have an injury and seven times more likely to have a fatal injury as other persons of comparable age and sex. Overwhelmingly, however, such injuries and fatalities were not work related, whereas those of nonalcoholic controls more often did occur at work.

They attribute this relative absence of work-related injuries to several protective factors. The problem drinker may (1) reduce his work to a routine he knows well, (2) become especially cautious of job hazards, (3) be protected by fellow workers, (4) stay away from work while incapacitated, (5) "steady" himself with small—and for him nonimpairing—amounts of alcohol while on the job, and (6) be assigned by supervisors to less hazardous work.

Roman and Trice review what little data there are about other drugs and conclude that although some anecdotes exist about drug-related injuries, the general consensus of studies is that experienced drug users, whether involving marihuana, amphetamines or other drugs, generally have no obvious impairment, or are impaired to a far less degree than with alcohol. Even Shain agrees that drug users very easily manage to "pass" as unimpaired, whereas the impairment of alcohol users is often obvious to fellow workers, including supervisors.

The last human factor is long-term personality patterns and response to stress. As early studies on so-called accident proneness have shown, a small group of individuals can be identified in industrial settings who do have more injury events in a given time frame than would be expected by chance. It has been suggested that some individual factor, either environmental or human or both, may explain this excess (which, however, still comprises only a minority of all injuries). Searchers for specific long-term personality factors, however, have been universally unsuccessful.

Several researchers, such as Behan and Hirschfeld, have identified what appear to be personal attributes in the pre-injury days or weeks that appear to make the individual more receptive to injury.[34] But these seem to be short-term traits, rather than long-term ones. The one trait most consistently associated with injury is excessive absenteeism, but, as with injury, this is an effect rather than a cause. One study found that this absentee/injury relationship held up for employess who sustained injuries in which they themselves were active rather than passive participants.[35] Furthermore, personality traits that might create a hazard in one work setting may conceivably represent an ideal worker/job fit for another occupation, time, or place of employment.

Thus, the conclusion of most research in this field is that one must look at the entire worker/occupation relationship rather than just at the worker him or herself. The "conventional wisdom" is that people who have wrong attitudes about safety are more likely to be injured. But one study of 493 farmers showed no difference in safety attitudes between farmers who had been injured and those who had not.[36]

Although most of the studies on the injury associations with life stresses such as pending divorce or money worries have not been carried out in the work setting, there is reasonable evidence that a relationship exists. It has been hypothesized that persons with severe off-the-job stresses may become so inward-directed during large portions of the day that they are less attentive to potential injury risks and thus avoid them less well during the period of the psychological crisis.

One stress that has been largely ignored in the literature is the effect of increased production expectations, especially for persons who are being paid on a piece-work basis. If top management states that it is placing great emphasis on safety but accompanies this with excessively demanding production schedules (especially where production is linked to personal income), the net result is that employees get a clear message that safety, after all, is of only secondary importance.[37,38] Under that stress, workers may knowingly take chances in order to put food on the table.

Environmental Factors in the Pre-Injury, Injury, and Post-Injury Phases

Several environmental issues have already been identified that determine frequency of work injury. One is management attitude and support for safety programs. Another is extent of supervision. Both appear to be involved in the fact that injury rates in small and very large places of employment are less than for middle-size plants. It is hypothesized that smaller businesses are more likely to have closer supervision, while larger ones are more likely to have formal safety programs.

The nature of the task—whether mobile and constantly changing or stable and repetitive—has also been noted as a factor, as well as the amount of clutter within the environment. Studies of ability to function in excessive heat and cold indicate that, especially if the individual is not acclimatized (and people vary in their ability to accomplish that process), there may be reduced capability to function effectively.[18] I have not seen any epidemiologic data, however, on injury rates in such uncomfortable climates.

Types of problems vary from industry to industry and sometimes between nations. However, several other generic types of environmental contribution can also be identified. As noted by Baker et al. and others, for example, about 40 percent of work-related fatalities in the United States involve motor vehicles. Earlier chapters delineate equipment and environmental factors commonly associated with those injuries. Gordon et al.,[13] however, also clearly indicate that vehicular injury may comprise little or none of the work injury in some other parts of the world. In those parts of the world, but in the developed nations as well, exposure to uncontrolled natural environment accounts for many injuries: contact with wild or domestic animals, falling objects, body strains, and falls involving uneven or slippery surfaces, and drowning.

Within the controlled environment, several major categories of environmental contribution deserve comment. One of these involves musculoskeletal pain from lifting, pulling, or pushing objects. It is usual in industry to assume that employees so injured have previous back problems that predispose them to injury or that they are not lifting in the manner that has been advised. Jones argues, however, that at least one of the prescribed methods for lifting actually can cause back injury,[39] while Freymoyer et al. have shown that constant exposure to vibration—a concomitant of many jobs—is closely associated with back pain.[21]

Lifting ability is a function not only of the lifter but of shape of object lifted.[40] Boxes with handles are far easier to lift than those without handles or than mailbags, and as size of mailbag increases so does the maximum acceptable weight. Back injury from uneven and slippery surfaces in the controlled environment is also an issue because employees may be forced to lift with their feet and bodies placed in awkward positions. A study of 163 small workplaces in Finland found poor lifting conditions in 29 percent of all lifting work.[41]

Much of the history of occupational safety in the United States and several other nations has been a story of identifying and protecting workers from equipment that has exposed cutting or tearing edges, pinch points, or similar hazards. This is a problem in both preindustrial and industrial societies. Gordon and associates[13] report, for example, that many of the injuries in rural Punjabi villages came from the chopping of feed for animals.

Gadalla notes a distinct increase in work-related injuries as farms become more and more mechanized.[42] However, there is a similar correlation with larger size of farm and other factors, and it is not clear which of the associations are causal and which not. Certainly, the hazards are well known of equipment such as the power takeoff, the corn picker, and similar mechanical devices that pull people in and literally tear them up.[43,44] Often this occurs, not during the work process per se but when the equipment becomes jammed and someone attempts to clear it. Booth observes that guarding and other devices to prevent injury often are designed to protect the operator but that others (setters, foremen, cleaners, apprentices, and passers-by) have to fend for themselves.[45]

A NIOSH study of 125 fatalities involving fixed machinery revealed that 31 resulted from activation of a stopped machine by an operator who was unaware that someone else was near, or in some cases actually inside, the machine.[46] Twenty-three were to workers who tried to clear a mixer or similar machinery without bothering to shut it off, while 21 were from equipment failure, and 41 from error in operating procedure. A survey of 163 small places of employment in Finland revealed that 20 percent of equipment had major defects and did not meet technical safety guides.[47]

McFarland's studies in the 1940s and 1950s documented that many injury events that apparently occur because workers misread dials or made errors of omission or comission were in fact attributable to equipment design that did not take human anatomy and physiology into account.[48] Thus, a dial may be misread because the letters or numbers are too small, the face of the dial is cluttered with excessive information, one dial moves in a clockwise direction while another does the opposite, or two dials (or knobs or other controls) that can be easily confused are placed very close together.

As an example of anatomical misfit, he and his colleagues found in a study of causal factors in truck crashes that in several truck models only 5 percent of drivers could reach and operate the handbrake comfortably. In others, clearance between the brake pedal and steering wheel was adequate for only 60 percent of drivers. In one model, the tallest 15 percent of the drivers were unable to raise the foot to the brake pedal when the shift lever was in either of the two left positions.

Locations of controls or switches frequently made operation difficult, and they emphasized the need for good dynamic, as well as static, data on human dimensions and biomechanics, including how persons are seated at the job, how far they can reach, and what forces they can apply. They emphasize the need for mockups of equipment to reveal design errors not apparent at the blueprint stage.

Over three decades later, design remains an issue in the occupational setting. Meagher observes, for example, that serious crash injuries still occur because workers unintentionally activate open-sided foot pedals that meet ANSI (American National Standards Institute) standards.[49] He attributes the reason that such a flagrant oversight in design could get into the standard to the fact that not one person trained in human factors engineering could be found among 324 members of 12 ANSI standards committees.

Worker/equipment misfit is also increasingly an issue because, in the United States at least, more women are joining the work force. Basic tools, machines, and safety equipment for many jobs have been designed only with the large-size male in mind, and this has been attributed as an important reason why female workers have more hand and wrist injuries than males.[50]

The problem is amply documented by Brooks, who found that small hand tools were too large and required too much grip force for most women employed as telephone installers, construction crew, and linesmen.[51] Larger hand tools, such as hoists and cable cutters, were extremely difficult to handle and demanded excesses of muscular activity to actuate. Leg-mounted climbing irons for pole climbing were developed for men in 1901 and were difficult for women to use because of the anatomical differences in male and female pelvic and muscle structures.

Under certain circumstances women took longer to drive trucks to their destination. The reason was that these trucks had long-travel stick shifts and heavy clutches, which were hard for women to operate. Therefore, the women chose travel routes with fewer hills or stop lights. They further found that the men then employed in outside-plant craft jobs were one standard deviation above average U.S. male civilian population, suggesting that any smaller-statured males in the work force (such as Spanish-speaking Americans) would also have difficulty in using both large and small hand tools.

The last generic environmental problem in the initiation of injury events is factors contributing to work-related falls. In one study, 20 percent of all injuries in the hotel industry involved falls on the same level, and 15 percent falls to a different level.[52] Contributory factors are not identified in a third of these, but environmental hazards (for example, slippery surface) are the single most common factors noted (23 percent).

Ladders and scaffolding are used in a wide range of industries. In another study of 116 fatalities with ladders, the types of industries in which they occurred were found to be quite diverse, but sixty-two were in construction and twenty-nine manufacturing.[53] Multiple factors contributed to over half the events. Only seven were from poor equipment. More common as primary factors were selection of the wrong type or design of ladder for the job at hand (sixteen cases), or setup of the ladder for a task to be carried out on it in such a way that it was unstable (twenty-six cases). Often in such cases, however, the worker may have limited options because the working surface may be such that it is extremely difficult to achieve stability. Another forty-nine involve incidental use of the ladder to get from one work location to another, with eighteen cases unclassified or unknown.

Obviously, characteristics of the environment may also contribute to the severity of injury during the energy transfer and post-injury phases. Where chemicals are released, severity depends on their inherent toxicity or explosive capability and on the extent to which the space is enclosed and has manually or automatically initiated ventilation. Presence and type of protective clothing must also be considered (such as masks, protective lenses, steel-tipped shoes, gloves and other clothing that can resist electricity, fire, or chemicals). Severity and survival may also depend on whether an affected worker is alone or near other workers and whether the place of work is near to definitive medical services or—as with forestry, some mineral extraction, farming, and some construction—located at a considerable distance from such care.

Countermeasures

All potential countermeasures against occupational injury require some form of commitment and action by management, which, as we have already shown, is one of the key factors in determining the success of occupational safety programs. Across the years, however, and no matter what the nation, employers not only have given extremely low priority to safety efforts but in some cases have actively fought against them.

Such commitment, therefore, has often been obtained through legislation compelling industry compliance, and it has often been at least moderately successful, especially in industries and situations where few safety efforts have yet been undertaken. Thus, for example, laws in the middle and late 1800s in both the British Isles and the United States that required guarding of exposed hazards on machinery, back-up exits in mines, and, more recently, compensation by the employer to injured workers are credited with bringing about substantial increases in levels of safety-related activity within industry. And these activities are generally credited with reducing the injury experiences within those occupations.[54] Ellis presents data, however, that casts at least some doubt on the role of workers' compensation as a motivating factor in the decrease in occupational injury.[55]

Union activity has also been identified as a force promoting not only better wages for workers but a safer work environment as well. While this perception may be true for specific times and specific places, data suggest that in general the trade-union movement has not been a very potent force in this regard.[56,57]

The most recent major safety legislation in the United States has been the Occupational Safety and Health Act of 1970 and its administrative child (OSHA), which has resulted in the issuance of multiple safety regulations primarily applicable to larger places of employment and the potential for unannounced inspection and the issuance of fines or other sanctions. The safety effects of this program, unfortunately, appear to be minimal.[58] Greenberg notes that the standards established are inflexible and often deal with issues that, while generally applicable, are irrelevant to potential causes of injury in specific places of employment.[59]

Concha argues that even where industry attempts to develop safety programs, the personnel available for carrying out these efforts usually are untrained or poorly trained and conversant only with outmoded health and safety concepts.[60] Among seventy-four companies with 100 to 1,500 employees, nineteen had only informal safety programs, and only 28 percent of either the formal or informal programs utilized personnel trained in safety to either the associate's or bachelor's degree level.[61] Fifty-nine percent had personnel with no safety training, and 12 percent of the companies that reported safety programs had no safety personnel!

Gleason and Barnum conclude that given OSHA's current record of frequency of inspections and the size of resultant fines, the economically astute employer should not attempt to comply with OSHA standards unless and until inspected and forced to correct safety deficits.[62] While these statements about safety legislation, its effects, and problems describe the situation in the United States, I believe they have wider generalizability to legislation in other nations as well.

Despite these negative comments about the apparent *current* effectiveness of compulsory occupational safety efforts, many of the past legislative and administrative requirements have been quite successful in reducing injury by removing many of the most blatant hazards, some of which still exist to a substantial degree in developing nations. Even now, easing of mine safety regulations in the United States under the Reagan administration appears to be associated with increases in injury and fatality patterns that had been brought under control with new regulations in 1966.[63] A major benefit of that 1966 legislation was the inclusion for the first time of standards for mines with fewer than fifteen employees.

Furthermore, beginning around 1910 a major voluntary occupational safety movement began in the United States, in large part associated with National Safety Council and to a substantial degree involving larger industries. These programs have often had outstanding successes resulting from integration of safety into the entire employment, manufacturing, and distribution process. Commonly, the factors that favor a high level of employee productivity are the same ones that promote a low injury experience.

What are those factors? They are presented in somewhat chronological order beginning with initiation of employment, rather than in order of importance, since all contribute importantly to safety. First, is care in the selection of new employees and in fitting them to the jobs most suited to their backgrounds, skills, and interests. This means, of course, that an employer has to start with a good knowledge of what the individual job requirements actually are. Many employers, unfortunately, lack this knowledge.

In larger industries that are able to afford medical departments, this selection and placement process includes a preplacement medical examination to obtain baseline employee health data as the beginning of a permanent medical record. In some communities, smaller employers as well are able to take advantage of these services by utilizing independent occupational health and safety facilities that offer medical, nursing, safety engineering, and industrial hygiene packages tailored in amount and type to the size and needs of the particular work place.

Adequacy of initial training and ongoing supervision of personnel are the next factors to be considered. As we have already noted, a majority of employers that have occupational safety programs are hampered in this particular area by having safety personnel who are totally lacking in safety training. Two other aspects are the training of supervisors themselves in the best motivational techniques to promote safety and the use of exercise classes for the purpose of strengthening key muscle groups among employees in occupations that require lifting or other forms of muscle strain.

An important part of adequate supervision is the development of a suitable feedback system that can record and identify the frequency and complete costs of all work injuries and permit analysis of causal factors. This requires establishment of formal record keeping and analysis systems for injury events and other mishaps and a formal review and decision mechanism to identify and deal with correctable problems.

Traditionally, much attention has been given to educating and motivating employees to act safely. In contrast to many of the unsuccessful educational and motivational programs described throughout this book, occupational efforts have greater likelihood of success. The population is truly captive, having been preselected. Of equal importance, employer satisfaction, raises, promotions, or even jobs are at risk if performance is not appropriate. Furthermore, in the work environment behavior can often be easily monitored. Several nations have specific legislation requiring training of all new employees in safety processes and methods relevant to their jobs.[64,65] The training materials and methods are often developed with a large degree of input by the workers themselves, thus helping to ensure teaching that is perceived by the workers as meeting their needs.

We have already noted that ambivalent messages, in which workers are told to pay attention to safety but simultaneously are forced to respond to pressures of piece-work payment schemes or similar production schedules, are likely to undermine safety efforts. Cunitz points out that "warning" signs and messages must not only be available when and where needed but must also be capable of attracting attention, motivating behavioral change, telling very specifically how to avoid harm, and, where necessary, how to provide specific first aid.[66] Furthermore, such warnings should be legible over the lifetime of the sign, be visible in difficult lighting conditions, be easy to understand, and not provide sensory overload. He further urges that signs be specifically tested before widespread use to ensure that they in fact are capable of doing what they allege to do.

A more basic approach is offered by Cohen, Smith, and Anger in an excellent review of both directive and nondirective methods to promote self-protective measures against work-place hazards.[67] They urge that workers do better when told how to promote safety and health rather than how to avoid unsafe or unhealthful situations through intensive fear techniques. Workers also need to be directly involved in safety efforts through techniques such as role playing rather than being "talked at."[68] Such education should be by immediate supervisors, who usually have good job-related credibility, as well as a high degree of personal control.

Feedback of behavioral change is absolutely essential.[67,69] In one study, for example, a worker group was found to have a 70 percent prevalence of safe job behavior. A 90 percent target was agreed upon by management and workers, and unannounced daily visits three or four times a week revealed that safe behavior increased to 98 percent of the time, a fact that was fed back to workers immediately and at regular intervals. After the level was maintained for twenty-five weeks, the posting of feedback data was stopped, at which point a drop in safety level began to occur. In response, management immediately began posting results again, and the safe behavior again rose to previous high levels.

Concurrent with this long-term increase in observed safe behavior was a drop from thirty-five to ten disabling injuries per million person-hours worked. Similar efforts involving feedback on wearing protective lenses and ear protection were also associated with marked and sustained increases in safety behavior and decreases in injuries.[67] Incentive programs of a more specific nature (money, merchandise, parking places, and so forth) have also proven successful, as have management efforts to include employees in decision-making processes involving safety programs.[67]

The approach to alcoholism in the working population that has been embraced by a few employers is another example of the advantages of an environment where strong social and economic sanctions can be applied and where behavior can be carefully observed. Thus, employer-sponsored alcoholism treatment programs are reported to have success rates as high as 90 percent.

These employee-assistance programs often are built around the concept of the "troubled employee": that is, the employee who, for whatever reason, is not functioning effectively. The demand to the employee, therefore, is to improve job performance rather than to treat the alcoholism per se. Since the abuse pattern is usually central to the work and other problems, however, the employee has little option but to seek and continue treatment if he wishes to keep his job. In a provocative paper, Walker and Shain seriously question whether improvements that occur in such employees result from the therapy they may enter into or from the confrontation process per se.[70] They further urge that such confrontation and advice be utilized for persons who are far earlier in their heavy drinking patterns than is usually the case.

Often forgotten is a consideration of worker placement and training in the area of rehabilitation. If an employer wishes to have a work force that has the advantages of long service and familiarity with the job, consideration must be given to the need to reassess and possibly retrain or carry out job modification for employees who seek to return after heart attacks or development of other health problems. The same principles apply here of task analysis and worker/task matching that were noted earlier for new employees.

Clearly, changes in the work-place tools and environment play a part in worker safety that is fully as important as worker selection, training, and motivation. A drop in musculoskeletal injuries among ambulance personnel, for example, was probably a result not only of selection of younger, stronger attendants and better training for them in lifting techniques but also of equipment's being changed from stretchers that had to be carried to gurneys that could be rolled when flat surfaces are available.[71]

Several types of environmental options are available for both the pre-injury and injury phases. Starting with the most general aspects, adequacy of lighting, temperature, humidity, and noise levels need to be examined and improved in those indoor environments where such changes are possible. Stabilizing of shift schedules where employees are on rotating shifts may also yield benefits measurable in both reduced injury and increased productivity.

Human factors engineering to ensure that equipment design and construction meets anatomical, physiological, educational, and behavioral attributes of the range of employees available is one of the most commonly overlooked options that is available and that, again, can bring improvements in both safety and productivity. Attention must be paid to tools and equipment designed to the needs of women and other employees who may be shorter and have different anatomical and musculature patterns than does the average male. In developing nations, illiteracy may be an important issue to be dealt with. Swain emphasizes the importance of actively involving workers themselves in the worker/task design process.[72]

Guarding and similar passive systems to prevent employees of all sorts as well as passersby from reaching actively moving machine parts or from inadvertently releasing or igniting hazardous chemicals or other materials are the next area for consideration. In some cases, automatic sensing and shutoff devices may be warranted to limit energy releases and thus reduce severity during the injury phase.

Personal protective equipment—restraining devices, helmets, protective shields and lenses, gloves, steel-tipped shoes, and so forth—is mentioned here rather than earlier because it is a less reliable method than are the more passive environmental measures already noted. Such equipment, by its very nature, often is cumbersome and uncomfortable, and it is often difficult to get employees to use it consistently. Therefore, such equipment should be perceived as a backup to other measures rather than as a primary method for injury reduction.

Finally, attention needs to be given to the use of early-warning devices in some occupational settings and to the availability of emergency medical services in the form of both appropriate equipment, trained personnel, and adequate plans of action to deal with the injured quickly and effectively. Some data suggest that first aid training programs for employees not only can prepare them for responding to injuries but can also provide motivation and education for prevention.[73]

27
Community Disasters

It is not my intention to cover exhaustively the field of disaster avoidance, preparedness, and response, which is now sufficiently large to have its own journal (*Disasters,* Pergamon Press) and which is extensively considered by those who deal with planning for emergency medical services. Some of the preventive or other aspects are discussed elsewhere in this book in chapters about rail, air and water transportation, fire, and hospitals. In this chapter I will review disasters involving "natural" events (earthquakes, volcanoes and avalanches, and flooding, tornadoes, and related weather phenomena) and disasters involving the built or designed environment, or so-called man-made disasters (collapse of dams and other structures, and the transport, storage and use of hazardous materials).

Each year about 250,000 people are killed in natural disasters that cost an estimated $25 billion in property damage.[1] Ninety-five percent of these deaths occur in developing nations, while most of the property damage is in developed countries. In the United States, for example, there have been 45,000 deaths in catastrophic events—that is, events in which five or more people died—over a thirty-five-year period from 1941 to 1975.[2] Only 8,300 (18 percent) of these, however, were from "natural" disasters (table 27–1).

The poorest nations are also likely to have vastly overcrowded and underprotected trucks, buses, trains, and water vessels used for public transportation, often converting simple mishaps into a substantial toll of life. For similar reasons of crowding and poor construction, fires and collapse of buildings in such nations may be especially costly in terms of lives lost.

Even if only natural disasters are considered, however, such events cost developing nations from 1 to 2 percent of their gross national product, while in developed countries the cost is generally less than 0.25 percent, or one-tenth as much.[1]

Closer examination of table 27–1 shows some interesting time trends that appear to be related to technological development. From 1941 to 1965, for example, catastrophic motor vehicle deaths increased as the number of cars on the roads grew but then declined as improved

Table 27–1
Deaths in Catastrophic Events by Type of Event, United States, 1941–75

								Total	
	1941–45	*1946–50*	*1951–55*	*1956–60*	*1961–65*	*1966–70*	*1971–75*	*Number*	*Percentage*
Motor vehicle[a]	916	1,069	1,732	2,305	2,045	1,508	941	10,516	23.3
Air transport	380	991	1,043	1,090	1,327	1,541	1,384	7,756	17.2
Water transport	594	380	421	298	212	204	117	2,226	4.9
Railroad	548	313	193	176	30	22	60	1,342	3.0
Fire and explosion	2,391	2,138	1,354	1,745	1,630	1,460	1,410	12,128	26.9
Weather	1,163	1,129	1,649	1,033	1,062	948	1,295	8,279	18.3
Mines and quarries	607	263	207	132	140	158	111	1,618	3.6
Other	202	129	170	242	156	70	283	1,252	2.8
Total	6,801	6,412	6,769	7,021	6,602	5,911	5,601	45,117	100.0

Source: Adapted from "Catastrophic Accidents: 35-Year Review," *Statistical Bulletin* 58 (March 1977):2–4 (New York: Metropolitan Life Insurance Co.).

[a]Includes motor vehicle versus train.

packaging and crash amelioration concepts were applied beginning about 1967. (An alternative, rather implausible, hypothesis is that the number of vehicle occupants increased between 1941 and 1965 and then decreased subsequently, thereby resulting in fewer crashes at risk for five or more deaths.) The progressive increase over time in air transport disasters probably reflects both greater numbers of flights and more passengers per flight, counterbalancing some improvements in packaging, while reductions in water and rail transport deaths are associated with reductions in passengers coupled with better safety programs.

Substantial changes in life safety codes, especially for public buildings, have occurred since 1941, which may explain the reduction in catastrophic deaths from fire and explosion. More stringent mine safety and occupational regulations, and some reductions in coal mining, account for the downward shift in deaths from disasters in mines and quarries. Catastrophies involving weather and "other" events show no change over time.

Natural Disasters

Quoting Burton et al., whose work is essential reading for anyone concerned with natural disasters, floods account for 40 percent of such events, tropical cyclones 20 percent, earthquakes 15 percent, and drought 15 percent. Earthquakes may be overestimated, whereas drought is underestimated because it is hard to define. Floods are the most frequent and do the most damage, while tropical cyclones cause most fatalities.[1]

One study of a tornado in Kansas reported that persons over age 60 were injured seven times more often than those under age 20. Above age 40, women had a greater risk of injury than men, and for persons over age 60 the risk for women was almost twice as great.[3] The deaths (and perhaps also the case fatality ratio) as well appeared to be higher for persons age 60 or older.

Another study, analyzing death rates in the 1976 Guatemalan earthquake that killed about 23,000, noted that risk of serious and fatal injury was greatest for the young and the elderly.[4] The youngest child usually slept with its mother and consequently had a low mortality rate. But the next to youngest had the highest rate, and the risk then decreased progressively, with the oldest (first born) having the lowest risk of death among the children. Also, the risk of injury was consistently greater for women than for men in almost all age groups.

The number of natural disasters has been about thirty per year for some time. Burton and his associates note that natural disasters have six features in common:

1. People do not choose vulnerability to hazard in ignorance but rather make a tradeoff between economic gain from land resources and social risk.
2. Increased hazard from extreme events results from interaction of natural systems and human-use systems, especially reliance upon single technologies, such as engineering works, to cope with extreme events. Such reliance leads to increased productivity but also to unprecedented disaster.
3. Courses of action chosen reflect a combination of community and individual decisions within a social structure that neither controls completely. For example, in describing two disastrous floods in Bangladesh and the United States, they note that by living where they did in high-risk locations, poor peasants and retired miners made personal decisions but did so within the limited options available to them because of public policy.
4. It is not by chance that the burden of disasters falls heavily on the poor.
5. Relatively inexpensive and reasonable preventive measures involving warning systems, building design, and land-use planning could markedly reduce property damage, deaths, and social disruption that far exceed the cost of such measures.
6. Each disaster generates measures to prevent its repetition.

Despite such measures, the outlook for avoiding major losses appears to be getting worse rather than better. Shifts of rural populations to cities, and especially cities on flood plains or in seismically active areas, result in increases in the number of people at risk, particularly if these people are in proximity to industrial hazards that may be released. In poor nations improved warning systems about weather are of little use because rapid evacuation becomes impossible. As population density increases in high hazard areas, some flood protection works actually increase river levels. Furthermore, as city residents move out into more rural areas, they may move to hazards (such as avalanches or flood plains) that their country neighbors know enough to avoid.[1]

In contrast to other chapters, this one will start with a discussion of environmental rather than human characteristics associated with natural disasters because to a large extent the events themselves cannot be prevented. By knowing, first, important characteristics of the events we are in a better position to understand how and why people respond as they do.

Seven components determine characteristics of potential disasters.[1] The first of these is the magnitude of the natural event. A flood may be measured by the number of feet or meters above the banks of a stream or river that the water rises and by the area covered or by the number of cubic feet or cubic meters per second of flow. Cyclones, tornadoes, and other storms are commonly measured by wind speed, which is equivalent to kinetic energy.

Earthquakes have at least eight currently popular scales of intensity. Two are the Richter and Modified Richter scales, which are based on energy released, and the Modified Mercalli scale, which is a measure of expected effects of damage to structures. These two scales are compared in table 27–2.

Other components of disaster are:

1. Frequency: varying in a particular location from several times a year for hurricanes and tornadoes to once every several centuries for large-intensity earthquakes and volcanic activity.
2. Duration: long in the case of droughts, intermediate with floods, and extremely brief with earthquakes.
3. Areal extent: widespread with droughts, floods, fog, and air pollution to very limited with some earthquakes and tornadoes.
4. Speed of onset: ranging from slow with droughts, cyclones, and

Table 27–2
Comparison of Richter and Modified Mercalli Scales for Measuring Earthquake Intensity

Mercalli Scale		*Richter Scale*	
Effect	*Modified Mercalli Number*	*Richter Number*	*Energy Release*
None	I	1–2	4.47×10^{12}
Felt by few people	II		
Felt by some people	III	3	7.94×10^{14}
Felt by many people	IV		
Felt by most people; damage to glass and plaster	V	4	2.51×10^{16}
Everyone feels; furniture and chimneys damaged	VI	5	7.94×10^{17}
Some poor structures damaged	VII		
Some ordinary structures damaged	VIII	6	2.51×10^{19}
Some resistant structures damaged	IX	7	7.94×10^{20}
Many structures damaged; some destroyed	X		
Most structures damaged; many destroyed	XI	8	2.51×10^{22}
All structures damaged; most destroyed	XII		

Source: Adapted from I. Burton, R.W. Kates, and G.F. White, *The Environment as Hazard* (New York: Oxford University Press, 1978).

flooding resulting from long, heavy rains and some volcanoes, to almost instantaneous with earthquakes.

5. Spatial dispersion: may be so diffuse as to be worldwide with the dust clouds resulting from volcanoes or quite concentrated with tornadoes and earthquakes.
6. Temporal spacing: maybe quite regular in their seasonal recurrence, as with cyclones and snowstorms, or may appear to be random, as with earthquakes and volcanoes.

Next, let us discuss human factors associated with avoidance of and response to natural disasters, emphasizing what controls actions by individuals. In order for actions to occur, there must be awareness that a given environmental situation represents a potential or actual disaster situation. The level of awareness varies from individual to individual and from culture to culture. Slovic et al. suggest that individuals go through four steps.[5] They (1) appraise the probability and magnitude of extreme events, (2) consider the range of possible alternative actions, (3) evaluate the costs and consequences of selected actions and finally, (4) choose one or a combination of actions. This process, however, appears to be one of "bounded rationality" or "satisficing," as discussed chapter 5 rather than being a truly rational process with examination of all risks and countermeasure possibilities.

It would appear that most people—including the experts—have difficulty in appraising the magnitude and frequency of extreme events and in evaluating more than a very small number of countermeasure options at any one time. They appear to deal with options in ordered sequence rather than simultaneously. Also, in general, individuals and groups respond more consistently and effectively to pervasive and repetitive phenomena that develop slowly enough to permit warning (such as storms, floods, and droughts) than they do to relatively uncommon and apparently random intensive events, such as earthquakes and volcanoes.[1]

What determines how a given individual is likely to act? No ready answer is available, but research offers some suggestions. Overall religious or other cultural attitudes regarding locus of control and expected response to "God's will" may play a roll. Tornadoes in southern United States take far more lives than do such storms in the northern tier of states despite no difference in frequency or in severity as measured by potential population at risk or property damage.[6] One explanation is that southerners exhibit more fatalism and lack of trust in organized systems of warning.

Some societies have supernatural explanations for hazardous natural events, and people simply accept their losses or try to get help from family, friends, and neighbors in recouping losses. Assuming that people are not relying on such explanations, however, substantial problems still remain.

Burton et al. note that people have trouble drawing valid conclusions from small samples and thus lean heavily on intuition. A person who has seen only one severe hurricane in twenty years, for example, is likely to have difficulty in estimating the future chances for damaging winds, especially if such events are ones that occur "once in a lifetime" or even less often.

In trying to understand past events, they are likely to use concrete pieces of information, such as from a neighbor, rather than more abstract or impersonal information sources. By trying to adjust to new information that they may be receiving from several sources, they believe they have a much better picture of the truth than they really do, and this commonly leads to underestimation of the hazard.

City dwellers or new arrivals to a rural area may be less accurate in their judgment of natural phenomena because they have received less information by personal experience or from others.[1] They lose this disadvantage, however, within relatively few years after moving to the new area. Tenants are less aware than are property owners.[1] In short, areas of high population mobility are likely to be areas where people have little experience on which to base their assessments. In fact, in such places people may be totally unaware of *any* risk of rare, extremely high-energy events. Urban residents, such as those in Tokyo or San Francisco, may be less concerned about events such as earthquakes because they view these natural events as only one of a set of hazards (such as traffic and crime) that threaten them.

Even if they have sufficient experience, people may misunderstand risk concepts. The sophisticated or probabilistic view of risk—which is more common in high-income areas—is that a catastrophic event with given probability has equal chance of occurring in any year, even if it has just occurred in the past year. But many people follow the deterministic view, or gambler's fallacy, that disasters come in runs or groups, to be followed by free intervals. This approach is more common in preindustrial societies.

Individuals also may be influenced—to their personal detriment—by governmental or other societal actions. The building of levees or similar earthworks to reduce high-frequency low-level flooding of flood plains in crowded nations such as Bangladesh may open up fertile land to peasants. While people are then protected from the more frequent events, they often do not realize that they are far more vulnerable to the less common high-intensity natural phenomena.[1] This problem of misplaced faith by individuals in single-technology solutions undertaken by government in flood plains is not limited to the developing nations. In the United States as well, the rare high-energy events may become truly catastrophic, in part because the very same retaining walls that keep out minor flooding serve to prevent serious floods from receding for days, weeks, or even months.

Finally, regarding individual actions, Burton et al. note that because people commonly have only limited perceptions of hazard and tend to maintain a short-term perspective, the chances are not very good that they will undertake appropriate preventive actions in the absence of strenuous effort by public agencies. To the extent that group or governmental influences are absent or are poorly designed, therefore, the outlook is good that there will be increasing suffering from rare events. But they observe that the record also suggests that as the risk of serious loss mounts, people do begin to take a variety of countermeasures that may retard or reverse destruction and enhance productivity. Despite general indifference to preventive action, evidence does exist that critical points may be reached beyond which the trend may be reversed.

What are the chances for convincing governmental units—whether local, national, or international—to take appropriate measures to prevent disasters or limit their effects? As the above comment suggests, at least some of the experts are hopeful. Somewhat less cheerful are conclusions of a series of studies edited, and in some cases undertaken, by Wright and Rossi.[7] Within the limits of location and study methods available to them, one of their reports found that except for statistically rare events there are no discernible long-term population and housing impacts on communities struck by natural disasters.

That's the good news. The bad news is that preventive legislation tends to be based on statistically rare, unusual events rather than on the average disaster. Furthermore, most communities give natural disasters extremely low priority among the many problems that require action. Even at state level, attention is not much greater because the other problems faced by communities are simply more urgent and more predictable than the *possible* consequences of low-probability events.

Wright and Rossi's surveys do suggest, however, that local officials and planners are not likely to look very sympathetically at suggestions that disaster effects be limited through land-use planning. Such planning to keep high-hazard industries and large populations away from flood plains, earthquake faults, or other high-risk locations cannot often stand up to the more immediate economic press for available land that faces most communities.

The major factor that influences severity of injury during the energy-transfer phase is the ability of structures surrounding the individual to resist collapse, the equivalent of packaging of occupants of motor vehicles and aircraft. Blass et al. showed that 60 percent of the deaths, and 51 percent of the serious injuries, in a tornado involved those few individuals who, contrary to instructions, attempted to flee the storm in their cars, which were badly buffeted by the winds.[3] Residents of apartment houses had a serious injury and death rate of 1.3 per 1,000 occupants. Persons hiding in single-family homes had a rate of 3.2, those in automobiles 23.2, while residents of mobile homes had 85.1 per 1,000 occupants, probably because small mobile homes are not designed for high impacts, as cars now are. In addition, the average home has furniture and other objects that can fly around.

In one village during the 1976 Guatemala quake, *all* of the deaths and serious injuries occurred in adobe houses, despite the fact that 15 percent of the homes were of other construction.[4] Virtually all buildings collapsed to some extent, but the heavy adobe ones did so completely, while in houses made with lightweight cornstalk walls supported on a wooden frame, the frame and the roof either remained intact or only partially collapsed.

Adobe homes more than seven years old have a 1.6 times greater risk of major injury compared to newer adobe homes. Adobe becomes brittle with age unless oil is added, which wasn't done in this area. Too much sand would also make the adobe more brittle with age.

The authors further note that adobe construction is relatively new to the Indian village they studied. In 1924, when another serious earthquake leveled all the houses, there were no deaths and few injuries. The next year, the first adobe home was built, representing the prestige associated with the Spanish culture of Guatemala City, and by 1971 the proportion of such structures had increased to 85 percent, shifting the risk of earthquake-related trauma from minimal to maximum in just forty years.

Prevention of natural events by eliminating or reducing energy buildup has not usually been a useful countermeasure option in the past. It may have some limited potential for the future, especially in the many areas of the world where flooding is becoming increasingly common and severe.

Population press has resulted in serious deforestation and water run off, leading to flooding or hillside avalanches that may bury entire villages.[8,9] Such disasters can be largely, if not totally, prevented by proper planting techniques with rapid growing vegetation that establishes deep roots. Seeding of tropical storms has been attempted to divert them or to reduce their intensity near large populations.[10] The results, however, do not appear to be outstandingly successful.

Much is being learned about the movement of the earth's tectonic plates, sections of the earth's crust whose constant motion against each other results in buildup of stress at the interfaces or "faults." At some point, the compacted plates release or "slip" to cause catastrophic earthquakes. Some fault areas have "gaps" that have not had large quakes for a number of years.

These silent areas, usually located between more active sections of fault, are now hypothesized to be the high-risk locations for high-energy quakes in the immediate future.[11,12,13] Such information may be useful for prediction and for timely warning to populations at risk. But it may also be possible to drill into these areas before they build up too much stress and to inject fluids that will defuse the hazard by causing numerous minor quakes.

This scheme is based on some interesting experience. As larger dams and their reservoirs have been built, as mines have been dug, and as subterranean atomic blasts have been carried out or atomic wastes have been buried in deep drill holes, nonrandom clusters of quakes have occurred surrounding these areas of human activity.[14] If it is thus possible to cause earthquakes, then well-placed efforts of this type may possibly be used to cause small, harmless tremors in order to defuse and avoid large, harmful ones.[14,15]

In similar fashion, strains in potential avalanche areas are now being monitored,[16–19]and in some cases small avalanches are intentionally triggered to prevent buildup of larger ones.[16,17] Factors that favor occurrence of avalanche are a slope of 30 to 40°, with ten to fifteen inches of snowfall in less than twenty-four hours, especially on a leeward slope.[18] Another report suggests that shaded and sheltered areas tend to slip in December to February, and sunny, exposed areas in March through May.[19] Slippage occurs because of weakening of the basal layer of snow.

A second approach, if the energy load cannot be reduced, is to try to prevent release of energy. Avalanches are avoided by installing deep-set snow fencing on unstable slopes in order to provide sufficient basal layer strength to deal with snow loads.

A far more common countermeasure is to channel the phenomenon away from areas where it can cause damage; for example, by building earthworks for flood waters, by land-use planning that keeps population and hazardous industry away from flood plains, and by building houses on raised platforms. In Florida, special sandy expanses of beach have been successful in breaking up and weakening waves in hurricanes before they reach more valuable structures.[20]

Another countermeasure—not common enough—is the strengthening of structures that might be damaged by high-energy loadings. Aseismic design of buildings keeps all parts tied together so that they float together like a ship on a seismic wave rather than shaking apart individually, as with brick, adobe, and masonry.[4] Buildings should not have overhanging parapets that can fall off onto people in the street. In cities, flexible connections between buildings and public utilities, such as gas and electricity, may be less likely to break under stress.[14]

In general, aseismic designs function pretty much as planned, and for this reason communities with high earthquake risk, such as in California, may have fairly stringent building codes for new structures and in some cases may require strengthening of existing structures as well. Because of their costs, however, especially for retrofitting older structures that are often in less affluent neighborhoods, such designs are sometimes rigorously resisted by those who are at greatest risk of injury and death.[21] Even such simple efforts as putting up protective shutters in hurricane areas may be ignored by as much as 80 percent of the population at risk.[1]

If strengthening structures may not be enough, one must resort to methods of predicting the event, or warning people, and of providing methods for timely evacuation from the areas of highest risk. New techniques, such as Doppler radar, permit prediction of violent weather more accurately,[22] while radiomonitoring can warn of impending avalanches up to hours before the event.[16] Use of long period seismic waves shows promise for better estimation of risk of Tsunamis, or tidal waves resulting from underwater earthquakes.[23]

Prediction has become increasingly successful with volcanoes, although with the Mount St. Helens eruption many deaths occurred both because the predictions were not totally correct[24] and apparently because state officials deviated somewhat from declaring an optimal "off limits" zone in order to avoid economic losses to logging companies.[25]

Every evacuation is costly in both time and money. If there are too many false alarms, people tend not to pay attention to the real events.[23] Both individuals and government, therefore, try to find a balance between being completely safe by taking action that only in retrospect may be found to be unnecessary or, on the other hand, ignoring warnings that in retrospect should have been heeded. There is no easy solution to this judgmental dilemma.

Attempts have been made to predict earthquakes to within as little as a few days' period. With at least two major Chinese quakes in 1975 and 1976, evacuating people to areas away from damagable structures is credited with saving many lives.[26] Some of the methods used to predict imminent quakes have been clustering of minor foreshocks, release of radioactive gases into deep wells, bulging of sections of land near or on an active fault, strange behavior of animals, and electrical discharges in the sky (or so-called earthquake lights).[26–30] These methods have failed at least as often as they have succeeded, however, perhaps because there may be more than one pattern of tectonic plate interaction.[31,32] Thus, methods successful for predicting a major tremor in one area may be irrelevant in other areas.[32]

Contrary to news media descriptions of evacuations allegedly involving mass hysteria and panic, people tend to remain almost too calm. Even when mass evacuations are carried out, the majority usually decide to stay behind.[10] Before doing anything, people tend to seek to validate warnings of impending disaster and requests for action. They are more likely to believe public messages only if they are repeated, are provided also by friends, neighbors, or others who they know, or are given personally by police officers and if people are asked to respond in ways that are mainly extensions of their normal, everyday behavior. Only rarely do people engage in unusual or unpredicatable behavior. If it is to succeed, therefore, warning advice must take into consideration normal human impulses and find ways to direct those impulses toward the desired action.[10]

Telling people not to use the telephone, for example, is futile. Instead, ways must be found to use such calls to advantage in order to improve dissemination of warning messages.[10] The design of messages to guide emergency response and evacuation is only now being recognized as a complex field that requires both extensive knowledge of human psychological responses *and* substantial pretesting of messages to be sure they will be understood.[33]

If damage does occur to people and property, its ultimate effects may still be limited to some extent through prompt and effective emergency and rehabilitative efforts. However, important aspects of response often are chaotic for far longer than has to be. Those people who themselves are in the disaster area tend to function in extremely calm, rational, and altruistic fashion during the immediate hours after the event. Panic is rare, as is looting in the various disasters that have been studied.[10] People first help family, then friends and neighbors, and then anyone else who needs help, doing "whatever needs to be done."[10,34] Contrary to common "wisdom," police, firefighters, and other officials do not abandon their tasks in order to find their families.[10]

While people bear up rather well under disasters, the organizations that respond often function poorly and, in extreme cases, may be more socially and psychologically disruptive than the actual physical disaster itself. Improved preparedness and response to disasters, it is concluded, will have to come through improvement in disaster organization,[10] especially if outside help is organized.

Usually there is not a great need for additional food and clothing, and supplies that arrive are often too much or materials are unneeded, inappropriate, and unusable. Attention must be diverted to dealing with these supplies, causing extra congestion at the disaster site.[10] Unless an entire area is totally destroyed, people in disaster zones in both developed and developing nations commonly depend far more on help from friends and neighbors—who willingly, and usually effectively, offer such help—than they do on organized help, such as from government, the Red Cross, or similar agencies.[10,34,35,36] Useful guidelines exist for planning and management of health services for both natural and man-made disasters.[37,38]

Man-Made Disasters

The factors in man-made disasters are similar to those associated with natural events, involving awareness and assessment of risk, decisions whether to take preventive action in advance, decisions regarding response if something begins to go wrong, and recovery once disaster strikes. We noted in an earlier chapter that in Cairo (and undoubtedly in other nations as well) people knowingly accept risks of living in houses that may collapse.[39] The uncomfortable choice is either to accept this risk or to live with no housing at all.

Philipson's article on hazardous material transportation references Chauncey Starr's work on public risk acceptance in relation to benefits.[40] He notes that risk acceptance increases in proportion to the cube root of the increase in benefits. People are willing to accept risks about three orders of magnitude greater if those risks are voluntary than if they are involuntary. These particular conclusions have since been disputed, however.

Philipson notes that three major philosophical problems exist with Starr's approach. First, for involuntary risks, the groups being asked or forced to accept the risks often differ from the groups receiving all or most of the benefits. Second, one must distinguish between low-probability/high-consequence risks and those with higher probability but lower consequence. The public and decision makers tend to be more concerned with the former. There is as yet no way to accurately measure the "disutility" of disasters, which appears to be nonlinear as disaster magnitude increases. Finally, the groups evaluating the risks of a hazardous activity often differ widely in their perceptions, both of benefits and of risk, and consequently of the acceptability of the activity.[40]

These issues are nowhere more apparent than in a discussion of the relative utility of dams, given the fact that they sometimes fail. Water impoundments are usually built for multiple purposes: to prevent downstream flooding and to provide water for irrigation, hydropower for electricity, and recreational facilities. Those who benefit usually are not the individuals whose lands and homes are appropriated for the project, and there usually are extensive arguments whether the total benefits to the larger public will exceed the costs of displacement and construction.

Between 1959 and 1965 the worldwide failure rate for dams was about 2×10^{-4} per dam-year, with most of the failures being major disasters.[41] In the United States between 1918 and 1958 the overall rate and major rates, respectively, were 5×10^{-4} and 0.8×10^{-4}. The median estimate is 1.5×10^{-4}, with the actual probability depending on many factors, such as project-specific engineering and construction, geologic setting, surface faulting and seismicity, type and age of dam, and flood frequency. The expected damage, should failure occur, depends on the property and population downstream.

Of particular importance is the occurrence of seismic activity *in response to* water impoundment, an occurrence we noted earlier. Moderate magnitude seismic activity occurred in less than 0.2 percent of reservoirs behind the world's approximately 11,000 large dams but in 10 percent of reservoirs over 90 meters deep and with water capacity of 10^3 cubic meters or more. The conclusion is that disasters involving dam failure, especially of larger dams, are probable enough so that the costs of these rare events must be included in all cost/benefit analyses. Were this done, far fewer dams would be built, even if the costs of lives were *not* included in the analysis.

With one exception—nuclear power—most people give little consideration to disasters in thinking about cost versus benefit in the built or designed environment. The fact that many current technologies (such as microcomputers) originally were developed for war has been largely forgotten by the public. Not so with nuclear power, whose first "practical" use at Hiroshima is indelibly imbedded in the minds of subsequent generations.[42] These fears certainly have not been put to rest with the disaster at Three Mile Island[43] or with newspaper reports such as "Atomic Plants had 2,835 Incidents in '78," which observed that a 1965 study linking leukemia to fallout from atomic bomb tests was withheld by anxious officials.[44]

It is not my intention here to discuss the pros and cons of nuclear power but rather to identify three factors shared between these facilities and other aspects of the built environment that contain risk of disaster. These factors are:

1. As a new technology is introduced the developers tend to play up its assets and to play down or ignore its problems.
2. Responsibility for regulating a new technology often is widely dispersed throughout both local and national governmental agencies.

Consequently, important checks and balances often fall between the cracks in planning for the prevention of hazard. With nuclear power this problem does not exist as much with respect to governmental agencies as it does with respect to coordination between multiple contractors and subcontractors.

3. Once a potential disaster is initiated, new technologies may present unique problems for which personnel who have traditional training or experience are unprepared.

Regarding the first issue, the very national agency that has responsibility for promoting nuclear power in the United States is the same one that has responsibility for regulating it. Consequently, the "dark side" of technological innovation has been largely ignored. Only now, for example, are the designers and operators of nuclear power plants beginning to realize that nuclear energy in these facilities introduces brittleness in metal to a degree never anticipated and thus creates hazards of failure also never foreseen.[45]

With other technologies, disasters with multiple deaths have occurred because foamed plastic materials have been promoted for bedding without awareness that their use in hospitals and jails could mean rapid dispersion in a fire of highly toxic gases to people who, through incarceration or impairment, would be unable to remove themselves.[46] Even with a more mobile population, these substances may prove lethal. The infamous Coconut Grove fire, which killed 491 people in Boston in 1942, was alleged to have taken so many lives because people panicked and therefore couldn't escape an inferno caused by plastic decorations. But the evidence suggests that many persons were asphyxiated before they even realized the danger.[10]

Use of heat-sensing controls for elevators in high-rise buildings was found in fires to draw cars full of passengers to the very floor where the conflagration was raging. In similar fashion, many hazardous materials have been stored and transported with little or no precaution because information about their hazards has not yet reached those who are ordering, transporting, and using these materials.

We turn next to diffusion of regulatory responsibility. As already commented, this does not exist with nuclear power plants. What does exist in this case, however, is an extremely complex facility whose structural and operational components have been parceled out to many different contractors and subcontractors. The result has been a human factors nightmare, so that even under normal conditions plant operators are functioning near the limits of their capabilities.[47,48] In some emergencies they may need to look simultaneously at two or more displays that have been designed and built by different contractors so that they are located back to back! Design failures such as these occur because no single person or group had authority and responsibility for taking—*and enforcing*—a system-analysis view of safety.

It is common for any single public building or hazardous material to fall under the purvue of several different local, regional, and federal agencies, which are overworked, underfunded, understaffed, and staffed with persons who sometimes lack appropriate training.[49] Consequently, especially with new technologies, it is hard for these personnel to be familiar with all of the potential hazards or to carry out all of the necessary inspections. For similar reasons, jails may remain hazardous because they were built many years ago, and, with low budgets, supervisory personnel are more concerned about security and other issues than they are about upgrading antiquated facilities for purposes of safety.[46]

As a result, what relevant rules and regulations do exist often are ignored by those who are supposed to be regulated. Among trucks in Virginia, 10 percent carried enough hazardous materials to require "placarding" or public warnings that such materials were present.[50] Four out of every ten of these trucks—which were usually traveling through highly populous areas—were in violation of the placard ordinance, and a quarter also failed to carry an appropriate freight bill to assist rescue personnel in an emergency.

Because of the complexities of governmental operation, it is perhaps too much to expect that all safety-related regulation would rest within the purvue of a single agency. Nor is it necessarily appropriate that such should be the case. What is appropriate, however, is periodic coordination of safety rules and resources to achieve a more unified, effective, and efficient approach, both to prevent disaster through standards and regulations and to respond effectively in emergencies.

Because required placarding often doesn't occur—but sometimes despite its occurrence—police and fire departments often have not known how to cope with toxic or other materials that are leaking or that catch fire. Or as happened at Three Mile Island or other nuclear power plants, operating personnel may be slow to realize that what appears to be a minor incident has very somber implications, and delays may occur in alerting others.

In the United States, at least, there has been increasing attention to providing specific training to alert all emergency personnel to certain hazards that require immediate and special action. Simultaneously, central advisory centers have been developed that are available "around the clock" to offer advice and other help. While I have not seen formal evaluation of this system, anecdotally within my own state the response to spillage of hazardous materials on the highways has become increasingly sophisticated in the past few years.

The Aftermath: Long-Term Effects

The data on the long-term effects of disasters are to some extent contradictory. As was already described, Wright and Rossi reported that except for statistically rare events, there are no discernible long-term population and housing impacts on communities struck by natural disasters.[7]

Frazier states that the last major urban area that failed to totally rebuild was Saint-Pierre in Martinique, which was destroyed when Mount Pelee erupted in 1902. A city, he notes, has symbolic value and is far more than just a collection of buildings and businesses.[10]

Haas et al., on the other hand, warn that if rebuilding is to be done in a manner that is less vulnerable to the next potential disaster, governmental officials must move quickly to study, design, and administer during the immediate post-disaster uncertainties and must not propose changes that are overly ambitious.[51] Grandiose plans lead to conflict and further delay, so that ultimately the plans are not executed. In particular, they suggest that relocation is rarely seen by residents and officials as an appropriate measure. The last relocation of which they are aware was the moving of Antigua, Guatemala, following an earthquake in 1773.

My own training in public health was under Dr. Henrik Blum, a practitioner who understood human nature well. At that time he was the health officer for Contra Costa County, California, an area at risk of earthquakes, floods, and explosions of a munitions plant and several oil refineries. When he came to the county Board of Supervisors with plans for disaster prevention or response they showed little interest—as he knew they would.

Undaunted, he filed the plans away for the time when a disaster or near disaster would occur and when they would then ask him to draw up plans to avert or deal with future hazard. Almost invariably, the anticipated problem eventually occurred, and the response was as expected. The fact that he already had plans, which had been developed without duress, also usually meant that those plans were accepted with minimal conflict.

Although communities appear to rebound well from disasters, many of the individuals involved, especially those who have lost relatives, friends, or neighbors, suffer from a sense of vulnerability and guilt because they survived whereas others did not.[52] The counterpart to guilt is blame, and survivors commonly try to find a scapegoat for disasters, especially if they are of the man-made variety.[10,52,53]

Logue et al. found that among the family members who suffered most distress after a flood, a third still had emotional distress and 47 percent physical distress over two years after the event.[54] For about a quarter, this distress lasted longer than four years. Others, too, have described this "post-disaster syndrome" as being common and long-lasting, no matter whether the precipitating event is natural or man-made.[55,56,57] Elderly survivors appear to be affected less by such events than are younger individuals, perhaps because their expectations are somewhat less than are those of younger persons, and at an age when loss of family and friends is the rule, they are more satisfied simply to survive without asking any probing questions about the how or why.[58]

Disasters in areas or communities already showing high unemployment, outmigration, and economic decline tend to be much more devastating to both the individuals and the community than are such events in communities that had been upbeat and economically vigorous previously.[55] Caplan's "crisis intervention" approach to psychiatry is based on the hypothesis that if people cope well with a given crisis, they are then that much stronger to cope with, and maybe even avert, subsequent crises.[59] Perhaps deteriorating communities respond so poorly to disaster because having coped poorly in the immediate past they are less able to cope effectively with the present event. In disaster planning, and in emergency and long-term rehabilitative efforts after a disaster, little attention is usually paid to the need for psychiatric and other support services. Experience suggests that such services must receive higher priority.

Part III
The Health and Safety Professions and High-Risk Populations

The basic thrust of all of the chapters that have preceded this section is to provide sufficient information about the occurrence and prevention or amelioration of injury under a range of circumstances to assist the health or safety professional—whether working with individual patients or clients, or at a community or public-health level—in making rational decisions about potential countermeasures. In the community or public-health setting examination and possibly regulation or modification of specific environments is often feasible and appropriate; for example, the work place, some aspects of homes and public buildings, camps, parks, carnivals, hospitals, and nursing homes.

For the physician, psychologist, social workers, nurse, or physical therapist, however, what presents itself is not an environment but rather an individual patient or client. As has been apparent throughout the entire book, certain groups are at higher-than-average risk of injury for a variety of reasons often associated with health or developmental issues that are in the purview of the health professional. It is appropriate, therefore, to examine the most important of these high-risk groups so that the health or safety professional, faced with an individual, can know what the high-risk problems are, why they are present, and what measures can be taken both at the individual and the community level to reduce the risk of injury and of disability or death.

Although this section deals only with high-risk segments of the population, I wish to emphasize that many, if not most, of the countermeasures that are useful for these groups are also beneficial to reducing the risk of injury, disability, and death for *all* individuals. No one of us is entirely immune from occasions when task demands of whatever activity we are engaged in become, for the moment at least, greater than our ability to cope. With some of us this happens relatively more often. But with everyone it happens. This section, therefore, in the broader sense is concerned with the health or safety professional's role in the prevention and amelioration of all injury.

28
"Accident" Proneness: Fact or Fiction?

For many years the public and substantial segments of the professionals directly concerned with injury-control activities have been under the impression that a majority of injury events occur to only a minority of the population. In one sense this is an absolutely accurate assessment, since injuries are rare events occurring only once in many thousands of exposures. In any one year period only a minority of the population will be involved in such events. The more important questions, however, are the following:

1. If one follows the injury experience of a population over a longer time frame (such as five years), are there individuals who are involved in repeated injury events, *and does this exceed the proportion of individuals in a population who purely by chance might be expected to have two or more such events in a similar time frame?*
2. If such individuals exist, do they account for more than a small minority of all injury events or of all serious injury events?
3. If so, can they be identified *before* the occurrence of repetitive trauma?
4. If they can be so identified, can anything useful be done to alter them or the nature of their interactions with potential hazards in their environments?

The first serious investigation of the frequency of injury events over a stated time period was undertaken by Greenwood and Woods[1] at a munitions factory in 1918. They found that the distribution of these events among individuals did not follow standard Poisson or random distribution but rather was consistent with negative binomial theory.

Bernacki says that after rejecting the random hypothesis Greenwood considered two others; namely, that an individual who randomly has one event then becomes nonrandomly more or less likely to incur another (the "single-biased" distribution) or that even with the first event individuals have unequal or nonrandom chance of injury ("unequally biased" distribution).[2] He has summarized the Greenwood data to show that 26 of 648 women had three or more mishaps in five weeks, in comparison to expected figures in Poisson distribution of 8 ($p < 0.0010$), single-biased distribution of 23 ($0.10 > p > 0.05$) and unequally biased distribution of 21 ($0.20 > p > 0.10$).

Haight observes that after Greenwood's purely statistical discovery, many investigators jumped to a far more radical assumption that every individual possesses a different *and relatively constant* risk of injury produced by his or her particular psychophysical makeup.[3] Among the earlier and most influential of these proponents was Flanders Dunbar, who described an "accident profile": namely, an individual who was impulsive, generally relaxed, and pleasure-dominated.[4]

Others, such as Karl Menninger,[5] Franz Alexander,[6] Rawson,[7] and Behan and Hirschfeld[8] have championed the idea that what appear to be unintentional injury events often have a distinct purposive component, serving such goals as self-inflicted punishment for guilt about hostile feelings, removal of the individual in a psychologically acceptable manner from untenable socioenvironmental or economic problems, and often simultaneously providing a means of economic compensation and perceived punishment for loved ones at whom they are angry. These individuals have also been referred to as "accident prone." An excellent and highly recommended review of the subject by Arbous and Kerrich observes that the term *accident proneness* has thus shifted from one that has statistical meaning to one that became a clinical diagnosis.[9]

In a much later study by a team with a high degree of statistical and research sophistication Mellinger and Manheimer identify at least two different populations of repeaters among children.[10] They note, however, that their explanation may be applicable only to children and not to adults. On the one hand, they find that several normal, healthy, and otherwise desirable personality traits are associated with high injury liability among boys who are active, extroverted, adventuresome, and curious. Such traits increase risk by increasing exposure to hazard. On the other hand, some children are so absorbed with inner problems and tensions that they cope poorly with their external environment. To the extent that such environment includes hazards, maladjustment thus increases liability of injury.

Waller and Whorton noted that persons who unintentionally shot themselves or others also had an excess of highway crashes and prior episodes involving deliberate violence.[11] But they stated that such individuals appear to comprise only a minority of persons in injury events and that even among the shooters several unrelated patterns of occurrence could be identified. There does, in fact, appear to be an association, as yet not explored in great depth, between persons who commit acts of deliberate violence—whether assault and homicide or suicide—and those who unintentionally injure themselves or others.[12,13] One characteristic that appears closely related to both forms of injury is abuse of alcohol.

The data presented so far in this book offer some interesting contradictions. On the one hand, as noted in chapter 8, if a population of drivers is followed beyond a single time frame, only a small minority of persons are to be found who have repeat events in successive periods. The substantial majority of the population who are in a first crash will not be involved in a second crash for many years to come but will be replaced in most subsequent time periods by other individuals who themselves were crash free in previous periods.

On the other hand, it has become equally clear that several subpopulations can be identified of individuals who for a variety of reasons are at increased risk of involvement in injury events. These include young children, teenagers and young adults (for highway and occupational injuries), persons who are heavy (and often addicted) users of alcohol, persons with certain forms of medical impairment, and some segments of the elderly population. In some cases (such as children and "poisoning") the increase in risk may be predominantly associated with minor injury. With the elderly or persons who are heavy users of alcohol, however, the increase in risk may be predominantly for events that cause serious injury or fatality.

Also in some cases, as with children, the increase in risk may be only temporary while the individual is passing through a particular developmental or learning phase. This was noted as long ago as 1936[14] by Vernon, who said that the "accident-proneness" of individuals is not a fixed quality but is influenced by changes in the environment and in physical and mental health.

In other cases, such with seizures, alcoholism, or cardiovascular disease, the impairment may be either repetitive or of much longer duration unless or until the individual becomes responsive to treatment that reduces the impairment. As we have also noted, some individuals may be at continual high risk of injury for socioeconomic reasons, such as inability to purchase appliances with safer characteristics or to live in safer environments. These may also be persons with young children, alcoholism, or medical impairment who thus are at risk for two reasons.

The previous chapters have identified that such groups of high-risk individuals may comprise a substantial percentage of persons involved in serious injury events. This does not mean, however, that we can with relative ease identify in advance which persons are likely to have large numbers of injury events. Even among the highest-risk groups—such as persons with alcoholism—only a minority may be injured or may injure others in a one- or two-year period, and only a small minority will do so repetitively in that time frame. In particular, removal of that small minority of repeaters will still leave the majority of injury events unaccounted for.

If the traits involved are strong enough, however, a sufficiently large minority of persons may be likely to be injured over even a short time frame, or—as in the case of alcoholics—the injury events may be so severe that intervention specific to this particular population becomes worth consideration. Thus, Mellinger and Manheimer note that their study may be useful to identify in advance traits associated with high injury liability and to offer the possibility of training in judgmental and decision-making skills, rather than psychotherapy, for prevention of repetitive injury.

In other cases, however, the traits may be of longer duration and thus warrant intervention because over the long time frame a very substantial minority or even a majority of such persons are likely to get into trouble. The next three chapters, therefore, deal specifically with three high-risk groups that often come to the attention of health professionals and examine countermeasures, both personal and environmental, that are of particular relevance to them. The reader must fully understand, however, that attention to these high-risk groups in no way precludes attention to environmental or other countermeasures—especially of a passive nature—that have wider relevance to preventing or ameliorating those occasions when, for whatever reason, even the most competent of us get into situations where task demands exceed our performance at a given moment in time.

It is probably surprising to some readers that, especially in the context of a chapter on "accident" proneness I have said almost nothing so far specifically about those individuals who clearly go out of their way to take risks: the Evel Knievals of the world. There can be no question from the data discussed in previous chapters that such individuals do exist and that their risk taking encompasses a wide variety of activities. Some individuals also appear to have injuries that are at least in part subintentional.

The question is whether either or both of these groups contribute an appreciable portion of injury events that occur, whether they can be identified before the fact, and whether their behavior can be modified with any acceptable degree of success. The answer to all three questions appears to be basically no.

Removal of such persons deletes only a relative minority of injury events. This is well documented in Bernacki's adaptation of Farmer and Chambers' data, which show that removal of drivers with three or more crashes in year one would remove 28 percent of drivers but reduce subsequent crashes by only 9 percent.[2] Removing persons with the worst 25 percent of driving tests would delete 23 percent of drivers but 7 percent of crashes, while removal of both groups would deny licenses to 44 percent of drivers to prevent 13 percent of crashes. Many high-risk drivers can be identified early, but the proportions of false negatives and false positives in such identification are unacceptably high for administrative programs. Furthermore, the recidivism rate among those who are identified also is quite substantial despite a wide range of programs aimed at behavioral modification.

To a very large extent such risk takers are to be found among the young and persons with problems associated with alcohol abuse. Therefore, the discussion of them is included in the chapters about these two groups.

29
Children and Youth

This and the next two chapters will not offer a complete review of the previous material but rather will focus on two issues: characteristics of members of the group that put them at high risk of injury and countermeasures currently or potentially available to limit the risk or ameliorate the results. In particular, where possible, attention will be paid to countermeasures that can be offered or applied at the individual level and that will, therefore, be useful for those health or safety personnel who are not in a position to initiate broader efforts. This emphasis is being placed in these three chapters, not because I believe such countermeasures are more important or more successful than are community-based environmental measures but rather because such individual efforts in some cases can alert the public to the need for more definitive approaches. In other cases they can supplement environmental approaches that have been discussed throughout this book.

Children under age 15 comprise a majority of the world's population and, as we have already documented, they are at increased risk of injury in and around the home setting, in various forms of recreation, and as pedestrians wherever motor vehicles are found throughout the world. Teenagers and young adults (age 20 to 24) on the other hand, have low injury risk as pedestrians in places like the United States but, as Baker[1] has documented, may be at high risk of such injuries in places such as Rio de Janeiro, where they find it necessary and are relatively more able and willing to take risks to cross inhospitable highways that lack pedestrian amenities. As drivers they are at extremely high risk of both injury and death, and they are also at greater than average risk of occupational injury. And because of their greater and more exuberant exposure to recreational activities, they are at high risk of injury here, too.

Unintentional injury is the single most frequent cause of death among children in the developed nations and is a major contributor to mortality in the developing countries as well. The differences in the distribution of injuries according to age, sex, and area of the world are shown in tables 29–1 and 29–2, reflecting both differences in types of activities for children of specific ages and sex and also the fact that the developed nations offer greater exposure to motor vehicles, while agrarian life in Asia and Oceania means greater proximity to bodies of water.[2]

Table 29–1
Mean Injury Mortality by Geographic Area for Children Age 1 to 4

	Europe	*North America*	*Latin America*	*Asia*	*Oceania*
Boys					
Injury deaths per 100,000 population	31.2	35.7	28.0	32.4	36.0
Percentage injury deaths are of all deaths	30.5	39.5	4.1	7.5	37.2
Percentage of all injury deaths by cause					
Motor vehicle	36.0	35.8	18.1	26.8	31.5
Other transport	1.6	1.3	1.3	3.7	1.4
Poisoning	4.9	4.7	4.8	1.8	2.7
Falls	6.3	3.8	6.3	4.2	5.0
Fire	5.9	17.0	16.9	3.1	4.1
Drowning	23.4	19.4	19.2	46.4	38.3
Firearms	0.4	1.8	0.5	0.1	2.3
Industrial type	7.5	6.3	4.3	6.4	5.4
Other	14.1	9.8	28.5	7.5	9.5
Girls					
Injury deaths per 100,000 population	19.4	26.3	21.5	21.3	25.7
Percentage injury deaths are of all deaths	23.4	34.4	3.1	5.6	32.2
Percentage of all injury deaths by cause					
Motor vehicle	51.7	46.6	36.9	37.6	55.6
Other transport	3.8	4.6	2.4	4.4	5.6
Poisoning	1.9	1.2	1.7	1.4	0.7
Falls	5.9	2.4	7.7	5.8	3.6
Fire	1.6	6.0	5.8	2.5	1.5
Drowning	18.7	20.0	16.4	30.6	16.3
Firearms	1.1	5.3	1.8	0.9	4.1
Industrial type	5.5	6.0	5.2	5.6	5.6
Other	9.8	7.8	22.0	11.2	5.9

Source: Adapted from H. Marcusson and W. Oehmisch, "Accident Mortality in Childhood in Selected Countries of Different Continents, 1950–1971," *World Health Statistical Report* 30 (1977):57–92.

Table 29–2
Mean Injury Mortality by Geographic Area for Children Age 5 to 14

	Europe	*North America*	*Latin America*	*Asia*	*Oceania*
Boys					
Injury deaths per 100,000 population	22.5	27.4	21.4	17.3	25.1
Percentage injury deaths are of all deaths	45.3	53.6	16.8	15.6	54.2
Percentage of all injury deaths by cause					
Motor vehicle	51.7	46.6	36.9	37.6	55.6
Other transport	3.8	4.6	2.4	4.4	5.6
Poisoning	1.9	1.2	1.7	1.4	0.7
Falls	5.9	2.4	7.7	5.8	3.6
Fire	1.6	6.0	5.8	2.5	1.5
Drowning	18.7	20.0	16.4	30.6	16.3
Firearms	1.1	5.3	1.8	0.9	4.1
Industrial type	5.5	6.0	5.2	5.6	5.6
Other	9.8	7.8	22.0	11.2	6.9
Girls					
Injury deaths per 100,000 population	10.5	12.9	10.3	8.3	10.0
Percentage injury deaths are of all deaths	32.7	38.7	9.6	9.4	37.0
Percentage of all injury deaths by cause					
Motor vehicle	63.5	57.9	33.7	36.7	73.8
Other transport	3.3	4.0	1.4	3.8	4.0
Poisoning	3.3	2.0	3.4	2.5	0.7
Falls	4.6	1.5	5.9	4.5	—
Fire	2.3	11.8	12.8	4.5	2.0
Drowning	9.2	11.4	11.8	31.4	12.8
Firearms	0.6	2.3	1.5	0.4	—
Industrial type	3.3	2.7	4.5	5.2	0.7
Other	9.9	6.3	25.0	11.0	6.0

Source: Adapted from H. Marcusson and W. Oehmisch, "Accident Mortality in Childhood in Selected Countries of Different Continents, 1950–1971," *World Health Statistics Report* 30 (1977):57–92.

Risk Factors

Over a dozen characteristics place the child at greater risk of involvement in injury events and, in some cases, of greater severity. Because of small size the young child cannot easily reach objects and thus may pull substances such as boiling water or grease onto itself. Also because of small size, spills of even modest amounts cover much of total body surface, increasing severity of injury. Small size also results in lesser visibility of a child to traffic, as well as lesser visibility of traffic to the child.

Limited mobility reduces ability to escape a rapidly approaching animal or motor vehicle or, especially for the very young, to escape from a burning or otherwise endangered structure. Lesser muscle strength limits capacity to escape from impending hazard (such as fire or a closed refrigerator) but may also result in initiation of hazard. A small child may be unable to hold up the heavy lid on a toy box, so that it falls onto the head or neck and causes asphyxiation. This lack of strength may prevent easy self-extrication when children fall into dug wells and pools or natural bodies of water or when infants are placed into excessively hot bath water by parents or older siblings.

Limited coordination is especially a problem for toddlers and for children who are beginning to use tools capable of cutting, piercing, or hammering. The fact that, especially when sitting, the center of gravity may be higher for young children than for older ones may combine with poor coordination to promote falling.

Two other anatomic and physiologic features unique to the young child are limited ability to judge distance and a sense of taste that permits it not only to initially try but also to continue to mouth substances that older children and adults find unacceptably bitter or sour.

The younger the child the greater the lack of experience. But as children get older and gain experience with specific tasks and situations, they tackle new ones. Thus, all the way into late teen years, when they begin driving motor vehicles, engage in more demanding recreational activities, and enter the work force, children and youths are on a continuing series of learning curves. This means greater number of errors per unit of exposure and consequently greater risk of injury unless specific safeguards have been built in so that error does not result in probable harm.

In their youngest years children must also cope with an innate but uneducated curiosity, a limited ability to handle more than one stimulus at a time, poorly developed concepts of hazard, limited ability to make appropriate and timely judgments, and an inability to postpone gratification. Some studies, in fact, have shown correlation between such factors as injury occurrence and high frustration level, hyperactivity, and impulsiveness.[3,4] Other studies, however, have not found behavioral differences,[5] while Mellinger and Manheimer have suggested that rather than being pathological some of the behavioral correlations that they observed are simply measures of normal, healthy development.[6]

Often it is not possible to parcel out relative contribution of each of these factors in increasing injury risk. The young child may seek to cross in the middle of a street rather than at the intersection, for example, because of limited experience and perception of hazard, poor judgment, impulsiveness, and limited willingness to wait until the intersection is reached. But the intersection also may be avoided because, unlike midblock, it provides too many simultaneous stimuli.

A few studies have also suggested that in some cases hazardous action by the young child may be one component of a child/parent struggle for control or may reflect disorganization in a family that is already beset by other physical or social stresses.[3] Injuries of children with psychiatrically disturbed mothers tend to clump during the weeks when the mother is coping most poorly.[7] Backett and Johnston suggest it is the family rather than the individual that is vulnerable.[8] One study suggests that not only mothers but their children, also, may have higher injury frequency during the mothers' paramenstrual days,[9] suggesting lesser ability of the mother at this time to attend to the child and keep it from danger.

Finally, a few children and youths are at increased risk of injury because of medical impairments, such as epilepsy or cerebral palsy.[10,11] These individuals get into trouble both because of a greater likelihood of falling and because once they have fallen, they are unable to remove themselves quickly if they have landed on an inhospitable surface.

In the teen years other problems as well place people at greater risk. In many societies these are the years of initial experimentation with alcohol and other drugs, especially under peer pressures. Problems of self-identification and related conflicts with parent figures may add to the willingness to take risks and to experiment with the extent to which one can push both the sociolegal and physical environment. For the young male such activities as fast or risky driving, athletics, and more ominous forms of confrontation, such as fighting, may be perceived as the only ways available to demonstrate success and prowess and obtain a sense of self-worth.[12,13]

Because of lack of training, skill, and experience, balanced by greater coordination and muscle strength, the young worker just entering the occupational marketplace often is given the hardest, dirtiest, most boring, and most hazardous jobs, which other workers are unwilling or no longer able to tackle. And, as entry-level workers, they receive the lowest pay. This means that unless there are requirements for safe cars and other equipment, they will be forced to begin their adult lives with tools for work, transportation, recreation, and home operation that are secondhand or otherwise least reliable and most prone to safety-related defects and problems. This combination of factors virtuallly ensures that the teenager and young adult—especially the males—will be at high risk of injury for reasons that are far broader than the well known and often discussed impatience and apparent devil-may-care attitude of youth. Further, if this young male has a wife and young children, it ensures that they too will be at greater risk of injury. Young women who enter the work force may receive even lower salaries than the men and may continue with lower wages for many years.

Countermeasures

The discussion of countermeasures must begin with some comments about what are reasonable expectations. Gustafssen, as quoted by Berfenstam,[14] states that preventive measures are unnecessary for 30 percent of injuries to children, since they represent learning experiences. Another 37 percent, he feels, could be prevented through rather simple measures, while 23 percent require extensive environmental changes.

While it appears to be true that many injuries to children are a result of learning experiences that will never be repeated, it is also essential to point out that, especially with children exposed to fire and youthful drivers and their equally young passengers, many of those learning experiences have extremely severe and long-lasting outcome, including death, permanent disfigurement, and head and spinal cord injuries with their lifelong consequences. The question, therefore, is how to uncouple inevitable judgment and behavioral errors of the learning process from the not-so-inevitable injury process.

Traditionally, education and guidance of parents and children has usually been viewed as the primary, and often the sole, countermeasure option. A report of an interesting program to train pediatric residents in concepts and methods of injury control has nicely documented both that in the absence of such training physicians tend not to ask appropriate questions and to give timely advice and that with such training their advisory behavior can be improved substantially.[15] Two well-designed countermeasure programs, however, based on community education must give one pause.

One of these programs involved organization of community discussion groups to promote understanding about child injury and the need for and types of preventive actions.[16] The other involved a twenty-minute safety discussion by a research assistant with mothers of children who were visiting a child health clinic.[17] Written material, electric outlet covers, and special cabinet locking devices were given to each mother. Neither project was associated with a decrease in child injuries.

On the other hand, efforts by physicians to promote infant seats have been moderately successful,[18] and the probability exists that direct advice by physicians is more persuasive than is that of other health workers. My own impression is that many of the safety recommendations discussed with parents in these and other campaigns are concerned with injuries that are relatively uncommon or are difficult to control through the countermeasures proposed.

Baker has stated that to be successful countermeasures to promote safety must be used, must be used properly, and must work when properly used.[18] Most effective, she notes, are those measures that never require any action by a child or his or her family. Next most effective are those measures that require one-time action. But she warns that many people will not undertake even a single effort. In Adelaide, only 18 percent of parents whose children had been poisoned subsequently made poisons less accessible. She further notes that the likelihood of success decreases as frequency of required action increases.

With this excellent admonition in mind, we will turn to a series of sections identifying potential countermeasures against injury for different age levels of children and youth. These countermeasures have been categorized according to their application by individual health and safety practitioners through counseling or individual action (I), through community-wide or group action (C) or both (B). Promotion of infant car seats, for example, can be carried out both through advice by physicians to individual parents as well as through efforts to pass laws requiring purchase and use of such devices. The countermeasures are also categorized according to the degree of individual action required by the person or the family of the person to be protected. As Baker has noted, a measure may require no individual effort (N), one-time or otherwise limited efforts (L), or frequent application (F) in order to be successful.

Some Preventive Measures for Injuries to Infants

In this age range injuries are largely of a passive nature, with children being injured because of the actions of others around them. As crawling begins, so does more active participation in their own injury events, resulting from chewing, pulling things onto themselves, or touching hazardous objects.

A. Thermal Injury

1. Reduce temperature of hot water heaters to 120°F (50°C). (B,L)
2. Use retractable or self-shortening appliance and extension cords so that young children can't as easily reach them and pull hot appliances down on themselves. Manufacturers could be convinced or required to provide cords of this type with appliances. (B, N, or L) Redesigning of electrical wires and plugs can also decrease the frequency of electrical burns to young children.[19]
3. Use fuel-operated lamps, coffee, and teapots with a low center of gravity and designed so that the lid or hot filter remains on if the pot topples over, thus reducing spillage of hot or flammable liquid.[19] If such designs are generally unavailable, manufacturers may need to be convinced or required to provide appropriate designs. (B, N, or L)
4. Use low-temperature humidifiers for children with respiratory problems. (I, L)
5. Select sleepwear and other clothing that is flame retardant. In the United States flame retardancy is required by law for all sleepwear. (C, N) Where such clothing is not already on the market it is possible to promote similar legislation or to impart a flame-retardant quality by using borax in the final wash rinse or by spraying a borax lotion on after the clothes have become dry. (I, F) This lotion is composed of 24 gm borax (sodium borate), 10 gm boric acid, and 280 ml warm tap water.[20] Wool and some synthetic fabrics are less flammable than are cotton and silk.
6. Portable or permanently placed space heaters should be designed to shut off if they fall over or if materials are placed on or against them, and should be located away from furniture and crawl or walk paths. Where these safeguards are not required by law (C, N), parents can be given advice about selection and placement. (I, L)
7. Educate parents about use of cold water for first aid treatment of burns. (B, F)
8. Install or require as part of construction fire and smoke alarm devices in all homes. (B, N/L)
9. Obviously, any requirements or technological improvements that reduce flammability and decrease toxicity of ignited materials in the home will benefit infants as well. (C, N)

B. Falls

1. Select high chairs, infant seats, and carriages that have wide base and low center of gravity. (I, L)

2. Counsel parents about the ease with which infants can roll and wiggle off if placed on high adult furniture, such as tables or chests. (I, F)
3. Select or convert tables and chairs to reduce injury resulting from striking sharp edges and corners in falls. (I, L)
4. Install protective gates or self-closing doors to prevent crawling infants from reaching and falling down stairs. (I, L)
5. Use protective head gear for children with seizures, cerebral palsy, or similar problems. (I, F)
6. Install protective bars or grates on windows that young children might be able to reach *and* place furniture away from windows so that childen can't crawl from furniture onto the window. (B, L) Where bars are used in windows, however, they should be designed for rapid and easy removal by an older child or adult to permit escape in case of fire.

C. Other Lacerations and Contusions

Select toys and child furniture that do not have sharp edges or surfaces and that cannot be easily broken to create such surfaces. (I, L) In the United States the Consumer Product Safety Commission (CPSC) has done much to limit this possibility through standards for toys, cribs, and so forth. Such legislation should be sought elsewhere, as well. (C, N)

D. Poisoning

This is a minor problem until the upper end of this age range unless infants are fed by older siblings or unless peeling or chewable paint is available for pica. Solutions to this latter problem are:

1. Alert parents—who often are not knowledgeable about this subject—to the specifics of what is pica, what are its implications, and what can be done about it. (B, L/F)
2. Counsel parents about use of nonlead paints and about cleanup of areas within the home that may have existing lead-based paints a child can reach and chew. If areas of peeling paint cannot be removed, they can sometimes be placed out of reach by moving furniture in front of them. (B, L) Periodic wet mopping can reduce the amount of lead available. Legislation to remove lead-based paints from the home environment is probably the best approach over the long range. (C, N)
3. Have poison control center facilities available to the community. (C, N)

E. Asphyxiation

1. Choose cribs and play pens with design (less than 60 mm between slats or rungs) that does not permit an infant to get its head caught. This is also a potential problem for infants crawling around banisters and similar railings. (I, L) Mattresses for cribs should fit snugly so an infant can't get caught between the crib wall and the mattress. CPSC regulations in the United States require child furniture to be of proper design (C, N), but hand-me-down equipment might not meet these standards.
2. Select toy boxes that have balanced lids that small children can open *and keep open* with minimal effort. (B, N/L)
3. Counsel parents about avoiding the use or availability to children of thin plastic sheets and bags. (B, F) Community campaigns and warning labels appear not to have reduced the frequency of deaths to young children from asphyxiation, and the only workable solution would seem to be legislation or regulation removing the thinnest and most dangerous material from the market. (C, N)
4. Baker and Fisher have documented the frequency with which infants die from aspiration of hot dogs or frankfurters that they have been given, often by slightly older siblings, and that they are unable to chew sufficiently.[21] The size, shape, and consistency of this food is almost "ideal" for creating problems. Parents need to be alerted to this problem, about which both parents and health professionals are currently unaware. (B, F) In all honesty, however, I have only limited hopes for resolution of the problem in this way, but I do not know of an acceptable better solution at this time, short of removing hot dogs from the market.

F. Drowning

1. Infants should not be bathed by siblings who are much younger than teenage. (I, F)
2. If families live on or near water, crawling infants should be kept on a tether that itself is designed not to cause asphyxiation. (I, F)

G. Highway Injury

1. Parents should be advised or required by law to obtain and use properly designed infant seats when children are transported by automobile. (B, F) Specific guidance must be provided as to proper methods for using these seats, since many of them are used improp-

erly.[22] Better design to reduce the likelihood of misapplication would resolve this problem. (C, N) Parents must especially be alerted that the best way to fatally crush a child in a crash is to hold the child in one's lap. Unfortunately, a few states in the United States have a child crusher clause that permits a parent who holds the child not to use an appropriate child seat. Such clauses should be removed because they increase, rather than decrease, the hazard to children. Seat belts should be used by mothers during all phases of pregnancy, since they cause far less harm to even a large fetus than does a crash to an unprotected mother.

2. In nations where children carried on their mother's backs are at risk as pedestrians, use of reflective materials by mothers might be of some benefit in decreasing risks. (B, F) Of greater benefit, but perhaps more difficult to attain, are pedestrian walk areas. (C, N)
3. Any efforts that improve the safety design and construction of vehicles and roads or the provision of emergency medical services will benefit children who are vehicle occupants. (C, N)

H. Other Injuries and Actions

1. Regulations or similar actions reducing electric current in houses from 220V to 110V and requiring electric sockets that are self-closing when not in use can reduce the frequency and severity of electrical injury (C, N)
2. Rat bites are a problem throughout the world in children of this age. Individual and community wide extermination efforts appear to be the only reasonable solution. (B, F)
3. Tetanus and diphtheria immunization must be provided to prevent infection by these organisms for any lacerations or other injuries that do occur. (B, L)
4. Child-care centers are needed for working mothers. (C, L)
5. Physicians and other health workers need to be alert to evidence of child abuse and to take appropriate steps to intervene. (I, F) Proper legal and social resources for intervention need to be available in the community. (C, F)

Some Preventive Measures for Injuries to Toddlers and Preschool Children

The increasingly mobile preschool child more actively explores its home environment and begins to move—sometimes with minimal supervision—outside the home. This, again, is reflected in the types of injuries that occur.

A. Thermal Injuries

1. All countermeasures noted in section A on infants are relevant in this age group.
2. Advise parents to (a) seek to use only those book matches that have the strike bar on the opposite side of the cover opening, (b) keep matches locked up, and (c) have children learn how to light matches only under close parental supervision. (I, F) Far better, however, is promotion through voluntary compliance of manufacturers (or, if necessary, through legislation) of matches that (a) have the strike bar as noted above and (b) burn with lower energy and self extinguish. Matches with such design are feasible and are available in a few places. (C, N)
3. Advise parents to choose stoves that have burner controls located toward the back of the stove, where fewer children can reach them. (B, L) Ideally, promote availability only of stoves that incorporate safer location of controls, as well as less error-prone control-burner linkage.[23] (C, N)
4. Urge parents to use less flowing and frilly designs for nightgowns and other clothing for young children. A recent decrease in burns to young girls in the United States at least in part reflects a shift from dresses to pants.[24] Use of pajamas instead of nightgowns reduces the likelihood that flammable material may brush against hot surfaces. (B, L)
5. Through legislation and regulations highly flammable solvents should be removed from the market and replaced by less flammable but equally efficacious substitutes. (C, N)

B. Falls

1. Countermeasures in section B on infants are relevant in this age group.
2. Public and private playground equipment should be anchored in soft, resilient material to reduce the severity of falls. (B, N/L)

C. Other Lacerations and Contusions

1. The countermeasure in section C on infants is relevant for toys used in this age group.

2. In developed nations window and door designs should follow recommendations noted in chapter 18. This can be accomplished with great difficulty by advising all parents what home changes need to be made (B, L), with a bit less difficulty (at least for new and remodeled housing) by educating building contractors and manufacturers about advantages of safer designs (C, N), and with least difficulty by including such designs as requirements in building codes and by enforcing their application. (C, N)
3. In developing nations the fact that children usually go without shoes results in many lacerations to soles of feet from stepping onto broken bottles and nails.[25] Promoting use of shoes is warranted here. (B, L) Bottle-return laws and reusable bottles can cut down on the availability of broken bottles at beaches and similar places where people are likely to walk with bare feet. (C, N)
4. Advise parents to select playground equipment without burrs or pinch points, with light, soft-seated swings and similar safer designs, and to place such equipment with sufficient space so that collisions are less likely to occur. (B, L) In the United States many of these design and construction issues are now covered by CPSC standards. (C, N)
5. Where wringer-type washing machines are still available and are not safety design—which should be required by law (C/N)—parents need to be warned about the hazards of letting children near them. (B, F)

D. Poisoning

1. For younger children in this age range recommendations 1 and 2 are applicable. Recommendation 3 is applicable across the entire age range.
2. Physicians should prescribe fewer doses per prescription for families with young children, thus limiting the possibility of massive overdose if a child consumes the entire contents of a prescription bottle. In nations where most medicines are available without prescription, the manufacturer or pharmacist should also limit the number of doses. Where possible, less toxic drugs should be substituted for more toxic ones. (B, N)
3. Medicines should be sold or prescribed in packages that discourage small children from opening them. This can be accomplished by using child-proof covers on bottles or by using single-dose packaging. (C, N)
4. As now required by CPSC, all household materials that are toxic or

caustic should be sold in containers that are demonstrated to be child-proof for the high-risk age range. (C, N)

5. Anticipatory education of parents at the individual health practitioner or community level should probably continue to be carried out. It appears to be of only limited effectiveness, however, and should not be seen as anything other than a minor supplementary method of prevention. Such education applies to (a) definition of what materials are hazardous, (b) avoiding use of substitute containers for hazardous materials (such as Coca-Cola bottles for gasoline), and (c) proper storage. (B, F)

E. Asphyxiation

1. For toddlers, the recommendations in section E on infants may still apply. In particular, plastic bags should not be made available for play. (B, F)
2. Parents should be warned about the hazards of letting children blow up balloons without close supervision or of letting them suck on balloons, since aspiration and death has occurred on occasion. (B, F)
3. Public education is required about abandonment of refrigerators or similar appliances without removal of the doors to avoid entrapment of young children. (B, L) Ideally, such appliances should be manufactured voluntarily or through compliance with the law so that the door can be opened from inside even by a toddler. (C, N)

F. Drowning

1. Dug wells, pools, and similar bodies of water in the built environment should have covers or fences with self-locking gates. (B, L)
2. The water level in pools should be kept high enough so that a small child can escape more easily without having to lift itself bodily to dry surface. (B, F)
3. Alarm mechanisms can be utilized for pools to alert people if an object the size of a child falls in. The devices can be set with a brief (for example, five-second) delay so they will activate only if whatever falls in begins to splash around. Unfortunately, such devices would need to be shut off when the pool is in use, with a possibility that at least some of the time people would forget to turn them back on when they leave the pool area. But even if used only half the time in areas with many pools, the potential for cost-effective application probably exists.

4. At this age, drownproofing lessons for children can begin. (B, L) While the concept of drownproofing is good, the actual effectiveness of this method in reducing the frequency of drowning is not known.
5. Rescue equipment should be available at high-hazard locations. (B, L)

G. Highway Injury

1. The recommendations in section G on infants are applicable here. As children get older they should be switched from infant seats to regular seat belts. In particular, many noncrash injuries occur to children who are loose occupants in vehicles,[26] and parents are usually unaware of this hazard.
2. Parents should be educated to push down door latches so that children are less able to open doors of moving cars. (B, F)
3. Parents and children should be educated about the safest way for children to cross the street. There is some evidence that children can be taught how to do so, even if they choose to cross in midblock.[27] (B, F)
4. Off-street play areas reduce frequency of pedestrian injuries to children.[28] These should be made available if possible in the home environment but also in the general community. (B, N/L)
5. Advise parents about the need to purchase first bicycles for their children that are of a size appropriate for the child at the time it is learning. The child should be able to touch the ground while sitting on the bike. (B, L)
6. Promote use of safety helmets for bicyclists. (B, F)

H. Other Injuries and Actions

1. All recommendations noted in section H on infants are relevant.
2. In many parts of the world there is exposure to rabid animals. Approaches to this problem are to educate parents and children about caution in approaching unfamiliar animals (B, F), require rabies immunization for all pets (B, L), and initiate and sustain rabies eradication programs at the community level (C, N)
3. Guns and fireworks are a constant source of injury in some areas. Properly enforced laws to limit their availability and type are one approach that has had some success. (C, N) Education of parents is recommended by some groups as the best approach to firearm safety in the United States. To date, however, there is little or no evidence that this approach has been of any value. (B, F)

Some Preventive Measures for Injuries to Primary-School Children

In this age range activities outside the home become much more important, in particular resulting in highway injuries to children as passengers, pedestrians, and bicyclists and—especially among males—injuries associated with recreation and competition.

A. Thermal Injuries

Countermeasures 2–5 listed in section A on toddlers and preschool children remain relevant, as do recommendations 1 and 4–9 in section A on infants.

B. Falls

Continue countermeasures 3 in section B on infants and 2 in section B on toddlers and preschool children.

C. Other Lacerations and Contusions

1. Countermeasures in section E on infants and 2 and 3 in section C on toddlers and preschool children continue in effect.
2. Toys designed for this age often include potentially hazardous projectiles, chemicals, and hot surfaces. Again, advice to parents on selection is indicated (B, L), but enforceable manufacturers' standards are far more effective (C, N).

D. Poisoning

This is only a minor problem in this age category.

E. Asphyxia

This also is now only a minor problem.

F. Drowning

1. Countermeasures 1–5 in section F on toddlers and preschool children continue to be useful.
2. Recommend use of high-contrast colors for bathing suits to increase

likelihood of quick discovery if a child gets into trouble in the water. (B, L)

3. Begin teaching children methods of mouth-to-mouth resuscitation as they reach the older ages in this category. (B, L)

G. Highway Injury

1. Continue countermeasure 3 in section G on infants and 2–6 in section G on toddlers and preschool children.
2. Where feasible, bicycle paths and lanes should be established. (C, N)
3. Develop bicycle rider training and testing programs for young children. (C, L)
4. School buses should meet standards for (a) driver qualifications, (b) ability to alert and stop other vehicular traffic in both directions when the bus is taking on or unloading passengers, (c) adequate maintenance, and (d) structural stability and egress in crash situations. (C, L) In addition, drivers need to be advised of the possibility of drawing in excessively high levels of carbon monoxide if buses are lined up nose to tail with their motors running in cold weather while waiting for children at the end of the school day. (C, F)

H. Other Injuries and Actions

1. Countermeasures 1, 2, 3, and 5 in section H on infants and 2 and 3 in section H on toddlers and preschool children continue in effect.
2. Formal school and community recreation programs hold potential for injury prevention. Components of such preventive programs include:

   a. Health standards for selection of participants. (B, L) In particular, attention needs to be given to the needs of children with history of prior head injury—which increases the likelihood of further head injury—and of children with history of seizures. At least one study suggests that there is little increase of drowning risk for children with epilepsy who are permitted to engage in swimming activities,[29] while other papers emphasize the importance of individual assessment of risks.[30,31]
   b. Selection and use of protective equipment, such as helmets and mouth and face guards. Children in body-contact sports should all be required to use individually fitted protective equipment, and equipment that they use should meet specific national stan-

dards for energy and injury attenuation. (C, L/F) If such standards have not been established, they should either be designed by a committee of coaches, physicians, and engineers familiar with energy-transfer issues or adopted from standards already existing elsewhere.

c. Examination of playing surfaces to remove hazards on the field and surrounding areas that players might crash into or otherwise contact. (C, N)

d. Review of playing rules to limit more hazardous actions by players. (C, L)

e. Review of potential injury and related emergency situations to ensure that potentially serious injuries are immediately identified and properly cared for *with primary attention to the needs of the injured child rather than those of the team.* (C, F)

3. In some school systems children begin to receive education about homemaking, shop, and occupational activities at this time. Such education should include the beginnings of education and training about occupational safety. (C, L)

Some Preventive Measures for Injuries to Teenagers

A. Thermal Injury

This is a relatively limited problem in this age range. Burns may occur from occupational exposures and use of hazardous solvents that have been discussed previously and from contact with the exhaust pipes of motorcycles, which are discussed below.

B. Falls

Ladders should meet minimum specifications for strength and have guidance regarding best position for placement, as now required in the United States by CPSC. (C, N)

C. Other Lacerations and Contusions

See countermeasures 2 and 3 in section C on toddlers and preschool children.

D. Poisoning

This is a relatively minimal problem in this age group with the exception of illicit use of drugs, discussed in chapter 31.

E. Asphyxia

Also a minimal problem in this age group.

F. Drowning

1. Alcohol, to be discussed in chapter 31, is an issue in drowning in this age group.
2. Countermeasures 4 and 5 in section F on toddlers and preschool children and 2 and 3 in section F on primary-school children continue to apply.

G. Highway Injury

1. Again, alcohol and drug abuse are major issues for consideration and will be covered in chapter 31.
2. Seatbelts and bicyclist helmet countermeasures remain relevant, as do bicycle lanes.
3. The prevention of trauma to motorcycle and moped riders is extremely important in this age range. If at all possible, parents and children should be advised about the extreme hazards associated with these and should be told to avoid or postpone this form of transportation. (B, L) If they will not do so, the importance of a good training program should be emphasized (B, L), as well as the absolute necessity of wearing a helmet and other protective clothing at all times when on these vehicles (B, F). Ideally, legislation requiring helmet use should be in place. (C, F) Such legislation should include standards for helmet performance in crash situations.

H. Other Injuries and Actions

Continue countermeasures 3 in section H on infants, and 3 in section H on toddlers and preschool children, and 2 and 3 in section H on primary-school children.

30
Medical Conditions and Aging

Old age can be considered as a biological state, a process, and a time of life when many individuals are beset by health conditions that are both more frequent and more severe than at other times. The first two of these considerations will be described as normative aging, the latter as pathological factors that are not necessarily associated with aging per se. In fact, the discussion of medical conditions that may increase injury risk is placed here primarily because these conditions are more common among the elderly and certainly not because they occur exclusively in this age category. Because both normative and pathological aging occur in the same person, it is sometimes difficult to decide which is which.

The process of aging that concerns us here may begin as early as the fourth and fifth decades for certain activities such as professional athletics and the fifth and sixth decades for some aspects of vision. In this chapter, however, old age is considered as beginning around age 60 or 65. The time of life known as "old old" is generally described as beginning somewhere between about age 75 and 85.

Issues Generally Associated with Normative Aging

Thirteen normative factors have been identified that may be associated with increases in injury risk. Of major importance, is the variability in these factors. *On average* the changes noted below increase linearly with age. Some individuals, however, can be expected to show only slight changes beginning late in life, while others will show extensive changes or changes that start while they are still relatively young. Equally important are changes that occur in reserve capacity to respond to more demanding task situations even though capacity to deal with usual task demands may not be altered.

1. Changes in vision. The lens becomes increasingly opaque and yellowed, especially in individuals exposed over the years to infrared

light through occupational or other activities. This reduces visual acuity and ability to distinguish colors. The average older person requires more lumens in order to see clearly, is more impaired by glare, and takes longer to adapt to dim light and to glare situations.[1] Visual fields may be reduced by folds of skin associated with aging of skin around the eyes, and depth perception deteriorates.[1] There is decreased dynamic visual acuity: that is, the ability to follow and identify an object during motion.[1,2] This probably is a reflection not only of visual changes but of reduced cervical mobility as well.

2. Changes in hearing. In general, ability to hear, unlike ability to see, does not appear to play a major role in the occurrence of most injury events. It may be a factor—although this is not well documented—in alerting people to avoid imminent hazards such as fire or an approaching emergency or other vehicle. Hearing does decrease with age, especially among men, who have more extensive occupational exposure to noise.[3]
3. Decrease in muscle mass and in muscle strength.[4] This is generally more apparent among women than men. It is not clear to what extent such reduced strength and mass reflect normative physiological changes per se versus reduced activity with increasing age or to what extent decreased activity leads to lesser strength, in turn leading to further decreases in activity.
4. Reductions in bone mass and increases in bone fragility. This is more severe in women, possibly because of endocrine factors involving menopause plus inadequate calcium intake and lack of exercise.
5. Normative reductions in overall stature and shifting forward of the center of gravity.[5]
6. Slowing of the walking pace because individuals are less sure footed.[6]
7. Decrease in stamina.[4,7] This reflects among other things changes in cardiovascular and respiratory function that are normal at this time of life.
8. Decrease in renal and hepatic function.[8] This is reflected in slower excretion and detoxification of many therapeutic drugs, consequently greater likelihood of toxic effect, measurable either directly as poisoning, or indirectly as psychomotor and sensory impairment that reduce ability to perform more demanding tasks and perhaps normal ones as well.
9. Slowing of reaction time.[4]
10. Decrease in sensitivity to temperature changes. There also is an increase in the pain threshold according to some, but not all, studies.[9] Reduced tactile and vibratory sensation can be measured as well.[9]

11. Changes in memory. There is no change in primary memory (which is more or less synonomous with short-term or immediate recall) but a distinct dropoff in secondary (or long term) memory.[10]
12. Decreases in learning and problem-solving ability. This occurs for a variety of reasons, at least some of which may reflect on the study methods used.[11]
13. Experiential history. An interesting bimodal situation may exist regarding the experiential history of the elderly. In agrarian societies, where relatively little change has occurred, the elderly person may be at some advantage over younger persons because of long years of experience with the community, the physical environment, and the home and occupational tasks to be performed. Where the society is in the process of rapid change, however, the older person may be at a disadvantage. This is likely to occur in developing nations involving traffic and occupational tools and methods and in specific occupational settings in developed nations.

Issues Involving Pathological Aspects of Aging

Many medical conditions theoretically can increase injury risk or are known to do so but only on rare occasions, either because the conditions themselves are rare or because sufficient impairment is rare. We will place emphasis here on those conditions that are relatively more common and that often cause enough impairment to make them important to safety. These conditions are cardiovascular diseases, diabetes, seizure disorders, Parkinsonism and other disorders of mobility, disorders of vision, senile dementias, and alterations of parasympathetic nervous system.

1. Cardiovascular diseases. The usual assumption is that individuals with C.V.D. may be at increased risk of injury because of loss of control during acute myocardial infarction. Probably more common but more subtle impairment, however, comes from attacks of angina (of which the individual is aware), alterations in cardiac efficiency and rhythm that may alter oxygenation of brain while carrying out more demanding tasks (of which the individual sometimes may be totally unaware), or transient ischemic attacks, and similar sudden alterations of consciousness or conscious control because of cerebral vascular deficiency.
2. Diabetes mellitus. In the younger person who may have a more

"brittle" diabetes, alteration of conscious control, especially because of hypoglycemic reaction, is the most serious problem. Such reactions are uncommon in the elderly. In that age range diabetes-associated problems of visual acuity and fields and of reduced peripheral sensation become the issues of concern.

3. Seizure disorders. While seizures are not uncommon among the elderly because of cerebral vascular disease, tumors, and so forth, the majority of persons so afflicted are under age 60. This condition poses a problem only if the seizures are poorly controlled. Firm data are not available, but it seems reasonable to assume that (a) the more frequent the seizures the higher the injury risk, (b) grand mal seizures carry a greater risk of injury than do petit mal and partial seizures, (c) an aura or warning may afford some protection compared to seizures not preceded by aura, and (d) persons with diurnal seizures are more likely to encounter difficulty than are those with nocturnal seizures only.
4. Disorders of mobility. The most frequent and probably most important of these are Parkinsonism, multiple sclerosis, stroke, and arthritis in its severe form. As we will discuss shortly, they may contribute to injury in a variety of ways.
5. Limited vision. Besides diabetic retinopathy, the major visual disorders of concern are cataract, hypertensive retinopathy, macular degeneration, and glaucoma. In some of the developing nations conditions such as trachoma may be much more important.
6. Senile dementias. The exact prevalence of the senile dementias (Alzheimer and others) is not known, but it increases substantially once the population reaches age 70 or 80. Even among persons age 90 or older, however, probably no more than a quarter to a third of the population is demented, and most of those are only mildly so and reside within the home environment.[12]
7. Disorders of parasympathetic nervous system. With old age, disorders of the parasympathetic nervous system increase markedly. Episodes of dizziness on rising rapidly, drop attacks, or dizzy spells on reaching upward or into deep shelves are not uncommon.[13] Some of these may be a result of pinching of vertebral or carotid arteries, and some from loss of balance because of changes in center of gravity and inadequate skeletal musculature to cope with sudden shifts. But the precise causation of many of these episodes remains unknown, they may in fact result from a combination of two or more of these conditions.
8. Trauma. Some of the disabilities described above are themselves traumatic in origin. This includes seizures, disorders of mobility, and some visual decrements.

9. Combinations. The possible combined effects of two or more conditions, neither of which may be sufficient in itself to cause serious impairment, must be considered.

Injury Results

Before noting actual relationships between injury and medical impairment and other factors associated with aging, mention should be made of alterations in amount and type of exposure to risk. It has sometimes been stated that the elderly are "safe" drivers because they have fewer crashes per hundred drivers than do persons of other ages. This difference, however, may be the net result of two conflicting tendencies. On the one hand, elderly persons often have problems just noted. On the other hand, because they often have retired from work, elderly drivers and pedestrians may be more able to control the amount and time of their excursions onto the roadway, thus limiting effects of greater impairment by reducing the types of exposure in which such impairment is likely to prove the most hazardous.

In one study, drivers with recent hospitalization for ischemic heart disease, most of whom were elderly, reduced both the total amount of driving and of driving in bad weather, at night, in heavy traffic, and for long distances.[14] Healthier persons of similar age and sex did not alter their driving in similar ways. Note that similar alterations in activity might not be possible for younger persons with impairment or for elderly persons who, despite impairment, must carry on outside activity. Nor would it apply to injury risks within the home if individuals are not in a position to reduce the pace of activities of daily living within the home environment. Supporting this admonition, excessive injury risk, either overall or per unit exposure, appears to exist for the elderly and for persons with medical impairment in four areas: falls, thermal injuries, poisoning, and highway injury.

The greater risk of falling reflects a number of the pre-injury phase factors noted above: reduced visual capability for both normative and pathological reasons, shifting forward of center of gravity accompanied by reduced muscle strength and muscle mass, altered mobility because of both normative and pathological changes, and alteration of consciousness and conscious control resulting from cardiovascular disease, seizures, drop attacks, temporary pinching off of cerebral blood flow, and altered parasympathetic response patterns. Add to this greater sensitivity to normal doses of drugs[8] and the fact that the elderly are acutely affected by alcohol to a greater extent than all the other adult groups except the very young[15] and also respond excessively to chronic effects.[16]

Bone fragility and reduced muscle mass increase the severity of falls for the elderly during the injury phase. Greater severity may result as well from altered consciousness or limitations of mobility that prevent a person, once fallen, from removing him or herself rapidly from hot surfaces or from submersion in water. In the post-injury phase, the fact that an elderly person may be living alone increases the likelihood of delayed discovery and treatment, while the pathological conditions to which the elderly are prone increase the chances for death from cardiovascular, pulmonary, renal, or hepatic complications.

Thermal injuries have similar causation if they result from a fall. Other thermal injuries are attributable to poor vision, dropping of matches or hot substances because of weakness, poor coordination or arthritis, slowed reaction time, and decreased sensitivity of peripheral nerve endings to heat. Inability to escape a fire and decreased reserve to cope with thermal trauma or combustion gases also play a role in greater severity. No data are available, but confusion and decreased problem-solving capability associated with senile dementia may be a factor in some cases both in initiation of injury events and in increased severity.

Poisoning in the elderly reflects in part their greater exposure to large numbers of prescription and over-the-counter drugs. It also often reflects forgetfulness of what drugs have been taken and increased sensitivity to toxic effects. Again, one can hypothesize about the roles of reduced vision, dementia, and so forth in these events, but hard data simply are not available.

Regarding highway injury there is little question but that the elderly are at high injury risk as pedestrians. Reduced vision and hearing, slowed mobility, confusion, and slowed response to rapidly changing and complex traffic situations all contribute. Greater tissue fragility and the likelihood of complications from organ failure due to preexisting disease add to severity.

It is more difficult to talk about aging and medical impairment and driving. Most, but not all, studies show increase in crash risk per unit drivers or per unit mile of driving for persons with medical conditions such as epilepsy, diabetes, ischemic heart disease, mental illness, and alcoholism, all of which involve potential changes in functional states from day to day and even from minute to minute.[17–20] In some studies static conditions, such as absence of a limb, appear not to be associated with increase in crash risk.[21] One study showed that elderly persons in essentially good health had no increase in crash risk over middle-age drivers in the same community.[22] Those older drivers, however, who had ischemic heart disease or episodes of forgetfulness or tremor did have higher crash rates, while drivers with both problems had much higher crash rates.

In almost all studies individuals have been defined entirely by the primary conditions being considered—such as ischemic heart disease—and there has been no attempt to determine the frequency with which other comorbid conditions may exist in a single individual or the extent to which such conditions may interact with the primary condition to cause more impairment than exists with the primary condition alone.[23] It is not at all uncommon, for example, to find that a person with ischemic heart disease also has diabetes, hypertension, cataracts, arthritis, and perhaps even early signs of senile dementia.[20]

Rather little is known about the effects of senile dementia on crash risk. Certainly, anecdotes abound about crashes involving elderly persons who are confused at intersections and who go through a traffic signal requiring them to stop or yield or who drive in the wrong direction on a one-way thoroughfare.

My own suspicions are that there is a substantial increase in crash risk for persons with early senile dementia. At this stage moments of confusion or forgetfulness may occur that can profoundly alter problem-solving capabilities in rapidly moving traffic, but the individual him or herself may not be aware of what is happening, nor may friends and relatives. Furthermore, full-scale diagnostic tests with sufficient sensitivity for diagnosis of early dementia do not exist, and heavy reliance must be placed on anecdotal data from relatives and friends.[12] Such individuals thus may be at high risk of crash involvement because their full exposure to the traffic environment continues at a time when their capabilities are failing but in an erratic and unpredictable fashion.

Countermeasures

We will again follow the countermeasure scheme used in chapter 29, identifying those actions that can be carried out by and with individuals (I), and those applicable through community agencies (C), or through both mechanisms (B). Measures may require no effort by the person at risk (N), limited, one-time, or occasional effort (L), or frequent personal participation (F).

Falls

1. Promote exercise programs in the elderly, or in younger persons with disorders of mobility in order to strengthen muscles, increase muscle mass, and bone strength, and improve general capabilities to move about in a flexible and assured manner. This countermeasure is based on results of community programs that suggest general

improvements in participating populations—all of whom have been volunteers—rather than on firm evidence at this point of capability to reduce the frequency or severity of falls. It appears to have broader benefits than safety alone, and warrants trial and evaluation for both purposes. (B, F)

2. Reduce dosage in prescriptions for the elderly, especially those with known renal or hepatic problems. (I, N)
3. For those elderly individuals who have fallen, search for correctable problems, such as excessive dosage of medications, vision changes requiring new prescription, early Parkinsonism, drop attacks, mechanical pinching off of cerebral blood supply, disorders of cardiac rhythm, and alcoholism. (I, L)
4. Recommend placement of most commonly used items in kitchen and elsewhere on shelves that require a minimum of reaching upward or outward into deep shelving.[24] This applies both for the elderly and for younger persons with disorders of mobility. (B, L) Communal or congregate housing should be originally constructed with narrower shelves to limit these risky movements. (C, N)
5. Recommend use of sufficient numbers of lamps and of brighter (such as 100-watt) light bulbs placed near eye level in homes. (B, L) Nursing homes, hospitals, and public or congregate housing should be designed to decrease glare by proper placement and nonglare coverage of any fluorescent fixtures that are used and use of nonglare surfaces and nongloss waxes on floors and walks.[6] Blinds, shades, or similar window covering can limit glare at specific times of day. Whether or not fluorescent lighting is used, there needs to be sufficient incandescent lighting at eye level for persons who are sitting or walking, and there should be no areas of uneven lighting: for example, on stepping from a hallway into a room or vice versa or on walking up or down stairs. (B, N)[6]
6. Buildings should be designed with stairs and ramps that provide adequate visual and tactile cues about changes in elevation through proper placement of handrails and steps that have well-delineated edges. Patterned rugs and runners, in particular, create a problem by obliterating cues to the location of stair edges. These characteristics are described in more detail in chapter 18. (B, N/L)
7. Choose or modify chairs so the rear of the seat is not lower than the front, making it difficult to rise from a sitting position. Modify chairs by slightly shortening the front legs or raising the rear ones. Armchairs provide better leverage than do chairs without arms. Hiatt recommends that the so-called geriatric wheelchair be abandoned in hospitals and nursing homes as particularly conducive to improper posture. (B, N/L)[25]

8. Select or modify furniture and floor covering in housing and nursing homes for the elderly, or for younger persons with impairment, to limit the severity of any falls that might occur. (B, N/L)
9. Establish networking systems for elderly persons living alone to ensure that they can get prompt help in emergencies.

Thermal Injury

1. Limit water temperature in hot water heaters to 120°F (49°C). (B, N/L)
2. Provide meal preparation and other homemaker services for individuals with severe impairments for whom congregate or other special housing is not available. (B, F)
3. Recommend, or require by law, stoves with burner-control linkage systems that lessen likelihood of turning on the wrong burner[26] or of touching a hot burner that looks cool. (B, N/L)
4. Provide adequate lighting around stoves. (B, N/L)
5. Require use of low-energy matches that do not flare up and are self-extinguishing after a relatively limited brief period of time. (C, N)
6. Recommend, or require by law, flame-retardant materials for clothing, bedding, and upholstery. (B, N/L)
7. Recommend or require flame and smoke warning devices in housing for the elderly. (B, N/L) Such devices may need to be modified for individuals who have limited hearing.
8. Where possible, place the elderly in housing that affords easy exit in case of fire. (B, N)
9. Advise elderly persons about methods for clothing themselves properly, getting adequate calories, and insulating homes to reduce chances of hypothermia. Community assistance can be provided especially for home repairs. (B, L/F)

Poisoning

1. Physicians should periodically review with their older patients all medications being taken in order to reduce the number and the dosage to the minimum necessary. Patients should be advised to dispose of all medications that are not being used. (I, F)
2. Providers of health services should assist older patients with methods for organizing their medication doses in order to avoid confusion. This may be particularly helpful for individuals with early dementia. (I,F)

Other Injuries

With lesser strength and lesser stability while standing, older people are particularly likely to have trouble opening windows and doors and run the risk of serious lacerations. The recommendations for window and doorway design and construction in chapter 18 should be followed either voluntarily or under building code laws and regulations. (B, N/L)

Highway Injury

1. In order to protect elderly and medically impaired pedestrians the primary and ultimate goal, wherever feasible, is to promote transportation systems that adequately separate pedestrian and motor vehicle traffic. Where this is not feasible—and, unfortunately, in most places it is not—other options must be tried, as follows.
2. Provide pedestrian walk cycles at intersections that (a) occur at reasonable distances to discourage crossing between intersections, (b) stop all vehicular traffic that can conflict with pedestrians, (c) are of sufficient duration to permit easy crossing by elderly persons, (d) do not keep pedestrians waiting too long between cycles, and (e) carry both a visual and auditory signal to alert persons with limited vision when the walk cycle has started and is ending. (C, N)
3. Provide elderly persons with reflective material to be worn on or over their clothing and encourage them to wear this material when they leave their homes. (B, F)
4. For more severely disabled persons, limit the need for shopping and other excursions by arranging for someone to provide these services for them. Arrange for vehicular transporation for those occasions when they must leave the house for medical care or other visits. These activities can be arranged individually but probably can be done more effectively and efficiently through community-based organization. (B, F)
5. As noted before, the most effective methods for reducing frequency of crashes that result from driver error are systemwide measures, such as ergonomic approaches to vehicular and roadway design. (C, N) These are particularly important with the elderly because of lesser ability as an aspect of normative aging to read signs at night, respond to glare, and see even moderate distances ahead. The reason for this last problem is that the older population tends to be female and of small stature. Especially in smaller cars that now comprise a substantial portion of the vehicular population, short drivers cannot scan as much of the road ahead of them as can taller drivers or drivers in middle-size and larger cars. To date, the highway and

vehicular systems simply have not been made with the average older driver in mind. Dr. Milton Halpern, former medical examiner for New York City, pointed out that drivers who die suddenly while operating a vehicle are significantly more likely to do so within 500 feet of an on or off ramp than anywhere else, suggesting he said, that the stress of the task demands contributed to their deaths.[27]

6. In the absence of passive restraint devices, elderly (and all other) occupants of motor vehicles should be advised to wear their seatbelts for all driving. (B, F) Unfortunately, many seat belts are designed so that it is difficult at best for an older person, especially with arthritis, to reach the belt easily and attach it. Thus, it is least available to those at greatest risk of serious injury and death in a crash.
7. Depending on the political jurisdiction, either advice can be given to patients and their families concerning whether they should attempt to drive a motor vehicle and under what circumstances, or laws may actually exist which require reporting of persons with certain medical conditions to the motor vehicle administration so that they can be evaluated for licensing purposes. The remainder of this chapter will be concerned with this issue of driver evaluation and the resulting medical advice or administrative action.

Evaluating Medical Impairment to Driving

Primary responsibility for bringing a potential medical impairment to the attention of a licensing agency lies with the person who seeks to be licensed. The physician's primary responsibility is to the patient and family, although this must be tempered by a responsibility as well as to the broader community if the patient's actions are likely to endanger others.

Most physicians feel extremely uncomfortable—and frankly unqualified—to make an assessment whether or not a person is sufficiently impaired to present a hazard on the highway. They feel equally "caught in between" by the requirement in some areas to report all persons with certain medical conditions because they believe that most individuals who get reported will lose their licenses and that patients consequently may avoid seeking medical care for fear of being reported. The facts are that, at least in the United States, relatively few persons who are reported lose their licenses after evaluation[28] and those who are evaluated usually show subsequent improvement in crash experience but not in violations. Furthermore, I am not aware of any real cases—only theoretical arguments—of medical care avoided because of fear of being reported.

Two major reasons exist for the confusion regarding evaluation of patients. In the first place, when considering severity most physicians tend to think in terms of amount of pathology *already existing* to specific organs, or of quantitative laboratory measurements available, rather than in terms of how well a person is likely to function *in the future* over a two- or three-year licensing period and over the range of driving situations he or she will probably encounter. This includes ability to deal with busy intersections, merges, travel at night or in bad weather along unfamiliar and poorly marked roads, or travel at night or in busy areas where the driver must pick out vehicles, pedestrians, and traffic signals from a background of neon lights and other illuminated surfaces.

Little guidance is provided to the physician—or the motor vehicle agency—in making these decisions. Measures of functional ability used in the field of rehabilitation medicine make no mention of ability to drive an automobile, and if a person is able to drive, even with a two- or threefold increase in crash risk, he or she is considered to be in the highest category of functional ability. But the needs of the physician or the motor vehicle agency in advising or regulating a driver demand ability to separate persons who can drive without increase in crash risk from those who cannot do so.

The second reason for confusion lies in our attitudes and their reflection in public policy regarding the degree to which we are willing to accept crash risk and consequences in order to promote mobility. The public continuously demands that something be done to remove "bad drivers" from the roads. Yet we permit licensing of teenagers, who have the highest crash risk of all age groups, and as individuals we prepare our own teenage children to drive at the first moment that they may do so legally, and sometimes even before that moment.

The basic stated policy concerning persons with medical impairment is that they should not be permitted to drive if they have an appreciable increase in risk of crashing as a result of their conditions. Although I have seen no specific statement, it would appear that the regulation of driving by this group—and especially of persons with seizure disorders—often is based not on this criterion of avoiding *increased risk* but rather on the criterion of avoiding if at all possible *all crashes attributable to impairment*. I suspect the reason for this extreme cautiousness is a fear that motor vehicle agencies have of adverse publicity, law suits, or both if anyone who they have licensed with a known medical condition gets into trouble because of that condition. In practice, therefore, a concept of risk management by balancing risk versus mobility sometimes gets converted into absolute risk avoidance.

Probably a reasonable series of questions that can be asked is the following. First, will the individual be engaged in (1) specialized driving tasks, such as operation of a truck, bus, or emergency vehicle that require greater attention to the demands of the task and to the protection of the public, (2) usual operation of a passenger vehicle for personal use, in which there will be a combination of elective driving and of driving in which the time, location, or amount is not entirely under control of the individual, or (3) limited driving that is predominantly or entirely of an elective nature, as may occur with an older person who has retired?

Second, what is the probable capability of the individual *at present* to (1) make a prompt and accurate determination what is encroaching in the path of his or her vehicle, from what direction, and at what rate of speed (input variables), (2) make a timely and appropriate decision what to do about it (assessment), and (3) convert that assessment into timely and appropriate actions? Furthermore, what is the probable capability of doing this, not in usual driving—for those are not the circumstances under which most crashes occur—but rather in conflict situations, such as busy intersections and merge maneuvers, unfamiliar roads, poor visibility, or confusing visual cues noted above?

With these questions in mind, we will consider several medical conditions, potential impairment associated with them, and appropriate decisions for different types of driving tasks. In each case greatest stringency will be applied to those individuals who must perform specialized driving tasks, and in general the recommendations will be similar to those I have published previously.[29]

Static and Slowly Progressive Conditions

These include amputations, congenital abnormalities that affect mobility, deafness, and most forms of visual impairment that alter fields or acuity. The probable effect on driving capability of the static disorders of mobility can usually be determined with reasonable accuracy through driving tests either with or without special equipment. Wherever possible, this should be done in conjunction with a program in rehabilitation medicine or through the driver education program of a department of education, which have individuals specially trained and knowledgeable in such evaluations and in selection and proper use of special vehicle control equipment, some of which, unfortunately, has not been well designed or of good quality. In those nations where specific exclusionary levels do not exist for drivers of special vehicles such as trucks or buses, attention must be paid not only to ability to perform the driving task on the specific type of vehicle to be driven and without special equipment but also to ability to carry out other special activities, such as dealing with passengers or loading and unloading a vehicle safely.

Visual impairment, such as diplopia, severe nystagmus, large central scotoma, corrected visual acuity below 20/70, or narrowing of visual fields of less than 110 degrees total field, should preclude any driving. Ability to carry out special driving tasks should require binocular vision with fields of 140° or greater and visual acuity of 20/40 or better with correction.

In recent years, telescopic devices have been touted to provide greater visual acuity, but at the expense of extremely narrow visual fields, for persons with macular degeneration and similar disorders. The driver is supposed to switch back and forth while driving between use of the device for clarity and nonuse for breadth of vision. So far, the very limited and largely anecdotal data available on the results of licensing such drivers suggest that, once licensed, these individuals engage in very limited driving. Despite little driving, they appear to have average or somewhat above-average crash experience, with an excess of crashes implicating visual fields as a problem. My own opinion at this time is that the added mobility gained through driving with these devices is not worth the additional risk to the public.

For general driving, even total deafness is not a serious handicap provided persons with over 50 decibels of loss (corrected) at 2,000 cycles per second in best ear are limited to daytime driving and use of special mirrors. Persons with over 40 dB loss after correction probably should not drive one of the special-task vehicles.

Seizures

The usual recommendation is that driving not be permitted or recommended until a person is seizure free for at least a year, as a prognostic indicator that the condition is under control and that future seizures are unlikely. This is an appropriate decision if the goal is to avoid any crashes involving seizures. If, however, the goal is simply to prevent an unacceptable excess of crashes (and what is defined as an unacceptable excess may vary from one political jurisdiction to another), then this standard is probably too stringent.

One must look at the probabilities that a seizure will occur, that it will occur while the person is operating a motor vehicle, that the driver will lose control as a result, and that serious harm will ensue. In my opinion, the special driving tasks require availability of sufficient skill at all times and carry high enough risk of serious injury or death to many so that these special licenses should not be permitted for persons who have not been seizure free for at least five years, the last two of which have been without antiepileptic medication.

For the average person driving up to 10,000 to 15,000 miles annually, I am now of the opinion that driving can probably be permitted for persons who are still having grand mal seizures, provided they are occurring less than every six months and provided the dose of medication is not sufficient to cause probable impairment. Persons with long histories (several years) only of nocturnal (sleep) seizures can probably be permitted to drive even if seizures are occurring relatively frequently. While they may have greater risk of injury from falling out of bed, they can be expected to show no increase in crash risk as drivers.

If aura is always present, and especially if it is a long one, that should provide an additional leeway for avoiding a crash. I am still uncomfortable, however, about permitting driving by individuals who always have auras but who also have seizures more often than every six months because some driving situations just do not permit easy and safe stopping even with a fairly long warning. Therefore, I still recommend that aura not be used as a factor in determining licensure.

Very brief lapses—one or two seconds—probably should not preclude limited driving even if they occur a few times daily. Nor should partial seizures that affect only a part of the body that is not essential to vehicular operation. Driving is contraindicated with longer lapses.

Cardiovascular Diseases

These tend to occur in groups, or in combination with other diseases such as diabetes. Assessment of risk, therefore, should be based on an evaluation of the entire person, rather than a single organ system.[20,29] Increased crash risk in cardiac disease may result from subtle alterations in ability to cope with demanding driving situations because of dysrhythmias and decreased cardiac output or, probably less often, from incapacity from severe angina or infarction.

For usual driving it is reasonable to tolerate mild or brief episodes of angina, even if occurring several times a week. But it is wise to suggest that angina sufficient to cause even brief cessation of daily activities is incompatible with usual driving if attacks of this severity occur as often as monthly. Elderly persons and others who are able to control the time and circumstances of their driving could be permitted to drive with a history of such episodes as often as once weekly provided they are advised to avoid times of day and circumstances with high-density traffic and to drive only during daylight hours and for short distances (less than half hour driving periods).

Evidence of cardiac failure in the absence of angina is not sufficient to preclude usual driving unless there are relatively marked symptoms.

Persons with one-flight dyspnea should be urged to restrict their driving in the manner noted above, while those with symptoms at rest should be advised not to drive.

No limitations are imposed per se by use of a pacemaker or by hypertension. If severe headaches are occurring weekly or more often, these should preclude driving. Other complications of hypertension are evaluated both on their immediate individual effects on functioning and on the basis of a worse prognosis because of the presence of the hypertension.

The major concern with stroke is its effects on visual skills and judgment. A driver may compensate for a weak arm or leg through use of special control devices on the vehicle. There is no substitute, however, for limited ability to perceive and assess traffic flow or to make and carry out appropriate judgments. These are complex areas of patient evaluation and require the assistance of specialists and staff in rehabilitation medicine. Persons with residua of stroke should be advised to limit their driving to the low-risk circumstances noted earlier.

The specialized driving tasks, of course, have more rigid requirements. No person who has had two or more strokes or heart attacks, even though subsequently symptom free, or who has any residual signs or symptoms following an initial stroke or heart attack should be permitted to drive a commercial vehicle. Nor should he drive such a vehicle if he has one-flight dyspnea, signs of congestive failure, or hypertension with any history of cerebrovascular damage, left ventricular hypertrophy, hypertensive retinal changes (Keith-Wagner retinopathy) stage II or greater, or proteinuria or abnormalities in urinary sediment.

Diabetes Mellitus

Mild hypoglycemic reactions that can be quickly aborted with carbohydrates are not incompatible with usual driving if they occur less often than weekly. On the other hand, reactions that are severe enough to interfere with usual activities even briefly are incompatible if they occur more often than once every six months. Because of the risk involved, persons with diabetes who require insulin should not be permitted to do specialized driving tasks. The cardiovascular and visual changes accompanying diabetes should be evaluated using the criteria already noted for driving with these conditions.

Senile Dementia and Other Disorders of Memory and Judgment

Among younger persons, schizophrenia, severe depression, and what are now called antisocial personality disorders (formerly, psychopathic personality patterns) are probably the most important disorders of judgment with potential relevance to safety. Among older persons, attention turns to the senile dementias, especially of the Alzheimer's type (SDAT).

Criteria for advice to or regulation of such drivers are hard to come by, perhaps being easiest for the specialized driving tasks. Such specialized driving is not considered appropriate for persons with two or more commitments to a mental institution or for persons who continue to require psychoactive drugs for more than three months after a single hospitalization or course of psychotherapy. An exception can be made if there had been excellent recovery since then, with no residual disability in coping, and at least two or three years have elapsed since last use of these medications. During the acute and early recovery phases of depression requiring medical attention, patients involved in such specialized driving tasks should also be disuaded from these activities.

Regarding usual driving activities, heavy dependence on psychoactive drugs is often sufficiently impairing in itself to recommend advice against driving. Persons who are actively hallucinating should also be disuaded or prevented from driving. Of particular concern are individuals with a history of acting out either violently or by jumping into their cars and driving when upset. Often, these are also the individuals most likely to use alcohol excessively when upset. Advice clearly is warranted, but unfortunately these people usually do not come first to the attention of health care providers, or if they do, they ignore the advice. They usually are known first to the police and motor vehicle agencies and only later are brought to medical care for the injuries they cause themselves and others.

Such is generally not the case with persons who have early senile dementia. These older individuals usually are under regular medical care, and they, their families, or both are usually receptive to medical advice. The more difficult question is what advice should be given.

Early dementia usually is not known to the physician until the individual or the family begins to complain of increasing frequency of brief memory losses, occasional episodes of confusion, driving the wrong way up a one-way street, or similar unexplicable behavior. The first sign may be an episode of "sundowning," or confusion on hospitalization for another unrelated illness. This is more likely to occur at night, and nurses should be advised to include such episodes, no matter how brief, in their nursing notes and to report them to the physician.

The patient may seem quite competent on superficial questioning in these early stages. Psychological testing, however, will often provide the correct diagnosis, even at this early date. If the episodes are relatively infrequent, the individual should be advised not to drive at night and to avoid more demanding times of day and types of roads. Using this approach, it may be possible to permit the person an additional two or three years of relatively risk-free driving. Even at these early stages, however, specialized driving tasks are no longer recommended.

If even a single crash or near crash results, however, that appears to be attributable to improper input or processing of traffic information, the individual should be advised—or compelled, if necessary—to stop driving entirely. The reasoning for such a stringent requirement is that the condition usually is progressive and the reported misadventures commonly turn out in retrospect to be only the tip of the iceberg.

After families have complained about erratic driving behavior, motor vehicle agencies then often give the person a driving test to determine ability to drive. But because the condition may vary from day to day, there is a fairly good chance that a single driving test will not uncover impairment that is occurring even a fair percentage of the time. Therefore, greatest attention should be paid to history from family members and to psychological tests rather than to successful completion of a single driving test.

31
Use of Alcohol and Other Drugs

> Make not thyself helpless in drinking in the beer shop. For will not the words of thy report repeated slip out from thy mouth without thy knowing that thou hast uttered them?
>
> Falling down thy limbs will be broken, and no one will give thee a hand to help thee up.
>
> As for thy companions in the swilling of beer, they will get up and say, "Outside with this drunkard."
>
> Egyptian papyrus

The drug, ethyl alcohol, has been known since antiquity and has been a subject of concern since then, as evidenced by the above Egyptian papyrus,[1] and a Hebrew blessing over wine that begins with a warning about the dangers of excessive consumption.[2] We will begin by briefly reviewing the metabolism and physiologic effects of this drug that increase injury risk. This will be followed by examination of other factors that affect risk and by consideration of possible countermeasures.

Metabolic and Physiologic Factors Increasing Injury Risk

After ingestion, alcohol is absorbed rapidly through the stomach and is distributed widely throughout the body. The greater the concentration of alcohol in the drink the more rapid the absorption.[3] Thus, a "straight shot" of 80- to 100-proof drink (40 to 50 percent alcohol) enters the blood stream more rapidly than does the same amount of alcohol ingested as a 5 percent solution diluted by water, soda, or the components of beer. Many people erroneously believe that beer causes less impairment and intoxication than does hard liquor, and some areas permit sale and advertisement of beer but not of hard liquor. The amount of alcohol in a standard drink—a 12-ounce bottle of 4 percent beer, a 5- to 6-oz glass of table wine, a 1-oz shot of 100-proof liquor, and a 1½-oz shot of 80-proof liquor—is about the same. Because the beer and wine are absorbed somewhat more slowly, the peak BACs with these drinks are slightly lower than for more concentrated drinks. But the difference is usually not enough to be of importance from the viewpoint of safety, and all alcoholic beverages should be viewed with equal caution.

Most alcoholic drinks contain small amounts of other materials called congeners. These are fusel oils, longer-chain alcohols, aldehydes, and esters. They are absorbed at the same rate as the ethyl alcohol and probably do not affect acute impairment significantly, but they may add to the severity of the hangover.

The amount of food in the stomach at the time alcohol reaches this organ also has an important effect on the rate of absorption.[3] Food eaten shortly before consumption of alcohol reduces the peak BAC by as much as a third. Food taken at the same time as the alcohol is associated with about a 25 percent reduction in peak BAC. Food taken even immediately after drinking, however, has no effect. Modest effects on distribution of alcohol and resultant peak BAC are related to amount of body fat (and consequently to gender).

Alcohol is detoxified predominantly through the liver. On the average, the rate of metabolism is about 0.015 percent of alcohol by weight per hour (15 mg per 100 ml), which is the rough equivalent to one standard drink per hour. It may be somewhat faster (up to 0.025 percent per hour) for persons who are usual heavy drinkers. This apparent advantage for the heavy drinker, however, is usually more than overwhelmed by much greater hourly and total consumption. Since other drugs, such as barbituates and tranquilizers, may use similar metabolic pathways, presence of these drugs in the body may slow the rate of alcohol detoxification, just as presence of alcohol may slow detoxification of the other drugs. Various solvents used in industry may have similar effect. Less than 5 percent is excreted without detoxification, predominantly through breath, urine, and skin.

Physiologic effects involve not only neurologic function but also the gastrointestinal system, prostate, and so forth. Most people think first of delayed reaction time as the major physiologic effect that increases injury risk. This is a rather late effect, seen only at higher BACs. While there is no way to state precisely which physiologic impairments contribute to which injury events, it is probable that other impairments play a more important role than does delayed reaction time.

Significant alteration of judgment begins to occur with the equivalent of only one or two drinks (under 0.05 percent BAC). In one study, bus drivers at 0.04 percent BAC were willing to drive their buses through a space that was as much as 12 inches narrower than the bus itself and were less capable than drivers without alcohol of accomplishing the task even if the space was wide enough to go through.[4]

Mood also is affected early, which is perhaps the major reason why we use alcohol. For years, the "loosening up" or loss of inhibition noted with small amounts of alcohol has been attributed by researchers to depression of higher brain centers that inhibit unsocial behavior rather than to stimulation of certain centers. Gitlow,[5] however, states that there is simultaneously a brief (two to three hour) rather substantial depressive effect and a far longer (ten to twelve hour) low-level stimulation effect. He attributes the wide-awake, nervous feeling that occurs several hours after drinking to this latter effect. Be that as it may, some people become happy, others sad, some withdraw into themselves, and others become belligerent and aggressive after consuming alcohol. Precisely what decides who acts in what way is not known, but the pattern seems to be fairly stable within individuals.

Also affected rather early is ability to maintain attention. Barmack and Payne[6] noted that drivers with alcohol in crashes very often described their surprise upon seeing an obstacle or other vehicle that "suddenly" appeared. These lapses of attention result in reduced ability to maintain proper visual search. Also affecting visual search is the fact that visual ability itself decreases in several ways. There is narrowing of visual fields, decreased glare resistance, and lesser visual acuity in dim light. Coordination and ability to do problem solving decrease at slightly higher BACs (about 0.05 percent).[3]

While some abilities do not show early impairment if tested alone, these same functions may be affected at rather low concentrations if one attempts to perform two tasks simultaneously. Thus, a driver may be able either to track a vehicle without weaving or to pay attention to all stop signals if each of these is the only task to be carried out. If he has to pay attention to both tracking and traffic lights, however, ability to perform one or the other or both decreases substantially.[7]

Also noted in previous chapters is the growing body of experimental evidence that alcohol may play a role during the injury phase in increasing tissue sensitivity to injury. Some of the possible explanations for this phenomenon are a greater bleeding tendency, altered blood vessel fragility, edema of brain and other neurologic tissues, and altered intracellular chemistry.

All of the above effects except increased tissue sensitivity may be modified by variables other than BAC per se. In 1874 it was noted that the amount of impairment at any given BAC is greater if the BAC is in the process of rising than if it is in the process of falling,[8] and the more rapid the rise the greater the impairment at a given BAC. This phenomenon was subsequently named the Mellanby phenomenon based on work done in 1919. Other mind-altering drugs may act additively or synergistically with alcohol to increase impairment.

It is essential to distinguish between the two terms *intoxication* and *impairment*. The former refers to the obvious appearance of alcohol effects, such as swaying, inability to walk a straight line, to stand on one leg, or to touch finger to nose with eyes closed. Other effects include slurred speech, watery eyes, disheveled clothes, broken conversation, and labile mood. Impairment means reduced ability to function at specific mental tasks *whether or not the above signs are present.*

Nowhere is the distinction between intoxication and impairment clearer than in a study carried out by the Royal Canadian Mounted Police of the ability to drive through a "gymkhana" course at various BACs.[9] In that study a physician identified sixty drivers whose driving he observed to be clearly impaired. All except two had BACs of 0.10 percent or greater. On standard clinical examination, however, he was able to identify only about 60 percent of these impaired drivers as intoxicated, and another physician who had not observed their driving found only a third to be intoxicated.

Goldberg[10] examined occasional, moderate, and heavy drinkers for objective signs of impairment to several tests of vision, coordination, and problem solving. At BACs of 0.05 percent or lower many of the occasional drinkers, few of the moderate drinkers, but none of the heavy ones showed significant impairment. At BACs between 0.05 percent and 0.10 percent all occasional drinkers, most moderate ones, and up to half of heavy ones showed impairment. But above 0.10 percent all the heavy drinkers as well showed wide ranging impairment. *There is thus clear and consistent evidence that significant impairment occurs even in heavy drinkers in the absence of intoxication.*

In many U.S. studies light drinking is defined as a modal quantity of one to two drinks per sitting, medium drinking as three to four drinks, and heavy drinking as five or more drinks per sitting. Teenagers, young adults, and elderly persons appear to get into trouble at lower BACs than do middle-age persons.[11,12] It is not clear whether among the young this reflects age per se or the fact that these young individuals generally have less experience with heavy drinking and with learned physiologic responses than do older persons.

Other Factors Affecting Injury Risk

Almost all studies of pre-injury phase risk according to BAC have been carried out in the highway setting. These show that, except for teenagers, there is no increase in risk at BACs below 0.05 percent. By the time 0.08 percent is reached there is a two- to threefold increase in risk of crashing. At 0.10 percent it has risen to six to eight times that of drivers with no alcohol, and by 0.15 percent the risk exceeds twenty-five times that of the nonalcoholic driver[13] and may be as high as forty times greater.

We have repeatedly noted also the effects of environmental factors. Drivers in heavy traffic, for example, show increase in crash risk at lower BACs than do those in less crowded circumstances,[14] and drivers generally do not wander off the road on straight stretches but rather on sharp curves, hills, or combinations of these more difficult driving tasks.[15] In the social environment we also noted that the alcoholic worker may be protected from injury by the actions of supervisors and other workers. Questions have been raised about the extent to which peer interaction among alcohol-impaired teenagers in an automobile or a swimming hole may serve to increase risk of inappropriate behavior such as excessive speed or swimming in unsafe locations or in unsafe ways. Nothing more than conjecture exists for these questions, however.

As noted earlier, people respond in different ways to the effects of alcohol as a mood modifier. Some evidence indicates that individuals with highway and certain alcohol-related injuries more often have previous histories of deliberate violence than do persons without injury.[16] Consequently, it has been suggested—but not yet definitively demonstrated—that the alcohol users most likely to be involved in injury events are not only those who are heavy frequent users but particularly those who tend to act out aggressively when they drink too much. Apparently acting to decrease risk are those tasks that are sufficiently simple and repetitive so that individuals can overlearn and thus perform effectively even while "under the influence."

In the injury phase we have already examined the question of increased risk of injury because of greater tissue sensitivity to damage. Also increasing severity is confusion among alcohol-impaired persons that affects ability to escape from a fire or car stalled on railroad tracks or a car or boat that has just become submerged in a body of water. The fact that heavy drinkers tend to be heavy smokers and thus have elevated carboxyhemoglobin levels may also compromise survivability from injuries involving blood loss or hypoxia.

In the post-injury phase several factors again work to the detriment of the person injured while impaired by alcohol. Because such injuries are likely to occur at night and on weekends, there may be delays in discovery and reduced availability and adequacy of emergency medical services, or both. Suspicion has existed that heavy drinkers are likely to postpone seeking medical care because, in their drunken stupor, they often are totally unaware of or underestimate the severity of their injuries. While anecdotes abound on this subject, however, the frequency with which such delay occurs, or the degree to which it affects ultimate outcome, are unknown.

Once medical care has been obtained, diagnosis of head and other injuries may be more difficult because of the effect of alcohol on sensorium. Furthermore, health workers may show considerable lack of patience with the intoxicated patient, who is sometimes outrageously noncooperative and belligerent. Finally, even if all of these obstacles have been overcome, medical personnel must remain alert to altered response to anesthetics and other drugs because of liver failure in the alcoholic, and to delerium tremens and delayed life-threatening withdrawal symptoms from barbituates and tranquilizers to which the alcoholic often is also addicted.

Countermeasures

Throughout this book we have considered, and urged that highest priority be given to, many specific countermeasures involving environmental modification that have profound implications for pre-injury and injury-phase benefits to all populations, including persons impaired by alcohol. These measures generally require intervention and action at the community level and, as such, are not usually considered by most health practitioners as the areas for direct activity on their part. This is unfortunate. The public and legislators still consider health professionals to be a highly creditable source of health and safety information and advice. Failure by health professionals to inform themselves and to provide such information and advice is abrogation of an important area in which they can and should be useful.

Included in the community-based environmental measures are efforts to reduce energy levels in specific types of activities, to apply principles and methods of ergonomics to transportation, home, recreational, and occupational activities, and to modify the energy-transfer phase through processes that decrease flammability, improve equipment guarding, provide better packaging for vehicle occupants, or alter the injury potential of home, recreational, and occupational tools and products. To date, and for the foreseeable future, these countermeasures appear to be the most effective approach for injuries involving alcohol.

Turning to behavioral countermeasures, a wide variety of community-based legal and regulatory efforts have also been undertaken. These include prohibition of the manufacture and sale of alcohol, or limitation of its use to specific types (such as beer), age groups, locations, time of day, or packaging (for example, sale only by the drink or establishment of package clubs in which individuals bring their own bottles). Generally, these countermeasures have not been evaluated or have been evaluated using inappropriate research methods. Little can be said, therefore, about their worth or effectiveness. There certainly is strong evidence that prohibition was not successful in the United States in preventing alcohol consumption, often in large quantity, and there is some evidence that it was not successful as an injury countermeasure either. Recent work suggests that increasing the minimum age for alcohol consumption from age 18 to 21 in the United States does reduce the highway injury rate in this age group.[17] Availability of fewer places to drink in a given geographic area is associated with higher crash fatality rates, presumably because people must drive further while impaired to get home.[18]

Laws concerning driving after alcohol consumption seem to be most successful if the high-risk segment of the public perceives a high likelihood of apprehension and punishment.[19] This has been shown to be more important in altering behavior than is increased severity of punishment.[19] As purveyors of information to legislators and the public, physicians and other health professionals need to emphasize this fact.

Education of the general public about specific aspects of alcohol and safety does seem to be worthwhile, based on studies that have identified areas about which the public is not knowledgeable and that have further shown that educational efforts can increase knowledge.[20] The studies, however, do not necessarily show that increased knowledge leads to safer actions or reduced frequency of injury. These areas of education include the following types of information:

1. The fact that a typical drink of beer or wine has as much alcohol as does a typical drink of hard liquor.
2. The fact that it takes about an hour to metabolize a single drink.
3. How much alcohol is likely to cause impairment, an illegal BAC, or both in a person. This information must simultaneously be easy to understand, considered reasonable by the high-risk segments of the population, and widely applicable to high-risk persons of different weights and sexes. In the United States, beer is the preferred beverage for a large segment of the high-risk population, and it is generally consumed by that population in multiples of the six-pack. Based on the 12-ounce bottle containing 4 percent alcohol, the average-size male would be approaching or at a BAC of 0.10 percent with one six-pack. An easy and relatively accurate message for this population, therefore, would be that a six-pack is too much for safety. Of course, in nations where the bottle is a liter in size, or where the alcohol concentration is higher, the message would need appropriate modification.
4. How one identifies who has an alcohol problem, and what should be done if there is suspicion that a problem does exist.

All of the above educational efforts can be applied at both the individual and community level. Unfortunately, all require frequent application by the population at risk of injury, thus limiting overall effectiveness.

We turn finally to perhaps the most important area of behavioral intervention for health and safety professionals. Substantial evidence exists from studies in a number of Western nations that the majority—and probably a substantial majority—of persons injured after consumption of alcohol are not simply social drinkers but rather have been in trouble previously because of alcohol and can be diagnosed as problem drinkers and alcoholics.[21,22,23] (So little data are available from Moslem nations about either the use of alcohol among the injured or characteristics of users that at this point it is impossible to know whether or not this assessment is applicable to those nations as well.)

The questions for the health and safety professions, therefore, are (1) the extent to which such individuals are identifiable in the course of treatment of injuries or, preferably, sooner; (2) what can be done to confront them with the correct diagnosis and to ensure that treatment will be initiated and completed; (3) what methods of treatment are warranted; and (4) what are reasonable expectations for success?

Without attempting to cover in depth a very large, often frustrating and extremely muddy field, several comments can be made about which many—but not all—experts on this subject would probably agree.

1. Alcoholism usually is defined as a condition characterized by frequent, excessive drinking sufficient to cause adverse health, social, or economic consequences. Some definitions also refer to a compulsive pattern of consumption. As a condition described by its manifestations rather than its causes, it is probable that what is called alcoholism is really a group of conditions that have similar manifestations but diverse causes. Furthermore, two or more causes may be at work in determining the illness of a single individual.

2. The diagnosis that a drinking problem exists has been one of the stumbling blocks for health workers, both because they often either fail to determine or else overlook either the presence or amount of alcohol in the injured and because even if alcohol is identified, they are loath to label a person as alcoholic.

If injury occurs in evening or nighttime hours in an adult, the chances are greater than even—and often considerably greater—that the person has been drinking. Thus, if only for management purposes, all adults injured at this time should have BAC determinations. Furthermore, no matter when they occur, single-vehicle crashes, drownings, and burns involve alcohol often enough so that BAC determinations should be undertaken in these cases also.

In the United States in recent years a BAC of 0.15 percent or greater has been utilized as a presumptive or screening level suggesting that a drinking problem is likely to exist and should be carefully sought. In 1972 the National Council on Alcoholism published guideline criteria for the definitive diagnosis of alcoholism.[24,25] According to these criteria—which are strongly recommended to the reader—a BAC of 0.30 percent or higher is adequate per se for an obligatory diagnosis of alcoholism, *as is a BAC above 0.15 percent without gross evidence of intoxication.*

A diagnosis of alcoholism does not depend on the individual being on skid row, since over 95 percent of alcoholics are not on skid row. Nor does it depend on the person always having a positive BAC, since many alcoholics drink or drink heavily only on weekends, or even less often. The Mortimer-Filkins test[26] and the Michigan Alcoholism Screening Test (MAST)[26] are also frequently used to assist in making a diagnosis.

3. Another stumbling block to treatment in those nations where fee-for-service patterns prevail is an assumption by physicians that they will not be paid by their alcoholic patients. This assumption has been directly refuted by Dr. Stanley Evans, an internist in Bangor, Maine, who treats many alcoholics and their families. He reports (personal communication) that the likelihood of being paid is a direct reflection of the attitudes and expectations of the treating physician. His own approach is to state that (a) treatment will require visits that are longer than usual visits to an internist, (b) he is willing to spend this greater amount of time with the patient and family, (c) his fees are based on the amount of time spent, and (d) his expectation is that he will be paid if the patient agrees to undertake treatment.

A recent trial program in California shows that when insurance companies are willing to reimburse a fair amount of in-patient and ambulatory care specifically for alcoholism, the subsequent overall costs of health care for both the alcoholic and his or her family drop spectacularly to levels similar to that of the rest of the population.[27] It is thus to the financial advantage of insurance programs to include reimbursement of treatment for alcoholism.

4. There is provocative evidence suggesting that with only minimal intervention, problem drinking and alcoholism may be a self-limited or reversible condition in some people, and perhaps in even a large number of persons.[28,31] Some of these persons do not stop drinking entirely but rather return to normative (light to medium) social drinking from a previous pattern of heavy drinking and increasingly deleterious consequences.

A few studies have documented that perhaps 5 to 10 percent of properly diagnosed alcoholics return to social drinking without further trouble.[25–31] These studies have been ferociously attacked by most members of the treatment community as heretical and dangerous. However, work by Cahalan et al.[32,33] shows that there is a peak of alcohol-related problems among persons in their twenties, with a substantial decrease in problems, but not in drinkers, in the decades immediately following.

Another study points to the fact that the cumulative incidence of new cases of alcoholism coming for treatment does not continue to rise continuously, as would be anticipated if it followed a typical pattern of progressive diseases.[34] Rather, it tapers off in about the sixth decade, suggesting a burnout phenomenon similar to what is seen with other drug addictions and with schizophrenia.

It is not clear how this reversal of problem patterns comes about. One possibility that fits within the concept of crisis intervention as a therapeutic approach[35] is that many problem drinkers and early alcoholics may in fact reach a health, economic, or social crisis that forces a decision. If the appropriate medical or other intervener is available and ready to act, such persons may be able to reverse the process with relatively minimal professional assistance.

Regarding the return by bona fide alcoholics to social drinking, one must distinguish between what actually happens in some cases and what sort of therapeutic guidance should be provided. There can be no question but that some individuals—even with profound alcoholism—do successfully go back to social drinking, just as there can be no question but that some individuals with well-documented untreated neoplasms have complete and total remission of their cancers. To suggest, however, that one should permit a person who has had an alcohol problem to try social drinking is as foolish as to suggest that cancers do not need early and rigorous treatment. But it is equally foolish to suggest that the phenomenon doesn't and can't exist just because it runs contrary to what should be recommended in wise medical practice.

5. Since alcoholism probably has at least several major etiologies, it follows that even if treatment is quite successful for each of the etiologies, no single method of treatment is likely to be successful for a majority of cases. The partial success of several different treatment modalities, but the absence of substantial success for any single one, therefore, may reflect our current inability to link the different etiologic routes to specific individuals who are being treated. While this means that a particular treatment mode that is chosen might not work in a specific patient, it also means that there is reasonable chance that another mode might work after the first one has failed or that combined modes might have greater chances for success.

6. Also not realized by many health professionals is that the rehabilitation process for the typical person with alcoholism takes up to approximately two years. Because they don't realize this, many health professionals are at first overly optimistic about chances for success and the speed with which it will occur. When relapse occurs after several

months—as it often does—they then become overly pessimistic, instead of realizing that they need both to consider several treatment modes and to allow enough time—as much as two years—for treatment to have its full effect.

7. The only place where rehabilitation of problem drinkers and alcoholics is being attempted as a safety measure is in the field of highway safety. At least in part as a result of my own work, there have been rather widespread efforts—often unevaluated or inadequately evaluated—throughout the United States to determine which persons arrested for driving while under the influence of liquor (DUIL or DWI) are alcoholics or prealcoholics and to refer them to treatment.

The effectiveness of these programs in preventing recidivism has been varied, in some cases rather successful, but in other cases no better and probably less effective than is suspension of the driver's license for several months.[26,36] Although originally one of the major advocates of such legal/medical system linkage, I have become one of the critics of the way it has been carried out because key components of the concept and method have been ignored.

As noted in chapter 26, it has been suggested that the process of confrontation, plus the ability to maintain close surveillance of and control over the alcoholic are key factors in the success of alcoholism treatment programs in the occupational setting.[27] The concept of crisis intervention as a psychiatric tool is that, when in acute crisis, an individual is both more receptive to accepting help and is more likely to benefit from a relatively minimal amount of knowledgeable intervention than he or she is after the immediate crisis has passed.

If a DWI arrest and conviction can be looked upon as a period of crisis in the life of the alcoholic individual, then knowledgeable intervention should have relatively greater chance for success *if the individual can be kept feeling that a crisis continues to exist during key early phases of the intervention process.*

It is well known that alcoholics very rapidly lose motivation until a certain amount of treatment has occurred unless the pressure can be kept on them, as occurs in industrial treatment programs with the confrontation and surveillance process and continued threat of job loss if treatment isn't completed. The original concept of legal/medical linkage for highway safety was to revoke or suspend the license of the person for DWI and not to return it until he or she is able to show that treatment has been followed and is succeeding. This is permitted in the United States under state laws and regulations that control licensing of persons with untreated medical conditions that are potentially hazardous to driving.

Instead of utilizing this carrot and stick approach, however, most rehabilitation programs have offered treatment in lieu of suspension or revocation, thus removing the critical crisis atmosphere and negating the treatment modality. Furthermore, the "treatment" that is offered very often is simply a series of classes on the effects of alcohol rather than a therapeutic program that is designed and carried out in accordance with what is known about alcoholism. In my opinion, the original crisis-intervention concept still has not been put to the test. This needs to be done before any conclusion can be reached about the effectiveness of rehabiliation for purposes of highway safety.

Other Drugs

In comparison to alcohol, rather little of a definitive nature can be said about the effects on safety of other drugs. The only exception is the role of drugs in falls among the elderly, an issue that has already been discussed in the preceding chapter.

Two types of situations need to be considered. The first involves individuals who are using drugs for therapeutic purposes. Such individuals may have (1) reduction in injury risk because of the beneficial effects of these drugs in reducing anxiety, angina, diabetic seizures, coma, problems of mobility associated with Parkinsonism, and so forth, (2) increase in injury risk because of soporific or other impairing effects of tranquilizers, insulin reactions, or other effects on sensorium, vision, or coordination, (3) no safety-related effect one way or the other, or, as in the case of severe seizure patterns, continued high injury risk despite treatment.

At present there is no evidence *overall* that therapeutic use of drugs is associated with increase of injury risk.[37,38] But an average effect may hide the fact that all three of the above phenomena may be occurring and overall may balance each other out. The onus falls on the health worker to assess whether a given drug is likely to reduce injury risk or to increase it in a given individual, and in the latter case to decide whether other beneficial effects outweigh this particular complication.

The second type of situation involves illicit use of drugs, such as amphetamines, cannabinols, opiates, and tranquilizers. Laboratory data indicate that some of these drugs often do have capability for causing impairment believed relevant to safety.[37,38] Occasional anecdotes of crashes involving drivers who are clearly impaired by drugs other than alcohol provide some support for these data.

But laboratory analyses of fatally injured drivers in the United States do not find very large proportions of persons with these or any other drugs, especially if one searches for their presence without the simultaneous presence of a high BAC.[37] No comparison samples are available of drugs in drivers not involved in crashes, but attempts to estimate what proportion of the general population of drivers are likely to have such drugs do not come up with figures that are substantially different from what is found in the fatalities.

Some studies suggest that illicit users of certain drugs, whether licit or illicit, have higher crash or citation rates or greater culpability in crashes than do nonusers.[39,40,41] Illicit use is often closely linked both to youth and to other specific attitudes and behaviors concerning society in general, while use of licit drugs may be for conditions that per se increase crash risk. It is not possible, therefore, to state whether any observed increase in highway or other injuries among such persons is a reflection of the effects of the drug per se, of characteristics of the person who uses it, or of the interaction between these two.[39,40,42]

The above comments suggest that in Western nations—where illicit drugs available on the street tend to be adulterated and weak—there is *in general* no appreciable increase in injury risk. It is not meant to suggest, however, that a similar absence of increased risk would also be found in nations or areas where the strength of such drugs is consistently greater. Currently there are insufficient data to argue strongly one way or the other.

What countermeasures are appropriate, given the above information (or, more appropriately, lack of information)? The data do not appear to urge that extensive programming is warranted *in the name of safety*. (It might, however, be warranted for other reasons that are more compelling.) In my opinion, the best approach from the viewpoint of safety, given the above data, is to promote the general ergonomic and other environmental countermeasures recommended under the alcohol-injury countermeasures. Educational approaches to counter illicit drug use appear to be only minimally effective, as do legal approaches and treatment programs. They do not deserve high priority for the purposes of promoting safety.

32
Injury Control and the Health Professional: Preparation for the Future

The ultimate question of this book is whether there can be any consistent way of providing the next generation of health and safety professionals with a more sophisticated view of injury control than past and current generations have had. Programs ranging from one or two hours up to several hours have been given in at least some medical schools in the United States but have generally been limited to traffic safety or poison ingestion as a problem among children.

It is my feeling that a different approach is needed that is brief enough to fit comfortably within the invariably tight curriculum of professional schools but also recognizes that injury control is not the only subject area slighted in such education. Several other subjects essential to understanding injury and its control also are poorly covered, and the inadequate understanding provided for each of these areas adds to the failure to understand the origin and control of trauma as well. These subjects are aging, alcohol abuse, forensic pathology, emergency medical care, occupational medicine, and rehabilitative medicine.

In similar manner, any discussion of injury control that is limited only to highway injury misses out on the possibility to link common human, environmental, and countermeasure issues that are applicable both to injury on the highway and in other activities. Besides relating injury issues to the broader practice of health care—whether it be medicine, nursing, physical or occupational therapy or other helping fields—it is also important that emphasis be placed on providing the same base of scientific conceptualization, data gathering, data testing, and synthesis of information from several sources into a feasible treatment plan. These are the same steps that are seen as relevant and essential in all other fields of health-care endeavor and all other courses in the health-care curricula.

Various courses in emergency medicine have been proposed for medical students and nurses.[1,2,3] Where possible, it is preferable that a program in injury control be given in addition to such courses. The curriculum proposed below, however, is based on an assumption that it might be possible to get twenty hours to cover both subject areas rather than a larger block of time to do each individually. This proposal draws extensively on a paper presented before the American Association for Automotive Medicine.[4] Briefly stated, the twenty hours are divided as follows:

1. introductory statistics and concepts (1 hr);
2. understanding and dealing with human factors (3 hrs);
3. environmental factors in the pre-injury phase (1 hr);
4. environmental factors in the injury phase (2 hrs);
5. the post-injury phase and training in emergency care (11 hrs); and
6. integrative exercises on highway and nonhighway injury events (2 hrs).

A more detailed description of each of these areas is given below.

Introductory Statistics and Concepts

Students should become familiar with the size of the injury problem in their particular country and its relationship to other health problems and should know its distribution according to type of event, age, sex, race, marital status, and place of residence. They should also be aware of factors that make so many injury data inaccurate. They must become familiar with modern concepts of injury occurrence, such as those promulgated by Haddon, Benner, and systems analysis specialists and described in chapter 3. Finally, in order to better understand the application of these concepts and to avoid provincialism, they should be exposed to comparative data from some other areas of the world and to possible explanations for differences that might exist.

Understanding and Dealing with Human Factors

Four broad subject areas can be identified here. First is the physiological and psychological limitations that people have at different stages of development. This includes youth, aging, learning processes, and various issues dealt with by human-factor specialists or ergonomists.

Second is temporary or permanent limitation of functions of information input, processing, and response brought about by various chronic medical conditions and rehabilitation strategies to prevent such limitation or reduce its effects on ability to perform activities of daily living.

Closely related is the subject of sociological, physiological, and medical factors in use of alcohol and other drugs, their effects upon safety in highway and nonhighway settings, the rationale of strategies to prevent or ameliorate the problem, and what is known about their success.

Finally, these three areas need to be integrated in a form useful to physicians and other health professionals with a discussion of patient and family counseling, legal issues related to impairment and safety, and how to interface with agencies such as departments of motor vehicles, Federal Aviation Agency, the Bureau of Motor Carrier Safety, social welfare agencies, industry management and unions, or their equivalents in the particular country where the course is being taught. Regarding what the physician can do in the area of patient counseling, the American Hospital Association has produced an excellent film called *Cause the Effect: Effect the Cause* that deals with the reactions of professional staff to an alcoholic patient in an emergency department and with their role in crisis intervention. This film would add substantially to student understanding of some of the issues involving alcohol and safety.

Environmental Factors in the Pre-Injury Phase

Building on what students have learned about physiological, psychological, and sociological frameworks of human behavior, they now need to integrate information about how the environment interacts with the human either to promote or reduce the degree of hazard in various everyday situations. At this point students should be introduced to the goals, methods, and limitations of national or regional agencies such as, in the United States, the Consumer Product Safety Commission (CPSC) and the Department of Transportation's (DOT's) strategies and standards in the precrash area. They should also learn what contribution they as practicing health professionals might make, either in alerting authorities to new environmental hazards or in helping to reduce those hazards that already are known to exist.

Environmental Factors in the Injury Phase

Here we touch upon several areas that, surprisingly, are totally unexplored in medical school or other professional programs. How long does it take and what happens during successive milliseconds of the injury event, whether we are talking about a crash or a thermal injury? What do we know about human thresholds to injury and what affects them?

What methods of injury scaling exist, how are they used, and what are the effects of different scaling philosophies and results of using, for example, the CPSC scale, and the Abbreviated Injury Scale and Injury Severity Score? Finally, how does crash investigation occur, with particular attention to the role of forensic pathology and of complete autopsies, including examination of head and neck, microscopic examination, testing for alcohol and other drugs, and actual examination at the scene of the causes of injury?

Prevention and amelioration strategies in the injury phase should be reviewed. This should be structured around steps 4 to 8 in Haddon's "Escape of Tigers" paper.[5] Coming out of this should be a description of the role that the individual physician or other health professional can play in affecting the injury phase. Here, too, useful films exist, such as *In the Crash,* produced by the Insurance Institute for Highway Safety in Washington, D.C.

Post-Injury Phase and Training in Emergency Care

This portion of the curriculum includes both general knowledge about issues in emergency care and specific training in skills that all medical and nursing school graduates should have. An hour should be devoted to what is known about inadequate emergency care as a cause of unnecessary death and disability, concepts and programs of emergency care organization in the prehospital and hospital settings, introduction to categorization of hospitals and other standards in common use, and minimal data recommended to ensure adequacy of record systems. Attention should also be given to differences of needs and methods in urban and rural settings. The remaining hours might be divided as follows:

1. triage at the scene (1 hr);
2. cardiopulmonary resuscitation and Heimlich maneuver (5 hrs);
3. issues in immobilization and extrication (3 hrs); and
4. common errors in initial diagnosis and treatment in the emergency department (1 hr).

This entire section, of course, can be expanded substantially if sufficient time can be found in the curriculum for more extensive training in emergency care concepts and methods. I have attempted here simply to indicate what relative emphasis I believe should be given within the context of a basic or absolute minimum course.

Integrative Exercises on Highway and Nonhighway Injury Events

Cases are presented that enable students to see how all of the previous materials fit together. As one possibility, each one-hour session could involve discussion before the entire class by three groups of students, each reviewing a different type of case. In the first hour one group could discuss a crash between a motorcycle and an automobile. A second could examine a single-vehicle motorcycle crash, while a third could dissect a truck versus automobile crash. In phase 1 or 2 nations, discussion might include a truck loaded with passengers. Some of the issues that could be elicited here include the effectiveness of driver education in general, specific environmental issues relevant to operation of a two-wheeled vehicle, such as conspicuity, vehicle stability, and the effect of potholes, environmental factors in the operation of very large vehicles such as trucks, and the effects of such human factors as experience, alcohol or other drugs, long hours of operation, or driver selection for operation of trucks.

Obviously, many factors are relevant to the injury phase, including total absence of protection for motorcycles, use of helmets, active and passive crash injury protection in automobiles, driver placement and protection in trucks, and issues of car underride in car versus truck crashes. Finally, extrication, immobilization, handling of hazardous cargo, and other aspects of emergency and long-term management can be discussed. While the specific items to be brought out depend on the specific circumstances of the cases chosen, I believe that the three general types of crashes suggested offer a maximum range of discussion.

During the second hour I would suggest consideration of thermal injuries in the nonhighway setting. Three possible cases might include a child whose clothing catches fire from an appliance that comes under jurisdiction of CPSC, a middle-age person who drops a cigarette onto a sofa or chair while dozing after ingestion of alcohol, and an elderly person who is scalded by excessively hot water from a faucet. These three cases touch upon developmental issues involving both the young and elderly, the role of alcohol and alcoholism, counseling considerations for parents, families of alcohol abusers, and the elderly, the role of products in initiation of injury events, and of fabric characteristics in the occurrence and severity of injury. Also relevant are the toxicity of gases produced as materials smolder, variations of temperature sensation and survivability related to age, and problems of management of care and regionalization of treatment facilities.

These types of injuries, I believe, are relevant to most, if not all, of the developed nations. The nonhighway problems may differ somewhat in some of the developing nations. In these areas other examples can be chosen that also cover a similar range of factors.

Mention should also be made of the possibilities for student projects, if time permits.[4] These might cover aspects of emergency care, the real versus apparent frequency or the outcome of specific injury types, assessment of factors involved in certain local injury events, or evaluation of possible countermeasures.

Organizing the Course

A course such as this should be developed by representatives of several departments, an approach that has worked successfully for courses on sexuality. Ideally, I would think the course should be given in the second or third year.

Suggested members for a schoolwide course committee in a medical school would include an emergency department surgeon, pathologist or medical examiner, a physician or other professional skilled in rehabilitation medicine or gerontology, an alcoholism specialist and/or a psychiatrist, an internist, an epidemiologist, and an engineer or other environmental-health specialist.

Final Words

Throughout this book I have tried to integrate information from the biological, physical, and social sciences to provide new explanations, insights, and options for professionals whose sources of reference have usually been limited to one or another of these fields. It is appropriate, therefore, to end with yet another view of the human being from a somewhat eclectic perspective. What is the human who so boldly challenges the environment?

> From the engineering viewpoint, he is a biological heat-engine with a limited fuel storage in the form of carbohydrates, glucose and fat, and an even more limited oxidizing capacity with virtually no storage of oxygen. He has a poorly supported hydraulic structure, with a built-in leak that needs constant replenishing. His structural materials are susceptible to damage by relatively small increments of heat, cold, pressure change, application of force, toxic chemicals, and radiant energy; his internal pumping systems, communication systems, and structural and motive systems are susceptible to the peculiar phenomena of aging and disease. His capacity to evaluate is time—and complexity—limited. From the design point of view, perhaps the most difficult of all problems to handle is his inconsistency—he is subject to marked biological variability, and his responses, abilities, and structure tend to vary from individual to individual, from circumstance to circumstance, and even from time to time in the same individual.[1]

This book has been about how to understand the human and how to keep him or her from falling apart during the exciting and frustrating process of challenging the environment over the duration of a lifetime.

Notes

Chapter 3

1. L. Benner, Jr., "Accident Theory and Accident Investigators," *Hazard Prevention* 13(4) (March/April 1977):18–21.

2. *Special Study: A Systematic Approach to Pipeline Safety* (Washington, D.C.: National Transportation Safety Board, Report NTSB-PSS-72-1, 1972).

3. L. Benner, Jr., "Accident Investigations: Multilinear Events Sequencing Methods," *Journal of Safety Research* 7 (1975):67–73.

4. J.J. Gibson, "Contribution of Experimental Psychology to the Formulation of the Problem of Safety: A Brief for Basic Research," in *Behavioral Approaches to Accident Research* (New York: Association for the Aid of Crippled Children, 1961), 77–89.

5. W. Haddon, Jr., "A Note Concerning Accident Theory and Research with Special Reference to Motor Vehicle Accidents," *Annals of New York Academy of Sciences* 107 (1963):635–646.

6. W. Haddon, Jr., "On the Escape of Tigers: An Ecologic Note," *American Journal of Public Health* 60 (1970):2229–2234.

7. K. Dalton, "Menstruation and Accidents," *British Medical Journal* 2 (1960):1425–1426.

8. G.G. Luce, *Biological Rhythms in Human and Animal Physiology* (New York: Dover Publications, Inc., 1971).

9. F.N. Platt, "Operations Analysis of Traffic Safety. Part 1: A Classification of Traffic Situations," *International Road Safety and Traffic Review* 6(2) (Spring 1958):1–8.

10. J. Mihalasky, "Whose Fault Is It: The Operator's or the Product's?," *Mechanical Engineering* 99(11) (November 1977):82. Quoted with permission.

11. Hippocrates, "On Injuries of the Head," in *The Genuine Works of Hippocrates,* translated by F. Adams (Baltimore: Williams and Wilkins Co. 1939).

12. H. DeHaven, "Mechanical Analysis of Survival in Falls from Heights of Fifty to One Hundred and Fifty Feet," *War Medicine* 2 (1942):586–596.

13. J.P. Stapp, "Effects of Mechanical Force on Living Tissue. I. Abrupt Deceleration and Windblast," *Journal of Aviation Medicine* 26 (1955):268–288.

14. E.S. Flamm, H.B. Demopoulos, M.L. Seligman, J.J. Tomasula,

V. DeCrescito, and J. Ransohoff, "Ethanol Potentiation of Central Nervous System Trauma," *Journal of Neurosurgery* 46 (1977):328–335.

15. L.I. Persson, L.E. Rosengren, and H.A. Hansson, "Ultrastructural Studies on Blood-Brain Barrier Dysfunction around Cerebral Stab Wounds, Aggravated by Acute Ethanol Intoxication," *Acta Neurologica Scandinavica* 57 (1978):405–417.

16. R.A. Brodner, J.C. Van Gilder, and W.F. Collins, "Experimental Spinal Cord Trauma: Potentiation by Alcohol," *Journal of Trauma* 21 (1981):124–127.

17. S.P. Baker, B. O'Neill, W. Haddon, Jr., and W.B. Long, "The Injury Severity Score: A Method for Describing Patients with Multiple Injuries and Evaluating Emergency Care," *Journal of Trauma* 14 (1974):187–196.

18. R.L. Somers, "The Probability of Death Score: An Improvement of the Injury Severity Score," *25th Proceedings of the American Association for Automotive Medicine* (Morton Grove, Ill.: American Association for Automotive Medicine, 1981), 281–290.

19. R.W. Carr, S.P. Desjardins, and T.L. Meador, *An Occupant Simulation Handbook* (Phoenix, Ariz.: Dynamic Science, Report 6910-75-123 on Contract N00014-71-C-0318, July 1975).

20. L.M. Patrick, "The Biomechanical Development of Injury-Attenuating Motor Vehicle Design," *Journal of Trauma* 10 (1970):220–229.

21. B.J. McGuire, J.R. Sorrells, and J.D. Moore, *Resistance of Human Skin to Puncture and Laceration* (Gaithersburg, Md.: National Bureau of Standards, Report NBSIR 73-123, 1973).

22. J.R. Sorrells and R.E. Berger, *Some Cutting Experiments on Human Skin and Synthetic Materials* (Gaithersburg, Md.: National Bureau of Standards, Report NBSIR 73-262, 1973).

23. R.E. Berger, "System for Assessing Eye Injury Potential of Propelled Objects," *Journal of Research of the National Bureau of Standards* 84 (1979):9–19.

24. R.I. Weiner, "An Evaluation of the Present Standards and Consumer Safety of Gas-Fired Gravity and Fan Type Floor Furnaces," in *National Commission on Product Safety Hearings, January–February 1969*, vol. 3B. (New York: Law-Arts Publications, 1970), 705–752.

25. A.M. Stoll, "Heat Transfer in Biotechnology," in J.P. Hartnett and T.F. Irvine (eds.): *Advances in Heat Transfer,* vol. 4 (New York: Academic Press, 1967), 65–141.

26. L.A. Marzetta, "A Thermesthesiometer: An Instrument for Burn Hazard Measurement," *IEEE Transactions on Biomedical Engineering,* vol. BME-21(5) (1974):425–427.

27. R.E. Gosselin, H.C. Hodge, R.P. Smith, and M.N. Gleason, *Clinical Toxicology of Commercial Products,* 4th ed. (Baltimore, Md.: Williams and Wilkins Co., 1976).

28. Y-C Wu, *Electrical Injuries: A Literature Review* (Gaithersburg, Md.: National Bureau of Standards, Report NBSIR 79-1710, 1979).

29. E. Browning, *Harmful Effects of Ionising Radiations* (Amsterdam: Elsevier Publishing Co., 1959).

30. E.P. Cronkite and V.P. Bond, *Radiation Injury in Man* (Springfield, Ill.: Charles C. Thomas Publishers, 1960).

31. C.E. Easterly, "Cancer Link to Magnetic Field Exposure: A Hypothesis," *American Journal of Epidemiology* 114 (1981):169–174.

32. C.F. Frey, D.F. Huelke, and P.W. Gikas, "Resuscitation and Survival in Motor Vehicle Accidents," *Journal of Trauma* 9 (1969):292–310.

33. M.W. Perrine, J.A. Waller, and L.S. Harris, *Alcohol and Highway Safety: Behavioral and Medical Aspects* (Burlington, Vt.: Psychology Department, University of Vermont, Final Report on Department of Transportation Contracts FH-11-6609 and FH-11-6899, 1971).

34. D.M. Bruser, "Emergency Care of Auto Crash Victims," in A.H. Keeney (ed.), *Proceedings of the 11th Annual Meeting of the American Association for Automotive Medicine* (Springfield, Ill.: Charles C. Thomas Publishers, 1970), 232–239.

35. J.A. Waller, "Factors Associated with Alcohol and Responsibility for Fatal Highway Crashes," *Quarterly Journal of Studies on Alcohol* 33 (1972):160–170.

36. D. Robinson, *The Face of Disaster* (Garden City, N.Y.: Doubleday and Co., 1959).

37. J.H. Sims and D.D. Baumann, "The Tornado Threat: Coping Styles of the North and South," *Science* 176 (1972):1386–1392.

Chapter 4

1. W. Haddon, Jr., "On the Escape of Tigers: An Ecologic Note," *American Journal of Public Health* 60 (1970):2229–2234.

2. W. Haddon, Jr., "The Basic Strategies for Reducing Damage from Hazards of All Kinds," *Hazard Prevention* 16(11) (September/October 1980):8–12.

Chapter 5

1. S.J. Segal and W.P. Mauldin, "The Tyranny of Numbers," *R.F. Illustrated* 5(3) (November 1981):19 (New York: Rockefeller Foundation).

2. W.W. Lowrance, *Of Acceptable Risk* (Los Altos, Calif.: William Kaufmann, Inc., 1976).

3. J.A. Waller, "Testimony before National Commission on Product Safety, February 19, 1969," in *National Commission on Product Safety Hearings,* vol. 3B (New York: Law-Arts Publishing, 1970), 654–681.

4. J.C. Mancuso, *The Concept of Fault in Moral Judgment Development: With Special Emphasis on the Morality of Roadway Use* (Albany, N.Y.: Department of Psychology, State University of New York at Albany, n.d.).

5. S.P. Baker, "Who Bought the Cars in Which People Are Injured? An Exploratory Study," *American Journal of Public Health* 69 (1979):76–78.

6. S.A. Merrill, "Political Determinants of Feasibility among Safety Standards: The Case of Occupant Restraint," *Proceedings of the 4th International Congress on Automotive Safety, July 14–16, 1975* (Washington, D.C.: National Highway Traffic Safety Administration, U.S. Department of Transportation, 1975), 519–536.

7. J.A. Waller and D. Klein, "Society, Energy, and Injury—Inevitable Triad?," in *Research Directions toward the Reduction of Injury in the Young and the Old* (Bethesda, Md.: National Institute of Child Health and Human Development, DHEW Publication (NIH) 73-124), 1–37.

8. A.B. Saunders and D.A. Benson, "The Practical Application of Social Costing in Road Safety Policy Making," *Proceedings of the 4th International Congress on Automotive Safety, July 14–16, 1975* (Washington, D.C.: National Highway Traffic Safety Administration, U.S. Department of Transportation, 1975), 591–604.

9. D. Okrent, "Comment on Societal Risk," *Science* 208 (1980):372–375.

10. K.B. Joscelyn and R.K. Jones, "Management of the Traffic Crash Risk: A Conceptual Framework," *Journal of Safety Research* 10 (1978):148–161.

11. R.A. Brown and C.H. Green, "Threats to Health or Safety: Perceived Risk and Willingness-to-Pay," *Social Science and Medicine* 15C (1981):67–75.

12. J.G. March, "The 1978 Nobel Prize in Economics," *Science* 202 (1978):858–861.

13. B.M. Faigin, "Societal Costs of Motor Vehicle Accidents for Benefit-Cost Analysis: A Perspective on the Major Issues and Some Recent Findings," *Proceedings of the 4th International Congress on Automotive Safety, July 14–16, 1975* (Washington, D.C.: National Highway Traffic Safety Administration, U.S. Department of Transportation, 1975), 155–172.

14. B. O'Neill, A.B. Kelley, and J. Wong, "Evaluating Motor Vehicle Safety Performance Standards," *Proceedings of the 4th International Congress on Automotive Safety, July 14–16, 1975* (Washington, D.C.: National Highway Traffic Safety Administration, U.S. Department of Transportation, 1975), 551–560.

15. D. Morganstein, "The Appropriate Role of Cost-Benefit Studies in the Formulation and Evaluation of Federal Safety Countermeasures," *Proceedings of the 4th International Congress on Automotive Safety, July 14–16, 1975* (Washington, D.C.: National Highway Traffic Safety Administration, U.S. Department of Transportation, 1975), 537–550.

16. R.B. Dyson, "Safety Versus Savings: An Essay on the Fallacy of Economic Costs of Accidents," *Proceedings of the 4th International Congress on Automotive Safety, July 14–16, 1975* (Washington, D.C.: National Highway Traffic Safety Administration, U.S. Department of Transportation, 1975), 145–154.

17. B. O'Neill and A.B. Kelley, *Costs, Benefits, Effectiveness and Safety: Setting the Record Straight,* paper presented at a meeting of the Society of Automotive Engineers, Toronto, October 21–25, 1974, SAE #740983 (Washington, D.C.: Insurance Institute for Highway Safety, 1974).

18. H.H. Wakeland, "An Array of Social Values for Use in Analyzing the Need for Safety Regulations," *Proceedings of the 4th International Congress on Automotive Safety, July 14–16, 1975* (Washington, D.C.: National Highway Traffic Safety Administration, U.S. Department of Transportation, 1975), 875–906. Reprinted with permission.

Chapter 6

1. L.A. Kaprio, "Death on the Road," *World Health* (October 1975):4–9.

2. *Road Traffic Accident Statistics,* report on a WHO Ad Hoc Technical Group, Prague, 26–28 September 1978 (Copenhagen: World Health Organization, 1979, EURO Reports and Studies 19).

3. R. Eastwood, "Suicide and Parasuicide," in J. Last (ed.), *Public Health and Preventive Medicine,* 11th ed. (New York: Appleton-Century-Crofts, 1980), 1359–1371.

4. N.L. Farberow, D.R. MacKinnon, and F.L. Nelson, "Suicide: Who's Counting?," *Public Health Reports* 92 (1977):225–232.

5. *Current Estimates from the Health Interview Survey: United States—1980* (Bethesda, Md.: National Center for Health Statistics, Department of Health and Human Services, National Health Survey Series 10 No. 139, 1981).

6. *Digest of Motor Laws 1981/1982* (Falls Church, Va.: American Automobile Association, 1981).

7. J.A. Waller, "Falls among the Elderly-Human and Environmental Factors," *Accident Analysis and Prevention* 10 (1978):21–33.

8. J. Sande and J. Thorson, "An Evaluation of the Official Swedish Statistics on Seriously Injured on Road Traffic Accidents," *Scandinavian Journal of Social Medicine* 3 (1975):5–11.

9. J.M. Ashi and M. El-Desouky, *Traffic Accidents in the Arab Gulf States* (Riyadh, Saudi Arabia: Secretariat General of Health for the Arab Countries of the Gulf Area, 1981).

10. R.N. Smith, "The Reporting Level of California State Highway Accidents," *Traffic Engineering* 36 (June 1966):20–25.

11. E.G. House, P.F. Waller, and G.G. Koch, *How Complete Are Driver Records? An Analysis Based on Insurance Claim Crashes* (Chapel Hill, N.C.: Highway Safety Research Center, University of North Carolina, 1974).

12. F.L. McGuire and R.C. Kersh, *An Evaluation of Driver Education* (Berkeley, Calif.: University of California Press, 1969).

13. G.S. Gregg and E. Elmer, "Infant Injuries: Accident or Abuse?," *Pediatrics* 44 (1969):434–439.

14. W. Haddon, Jr., P. Valien, J.R. McCarroll, and C.J. Umberger, "A Controlled Investigation of the Characteristics of Adult Pedestrians Fatally Injured by Motor Vehicles in Manhattan," *Journal of Chronic Diseases* 14 (1961):655–678.

15. P.F. Waller, D.W. Reinfurt, J.L. Freeman, and P.B. Imrey, "Methods for Measuring Exposure to Automobile Accidents" (Chapel Hill, N.C.: Highway Safety Research Center, University of North Carolina, paper presented at the Annual Meeting of the American Public Health Association, 8 November 1978).

16. F.A. Haight, "Induced Exposure," *Accident Analysis and Prevention* 5 (1973):111–126.

17. J.A. Gardiner, "Police Enforcement of Traffic Laws: A Comparative Analysis," in J.Q. Wilson (ed.), *City Politics and Public Policy* (New York: John Wiley and Sons, 1968).

18. F.K. Heussenstamm, "Bumper Stickers and the Cops," *Trans-Action* 8(4) (February 1971):32–33.

19. R.S. Coppin, A. Lew, and R.C. Peck, *The 1964 California Driver Record Study, Part 7: The Relationship between Types of Convictions and Accidents* (Sacramento, Calif.: Research and Statistics Section, California Department of Motor Vehicles, Report 20, 1966).

20. J. O'Day, A. Wolfe, and R. Kaplan, *Design for NASS: A National Accident Sampling System*, vol. 1 (Ann Arbor, Mich.: Highway Safety Research Institute, University of Michigan, Report UM-HSRI-SA-75-14-1, 1975).

21. *Optimum Recall Period for Reporting Persons Injured in Motor Vehicle Accidents* (Bethesda, Md.: National Center for Health Statistics, Department of Health and Human Services, Vital and Health Statistics, Series 2 No. 50, 1972).

22. John States, personal communication (Rochester, N.Y.: Department of Orthopedic Surgery, University of Rochester, 1978).

23. Committee on Injury Scaling, *The Abbreviated Injury Scale: 1980 Revision* (Morton Grove, Ill.: American Association for Automotive Medicine, 1980; previous versions published in 1971 and 1976).

24. J.I. Barancik and B.F. Chatterjee, "Methodological Considerations in the Use of the Abbreviated Injury Scale in Trauma Epidemiology," *Journal of Trauma* 21 (1981):627–631.

25. S.P. Baker, B. O'Neill, W. Haddon, Jr., and W.B. Long, "The Injury Severity Score: A Method for Describing Patients with Multiple Injuries and Evaluating Emergency Care," *Journal of Trauma* 14 (1974):187–196.

26. J.P. Bull, "The Injury Severity Score of Road Traffic Casualties in Relation to Mortality, Time of Death, Hospital Treatment Time and Disability," *Accident Analysis and Prevention* 7 (1975):249–255.

27. R.L. Somers, "The Probability of Death Score: An Improvement of the Injury Severity Score," *25th Proceedings of the American Association for*

Automotive Medicine (Morton Grove, Ill.: American Association for Automotive Medicine, 1981):281–290.

28. "National Electronic Injury Surveillance System, Estimated Mean Severity" (12 April 1979); "Summary of Severity Index" (n.d); "Priority Index for Injury Classification" (rev. October 1970) (Washington, D.C.: National Injury Information Clearinghouse, Consumer Product Safety Commission, mimeographed documents).

29. *Vehicle Damage Scale for Traffic Accident Investigators* (Chicago, Ill.: National Safety Council, TAD Project Technical Bulletin No. 1, 1971).

30. F.J. Vilardo, *Vehicle Damage Scale for Traffic Accident Investigators: An Investigation of Its Use and Potential for Predicting Driver Injury* (Chapel Hill, N.C.: Highway Safety Research Center, University of North Carolina, 1972).

31. L.I. Griffin III, *Bias in the TAD Severity Score* (Chapel Hill, N.C.: Highway Safety Research Center, University of North Carolina, 1973).

32. *The National Accident Sampling System: A Status Report,* vol. 3, *Implementation of NASS Subsystems* (Washington, D.C.: National Highway Traffic Safety Administration, U.S. Department of Transportation, 1978).

33. J.A. Waller and E.B. Whorton, unpublished observations based on "Unintentional Shootings, Highway Crashes and Acts of Violence: A Behavior Paradigm," *Accident Analysis and Prevention* 5 (1973):351–356.

34. J.A. Waller, "Factors Associated with Police Evaluation of Drinking in Fatal Highway Crashes," *Journal of Safety Research* 3 (1971):35–41.

35. G.W. Brown, "Analysis of 104 Eastern Iowa Motor Vehicle Casualty Accidents," *Proceedings of the 3rd Triennial Congress on Medical and Related Aspects of Motor Vehicle Accidents, International Association for Accident and Traffic Medicine, New York, 29 May–4 June 1969* (Ann Arbor, Mich.: Highway Safety Research Institute, University of Michigan, 1971), 216–218.

36. S.T. McDonald and R.A. Romberg, "Driver/Vehicle Characteristics Related to Accident Vehicle Condition and an Assessment of Indiana PMVI Effectiveness," *Proceedings of the American Association for Automotive Medicine, 22d Conference and the International Association for Accident and Traffic Medicine VII Conference* (Morton Grove, Ill.: American Association for Automotive Medicine, 1978), 1:98–111.

37. J. Thorson, "The 'Human Factor'—Explanation or Rationalization?," *Laekartidningen* 70 (1973):3911. Quoted with permission.

38. *The National Accident Sampling System: A Status Report,* vol. 1 *Objectives of the National Accident Sampling System* (Washington, D.C.: National Highway Traffic Safety Administration, U.S. Department of Transportation, 1978).

Chapter 7

1. L. Gordis, "An Epidemiologist Views the Evaluation of Alcoholism Treatment," *Alcoholism: Clinical and Experimental Research* 5 (1981):483–488.

2. J.A. Waller, "A Systems Model for Safety Program Evaluation," *Accident Analysis and Prevention* 12 (1980):1–5.

3. D. Morganstein, "The Appropriate Role of Cost-Benefit Studies in the Formulation and Evaluation of Federal Safety Countermeasures," *Proceedings of the 4th International Congress on Automotive Safety, July 14–16, 1975* (Washington, D.C.: National Highway Traffic Safety Administration, U.S. Department of Transportation, 1975), 537–550.

4. D. Klein and J.A. Waller, *Causation, Culpability and Deterrence in Highway Crashes* (Washington, D.C.: Automobile Insurance and Compensation Study, U.S. Department of Transportation, 1970).

5. J.J. Conger, W.C. Miller, and R.V. Rainey, "Effects of Driver Education: The Role of Motivation, Intelligence, Social Class, and Exposure," *Traffic Safety Research Review* 10 (September 1966):67–71.

6. J.W. Asher, "Do Driver Training Courses Produce Better Drivers? An Alternative Hypothesis," *Traffic Safety Research Review* 12 (March 1968):2–6.

7. T.D. Cook and D.T. Campbell, *Quasi-Experimentation: Design and Analysis Issues for Field Settings* (Chicago, Ill.: Rand McNally Publishing Company, 1979).

8. B.J. Campbell and D.W. Reinfurt, "The Degree of Benefit of Belts in Reducing Injury: An Attempt to Explain Study Discrepancies," paper presented at meeting of Society of Automotive Engineers (Warrendale, Pa.: Society of Automotive Engineers, SAE Technical Paper Series 790684, 1979).

9. L.W. Green, "Evaluation and Measurement: Some Dilemmas for Health Education," *American Journal of Public Health* 67 (1977):155–161.

10. J.A. Waller and J.K. Worden, "Strategies for Safety Program Planning and Evaluation: Lessons from the Vermont Alcohol and Highway Safety Campaign," *Proceedings of a Symposium on Traffic Safety Effectiveness (Impact) Evaluation Projects, May 18–20, 1981* (Chicago, Ill.: National Safety Council, 1981), 117–131.

Chapter 8

1. *Current Estimates from the National Health Interview Survey: United States, 1980* (Hyattsville, Md.: U.S. Department of Health and Human Services, National Health Survey Series 10 No. 139, 1981).

2. *Persons Injured and Disability Days by Detailed Type and Class of Accident, United States 1971–1972* (Hyattsville, Md.: National Health Survey, U.S. Department of Health and Human Services, National Health Survey Series 10 No. 105, 1976).

3. J.E. Gordon, P.V. Gulati, and J.B. Wyon, "Traumatic Accidents in Rural Tropical Regions: An Epidemiological Field Study in Punjab, India," *American Journal of Medical Sciences* 243 (1962):382–402.

4. *World Health Statistics Annual,* vol. 1, *1978: Vital Statistics and Causes of Death* (Geneva: World Health Organization, 1978).

5. A.M. Gittelsohn, "On the Distribution of Underlying Causes of Death," *American Journal of Public Health* 72 (1982):133–140.

6. N.S. Hartunian, C.N. Smart, and M.S. Thompson, "The Incidence and Economic Costs of Cancer, Motor Vehicle Injuries, Coronary Heart Disease and Stroke: A Comparative Analysis," *American Journal of Public Health* 70 (1980):1249–1260.

7. J. Thorson, "Long-Term Effects of Traffic Accidents," (Lund, Sweden: Hakan Ohlssons, 1975).

8. C.N. Smart and C.R. Sanders, *The Costs of Motor Vehicle Related Spinal Cord Injuries* (Washington, D.C.: Insurance Institute for Highway Safety, 1976).

Chapter 9

1. G.M. Mackay, University of Birmingham, England, personal communication.

2. *MVMA Motor Vehicle Facts and Figures, 1981* (Detroit, Mich.: Motor Vehicle Manufacturers Association of the United States, 1981).

3. P. Anderson, "Picturesque Outlook of Chinese Traffic," *Mexico City Daily Bulletin,* November 11, 1981, p. 4.

4. *Accident Facts, 1981 Edition* (Chicago, Ill.: National Safety Council, 1981).

5. B.J. Campbell, Highway Safety Research Center, University of North Carolina, Chapel Hill, N.C., personal communication, January 1976.

6. B. Sabey, "Nature and Scale of the Problem" (Crowthorne, Berkshire, U.K.: Transport and Road Research Laboratory, Department of Environment, 1981). Remarks presented at the World Health Organization Conference on Road Traffic Accidents in Developing Countries, Mexico City, 9–13 November 1981.

7. "Kuwait-Epidemic on Wheels," *World Health* (October 1975):16.

8. F.A. Haight, "Traffic Safety in Developing Countries," *Journal of Safety Research* 12 (1980):50–58.

9. *National Accident Sampling System—NASS—Report on Traffic Accidents and Injuries for 1979* (Washington, D.C.: National Highway Traffic Safety Administration, U.S. Department of Transportation, 1980).

10. A.F. Williams and S.E. Goins, "Fatal Falls and Jumps from Motor Vehicles," *American Journal of Public Health* 71 (1981):275–279.

11. G.D. Jacobs, M.N. Bardsley, and I. Sayer, *Road Accident Data Collection and Analysis in Developing Countries* (Crowthorne, Berkshire, U.K.: Transport and Road Research Laboratory, Department of Environment, TRLL Laboratory Report 676, 1979).

12. G.D. Jacobs and P.R. Fouracre, *Further Research on Road Accident Rates in Developing Countries* (Crowthorne, Berkshire, U.K.: Transport and

Road Research Laboratory, Department of Environment, TRRL Supplementary Report 270, 1977).

13. G.D. Jacobs and P. Hutchinson, *A Study of Accident Rates in Developing Countries* (Crowthorne, Berkshire, U.K.: Transport and Road Research Laboratory, Department of Environment, TRRL Report LR546, 1973).

14. G.D. Jacobs and W.A. Hards, *Further Research on Road Accident Rates in Developing Countries (Second Report)* (Crowthorne, Berkshire, U.K.: Transport and Road Research Laboratory, Department of Environment, TRRL Supplementary Report 434, 1978).

15. P.R. Fouracre and G.D. Jacobs, *Comparative Accident Costs in Developing Countries* (Crowthorne, Berkshire, U.K.: Transport and Road Research Laboratory, Department of Environment, TRRL Supplementary Report 206UC, 1976).

16. J.D. Jacobs and I.A. Sayer, *An Analysis of Road Accidents in Kenya in 1972* (Crowthorne, Berkshire, U.K.: Transport and Road Research Laboratory, Department of Environment, TRRL Supplementary Report 227UC, 1976).

17. A. Bayoumi, "The Epidemiology of Fatal Motor Vehicle Accidents in Kuwait," *Accident Analysis and Prevention* 13 (1981):339–348.

18. A. Bayoumi, "The Epidemiology of Injury Motor Vehicle Accidents in Kuwait," (Kuwait: Department of Community Medicine, Kuwait University Faculty of Medicine, unpublished paper, 1979).

19. M.E. Abulfotooh, "Road Traffic Accidents in Qatar: The Size of the Problem," *Accident Analysis and Prevention* 12 (1980):287–298.

20. *Alcohol and Highway Safety: Report to the U.S. Congress* (Washington, D.C.: U.S. Department of Transportation, 1968).

21. R.K. Jones and K.B. Joscelyn, *Alcohol and Highway Safety 1978: A Review of the State of Knowledge* (Ann Arbor, Mich.: Highway Safety Research Institute, University of Michigan, Report DOT HS-803 764, 1978).

22. J.M. Ashi and M. El-Desouky, *Traffic Accidents in the Arab States* (Riyadh, Saudia Arabia: Secretariat General of Health for the Arab Countries of the Gulf Area, 1981).

23. H.W. Smith and R.E. Popham, "Blood Alcohol Levels in Relation to Driving," *Canadian Medical Association Journal* 65 (1951):325–328.

24. M.W. Perrine, J.A. Waller, and L.S. Harris. *Alcohol and Highway Safety: Behavioral and Medical Aspects* (Burlington, Vt.: Project ABETS, Psychology Department, University of Vermont, Final Report on Department of Transportation Contracts FH-11-6609 and FH-11-6899, 1971).

25. M.M. Hyman, "Accident Vulnerability and Blood Alcohol Concentrations of Drivers by Demographic Characteristics," *Quarterly Journal of Studies on Alcohol* 29(Supplement 4) (1968):34–57.

26. R.F. Borkenstein, R.F. Crowther, R.P. Shumate, W.B. Ziel, and R. Zylman, *The Role of the Drinking Driver in Traffic Accidents* (Bloomington, Ind.: Department of Police Administration, Indiana University, 1964).

27. J.A. Waller, "Factors Associated with Alcohol and Responsibility for Fatal Highway Crashes," *Quarterly Journal of Studies on Alcohol* 33 (1972):160–170.

28. S. Encel and K. Kotowicz, "Heavy Drinking and Alcoholism, Preliminary Report," *Medical Journal of Australia* 1 (1970):607–612.

29. F.A. Whitlock, J.L. Armstrong, J.I. Tonge, M.J.J. O'Reilly, A. Davison, N.G. Johnston, and R.P. Biltoft, "The Drinking Driver or the Driving Drinker," *Medical Journal of Australia* 2 (1971):5–16.

30. K.B. Joscelyn and R.P. Maickel, *Drugs and Driving: A Research Review* (Bloomington, Ind.: Indiana University, Final Report on U.S. Department of Transportation Contract DOT-HS-4-00994, 1977).

31. K.B. Joscelyn, A.C. Donelson, R.K. Jones, J.W. McNair, and P.A. Ruschmann. *Drugs and Highway Safety 1980* (Ann Arbor, Mich.: Highway Safety Research Institute, University of Michigan, Final Report on U.S. Department of Transportation Contract DOT-HS-7-01530, 1980).

32. J.A. Waller, "Drugs and Highway Crashes: Can We Separate Fact from Fancy?" *Journal of the American Medical Association* 215 (1971):1477–1482.

33. J.A. Waller, "Hunting the Evasive Solutions to Medical Impairment and Highway Crashes," *Physician Reporting of Driver Limitation, Proceedings of Regional Conferences 1975–1976* (Chicago, Ill.: American Medical Association and American Association of Motor Vehicle Administrators, 1976), 15–25.

34. J.A. Waller, "Chronic Medical Conditions and Traffic Safety: A Review of California Experience," *New England Journal of Medicine* 273 (1965):1413–1420.

35. J.A. Waller and J.T. Goo, "Highway Crash and Citation Patterns of Drivers with Chronic Medical Conditions," *Journal of Safety Research* 1 (1968):13–27.

36. L. Ysander, "The Safety of Physically Disabled Drivers," *British Journal of Industrial Medicine* 23 (1966):173–180.

37. N.E. Liskey, "Accidents: Rhythmic Threat to Females," *Accident Analysis and Prevention* 4 (1972):1–12.

38. J.A. Waller, "Cardiovascular Disease, Aging, and Traffic Accidents," *Journal of Chronic Diseases* 20 (1967):615–620.

39. D.C. Pelz and S.H. Schuman, "Are Young Drivers Really More Dangerous After Controlling for Exposure and Experience?" *Journal of Safety Research* 3 (1971):68–79.

40. L.G. Goldstein, "Youthful Drivers as a Special Safety Problem," in P. Waller (ed.), *The Young Driver: Reckless or Unprepared? North Carolina Symposium on Highway Safety* (Chapel Hill, N.C.: Highway Safety Research Center, University of North Carolina, 1971), 5:37–101.

41. D. Klein, "Adolescent Driving as Deviant Behavior," in P. Waller (ed.), *The Young Driver: Reckless or Unprepared? North Carolina Symposium on Highway Safety* (Chapel Hill, N.C.: Highway Safety Research Center, University of North Carolina, 1971), 5:3–19.

42. "Rapid Police Pursuit Causes Highway Deaths" (Springfield, N.J.: Physicians for Automotive Safety, 17 June 1968).

43. D.C. Pelz and S.H. Schuman, "Motivational Factors in Crashes and Violations of Young Drivers" (Ann Arbor, Mich.: University of Michigan, paper presented at the Annual Meeting of American Public Health Association, 13 October 1971).

44. C.A. Williams, *Traffic Accidents* (Springfield, Ill.: Charles C. Thomas Publishers, 1954).

45. R.S. Coppin, A. Lew, and R.C. Peck, *The 1964 California Record Study,* pt. 7, *The Relationship Between Types of Convictions and Accidents* (Sacramento, Calif.: California Department of Motor Vehicles, Report No. 20, 1966).

46. "Who Really Causes the Accidents?" *Signal 99* 1(2) (Spring 1971):3–5 (Raleigh, N.C.: North Carolina Governor's Highway Safety Program).

47. J.W. Hutchinson, C.S. Cox, and B.R. Maffet, "An Evaluation of the Effectiveness of Televised, Locally Oriented Driver Reeducation," *Highway Research Record* 292 (1969):51–63 (Washington, D.C.: Highway Research Board).

48. D.R. Dreyer, *An Evaluation of California's Drivers Licensing Examination* (Sacramento, Calif.: California Department of Motor Vehicles, 1976).

49. J.A. Waller and J. Goo, "Accident and Violation Experience and Driving Test Score," *Highway Research Record* 225 (1968):1–8 (Washington, D.C.: Highway Research Board).

50. P. Babarik, "Automobile Accidents and Driver Reaction Pattern," *Journal of Applied Psychology* 52 (1968):49–54.

51. L.S. Robertson and S.P. Baker, "Prior Violation Records of 1,447 Drivers Involved in Fatal Crashes," *Accident Analysis and Prevention* 7 (1975):121–128.

52. L. Evans and P. Wasielewski, "Do Accident-Involved Drivers Exhibit Riskier Everyday Driving Behavior?" *Accident Analysis and Prevention* 14 (1982):57–64.

53. D. Solomon, *Accidents on Main Rural Highways Related to Speed, Driver and Vehicle* (Washington, D.C.: U.S. Bureau of Public Roads, 1964).

54. M.A.O. Malik and H.A. Hakim, "Road Traffic Accidents in a Developing Country," paper presented at the *5th International Conference of the International Association for Accident and Traffic Medicine,* London, 1–5 September 1975.

55. F.A.O. Owasina, *The Traffic Scene in Nigeria: An African Example* (Igbobi, Lagos, Nigeria: National Orthopedic Hospital, 1981).

56. M.W. Brown, "Yugoslavia Combats View That Her Jammed Roads Are Driver's Death Trap," *New York Times,* 8 September 1974, p. 12.

57. G.D. Jacobs, I.A. Sayer, and A.J. Downing, *A Preliminary Study*

of Road-User Behaviour in Developing Countries (Crowthorne, Berkshire, U.K.: Transport and Road Research Laboratory, Department of Environment, TRRL Supplementary Report No. 646, 1981).

58. R. Nader, *Unsafe at Any Speed* (New York: Grossman Press, 1965).

59. J.R. Treat and K.B. Joscelyn, "Results of a Study to Determine Accident Causes" (Warrendale, Pa.: Society of Automotive Engineers, SAE Paper No. 730230, 1973).

60. *Automotive Repair Industry, Hearings before the Subcommittee on Antitrust and Monopoly of the Committee on the Judiciary, United States Senate, 90th Cong. 2d Sess., Pursuant to Senate Resolution 233, Part 1, 3–5 December 1968* (Washington, D.C.: U.S. Government Printing Office, 1969).

61. "Eleven of 24 Auto-Repair Shops Pass a Test on Honesty," *New York Times,* December 8, 1975:1,50.

62. J.S. Creswell, Jr., "Driver Characteristics Affecting Vehicle Condition and Response to a Motor Vehicle Inspection Program," *HIT LAB Reports* 4(6) (February 1974):1–13 (Ann Arbor, Mich.: Highway Safety Research Institute, University of Michigan).

63. "Report Issued on Israel Auto Safety," *Quarterly/1* (March 1976):15 (Morton Grove, Ill.: American Association for Automotive Medicine).

64. W. E. Woodson, D.W. Conover, G.E. Miller, and P.H. Selby, *Motor Vehicle Instrument and Control Location, Accessibility, and Identification* (San Diego, Calif.: Man Factors, Inc., Report on Department of Transportation Contract DOT-11-6907, 1969).

65. A. Chapanis (ed.), *Ethnic Variables in Human Factors Engineering* (Baltimore, Md.: Johns Hopkins University Press, 1975).

66. J.L. Barnoski, M.R. Maurer, and B.A. Kugler, *Evaluation of Direct Visibility for Automotive Passenger Vehicles by a Figure of Merit* (Marina del Rey, Calif.: Measurement Analysis Corporation, Report on Department of Transportation Contract DOT-FH-11-6893, 1969).

67. C.R. Kelley and D.J. Prosin, *Motor Vehicle Rear Vision* (Santa Monica, Calif.: Dunlap and Associates, Inc., Report PB 186228 on DOT Contract FH-11-6951, 1969).

68. *Tires: A Comparison of Tire Reserve Load for 1976 Passenger Cars* (Washington, D.C.: National Highway Traffic Safety Administration, U.S. Department of Transportation, Consumer Aid Series, vol. 6, pt. 2, 1976).

69. *Brakes: A Comparison of Braking Performance for 1976 Passenger Cars and Motorcycles* (Washington, D.C.: National Highway Traffic Safety Administration, U.S. Department of Transportation, Consumer Aid Series, vol. 6, pt. 1, 1976).

70. *Acceleration and Passing Ability: A Comparison of Acceleration and Passing Ability for 1976 Passenger Cars and Motorcycles* (Washington, D.C.: National Highway Traffic Safety Administration, U.S. Department of Transportation, Consumer Aid Series, vol. 6, pt. 3, 1976).

71. *Incompatability of Standards Used in: Qualifying Drivers, Building*

Highways, Designing Vehicles (Washington, D.C.: National Highway Safety Advisory Committee, Report to the Secretary of Transportation, 17 June 1980).

72. H.W. Case, A. Burg, and J.D. Baird, "Vehicle Size and Accident Involvement: A Preliminary Study," *Journal of Safety Research* 5 (March 1973):26–35.

73. D.W. Reinfurt and B.J. Campbell, *Mileage Crash Rates for Certain Car Make and Model Year Combinations: A Preliminary Study* (Chapel Hill, N.C.: Highway Safety Research Center, University of North Carolina, 1974).

74. *Hearing before the Senate Committee on Commerce, 92d Cong., 1st Sess., Auto Safety Oversite Hearing: Corvair Heater, February 16, 1972* (Washington, D.C.: U.S. Government Printing Office, Serial No. 92-62, 1972).

75. "Tail Pipe Problems Significant in Carbon Monoxide Deaths," *Status Report* 8(2) (January 1973):6–7 (Washington, D.C.: Insurance Institute for Highway Safety).

76. T.C. Doege and P.S. Levy, "Injuries, Crashes, and Construction on a Superhighway," *American Journal of Public Health* 67 (1977):147–150.

77. *Special Study: Fatal Highway Accidents on Wet Pavement—The Magnitude, Location, and Characteristics* (Washington, D.C.: National Transportation Safety Board, Report NTSB-HSS-80-1, 1980).

78. R.A. Olsen, "The Driver as Cause or Victim in Vehicle Skidding Accidents," *Accident Analysis and Prevention* 10 (1978):61–68.

79. J.A. Blatnik, "Introductory Comments," *Highway Safety, Design and Operations: Freeway Signing and Related Geometrics, Hearings before the Special Subcommittee on the Federal-Aid Highway Program of the House Committee on Public Works, 90th Cong., 2nd Sess., 7–9 May and 9–11, 16–18 July 1968* (Washington, D.C.: U.S. Government Printing Office):2.

80. *Traffic Control and Roadway Elements* (Washington, D.C.: Automotive Safety Foundation and U.S. Bureau of Public Roads, 1963).

81. G.J. Alexander and H. Lunenfeld, *Positive Guidance in Traffic Control* (Washington, D.C.: Federal Highway Administration, U.S. Department of Transportation, 1965).

82. T.N. Tamburri, "Wrong-Way Driving Accidents Are Reduced," *Highway Research Record* 292 (1969):24–50 (Washington, D.C.: Highway Research Board).

83. A.B. Clayton, "An Accident-Based Analysis of Road-User Errors," *Journal of Safety Research* 4 (1972):69–74. Quoted with permission of *Journal of Safety Research*, a joint publication of National Safety Council and Pegamon Press.

84. R.A. McFarland, G.S. Tune, and A.T. Welford, "On the Driving of Automobiles by Older People," *Journal of Gerontology* 19 (1964):190–197.

85. R.A. Brodner, J.C. Van Gilder, and W.F. Collins, "Experimental Spinal Cord Trauma: Potentiation by Alcohol," *Journal of Trauma* 21 (1981):124–129.

86. J.O. Moore and B. Tourin, *A Study of Automobile Doors Opening under Crash Conditions: The Relationship between the Opening of Front Doors*

and the Area of Passenger Automobile Sustaining the Principal Impact (New York: Automotive Crash Injury Research of Cornell University, 1954).

87. J.W. Garrett and A. Stern, "A Study of Volkswagen Accidents in the United States," *Journal of Safety Research* 1 (1969):115–126.

88. G.M. Mackay, "Some Features of Traffic Accidents," *British Medical Journal* 4 (1969):799–801.

89. G.A. Ryan and G.M. Mackay, "Comparisons of Car Crashes in Three Countries," *Proceedings of the 13th Stapp Car Crash Conference, Boston, Mass., 2–4 December 1969* (Warrendale, Pa.: Society of Automotive Engineers, Paper 690813), 336–353.

90. D.F. Mela, *A Statistical Relation between Car Weight and Injuries* (Washington, D.C.: Office of Statistics and Analysis, National Highway Traffic Safety Administration, U.S. Department of Transportation, NHTSA Technical Note, DOT HS-801-629, 1975).

91. W. Haddon, Jr., "Reducing the Damage of Motor-Vehicle Use," *Technology Review* 77(8) (July/August 1975):1–9.

92. L. Ricci, *National Crash Severity Study Statistics* (Ann Arbor, Mich.: Highway Safety Research Institute, University of Michigan, Special Report on National Highway Traffic Safety Administration Contract DOT HS-8-01944, 1979).

93. K.A. Stonex, "Relation of Cross-Section Design and Highway Safety," *Traffic Safety Research Review* 7(4) (December 1963):2–14.

94. J.F. Fitzpatrick, M.N. Sohn, T.E. Silfen, and R.W. Wood, *The Law and Roadside Hazards* (Charlottesville, Va.: Michie Co., 1974).

95. J.A. Waller, L.S. Harris, and J.J. Oprendek, Jr., *Booby Trapped Highways in the Beckoning Country* (Burlington, Vt.: Associates in Community Medicine, 1975).

96. *Fatal and Injury Accident Rates on Federal-Aid and Other Highway Systems, 1968* (Washington, D.C.: Bureau of Public Roads, 1969).

97. " 'Priorities' Identified for Hazard Correction," *Status Report* 11(4) (3 March 1976):1–3 (Washington, D.C.: Insurance Institute for Highway Safety).

98. J.H. Davis and A.J. Fisk, "The Dade County, Florida Study on Carbon Monoxide, Alcohol and Drugs in Fatal Single Vehicle Automobile Accidents, Dade County, Florida Coroner's Office," *Proceedings of the National Association of Coroners 1964–1966*, Perlmuter Printing Co., Cleveland: 197–204.

99. P. Cooley, "Fire in Motor Vehicle Accidents," *Proceedings of the Fourth International Congress on Automotive Safety, San Francisco, Calif., 14–16 July 1975* (Washington, D.C.: National Highway Traffic Safety Administration, U.S. Department of Transportation, 73–138.

100. C.F. Scheffey, "Research into Driver-Roadway Interaction" (Washington, D.C.: U.S. Department of Transportation, Presentation to National Highway Safety Advisory Committee, Ann Arbor, Mich., 14 June 1971).

101. D. Klein, "Social Aspects of Exposure to Highway Crash," *Human*

Factors 18 (1976):211–220. Copyright 1976 by The Human Factors Society, Inc., and reproduced by permission.

102. "State Highway Safety Standards' Costs," *National Traffic Safety Newsletter* (April 1976):12 (Washington, D.C.: National Highway Traffic Safety Administration, U.S. Department of Transportation).

103. D.E. Payne and J.E. Barmack, "An Experimental Field Test of the Smith-Cummings-Sherman Driver Training System," *Traffic Safety Research Review* 7(1) (March 1963):10–14.

104. D.H. Schuster, "A Short-Term Evaluation of a Driver Improvement Course for Military Drivers," *Traffic Safety Research Review* 11(1) (March 1967):25–26.

105. A.F. Williams and B. O'Neill, "On-the-Road Driving Records of Licensed Race Drivers," *Accident Analysis and Prevention* 6 (1970):263–270.

106. A.F. Williams, R.S. Karpf, and P.L. Zador, "Variations in Minimum Licensing Age and Fatal Motor Vehicle Crashes," *American Journal of Public Health* 73 (1983):1401–1403.

107. J.K. Williams, "Transportation Safety in the 1970s: A Situation Report," *Transportation Research News* 55 (Summer 1974):15 (Washington, D.C.: Transportation Research Board, National Academy of Sciences). Reprinted with permission.

108. R.S. Coppin and G. Van Oldenbeek, *Driving under Suspension and Revocation* (Sacramento, Calif.: California Department of Motor Vehicles, 1965).

109. R.C. Peck, "Toward a Dynamic System of Driver Improvement Program Evaluation," *Human Factors* 18 (1976):493–506.

110. R.S. McBride and R.C. Peck, "Modifying Negligent Driving Behavior through Warning Letters," *Accident Analysis and Prevention* 2 (1970):147–174.

111. W.V. Epperson and R.M. Harano, "An Evaluation of Some Additional Factors Influencing the Effectiveness of Warning Letters," *Accident Analysis and Prevention* 7 (1975):239–247.

112. N. Kaestner and E.M. Syring, "Accident and Violation Reduction through Brief Driver Improvement Interviews," *Traffic Safety Research Review* 11 (1967):99, 121–124.

113. N. Kaestner and E.M. Syring, "Follow-up of Brief Driver Improvement Interviews in Oregon," *Traffic Safety Research Review* 12 (1968):111–117.

114. "NSC 'Driving' Evaluation Fails to Support Claims" *Status Report* 8(7) (26 March 1973):7–8 (Washington, D.C.: Insurance Institute for Highway Safety).

115. R.M. Harano and R.C. Peck, "The Effectiveness of a Uniform Traffic School Curriculum for Negligent Drivers," *Accident Analysis and Prevention* 4 (1972):13–45.

116. J.C. Prothero, "Evaluation of an Experimental Treatment for Problem Drivers," *Human Factors* 20 (1978):489–493.

117. R.S. Coppin, *A Controlled Evaluation of Group Driver Improvement Meetings* (Sacramento, Calif.: California Department of Motor Vehicles, 1961).

118. L.I. Li and P.F. Waller, *Evaluation of the North Carolina Habitual Offender Law* (Chapel Hill, N.C.: Highway Safety Research Center, University of North Carolina, 1976).

119. "Facts on Vital Issues: The 55 MPH Speed Limit," *Highway Users Federation Reporter* (November 1975):3–4.

120. "55 MPH Speed Limit Enforcement by All 50 States" (Washington, D.C.: Office of the Secretary, U.S. Department of Transportation, 18 February 1976, press release).

121. D.A. Pocock and A.A. Landauer, "The Severity of Drunken Driving as Perceived by Drunken Drivers," *Accident Analysis and Prevention* 12 (1980):105–111.

122. J.A. Waller, *Determining Strategies and Expectations Regarding Increased Enforcement against Alcohol Impaired Driving in Rural Areas* (Waterbury, Vt.: Project CRASH, Vermont Department of Mental Health, CRASH Report III-3, 1973).

123. J.A. Gardiner, "Police Enforcement of Traffic Laws: A Comparative Analysis," in J.Q. Wilson (ed.), *City Politics and Public Policy* (New York: John Wiley and Sons, 1968), 151–172.

124. L.S. de S. Lohman, E.C. Leggett, J.R. Stewart, and B.J. Campbell, *Identification of Unsafe Driving Actions and Related Countermeasures* (Chapel Hill, N.C.: Highway Safety Research Center, University of North Carolina, 1976).

125. V.L. Streib, "Classifying Traffic Law Systems According to Jurisprudential Policy," *Journal of Safety Research* 6 (1974):52–59.

126. "NATO Countries Report Dramatic Progress in Highway Safety" (Washington, D.C.: National Highway Traffic Safety Administration, U.S. Department of Transportation, 27 April 1976, press release).

127. H.L. Ross, *Deterring the Drinking Driver* (Lexington, Mass.: Lexington Books, 1981).

128. V. Ahola, K. Eklund, U. Leppänen, and L. Oranen, "Traffic Week in Kouvola in 1968" (Helsinki: Liikenneturva, Central Organization for Traffic Safety in Finland, 1972).

129. P. Zador, "Statistical Evaluation of the Effectiveness of 'Alcohol Safety Action Projects,' " *Accident Analysis and Prevention* 8 (1976):51–66.

130. P. Zador, "A Rejoinder to A Critique of the Paper 'Statistical Evaluation of the Effectiveness of Alcohol Safety Action Projects' by Johnson et al.," *Accident Analysis and Prevention* 9 (1977):15–19.

131. J.A. Waller and J.K. Worden, "Strategies for Safety Program Planning and Evaluation: Lessons from the Vermont Alcohol and Highway Safety Campaign," *Proceedings of Symposium on Traffic Safety Effectiveness (Impact) Evaluation Projects, Chicago, Ill., 19–21 May 1981* (Chicago, Ill.: National Safety Council, 1981), 117–131.

132. R.E. Mann, G. Leigh, E.R. Vingilis, and K. deGeneva, "A Critical

Review on the Effectiveness of Drinking-Driving Rehabilitation Programs," *Accident Analysis and Prevention* 15 (1983):441–462.

133. Mini Guide to the Federal Motor Vehicle Safety Standards (Washington, D.C.: Truck Body and Equipment Association, 1982).

134. L.S. Robertson, *The Effects of New-Car Safety Regulation on Fatality Rates* (Washington, D.C.: Insurance Institute for Highway Safety, 1976).

135. A. Nahum and A.W. Siegel, "Testimony at Hearing on Implementation of the National Traffic and Motor Vehicle Safety Act of 1966 before the U.S. Senate Committee on Commerce," 90th Cong., 2nd Sess., Washington, D.C., 25 April 1968.

136. B. O'Neill, W. Haddon, Jr., A.B. Kelley, and W.W. Sorenson, "Automobile Head Restraints: Frequency of Neck Injury Claims in Relation to the Presence of Head Restraints," *American Journal of Public Health* 62 (1972):399–406.

137. D.F. Huelke and J. O'Day, "The Federal Motor Vehicle Safety Standards: Recommendations for Increased Occupant Safety," *Proceedings of 4th International Congress on Automotive Safety, San Francisco, Calif., 14–16 July 1975* (Washington, D.C.: National Highway Traffic Safety Administration, U.S. Department of Transporation), 275–292.

138. R.W. McCutcheon and H.W. Sherman, "The Influence of Periodic Motor Vehicle Inspection on Mechanical Condition," *Journal of Safety Research* 1 (1969):184–193.

139. T. Colton and R.C. Buxbaum, "Motor Vehicle Inspection and Motor Vehicle Accident Mortality," *American Journal of Public Health* 58 (1968):1090–1099.

140. B.J. Schroer and W.F. Peyton, "The Effects of Automobile Inspections on Accident Rates," *Accident Analysis and Prevention* 11 (1979):61–68.

141. B. Tourin and J.W. Garrett, *Safety Belt Effectiveness in Rural California Automobile Accidents: A Comparison of Injuries to Users and Non-Users of Safety Belts* (Buffalo, N.Y.: Automotive Crash Injury Research of Cornell University, 1960).

142. "New DOT Study Finds Only 14% of Drivers Use Auto Safety Belts" (Washington, D.C.: Office of Public and Consumer Affairs, U.S. Department of Transportation, news release, 15 December 1978).

143. WHO Technical Group, *Seat Belts and Other Devices to Reduce Injuries From Traffic Accidents* (Copenhagen: World Health Organization Regional Office for Europe, EURO Reports and Studies 40, 1981).

144. "Facts on Vital Issues. Safety Belt Use," *Highway Users Federation Reporter* (December 1975):3–4 (Washington, D.C.: Highway Users Federation).

145. L.S. Robertson, "The Seat Belt Use Law in Ontario: Effects On Actual Use," *Canadian Journal of Public Health* 69 (1978):154–157.

146. L. Evans, P. Wasielewski, and C.R. von Buseck, "Compulsory Seat Belt Usage and Driver Risk-Taking Behavior," *Human Factors* 24 (1982):41–48.

147. W. Coleman, Jr., "Statement at News Conference, December 6, 1976, on the Announcement of a Proposed Demonstration Program of Passive Restraints (Washington, D.C.: Office of the Secretary, U.S. Department of Transportation, 1976).

148. H.M. Bunch, "Smaller Cars and Safety: The Effect of Downsizing on Crash Fatalities in 1995," *The HSRI Research Review* 9(3) (November/December 1978):1–5 (Ann Arbor, Mich.: Highway Safety Research Institute, University of Michigan).

149. *Problems in Implementing the Highway Safety Improvement Program, Federal Highway Administration, Department of Transportation* (Washington, D.C.: Comptroller General of the United States, Report to the House Subcommittee on Investigations and Oversight Committee on Public Works, 92nd Cong., 2nd Sess. (26 May 1972)).

150. R.N. Smith and T.N. Tamburri, "Direct Costs of California State Highway Accidents," *Highway Research Record* 225 (1968):9–29 (Washington, D.C.: Highway Research Board).

151. "Annual Evaluation of California's Traffic Safety Program," *FHWA Notice,* 1 February 1971 (Washington, D.C.: Federal Highway Administration, U.S. Department of Transportation).

152. J.G. Viner, "Vehicle Downsizing and Roadside Safety Hardware," *Proceedings of the 23rd Conference of the American Association for Automotive Medicine, Louisville, Ky., October 4–6, 1979* (Morton Grove, Ill.: American Association for Automotive Medicine), 348–360.

153. *Handbook of Highway Safety Design and Operating Practices* (Washington, D.C.: Bureau of Public Roads, U.S. Department of Transportation, 1968).

154. F. Council and W. Hunter, *Implementation of Proven Technology in Making the Highway Environment Safe* (Chapel Hill, N.C.: Highway Safety Research Center, University of North Carolina, 1976).

155. M. Livneh and A.S. Hakkert, "Some Factors Affecting the Increase of Road Accidents in Developing Countries, with Particular Reference to Israel," *Accident Analysis and Prevention* 4 (1972):117–134.

156. *Emergency Care and Transportation of the Sick and Injured, 3d ed.* (Chicago, Ill.: American Academy of Orthopedic Surgeons, 1981).

157. J.A. Waller and C.E. Gettinger, "Rural EMS, The Other Pickwickian Syndrome and the Pooh Bah Dilemma," *EMT Journal* 1(3) (September 1977):31–35.

158. *Federal Specification Ambulance* (Washington, D.C.: General Services Administration, 1980, Federal Specification KKK-A-1822A).

159. "Essential Equipment for Ambulances," *Bulletin of the American College of Surgeons:* 62(9) (September 1977):7–12.

160. Education Committee, *Emergency Department Nurses Association Core Curriculum, 2d ed.* (Chicago, Ill.: Emergency Department Nurses Association, 1980).

161. E.J. McKenzie and J.A. Waller, "Epidemiologic Factors in Emergency Care," in G.R. Schwartz (ed.): *Principles and Practices of Emergency Medicine, 2d ed.* (Philadelphia, Pa.: W.B. Saunders and Co., in press).

162. M.A. Gaber and J.S. Yerrell, "Road Safety Research in Egypt," paper presented at the *9th International Congress on Medicine and Accidents in Traffic of the International Association for Accident and Traffic Medicine, Mexico City, 26–29 September 1983* (Cairo, Egypt: Assistant Minister of the Interior, and Crowthorne, Berkshire, U.K.: Transport and Road Research Laboratory, Department of Environment, 1983).

Chapter 10

1. "Facts on Vital Issues: Truck Transportation," *Highway Users Federation Reporter* (October 1975):3–4 (Washington, D.C.: Highway Users Federation).

2. *Fact Book, Statistical Information on Highway Safety* (Washington, D.C.: Office of Statistics and Analysis, National Highway Traffic Safety Administration, U.S. Department of Transportation, 1980).

3. K.L. Pierson, *Remarks before a Seminar on Key Issues in Heavy Truck Safety,* Washington, D.C., 12 July 1976 (Washington, D.C.: National Motor Vehicle Safety Advisory Council, U.S. Department of Transportation, 1976).

4. L.S. deS. Lohman and P.F. Waller, *Trucks: An Analysis of Accident Characteristics by Vehicle Weight* (Chapel Hill, N.C.: Highway Safety Research Center, University of North Carolina, 1975).

5. *Fatal Accident Reporting System 1980* (Washington, D.C.: National Highway Traffic Safety Administration, U.S. Department of Transportation, Report DOT-HS-805-953, 1981).

6. G.G. Parsons, "Statistics on Heavy Truck Accidents," paper presented at a seminar on *Key Issues in Heavy Truck Safety,* Washington, D.C., 12 July 1976 (Washington, D.C.: National Motor Vehicle Safety Advisory Council, U.S. Department of Transportation).

7. S.P. Baker, J. Wong, and W.C. Masemore, "Fatal Tractor Trailer Crashes: Considerations in Setting Relevant Standards," *Proceedings of the 4th International Congress on Automotive Safety, San Francisco, Calif., 14–16 July 1975* (Washington, D.C.: U.S. Department of Transportation, 1975), 25–36.

8. T.A. Karlson and S.P. Baker, "Fatal Occupational Injuries Associated with Motor Vehicles," *Proceedings of American Association for Automotive Medicine, 22d Conference and International Association for Accident and Traffic Medicine 7th Conference, Ann Arbor, Mich., 10–14 July 1978,* vol. 1 (Morton Grove, Ill.: American Association for Automotive Medicine), 229–241.

9. *Accident Facts, 1981 Edition* (Chicago, Ill.: National Safety Council, 1981).

10. R. Lindsey, "Risk Factor Cited in Mobile Homes," *New York Times*, September 2, 1973, p. 8.

11. "We Hear . . . ," *Arizona Safety Sad-istics* (Phoenix, Ariz.: Arizona Department of Highways (January/February 1973)), 2.

12. T.N. Herzog, *Injury Rate as a Function of Truck Weights in Car-Truck Accidents* (Washington, D.C.: Office of Statistics and Analysis, National Highway Traffic Safety Administration, U.S. Department of Transportation, Report DOT-HS-801-472 Technical Note 43-31-7, rev. 1976).

13. G.D. Jacobs and I.A. Sayer, *An Analysis of Road Accidents in Kenya in 1972* (Crowthorne, Berkshire, U.K.: Transport and Road Research Laboratory, Department of Environment, TRRL Supplementary Report 227 UC, 1976).

14. J.B. Gregory, "Safety of Double Bottom Trucks" (Washington, D.C.: U.S. Department of Transportation, Memorandum #N43-31 to Assistant Secretary for Environmental Safety and Consumer Affairs, 19 April 1976).

15. D.B. Brown and J. Owens, *Heavy Truck Study (Update-1)* (Auburn, Ala.: Auburn University, Alabama Office of Highway and Traffic Safety, Report 300-76-002-001-028, 1975).

16. *Traffic Control and Road Elements* (Washington, D.C.: U.S. Bureau of Public Roads, 1963).

17. J.V. Roberts, *Recreational Vehicle Accident Research* (Washington, D.C.: Motor Vehicle Safety Advisory Council, U.S. Department of Transportation, Report on Contract DOT-HS-201-3-766, 1976).

18. J. O'Day and R.E. Scott, "An Analysis of Truck Accident Involvement," *HIT Lab Reports* 4(8) (April 1974):1–16 (Ann Arbor, Mich.: Highway Safety Research Institute, University of Michigan).

19. J. McMichael, *School Bus Accidents and Driver Age* (Chapel Hill, N.C.: Highway Safety Research Center, University of North Carolina, 1974).

20. R.G. Vaughan, *Caravans in Traffic Crashes* (Sydney, New South Wales, Australia: Traffic Accident Research Unit, Department of Motor Transport, 1974).

21. S.P. Baker, "Alcohol in Fatal Tractor Trailer Crashes," *Proceedings of the 19th Annual Meeting of the American Association for Automotive Medicine, San Diego, Calif., 20–22 November 1975* (Morton Grove, Ill.: American Association for Automotive Medicine), 234–243.

22. "India, A Lack of Discipline," *World Health* (October 1975):26–27.

23. W. Harris, R.R. Mackie, et al., *A Study of the Relationships Among Fatigue, Hours of Service, and Safety of Operations of Truck and Bus Drivers* (Goleta, Calif.: Human Factors Research, Inc., Contract DOT-FH-11-7777, 1972).

24. L.G. Norman, "Medical Aspects of Road Safety," *Lancet* 1 (1960):1038–1045.

25. P.F. Waller and L.K. Li, *Truck Drivers: Licensing and Monitoring. An Analysis With Recommendations. Summary Report* (Chapel Hill, N.C.: Highway Safety Research Center, University of North Carolina, 1979).

26. F.A.O. Owosina, *The Traffic Scene in Nigeria: An African Example* (Igbobi, Lagos-Nigeria: National Orthopedic Hospital, Report Prepared for World Health Organization Conference on Road Traffic Accidents in Developing Countries, Mexico City, 9–13 November 1981).

27. I.D. Brown, "Some Alternative Methods of Predicting Performance Among Professional Drivers in Training," *Ergonomics* 11 (1968):13–21.

28. J.E. Thompson and A.T. Fry, "Major Findings of a Study of Heavy Vehicle Speed and Operational Safety in Victoria," *Traffic Quarterly* 34 (1980):377–395. Reprinted with permission.

29. M.A.O. Malik and H.A. Hakim, "Road Traffic Accidents in a Developing Country," paper presented at the *5th International Conference of the International Association for Accident and Traffic Medicine*, London, U.K., 1–5 September 1975 (Khartoum, Sudan: Faculty of Medicine, University of Khartoum).

30. G.W. Brown, "Iowa Trucking Legislation" (Solon, Iowa: Statement submitted to the Iowa Legislature, 1969).

31. D.H. Weir, R.H. Hoh, and G.L. Teper, "Driver-Vehicle Control and Performance in the Presence of Aerodynamic Disturbances from Large Vehicles," *Driver Performance: Transportation Research Record No. 520* (Washington, D.C.: Transportation Research Board, 1974), 1–12.

32. J. Gustafson, *Report on Truck Safety* (Washington, D.C.: National Motor Vehicle Safety Advisory Council, U.S. Department of Transportation, 28 January 1976).

33. J.B. Gregory, *Summary Statement: Trucks and Trailer Air Brake Systems—DOT/NHTSA Revises Performance, Dynamometer and Parking Brake Requirements, and Delays Applicability for Certain Vehicles, Effective Date February 26, 1976* (Washington, D.C.: U.S. Department of Transportation, 1976).

34. R.D. Ervin, "Unintended Responses of Heavy Trucks to Braking or Steering Inputs," *The HSRI Research Review* 10(5) (March/April 1980):1–11 (Ann Arbor, Mich.: Highway Safety Research Institute, University of Michigan).

35. R.D. Ervin, "Tire Properties and Truck Handling: Some Surprising New Findings," *HSRI Research* 7(10) (July/August 1976):3–12 (Ann Arbor, Mich.: Highway Safety Research Institute, University of Michigan).

36. "Tip Prone Army Truck Faces National Safety Bureau Inquiry," *New York Times*, May 29, 1969, p. 14.

37. M.L. Reiss, H. Lunenfeld, and G.W. Morton, *Field of View Requirements Directly Behind Trucks and Buses* (Deer Park, N.Y.: AIL, Division of Cutler-Hammer, Contract DOT-HS-112-1-162, 1972).

38. R.A. McFarland, J.W. Dunlap, W.A. Hall, and A.L. Moseley, *Human Factors in the Design of Highway Transport Equipment: A Summary*

Report of Vehicle Evaluation (Boston, Mass.: School of Public Health, Harvard University, 1953).

39. D.F. Dunlap and J. O'Day, "Large-Truck Accidents Involving Tire Failure," *HIT Lab Reports* 5(6) (February 1975):1–17 (Ann Arbor, Mich.: Highway Safety Research Institute, University of Michigan).

40. *Federal Size and Weight Update* (San Bruno, Calif.: Western Highway Institute, 1975).

41. G.W. Brown, "Trucking Legislation" (Solon, Iowa: Statement to the 1971 Alabama Legislature).

42. *Review of Safety and Economic Aspects of Increased Vehicle Sizes and Weights* (Washington, D.C.: Federal Highway Administration, U.S. Department of Transportation, 1969).

43. J.A. Waller, Letter to Associate Director for Traffic Safety Programs, National Highway Safety Bureau, U.S. Department of Transportation, 7 May 1970 (Washington, D.C.: National Highway Safety Advisory Committee, U.S. Department of Transportation).

44. D.J. Minahan and J. O'Day, "Fatal Car-Into-Truck/Trailer Underride Collisions," *HSRI Research Review* 8(3) (November/December 1977):1–16 (Ann Arbor, Mich.: Highway Safety Research Institute, University of Michigan).

45. J.G. Viner, "Vehicle Downsizing and Roadside Safety Hardware," *Proceedings of the 23d Conference of the American Association for Automotive Medicine, Louisville, Ky. 4–6 October 1979* (Morton Grove, Ill.: American Association for Automotive Medicine), 348–360.

46. S. Charles and A. Shelness, "How Safe Is Pupil Transportation?" *Pediatrics* 45(1) (pt. 2) (1970):166–187.

47. K.L. Campbell, "Assessing the Safety Effects of Federal Motor Vehicle Safety Standard 121," *HSRI Research Review* 12(4) (January/February 1982):1–8 (Ann Arbor, Mich.: Highway Safety Research Institute, University of Michigan).

48. "Braking Bigger Trucks," *Status Report* 10(19) (24 November 1975):9 (Washington, D.C.: Insurance Institute for Highway Safety).

49. E.D. Ervin, "Improving Anti-Roll Properties of Semitrailers, Road Tractors, and Heavy Trucks," *HSRI Research Review* 9(5) (March/April 1979):7–8 (Ann Arbor, Mich.: Highway Safety Research Institute, University of Michigan).

50. R.D. Ervin, R.L. Nisonger, and C. Mallikarjunarao, "Eliminating Yaw Instability in Tractor-Semitrailers During Cornering," *HSRI Research Review* 10(1) (July/August 1979):1–17 (Ann Arbor, Mich.: Highway Safety Research Institute, University of Michigan).

51. Mr. Urban, Microflex Corporation, presentation before the National Motor Vehicle Safety Advisory Council, 28 April 1976 (Washington, D.C.: National Highway Traffic Safety Administration, U.S. Department of Transportation).

52. C.J. Johnson, J. Moran, and R. Pekich, "Carbon Monoxide in School Buses," *American Journal of Public Health* 65 (1975):1327–1329.

53. W.W. Hunter, N.C. Crowe, Jr., and D.G. Cole, "An Examination of Runaway Truck Escape Ramps," *Proceedings of the 22d Conference of the American Association for Automotive Medicine and the 7th Conference of the International Association for Accident and Traffic Medicine, Ann Arbor, Mich., 10–14 July 1978,* vol. 2 (Morton Grove, Ill.: American Association for Automotive Medicine), 15–22.

54. R.D. Ervin, "Safer Gasoline Tankers for Michigan," *HSRI Research Review* 11(5) (March/April 1981):1–11 (Ann Arbor, Mich.: Highway Safety Research Institute, University of Michigan).

55. J.W. Schmidt and D.L. Price, "The Flow of Hazardous Materials on Virginia Highways," *Journal of Safety Research* 11 (1979):109–114.

56. G.W. Brown, "Interstate Trucking Subsidy" (Solon, Iowa: n.d.).

57. *Accident Facts, 1975 Edition* (Chicago, Ill.: National Safety Council, 1975).

58. P. Gad, "Traffic Accidents with Personal Injury During Emergency Driving," *Danish Medical Bulletin* 18(3) (1971):57–61.

59. R.W. Nichols, *The Call of the Sirens* (Albany, N.Y.: Bureau of Emergency Health Services, New York State Department of Health, 1973).

60. B.C. MacLean, "Introductory Remarks," *Canadian Services Medical Journal* 11 (1955):564–565.

61. "Ford Lower Control Arm Probe," *Status Report* 5(10) (16 June 1970):4 (Washington, D.C.: Insurance Institute for Highway Safety).

62. "DOT Ford Lower Control Arm Finding Questioned," *Status Report* 9(6) (26 March 1974):3–5 (Washington, D.C.: Insurance Institute for Highway Safety).

63. "Chrysler Limits Recall to Police Cars," *Status Report* 10(20) (10 December 1975):1–2 (Washington, D.C.: Insurance Institute for Highway Safety).

64. S.P. Baker, Personal communication (Baltimore, Md.: School of Public Health and Hygiene, Johns Hopkins University).

65. "Tail Pipe Problems Significant in Carbon Monoxide Deaths," *Status Report* 8(2) (15 January 1973):6–7 (Washington, D.C.: Insurance Institute for Highway Safety).

66. F.J. Lewis, Jr., "Safe Operations of Ambulances," *Emergency Medical Services* 4(5) (September/October 1975):51–55,58–59,62,96. Reprinted with permission.

Chapter 11

1. "Motorcycle," *New Columbia Encyclopedia* (New York, N.Y.: Columbia University Press, 1975), 1847.

2. H. Cairns, "Head Injuries in Motor-Cyclists," *British Medical Journal* 2 (1941):465–471.

3. W. Lewin and W.F.C. Kennedy, "Motor-Cyclists, Crash Helmets, and Head Injuries," *British Medical Journal* 1 (1956):1253–1259.

4. *Motorcycles in the United States* (Cincinnati, Ohio: Injury Control Program, Public Health Service, U.S. Department of Health, Education and Welfare, PHS Publication 999-UIH-7, 1967).

5. P.W. Bothwell, "The Problem of Motorcycle Accidents," *Practitioner* 188 (1962):474–488.

6. W. Hunter and J.C. Stutts, *An Analysis of Mopeds as a Potential Safety Problem in the United States,* vol 1: *Report of the Literature and Data Search. Final Report* (Chapel Hill, N.C.: Highway Safety Research Center, University of North Carolina, Report DOT-HS-805-035, 1979).

7. T.L. McDole, "Motorcycles: Random Particles in the Traffic Stream," *HIT Lab Reports* (Ann Arbor, Mich.: Highway Safety Research Institute, University of Michigan, December 1970), 1–8.

8. W.W. Hunter and J.C. Stutts, *Exposure Characteristics of North Carolina Moped Riders* (Chapel Hill, N.C.: Highway Safety Research Center, University of North Carolina, 1980).

9. H.H. Hunter, Jr., *Motorcycle Accident Factors Study: Summary of Results* (Los Angeles, Calif.: Traffic Safety Center, University of Southern California, Materials for Final Briefing on Contract DOT-HS-5-01160, 1980).

10. L. Ricci, *National Crash Study Statistics* (Ann Arbor, Mich.: Highway Safety Research Institute, University of Michigan, Special Report DOT-HS-805227, 1979).

11. *Accident Facts, 1981 Edition* (Chicago, Ill.: National Safety Council, 1981).

12. R.S. Riggins, J.F. Kraus, C.E. Franti, and W.F. Drysdale, "Motorcycle Collision Injuries," *Proceedings of the 3d International Congress on Automotive Safety, San Francisco, 15–17 July 1974,* vol. 1, *Supplement* (Washington, D.C.: National Highway Traffic Safety Administration, U.S. Department of Transportation, Report DOT-HS-801-480, 1975), 4-1 to 4-22.

13. C.W. Van Rooy, "Minibikes," *Pediatrics* 67 (1981):154.

14. G.D. Jacobs and P. Hutchinson, *A Study of Accident Rates in Developing Countries* (Crowthorne, Berkshire, U.K.: Transport and Road Research Laboratory, Department of Environment, TRRL Report LR 546, 1973).

15. P.Z. Barry, "The Role of Inexperience in Motorcycle Crashes," *Journal of Safety Research* 2 (1970):229–239.

16. G.F. Messiter, *An Assessment of Measures to Reduce Cyclist and Motorcyclist Accidents* (Sydney, New South Wales, Australia: Traffic Accident Research Unit, Department of Motor Transport, 1972).

17. R.M. Harano and R.C. Peck, *An Abstract of the California Motorcycle Study: Driver and Accident Characteristics* (Sacramento, Calif.: California Department of Motor Vehicles, 1968).

18. R.B. Gustilo, D.L. Foss, W.R. Leslie, and R.L. Telander, "Motorcycle Injuries," *Minnesota Medicine* 48 (1965):489–491.

19. P.F. Waller, *An Analysis of Motorcycle Accidents with Recommendations for Licensing and Operation* (Chapel Hill, N.C.: Highway Safety Research Center, University of North Carolina, 1972).

20. L.I. Griffin III, *Motorcycle Accidents: Who, When, Where, and Why* (Chapel Hill, N.C.: Highway Safety Research Center, University of North Carolina, 1974).

21. M.J. Williams and E.R. Hoffman, "Conspicuity of Motorcycles," *Human Factors* 21 (1979):619–626.

22. J.W. Graham, "Fatal Motorcycle Accidents," *Journal of Forensic Science* 14 (1969):79–86.

23. J.A. Waller, E.M. King, G. Nielson, and H.W. Turkel, "Alcohol and Other Factors in California Highway Fatalities," *Journal of Forensic Science* 14 (1969):429–444.

24. S.P. Baker and R.S. Fisher, "Alcohol and Motorcycle Fatalities," *American Journal of Public Health* 67 (1977):246–249.

25. A.M. Nicholi, "The Motorcycle Syndrome," *American Journal of Psychiatry* 126 (1970):1588–1595.

26. P.F. Waller, D.W. Reinfurt, C.B. Reifler, and G.G. Koch, *Motorcycles versus Automobiles: How Do Their Owners Differ?* (Chapel Hill, N.C.: Highway Safety Research Center, University of North Carolina, 1969).

27. W. King, "Motorbike Racing Starts at Age 6," *New York Times*, 13 July 1975, p. 1,36.

28. J.M. Munden, "The Variation of Motorcycle Accident Rates with Age of Rider and Size and Age of Machine," *International Road Safety and Traffic Review* 12(1) (Winter 1964):12–16.

29. D. Bischoff, Testimony before Motorcycle Committee, National Motor Vehicle Safety Advisory Council, Washington, D.C., 22 October 1975 (Washington, D.C.: National Highway Traffic Safety Administration, U.S. Department of Transportation).

30. L.S. Buchanan, "Problems in Motorcycle Safety," paper presented at the 45th Annual Meeting of the Institute of Traffic Engineers, Seattle, Wash., 20 August 1975 (Washington, D.C.: National Highway Traffic Safety Administration, U.S. Department of Transportation).

31. M.L. Reiss, W.G. Berger, and G.R. Vallette, *Analysis of Motorcycle Accident Reports* (Falls Church, Va.: Biotechnology, Inc., 1974).

32. K.H. Bauer, *CIBA Symposia* 5 (1957):148, as quoted by P.W. Bothwell in "The Problems of Motorcycle Accidents," *Practitioner* 188 (1962):474–488.

33. C.E. Dare, J.C. Owens, and S. Krane, *Impact of Motorcycle Helmet Usage in Colorado. Executive Summary* (Denver, Colo.: Division of Highway Safety, Colorado Department of Highways, Final Report DOT-HS-803-679, 1978).

34. P.W. Bothwell, "Motor-Cycle Accidents," paper presented before the Royal College of Surgeons, England, *Convention on Accident Prevention and Life Saving,* London, 1963.

35. I.J. Wagar, San Pedro, Calif., personal communication.

36. "Motorcycle Licensing across the U.S.," *Highway Safety Highlights* 8(5) (September 1974) (Chapel Hill, N.C.: Highway Safety Research Center, University of North Carolina).

37. J. Anderson, J.L. Ford, and R.C. Peck, *Improved Motorcyclist Licensing and Testing Project. Executive Summary* (Sacramento, Calif.: California Department of Motor Vehicles, Final Report DOT-HS-805-599, 1980).

38. *Motorized Bicycle (Moped): Findings of a Survey* (Washington, D.C.: National Highway Traffic Safety Administration, U.S. Department of Transportation, 1976).

39. "Information of Laws Requiring the Daytime Use of Motorcycle Headlights" (Washington, D.C.: National Highway Traffic Safety Administration, U.S. Department of Transportation, background material for a meeting of the Motorcycle Committee, National Motor Vehicle Safety Advisory Council).

40. *Daytime Motorcycle Headlight and Tail Light Operation: Executive Summary* (Philadelphia, Pa.: Franklin Institute Research Laboratories, Report on Contract DOT-FH-11-7311, 1970).

41. R.D. Hazlett, G.R. Courtney, L.A.F. Stockley, and M.J. Allen, "Motorcycle Helmet Visibility and Retro-Reflectorization," *American Journal of Optometry and Archives of the American Academy of Optometry* 46 (1969):666–675.

42. P.L. Olson, R. Halstead-Nussloch, and M. Sivak, "The Effect of Improvements in Motorcycle/Motorcyclist Conspicuity on Driver Behavior," *Human Factors* 23 (1981):237–248.

43. I.J. Wagar, "Report to the Motorcycle Committee, National Motor Vehicle Safety Advisory Committee on 2nd International Motorcycle Safety Conference" (Washington, D.C.: National Highway Traffic Safety Administration, U.S. Department of Transportation, 16–17 December 1975).

44. *Standards for Protective Headgear* (Sacramento, Calif.: Snell Memorial Foundation, 1962).

45. J.F. Kraus, R.S. Riggins, and C.E. Franti, "Some Factors Associated with Severity of Injuries in Motorcycle Collisions," *International Congress on Automotive Safety (3d) Proceedings, San Francisco, July 15–17, 1974,* vol. 1, *Supplement* (Washington, D.C.: National Highway Traffic Safety Administration, U.S. Department of Transportation, Report No. DOT-HS-801-480, 1975):5-1 to 5-25.

46. *A Report to the Congress on the Effect of Motorcycle Helmet Use Law Repeal: A Case for Helmet Use* (Washington, D.C.: National Highway Traffic Safety Administration, U.S. Department of Transportation, 1980).

47. S. Gordon and J. Prince, *Field of View with and without Motorcycle Helmets* (Washington, D.C.: Safety Research Laboratory, National Highway Traffic Safety Administration, U.S. Department of Transportation, 1975).

48. A. Muller, "Evaluation of the Costs and Benefits of Motorcycle Helmet Laws," *American Journal of Public Health* 70 (1980):586–592.

49. S.E. Asogwa, "The Crash Helmet Legislation in Nigeria: A Before-and-After Study," *Accident Analysis and Prevention* 12 (1980):213–216.

50. B. Aldman, I. Cacciola, H. Gustafsson, A. Nygren, and J. Wersäll, "The Protective Effect of Different Kinds of Protective Clothing Worn by Motorcyclists," *Journal of Traffic Medicine* 9 (1981):57–58.

Chapter 12

1. "Bicycle," *New Columbia Encyclopedia* (New York: Columbia University Press, 1975).

2. *Accident Facts, 1981 Edition* (Chicago, Ill.: National Safety Council, 1981).

3. *NEISS Data Highlights* 5(4) (October/December 1981) (Washington, D.C.: Consumer Product Safety Commission).

4. J.D. Flora and R.D. Abbott, "National Trends in Bicycle Accidents," *Journal of Safety Research* 11 (1979):20–27.

5. *Hazard Analysis: Bicycles* (Washington, D.C.: Consumer Product Safety Commission, July 1973).

6. "Cycling Accidents in the United States," *Statistical Bulletin* 62(4) (October/December 1981):4–6 (New York: Metropolitan Life Insurance Co.)

7. J.A. Waller, "Bicycle Ownership, Use and Injury Patterns among Elementary School Children," *Pediatrics* 47 (1971):1042–1050.

8. E.A. Pascarella, *A Study of Youthful Bicycle Riders in an Urban Community* (Chapel Hill, N.C.: Highway Safety Research Center, University of North Carolina, 1971).

9. T.W. Chlapecka, S.A. Schupack, T.W. Planek, N. Klecka, and G.J. Driessen, *Bicycle Accidents and Usage among Elementary School Children in the United States* (Chicago, Ill.: National Safety Council, 1975).

10. F.J. Vilardo and J.H. Andersen, *Bicycle Accidents to School Aged Children* (Chicago, Ill.: National Safety Council, Report No. 169, 1969).

11. S.A. Schupack and G.J. Driessen, "Bicycle Accidents and Usage among Young Adults: A Preliminary Study," *Highway Safety Literature* HSL No. 76-10, (Washington, D.C.: National Highway Traffic Safety Administration, U.S. Department of Transportation, October 1976), A1–A25.

12. J. Thorson, "Pedal Cycle Accidents," *Scandinavian Journal of Social Medicine* 2 (1974):121–128.

13. A.F. Williams, "Factors in the Initiation of Bicycle-Motor Vehicle Collisions," *American Journal of Diseases of Children* 130 (1976):370–377.

14. K.D. Cross and G. Fisher, *A Study of Bicycle/Motor Vehicle Accidents: Identification of Problem Types and Countermeasure Approaches*, vol. 1 (Santa Barbara, Calif.: Anacapa Sciences, Inc., NHTSA Contract DOT-HS-4-00982, Report DOT-HS-803-313, 1977).

15. E. Brezina and M. Kramer, "An Investigation of Rider, Bicycle, and Environmental Variables in Urban Bicycle Collisions," *Proceedings of the 14th Annual Conference of the American Association for Automotive Medicine, Ann Arbor, Mich., 19–20 November 1970* (Ann Arbor, Mich.: University of Michigan, 1971), 139–165.

16. T.R. Howell, "Accidents and Those Bizarre Bicycles," *Pediatrics* 42 (1968):214.

17. L. Gonski, W. Southcombe, and D. Cohen, "Bicycle Accidents in Childhood," *Medical Journal of Australia* 2 (1979):270–271.

18. H.L. Kravitz, "Preventing Injuries from Bicycle Spokes," *Pediatric Annals* 6 (1977):713–716.

19. P.C. Noordzi, "Cycling in the Dark: An Analysis of Fatal Bicycle Accidents in the Netherlands," *Journal of Safety Research* 8 (1976):73–76.

20. P.F. Waller and D.W. Reinfurt, *Bicycles: An Analysis of Accidents in North Carolina* (Chapel Hill, N.C.: Highway Safety Research Center, University of North Carolina, 1969).

21. "Bicycle Spoke Injuries," *British Journal of Medicine* 4 (1969):182.

22. *National Commission on Product Safety: Final Report* (Washington, D.C.: National Commission on Product Safety, June 1970).

23. D.L. Kruse and A.A. McBeath, "Bicycle Accidents and Injuries," *American Journal of Sports Medicine* 8 (1980):342–344.

24. M.G. Lind and S. Wollin, "Bicycle Accidents in Stockholm. III. Drug Intoxication," paper presented at the 9th International Congress of Accident and Traffic Medicine, Mexico City, 26–29 September 1983 (Stockholm, Sweden: Department of Otology, Karolinska Hospital).

25. B. Preston, "Child Cyclist Accidents and Cycling Proficiency Training," *Accident Analysis and Prevention* 12 (1980):31–40.

26. C.G. Drury, "The Law and Bicycle Safety," *Traffic Quarterly* 32 (1978):599–620.

27. R.E. Dewar, "Bicycle Riding Practices: Implications for Safety Campaigns," *Journal of Safety Research* 10 (1978):35–42.

28. A. Burg and J. Beers, "Reflectorization for Nighttime Conspicuity of Bicycles and Motorcycles," *Journal of Safety Research* 10 (1978):69–77.

29. D.F. Lott and D.Y. Lott, "Effect of Bike Lanes on Ten Classes of Bicycle-Automobile Accidents in Davis, California," *Journal of Safety Research* 8 (1976):171–179.

30. T. Balderston, "Bicycle Helmets. Which One?" *Bicycling* 24 (1983):125–145.

31. M.G. Lind and S. Wollin, "Bicycle Accidents in Stockholm. IV. Skull Injuries," paper presented at the 9th International Congress of Acci-

dent and Traffic Medicine, Mexico City, 26–29 September 1983, (Stockholm, Sweden: Department of Otology, Karolinska Hospital).

Chapter 13

1. *Accident Facts, 1981 Edition* (Chicago, Ill.: National Safety Council, 1981).

2. *National Accident Sampling System: Report on Traffic Accidents and Injuries for 1979* (Washington, D.C.: National Highway Traffic Safety Administration, U.S. Department of Transportation, 1981).

3. A. Bayoumi, "The Epidemiology of Fatal Motor Vehicle Accidents in Kuwait," *Accident Analysis and Prevention* 13 (1981):339–348.

4. A. Bayoumi, "The Epidemiology of Injury Motor Vehicle Accidents in Kuwait" (Kuwait: Department of Community Medicine, Kuwait University, data presented at the annual meeting of the American Association for Automotive Medicine, Louisville, Ky. 1978).

5. S.E. Asogwa, "Deaths and Injuries on Nigerian Roads: A Study of 1590 Casualties," *Journal of Traffic Medicine* 6 (1978):52–54.

6. J.F. Silva, "A Comparative Study of Road Traffic Accidents in West Malaysia," *Annals of the Royal College of Surgeons of England* 60 (1978):457–463.

7. K. Rumar, "Road Safety in Sweden," *Hazard Prevention* 15(7) (November/December 1979):20–23.

8. W. Haddon, Jr. and S.P. Baker, "Injury Control," in D.W. Clark and B. MacMahon (eds.), *Preventive and Community Medicine,* 2d ed. (Boston, Mass.: Little Brown & Co., 1981), 109–140.

9. R.J. Smeed, "Pedestrian Accidents" (London: University College, n.d.).

10. G.D. Jacobs and P.R. Fouracre, *Further Research on Road Accident Rates in Developing Countries* (Crowthorne, Berkshire, U.K.: Transport and Road Research Laboratory, Department of Environment, TRRL Supplementary Report 270, 1977).

11. S.P. Baker, "Pedestrian Deaths in Rio de Janeiro and Baltimore," *Accident Analysis and Prevention* 9 (1977):113–118, and paper presented at a meeting of the American Public Health Association, San Francisco, 6 November 1973.

12. J.D.J. Havard, "Child Pedestrian Casualties as a Public Health Problem," *Medicine, Science and the Law* 14 (1974):168–179.

13. *The Skandia Report: A Report on Children in Traffic* (summary in English) (Stockholm, Sweden: Skandia Insurance Co., Ltd., 1971).

14. M.P. Vinjé, "Children as Pedestrians: Abilities and Limitations," *Accident Analysis and Prevention* 13 (1981):225–240.

15. M. Limbourg, "Das Verhalten von 4–9 Jähringen Kindern bei der Strassenüberquerung," *Zeitschrift für Experimentelle und Angewandte Psychologie* 23 (1976):666–677.

16. W. Haddon, Jr., personal communication concerning Reference 13–20 (Washington, D.C.: Insurance Institute for Highway Safety, 1967).

17. M.B. Snyder and R.L. Knoblauch, *Pedestrian Safety: The Identification of Precipitating Factors and Possible Countermeasures,* (Silver Spring, Md.: Operations Research, Inc., Report DOT-HS-800-403, 1971).

18. G. Bako, W.C. Mackenzie, and E.S.O. Smith, "The Passenger and Pedestrian Contribution to the Highway Accident Toll in Alberta, Canada, 1970–1972," *Journal of Traffic Medicine* 4 (1976):48–52.

19. W. Haddon, Jr., P. Valien, J.R. McCarroll, and C.J. Umberger, "A Controlled Investigation of the Characteristics of Adult Pedestrians Fatally Injured by Motor Vehicles in Manhattan," *Journal of Chronic Diseases* 14 (1961):655–678.

20. *1968 Alcohol and Highway Safety Report* (Washington, D.C.: National Highway Traffic Safety Administration, U.S. Department of Transportation, 1968).

21. "Reports: USSR," *Journal of Traffic Medicine* 9 (1981):49.

22. S.P. Baker, L.S. Robertson, and B. O'Neill, "Fatal Pedestrian Collisions," *American Journal of Public Health* 64 (1974):318–325.

23. R.D. Blomberg, D.F. Preusser, A. Hale, and R.G. Ulmer, *A Comparison of Alcohol Involvement in Pedestrians and Pedestrian Casualties* (Norwalk, Conn.: Dunlap and Associates East, Final Report on Contract DOT-HS-94-00946, 1979).

24. J.A. Waller, "Factors Associated with Alcohol and Responsibility for Fatal Highway Crashes," *Quarterly Journal of Studies on Alcohol* 33 (1972):160–170.

25. R.T. Johnson, *Freeway Pedestrian Accidents 1958–1962* (Sacramento, Calif.: Department of Public Works, California Highway Transportation Agency, Traffic Bulletin 9, 1964).

26. J.A. Waller, E.M. King, G. Nielson, and H.W. Turkel, "Alcohol and Other Factors in California Highway Fatalities," *Journal of Forensic Science* 14 (1969):429–443.

27. F.A. Haight and R.A. Olsen, "Pedestrian Safety in the United States: Some Recent Trends," *Accident Analysis and Prevention* 13 (1981):43–54.

28. G.D. Jacobs, I.A. Sayer, and A.J. Downing, *A Preliminary Study of Road-User Behaviour in Developing Countries* (Crowthorne, Berkshire, U.K.: Transport and Road Research Laboratory, Department of Environment, TRRL Supplementary Report 646, 1981).

29. B.F. Herms, "Pedestrian Crosswalk Study: Accidents in Painted and Unpainted Crosswalks," *Highway Research Record No. 406: Pedestrian Protection* (Washington, D.C.: Highway Research Board, 1972), 1–13.

30. M.J. Allen, R.D. Hazlett, H.L. Tacker, and B.V. Graham, "Actual Pedestrian Visibility and the Pedestrian's Estimate of His Own Visibility," *American Journal of Optometry and Archives of the American Academy of Optometry* 47 (1970):44–49.

31. B. Preston, "Statistical Analysis of Child Pedestrian Accidents in

Manchester and Salford," *Accident Analysis and Prevention* 4 (1972):323–332.

32. H.H. Wakeland, "Systematic Automobile Design for Pedestrian Injury Prevention," *Fifth Stapp Automotive Crash and Field Demonstration Conference, 14–16 September 1962* (Minneapolis, Minn.: University of Minnesota, 1961):193–218.

33. H. Appel, A. Kuehnel, G. Stuertz, and H. Gloeckner, "Pedestrian Safety Vehicle-Design Elements: Results of In-Depth Accident Analysis and Simulation," *Proceedings of the American Association for Automotive Medicine 22d Conference and the International Association for Accident and Traffic Medicine VII Conference, Ann Arbor, Mich., 10–14 July 1978,* vol. 2 (Morton Grove, Ill.: American Association for Automotive Medicine), 132–153.

34. D.F. Huelke and R.A. Davis, *A Study of Pedestrian Fatalities in Wayne County, Michigan* (Ann Arbor, Mich.: Highway Safety Research Institute, University of Michigan, HSRI Report Bio-9, 1969).

35. J.A. Waller, "Emergency Care for Fatalities from Injury and Illness in the Nonhighway Setting," *Journal of Trauma* 12 (1973):54–60.

36. J. Schreiber and J. Lukin, *Communicating Road Safety to the Young. Volume 1. An Exploratory Research Programme* (Sydney, N.S.W., Australia: Traffic Accident Research Unit, Department of Motor Transport, New South Wales, 1978).

37. J. Schreiber and C. Berry, *Communicating Road Safety to the Young Pedestrian: Evaluation of Road Safety Resource Material for Infants Schools* (Sydney, N.S.W., Australia: Traffic Accident Research Unit, Department of Motor Transport, New South Wales, 1978).

38. J.A. Rothengatter, "The Influence of Instructional Variables on the Effectiveness of Traffic Education," *Accident Analysis and Prevention* 13 (1981):241–253.

39. R.D. Blomberg, D.F. Preusser, A. Hale, and W.A. Leaf, *Experimental Field Test of Proposed Pedestrian Safety Messages,* vols. 1–3 (Norwalk, Conn.: Dunlap and Associates East, Contract DOT-HS-4-00952, 1983).

40. E.L. Wiener, "The Elderly Pedestrian: Response to An Enforcement Campaign," *Traffic Safety Research Review* 12 (1968):100–110.

41. R.D. Blomberg, A. Hale, and E.F. Kearney, *Development of Model Regulations for Pedestrian Safety* (Darien, Conn.: Dunlap and Associates, Inc., Report DOT-HS-801-287, 1974).

42. W.M. Bartholomew, "Pedestrian Accidents in Service Areas of Selected City Recreation Facilities," *Traffic Safety Research Review* 11 (1967):117–124.

43. R.D. Hazlett and M.J. Allen, "The Ability to See a Pedestrian at Night: The Effects of Clothing, Reflectorization and Driver Intoxication," *American Journal of Optometry and Archives of the American Academy of Optometry* 45 (1968):246–258.

44. A. Polus and A. Katz, "An Analysis of Nighttime Pedestrian Accidents at Specially Illuminated Crosswalks," *Accident Analysis and Prevention* 10 (1978):223–228.

45. A. Hale, R.D. Blomberg, and D.F. Preusser, *Experimental Field Test of the Model Ice Cream Truck Ordinance in Detroit* (Darien, Conn.: Dunlap and Associates, Report DOT-HS-803-410, 1978).

Chapter 14

1. *Transportation Facts and Trends,* 11th ed. (Washington, D.C.: Transportation Association of America, 1974).
2. "Rail Accident Fatalities," *Statistical Bulletin* 62(3) (July/September 1981):4–7, (New York: Metropolitan Life Insurance Co.).
3. R.D.H. Jones, "A Historical Note on U.S. Railroad Train Collisions," *Accident Analysis and Prevention* 3 (1971):277–279.
4. *Accident/Incident Bulletin No. 149: Calendar Year 1980* (Washington, D.C.: Federal Railroad Administration, U.S. Department of Transportation, 1981).
5. *Accident Facts, 1981 Edition* (Chicago, Ill.: National Safety Council, 1981).
6. "Drunk in Charge of a Train," *Journal of Alcoholism* 11(1) (Spring 1976):3–5.
7. *Railroad Accident Investigation, Ex Parte No. 229, 1962 and No. 4086, 1966* (Washington, D.C.: Interstate Commerce Commission).
8. A. Lomax, *The Folk Songs of North America* (Garden City, N.Y.: Doubleday and Co., 1960), 553–555.
9. E.C. Wigglesworth, "The Effects of Local Knowledge and Sight Restrictions on Driver Behavior at Open Railway Crossings," *Journal of Safety Research* 10 (1978):100–107.
10. J. Thorson, *Warning of Trains! Collisions Between Road and Railway Vehicles* (Umeå, Sweden: Department of Hygeine, University of Umeå, 1976).
11. J.A. Waller, "The Role of Alcohol in Fatal Collisions with Trains," *Northwest Medicine* 67 (1968):852–856.
12. E.C. Wigglesworth, "The Epidemiology of Road-Rail Crossing Accidents in Victoria, Australia," *Journal of Safety Research* 11 (1979):162–171.
13. J.A. Green, "Fatal Train-Vehicle Collisions in Michigan," *HIT Lab Reports,* (Ann Arbor, Mich.: Highway Safety Research Institute, University of Michigan, April 1972), 1–4.
14. *Rail-Highway Crossing Accident/Incident and Inventory Bulletin No. 3 Calendar Year 1980* (Washington, D.C.: Federal Railroad Administration, U.S. Department of Transportation, 1981).
15. W.D. Berg and J.C. Oppenlander, "Accident Analysis at Railroad-Highway Grade Crossings in Urban Areas," *Accident Analysis and Prevention* 1 (1969):129–141.
16. D.A. Zalinger, B.A. Rogers, and H.P. Johri, "Calculation of

Hazard Indices for Highway-Railway Crossings in Canada," *Accident Analysis and Prevention* 9 (1977):257–273.

17. V. Cummings and G. Molnar, "Traumatic Amputation in Children Resulting from Train-Electric-Burn Injuries: A Social-Environmental Syndrome?," *Archives of Physical Medicine and Rehabilitation* 55 (1974):71–73.

18. *Special Study of Rail Rapid Transit Safety* (Washington, D.C.: National Transportation Safety Board, Report NTSB-RSS-71-1, 1971).

19. G.E. Braden, "Aircraft-Type Crash Injury Investigation of a Commuter Train Collision," *Aviation, Space, and Environmental Medicine* 46 (1975):1157–1160.

20. G. Braden, "Application of Commercial Aircraft Accident Investigation Techniques to a Railroad Derailment," *Aerospace Medicine* 45 (1974):772–779.

21. R.S. Prosser, "How Safe Were the Motor Trains?," *Traffic Quarterly* 27 (1973):601–618.

22. *Special Investigation Report: The Accident Performance of Tank Car Safeguards* (Washington, D.C.: National Transportation Safety Board, Report NTSB-HZM-80-1, 1980).

23. J.E. Tyworth and A.J. Reinschmidt, "Role of Safety and Train Speed in Track Maintenance Spending Decisions: A Case Analysis," *Traffic Quarterly* 31 (1981):43–67.

24. "How Did They Get Hurt? What Were the Dangerous Jobs?," *National Safety News* 87(5) (May 1963):42–43.

25. W. Hammer, comments made at a workshop on Rare Event/Accident Research Methodology, National Bureau of Standards, Gaithersburg, Md., 26–28 May 1976.

Chapter 15

1. *Merchant Marine Safety: A Study of the United States Merchant Marine Safety Regulatory System* (Washington, D.C.: Ship Safety Panel of the Ship Operations Committee, Maritime Transportation Research Board, National Academy of Sciences, 1970).

2. S. Tomaszunas, "The Health of Seafarers: 2. International Aspects," *WHO Chronicle* 29 (1975):393–396.

3. F.J. Vilardo and R.J. Ripberger, "A Review of Selected State Recreational Boating Accident Reporting Systems," *Journal of Safety Research* 9 (1977):68–76.

4. "Hazards in Recreational and Commercial Boating," *Statistical Bulletin* 58(9) (September 1977):5–8 (New York: Metropolitan Life Insurance Co.).

5. *Annual Report to Congress, 1974* (Washington, D.C.: National Transportation Safety Board).

6. *Annual Statistics of Casualties, 1975* (Washington, D.C.: U.S. Coast Guard).

7. *Accident Facts, 1981 Edition* (Chicago, Ill.: National Safety Council, 1981).

8. E. Hale, "Analysis of Fatal Drowning Accidents Which Occurred in 1961," *Royal Naval Medical Services Journal* 49 (1963):233–236.

9. V.D. Pleuckhahn, "The Aetiology of 134 Deaths Due to 'Drowning' in Geelong During the Years 1957–1971," *Medical Journal of Australia* 2 (1972):1183–1187.

10. "Accidental Drownings by Age and Activity," *Statistical Bulletin* 58(5) (May 1977):2–5 (New York: Metropolitan Life Insurance Co.).

11. "Insurer Advises More Care to Reduce Deaths in Boating," *Hospital Tribune*, 25 September 1967, p. 19.

12. E. Pace, "Uncertain Crosswinds for 'Flags of Convenience,' " *New York Times*, 16 May 1982, p. E3.

13. A.H. Schuyler, Jr., "Tanker Safety: Vessel Traffic Control?" *Science* 201 (1978):398.

14. J.C. Giertsen, "Drowning While under the Influence of Alcohol," *Medicine, Science and the Law* 10 (1970):216–219.

15. I. Mackie, "Alcohol and Aquatic Disasters," *Medical Journal of Australia* 1 (1978):652–653.

16. J.A. Waller, "Nonhighway Injury Fatalities: I. The Role of Alcohol and Problem Drinking, Drugs and Medical Impairment," *Journal of Chronic Diseases* 25 (1972):33–45.

17. A. Ponttila, J. Pikkarainen, and S. Piipponen, "Drunken Driving with Motorboat in Finland: A Pilot Study on the Southern Seacoast in Summer 1978," *Accident Analysis and Prevention* 11 (1979):237–239.

18. O. Arner, "The Role of Alcohol in Fatal Accidents Among Seamen," *British Journal of Addiction* 68 (1973):185–189.

19. P.E. Dietz and S.P. Baker, "Drowning Epidemiology and Prevention," *American Journal of Public Health* 64 (1974):303–312.

20. D. Hitz, "Drunken Sailors and Others," *Quarterly Journal of Studies on Alcohol* 34 (1973):496–505.

21. S. Brun-Gulbrandsen and O. Irgens-Jensen, "Abuse of Alcohol Among Seamen," *British Journal of Addiction* 62 (1967):19–27.

22. L.J. Carter, "Amoco Cadiz Incident Points Up the Elusive Goal of Tanker Safety," *Science* 200 (1978):514–516.

23. A. McKenzie, "Tanker Losses," *Hazard Prevention* 15(3) (January/February 1979):4–5.

24. "Youths in More Boat Accidents," *Oakland (Calif.) Tribune*, 12 December 1962, p. 38X.

25. "Boating and Health," *New England Journal of Medicine* 289 (1973):1038–1039.

26. "Iceberg Patrol: A Prophylaxis against Collision," *Medical News,* 1 May 1967, p. 20.

27. "Lifesaving Devices for Boats," *Consumer Reports* 34 (1969):450–456.

28. W.R. Keatinge, "Death After Shipwreck," *British Medical Journal* 2 (1965):1537–1541.

29. R.M. Harnett and M.G. Bijlani, *The Involvement of Cold Water in Recreational Boating Accidents* (Clemson, S.C.: Clemson University, Report DOT-CG-72074A, 1979).

30. A. Hutchison, "The Health of Seafarers: I. Historical Background and Present Situation," *WHO Chronicle* 29 (1975):387–392.

31. H.E. Mayer, Jr., "Hazards at Sea," *Accident Analysis and Prevention* 6 (1974):83–84.

32. E. Sager, K. Geissler, B. Hayes, and J. Berman, *Educational Alternatives for Boating Safety Programs* (Huntsville, Ala.: Wyle Labs, Report DOT-CG-40672-A, 1978).

33. " 'Survival Suit' is Aiding Mariners in Fight for Life in Chilly Water," *New York Times,* 29 April 1979, p. 53.

Chapter 16

1. *Accident Facts, 1981 Edition* (Chicago, Ill.: National Safety Council, 1981).

2. G. Fromm, *Aviation Safety* (Washington, D.C.: Brookings Institute, 1969).

3. J.R. Wiley, *Airport Administration* (Westport, Conn.: Eno Foundation for Transportation, 1981).

4. C.C. Singh, Personal Communication (Montreal: International Civil Aviation Organization, 23 June 1981).

5. *Annual Review of Aircraft Accident Data: U.S. Air Carrier Operations 1979* (Washington, D.C.: National Transportation Safety Board, Report NTSB-ARC-81-1, 1981).

6. *Annual Review of Aircraft Accident Data: U.S. General Aviation, Calendar Year 1979* (Washington, D.C.: National Transportation Safety Board, Report NTSB-ARG-81-1, 1981).

7. *Special Study: In-Flight Safety of Passengers and Flight Attendants Aboard Air Carrier Aircraft* (Washington, D.C.: National Transportation Safety Board, Report NTSB-AAS-73-1, 1973).

8. J. Lederer, "Operational Failures: Subjective External and Internal Influences," *Hazard Prevention* 14(5) (May/June 1978):28–30.

9. L. Gonzales, "Etc. Etc. and Oh Yes, Passengers Die,"*New York Times,* 28 April 1977, p. A29.

10. R.L. Wick, "General Aviation Safety," *Archives of Environmental Health* 21 (1970):203–205.

11. G.B. Parker, "Why Doesn't Aircraft Accident Investigation Prevent Accidents?," *Proceedings of 9th International Seminar of the International Society of Air Safety Investigators, Seattle, Wash., 3–5 October 1978,* pp. 6–9.

12. J.E. Brody, "Pilots' Role in Accidents Draws Increasing Attention in Research," *New York Times,* 23 June 1980, pp. A1, A8.

13. C.R. Harper and W.R. Albers, "Alcohol and General Aviation Accidents," *Aerospace Medicine* 35 (1964):462–464.

14. D.J. Lacefield, P.A. Roberts, and C.W. Blossom, "Toxicological Findings in Fatal Civil Aviation Accidents, Fiscal Years 1968–1974," *Aviation, Space and Environmental Medicine* 46 (1975):1030–1032.

15. "General Aviation Accidents: Alcohol a Significant Factor," *Medical Tribune* 7(65) (30 May 1966):1, 16.

16. J.R. Dille, "Drug and Alcohol Findings and Effects in Civil Aviation: 1978 Update," *ISASI Forum* 11(4) (Winter 1978):49–50.

17. J.R. Dille, "Tangible Evidence of Human Factors Involvement in Fatal General Aviation Accidents," *Proceedings of 2d Annual Seminar of International Society of Air Safety Investigators, Los Angeles, Calif., 26–28 October 1971* (Washington National Airport, Alexandria, Va.: International Society of Air Safety Investigators).

18. A.R. Hricko, "Alcohol Has Menacing Role in Flight Safety as on Highways," *National Underwriter* (7 August 1970):1, 38–39, and (14 August 1970):10–13.

19. D.J. Lacefield, P.A. Roberts, and C.W. Blossom, *Agriculture Aviation versus Other General Aviation: Toxicological Findings in Fatal Accidents* (Oklahoma City, Okla.: Federal Aviation Administration Civil Aeromedical Institute, Report FAA-AM-78-31, 1978).

20. A. Ebneter, "Aircrew Error Rate Determination," *Hazard Prevention* 13(3) (January/February 1977):17–19.

21. G.J. Kidera, "Clinical Aspects of Commercial Aviation Medicine," *Journal of American Medical Association* 201 (1967):242–246.

22. L.E. Buley, "Incidence, Causes and Results of Airline Pilot Incapacitation While on Duty," *Aerospace Medicine* 40 (1969):64–70.

23. J.C. Lane, "Risk of In-Flight Incapacitation of Airline Pilots," *Aerospace Medicine* 42 (1971):1319–1321.

24. P.J.C. Chapman, "Aircraft Accidents," *Practitioner* 222 (1979):783–790.

25. J.H. Grosslight, H.J. Fletcher, R.B. Masterton, and R. Hagen, "Monocular Vision and Landing Performance in General Aviation Pilots: Cyclops Revisited," *Human Factors* 20 (1978):27–33.

26. D.S. Kochhar and T.M. Fraser, "Monocular Peripheral Vision as a Factor in Flight Safety," *Aviation, Space and Environmental Medicine* 49 (1978):698–706.

27. H.B. Mayer and J.C. Lane, "Monocular Pilots: A Follow up Study," *Aerospace Medicine* 44 (1973):1070–1074.

28. J.R. Dille and C.F. Booze, "1975 Accident Experience of Civilian

Pilots with Static Physical Defects," *Aviation, Space and Environmental Medicine* 49 (1978):422–425.

29. C.F. Booze, Jr., "Epidemiologic Investigation of Occupation, Age, and Exposure in General Aviation Accidents," *Aviation, Space and Environmental Medicine* 48 (1977):1081–1091.

30. M.G. Sanders and M.A. Hoffman, "Personality Aspects of Involvement in Pilot-Error Accidents," *Aviation, Space and Environmental Medicine* 46 (1975):186–190.

31. J.R. Levine, W.B. McHugh, J.O. Lee, and R.H. Rahe, "Recent Life Changes and Accidents Aboard an Attack Carrier," *Military Medicine* 142 (1977):469–471.

32. C.N. Kurucz and T.M. Khalil, "Probability Models for Analyzing the Effects of Biorhythms on Accident Occurrence," *Journal of Safety Research* 9 (1977):150–158.

33. J.H. Wolcott, R.R. McMeekin, R.E. Burgin, and R.E. Yanowitch, "Correlation of General Aviation Accidents with the Biorhythm Theory," *Human Factors* 19 (1977):283–293.

34. D.P. Phillips, "Airplane Crash Fatalities Increase Just after Newspaper Stories about Murder and Suicide," *Science* 201 (1978):748–749.

35. E.L. Wiener, "Special Issue Preface," *Human Factors* 22 (1980):517–519.

36. E.L. Wiener, "Controlled Flight into Terrain Accidents: System Induced Errors," *Human Factors* 19 (1977):171–181.

37. J.W. Danaher, "Human Error in ATC System Operations," *Human Factors* 22 (1980):535–545.

38. E.L. Wiener, "Midair Collisions: The Accidents, the Systems, and the Realpolitik," *Human Factors* 22 (1980):521–533.

39. *Special Study: Accidents Involving Engine Failure/Malfunction, U.S. General Aviation 1965–1969* (Washington, D.C.: National Transportation Safety Board, Report NTSB-AAS-72-10, 1972).

40. *Special Study: Carburetor Ice in General Aviation* (Washington, D.C.: National Transportation Safety Board, Report NTSB-AAS-72-1, 1972).

41. *Improving Aircraft Safety* (Washington, D.C.: Committee on FAA Airworthiness Certification Procedures, National Research Council, National Academy of Sciences, 1980).

42. "3.5 Million Awarded in Product Liability Case," *Human Factors Society Bulletin* 23(3) (March 1980):2.

43. R.L. Thorndike, *The Human Factor in Accidents with Special Reference to Aircraft Accidents* (Randolph Field, Tenn.: U.S. Air Force School of Aviation Medicine, Project 21-30-001 Report 1, 1951).

44. M.I. Bullock, "Cockpit Design-Pilot Accommodation and Accessibility to Controls," *Aerospace Medicine* 44 (1973):1295–1299.

45. A.M. Stave, "The Effect of Cockpit Environment on Long-Term Pilot Performance," *Human Factors* 19 (1977):503–514.

46. F.E. Gomer and R.G. Eggleston, "Perceived Magnitudes of Distortion, Secondary Imaging, and Rainbowing in Aircraft Windshields," *Human Factors* 20 (1978):391–400.

47. G.A. Ryan and J.D. Dougherty, "Epidemiology of Aerial Application Accidents," *Aerospace Medicine* 40 (1969):304–309.

48. *Special Study: Jet Blast Hazards* (Washington, D.C.: National Transportation Safety Board, Report NTSB-AAS-72-7, 1972).

49. R.W. Doughty, "Competition for Airspace: Bird Strikes and Aircraft Operations," *Traffic Quarterly* 30 (1976):449–467.

50. S.N. Roscoe, "When Day Is Done and Shadows Fall, We Miss the Airport Most of All," *Human Factors* 21 (1979):721–731.

51. J.N. Wilford, "Air Control Technology Refined to Meet Hazards," *New York Times,* 22 January 1980, pp. C1, C3.

52. R. Lindsey, "Pilots and FAA Clash on Safety," *New York Times,* 19 December 1971, p. 58.

53. G.B. Kolata, "FAA Plans to Automate Air Traffic Control," *Science* 213 (1981):845–846.

54. *Special Study of Fatal, Weather-Involved, General Aviation Accidents* (Washington, D.C.: National Transportation Safety Board, Report NTSB-AAS-74-2, 1974).

55. *Study of Lessons to Be Learned from Accidents Attributed to Turbulence* (Washington, D.C.: National Transportation Safety Board, Report NTSB-AAS-71-1, 1971).

56. P. Kuhn and F. Caracera, "Clear Air Turbulence: Detection by Infrared Observations of Water Vapor," *Science* 196 (1977):1099–1100.

57. L.P. Stearns, P.M. Kuhn, R.L. Kurkowski, and F. Caracera, "Clear Air Turbulence: an Airborne Alert System," *Science* 213 (1981):1007–1008.

58. H. DeHaven, *Comments at the 19th Annual Meeting of the American Association for Automotive Medicine,* San Diego, Calif., 20–22 November 1975.

59. H. DeHaven, "Mechanical Analysis of Survival in Falls From Heights of Fifty to One Hundred and Fifty Feet," *War Medicine* 2 (1942):586–596.

60. D. Fife, B. Rosner, and W. McKibben, "Relative Mortality of Unbelted Infant Passengers and Belted Non-Infant Passengers in Air Accidents With Survivors," *American Journal of Public Health* 71 (1981):1242–1246.

61. "Private-Plane Safety Measures Found Lagging," *Status Report* 13(8) (15 January 1978):1, 10 (Washington, D.C.: Insurance Institute for Highway Safety).

62. R.G. Snyder, "Occupant Impact Injury Tolerances for Aircraft Crashworthiness Design," *Dynamic Science Report, 2d quarter* (Newport Beach, Calif.: Ultrasystems, Inc., 1972).

63. R.J. Smith, "FAA is Cool to Cabin Safety Improvements," *Science* 211 (1981):557–558, 560.

64. C. Holden, "Pilots Take Unilateral Action on Flying Hazardous Cargo," *Science* 187 (1975):630.

65. D.W. Pollard, *Injuries in Air Transport Emergency Evacuation* (Okla-

homa City, Okla.: Federal Aviation Administration Civil Aeromedical Institute, Report FAA-AM-79-6, 1979).

66. *Special Study: Safety Aspects of Emergency Evacuations from Air Carrier Aircraft* (Washington, D.C.: National Transportation Safety Board, Report NTSB-AAS-74-3, 1974).

67. H.B. Altman, "Some Highlights of Aircraft Passenger Behavior Research," *Aviation, Space and Environmental Medicine* 46 (1975):89–91.

68. "FAA Proposes Upgrading of Airport Medical Services" (Washington, D.C.: Federal Aviation Administration, Press Release, 22 April 1976).

69. J.C. Duffy, "Emergency Mental Health Services during and after a Major Aircraft Accident," *Aviation, Space and Environmental Medicine* 49 (1978):1004–1008.

70. J.C. Lane and T.C. Brown, "Probability of Casualties in an Airport Disaster," *Aviation, Space and Environmental Medicine* 46 (1975):958–961.

71. H.H. Valverde, "A Review of Flight Simulator Transfer of Training Studies," *Human Factors* 15 (1973):510–523.

72. A.S. Blaiwes, J.A. Puig, and J.J. Regan, "Transfer of Training and the Measure of Training Effectiveness," *Human Factors* 15 (1973):523–533.

73. D.O. Weitzman, M.L. Fineberg, P.A. Gade, and G.L. Compton, "Proficiency Maintenance and Assessment in an Instrument Flight Simulator," *Human Factors* 21 (1979):701–710.

74. R.S. Jensen, "Pilot Judgment: Training and Evaluation," *Human Factors* 24 (1982):61–73.

75. "Commercial Pilot Exams Debated," *American Medical News,* 27 March 1972, pp. 1, 6.

76. R.C. Leighton-White, "Airline Pilot Incapacitation in Flight," *Aerospace Medicine* 43 (1972):661–664.

77. P.J.C. Chapman, "Aircraft Accidents," *Practitioner* 222 (1979):783–790.

78. J.P. Loomis and R.F. Porter, "The Performance of Warning Systems in Avoiding Controlled-Flight-into-Terrain (CFIT) Accidents," *Hazard Prevention* 17(4) (September/October 1981):27–31.

79. S.P. Desjardins, "Design for Crash Survival in Light Fixed-Wing Aircraft," *Dynamnic Science Report,* 2d Quarter (Phoenix, Ariz.: Ultrasystems, Inc., 1973).

80. G.A. Peters, "How to Design a Safe Aircraft," *Hazard Prevention* 15(4) (March/April 1979):6–11.

81. L.C. Abelson, L.D. Star, and J.X. Stefanki, "Passenger Survival in Wide-Bodied Jet Aircraft Accidents vs. Other Aircraft: A Comparison," *Aviation, Space and Environmental Medicine* 51 (1980):1266–1269.

Chapter 17

1. S.J. Segal and W.P. Mauldin, "The Tyranny of Numbers," *R.F. Illustrated* 5(3) (November 1981):19 (New York: Rockefeller Foundation).

2. *Accident Facts, 1981 Edition* (Chicago, Ill.: National Safety Council, 1981).

3. *Current Estimates from the National Health Interview Survey: United States, 1980* (Hyattsville, Md.: National Center for Health Statistics, U.S. Department of Health and Human Services, Series 10, No. 139, 1981).

4. *Persons Injured and Disability Days by Detailed Type and Class of Accident: United States, 1971–1972* (Rockville, Md.: U.S. Department of Health, Education and Welfare, Vital and Health Statistics Series 10, No. 105, 1976).

5. *Accident Facts, 1961 Edition* (Chicago, Ill.: National Safety Council, 1961).

6. *Health Statistics from the U.S. National Health Survey: Persons Injured by Detailed Type and Class of Accident. United States July, 1959–June, 1960* (Washington, D.C.: U.S. Department of Health, Education and Welfare, Series B-No. 37, 1962).

7. "Accidents in the Home," *WHO Chronicle* 20 (1966):3–19.

8. J.D.F. Lockhart, G.I. Forbes, and R.K. Bowman, "A Survey of Domestic Accidents in Hong Kong During May 1966," *Canadian Journal of Public Health* 58 (1967):249–256.

9. J.A. Waller, "Nonhighway Injury Fatalities: I. The Roles of Alcohol and Problem Drinking, Drugs and Medical Impairment," *Journal of Chronic Diseases* 25 (1972):33–45.

10. H. Wechsler, E.H. Kasey, D. Thum, and H.W. Demone, "Alcohol Level and Home Accidents," *Public Health Reports* 84 (1969):1043–1053.

11. J.A. Waller, "Nonhighway Injury Fatalities: II. Interaction of Product and Human Factors," *Journal of Chronic Diseases* 25 (1972):47–52.

12. *1979 Annual Report: Part Two* (Washington, D.C.: Consumer Product Safety Commission, 1979), app. D, pp. 45–59.

Chapter 18

1. "Cairo's Housing Crisis: 100,000 Live in Cemetery," *Montreal Gazette* 27 September 1978, p. 32.

2. *NEISS Data Highlights: Hazard Identification and Analysis* 4(4) (October–December 1980) (Washington, D.C.: Consumer Product Safety Commission).

3. R. Neutra and R.A. McFarland, "Accident Epidemiology and the Design of the Residential Environment," *Human Factors* 14 (1972):405–420.

4. J. Archea, B.L. Collins, and F.I. Stahl, Guidelines for Stair Safety (Washington, D.C.: National Bureau of Standards, U.S. Department of Commerce, NBS Building Science Series 120, 1979).

5. R.H. Shuford, Jr. (ed.), *Home Accident Causes and Recommended Remedial Measures: Summary Report, Phase I Study* (Huntsville, Ala.: Brown Engineering Co., Inc., Report IESD-HUD-1064, 1970).

6. D. Alessi, M. Brill, C. Brady, K. Hammond, A. Schubert, and M. Wigglesworth, *Home Safety Guidelines for Architects and Builders* (Buffalo, N.Y.: Buffalo Organization for Social and Technological Innovation (BOSTI), Report NBS GCR 78-156, 1978).

7. M.N. Tempest, "A Survey of Domestic Burns and Scalds in Wales during 1955, *British Medical Journal* 1 (1956):1387–1392.

8. J.P. Bull, D.M. Jackson, and C. Walton, "Causes and Prevention of Domestic Burning Accidents," *British Medical Journal* 2 (1964):1421–1427.

9. "Accidents in the Home," *WHO Chronicle* 20 (1966):3–19.

10. R.K. Wright and J.H. Davis, "The Investigation of Electrical Deaths: A Report of 220 Fatalities," *Journal of Forensic Science* 25 (1980):514–521.

11. *Accident Facts, 1981 Edition* (Chicago, Ill.: National Safety Council, 1981).

12. S. Ducic and H.R. Ghezzo, "Epidemiology of Accidental Home Fires in Montreal," *Accident Analysis and Prevention* 12 (1980):67–73.

13. *Hazard Analysis: Appliance Cords, Extension Cords and Replacement Wire* (Washington, D.C.: Consumer Product Safety Commission, November 1974).

14. J.H. Foley, "Ground-Fault Protection," *Fine Homebuilding* (December 1981/January 1982):39–41.

15. *Hazard Analysis: Aluminum Wiring* (Washington, D.C.: Consumer Product Safety Commission, April 1975).

16. P.M. Fulcomer, *Temperature Measurement on Operating Recessed Lighting Fixtures* (Washington, D.C.: Center for Consumer Product Technology, National Bureau of Standards, U.S. Department of Commerce, Report NBSIR 79-1913, 1979).

17. P.M. Fulcomer, *Temperature Measurement on Operating Surface Mounted Lighting Fixtures* (Washington, D.C.: Center for Consumer Product Technology, National Bureau of Standards, U.S. Department of Commerce, Report NBSIR 79-1912, 1979).

18. J.S. McConnaughey, Jr., *An Economic Analysis of Building Code Impacts: A Suggested Approach* (Washington, D.C.: Center for Building Technology, National Bureau of Standards, U.S. Department of Commerce, Report NBSIR 78-1528, 1978).

19. F.T. Ventre, *Social Control of Technological Innovation: The Regulation of Building Construction* (Cambridge, Mass.: Massachusetts Institute of Technology, submitted toward fulfillment of the Ph.D. requirements, June 1973).

20. "Study Faults Kansas City Building Inspection," *New York Times*, 21 March 1982, section i, p. 29.

Chapter 19

1. *NEISS Data Highlights: Hazard Identification and Analysis* 4(4) (October–December 1980) (Washington, D.C.: Consumer Product Safety Commission).

2. F.P. Rivara and L.R. Berger, "Consumer Product Hazards: Setting Priorities for Research and Regulatory Action," *American Journal of Public Health* 70 (1980):701–704.

3. J.F. McAllister, "Analysis of Risk Associated with a User-Discoverable Defect," *Journal of Safety Research* 8 (1976):2–7.

4. D. Klein, "Societal Influences on Childhood Accidents," *Accident Analysis and Prevention* 12 (1980):275–281.

5. G.K. Tokuhata, V. Colflesh, M. Smith, K. Ramaswamy, and E. Digon, "Consumer Behavior and Product Injuries," *Journal of Safety Research* 8 (1976):116–125.

6. A. Zavala, "Consumerism Problems from Consumers' Viewpoints," *Human Factors Society Bulletin* 16(5) (May 1973):3–5.

7. J.G. March, "The 1978 Nobel Prize in Economics," *Science* 202 (1978):858–861.

8. C.C. Clark, "Safety System Dynamics for Consumer Products: Some Factors Affecting Decisions About Safety," paper presented at the 21st Annual Appliance Technology Conference, Institute of Electrical and Electronic Engineers, Mansfield, Ohio, 5 May 1970, IEEE Paper 70 CP 351-IGA.

9. J.P. Bull, D.M. Jackson, and C. Walton, "Causes and Prevention of Domestic Burning Accidents," *British Medical Journal* 2 (1964):1421–1427.

10. A. Crittenden, "U.S. Won't Ban Export of Unsafe Products," *New York Times* 30 September 1980, p. D8.

11. "CPSC Working with International Organization to Share Information on Hazardous Exports and Imports" (Washington, D.C.: Consumer Product Safety Commission, Press Release, 12 June 1980).

12. *Product Advertising and Consumer Safety* (New York: National Advertising Review Board, June 1974).

13. *Hazard Analysis: High Chairs* (Washington, D.C.: Consumer Product Safety Commission, July 1974).

14. *Summarization of 64 In-Depth Investigations of Product-Related Injuries: Strollers (1522)* (Washington, D.C.: Consumer Product Safety Commission, June 1974).

15. *Hazard Analysis: Infant Seats* (Washington, D.C.: Consumer Product Safety Commission, March 1974).

16. *Summarization of 25 In-Depth Investigations of Product-Related Injuries: Beach Chairs, Folding Furniture, Multiple Use Patio Furniture (0643)* (Washington, D.C.: Consumer Product Safety Commission, 12 February 1974).

17. J.D. Ramsey, "Product Safety and Liability: Home Furnishings," *Proceedings, 6th Congress of the International Ergonomics Association, July 1976*, 498–506.

18. *Hazard Analysis: Cribs* (Washington, D.C.: Consumer Product Safety Commission, December 1975).

19. M. Bass, "Asphyxial Crib Deaths," *New England Journal of Medicine* 296 (1977):555–556.

20. *Summary Analysis of Playpen Injuries (1513)* (Washington, D.C.: Consumer Product Safety Commission, 27 September 1973).

21. "Crib Injuries Are Declining," *CPSC Memo* (Washington, D.C.: Consumer Product Safety Commission, May 1979), 5.

22. *Hazard Analysis: Toy Chest Related Injuries* (Washington, D.C.: Consumer Product Safety Commission, January 1975).

23. W.Q. Sturner, F.G. Spruill, R.A. Smith, and W.J. Lene, "Accidental Asphyxial Deaths Involving Infants and Young Children," *Journal of Forensic Sciences* 21 (1976):483–487.

24. *Hazard Analysis: Bunk Beds* (Washington, D.C.: Consumer Product Safety Commission, January 1975).

25. J.D.F. Lockhart, G.I. Forbes and R.K. Bowman, "A Survey of Domestic Accidents in Hong Kong During May 1966," *Canadian Journal of Public Health* 58 (1967):249–256.

26. L. Hiatt, Comments at Workshops on *Environmental Factors and the Elderly* at Brattleboro Retreat, Brattleboro, Vt., 1980 and 1981 (New York: American Foundation for the Blind, Inc.).

27. D. Zohar, "Why Do We Bump Into Things While Walking," *Human Factors* 20 (1978):671–679.

28. *Hazard Analysis: Space Heaters* (Washington, D.C.: Consumer Product Safety Commission, February 1975).

29. "Portable Electric Fans," *NEISS News* 3(1) (July 1974):1–2 (Washington, D.C.: Consumer Product Safety Commission).

30. *Summary Analysis of Electric Mixers (0231)* Washington, D.C.: Consumer Product Safety Commission, 8 August 1973).

31. J.H. McCulloch, J.A. Boswick, and R. Jonas, "Household Wringer Injuries: A Three-Year Review," *Journal of Trauma* 13 (1973):1–8.

32. *Summary Analysis of Wringer Washer Injuries (0102)* (Washington, D.C.: Consumer Product Safety Commission, 26 September 1973).

33. C.S.B. Galasko, "Spin Dryer Injuries," *British Medical Journal* 4 (1972):646.

34. *Summarization of 124 In-Depth Studies of Electrical Coffeemakers and Tea Pots-Associated Injuries (October 1965 through May 1972)* (Washington, D.C.: Consumer Product Safety Commission, 1972).

35. M.N. Tempest, "A Survey of Domestic Burns and Scalds in Wales during 1955," *British Medical Journal* 1 (1956):1387–1392.

36. "Fact Sheet No. 76: Electric Irons" (Washington, D.C.: Consumer Product Safety Commission, March 1975).

37. D.P. Barich, "Steam Vaporizers: Therapy or Tragedy?," *Pediatrics* 49 (1972):131–132.

38. P.M. Fulcomer, *Possible Fire and Electric Shock Hazards from Hot Lights in Minature Christmas Tree Light Strings and Decorations* (Washington, D.C.: National Bureau of Standards, U.S. Department of Commerce, Report NBSIR 79-1716, 1979).

39. "Hair Dryers and Electric Combs," *NEISS News* 5(3) (October 1976):1, 3 (Washington, D.C.: Consumer Product Safety Commission).

40. "CPSC Warns of Severe Electric Shock Hazard in Lamp" (Washington, D.C.: Consumer Product Safety Commission, Press Release, 6 February 1974).

41. N. Kreitman, "The Coal Gas Story," *British Journal of Preventive and Social Medicine* 30 (1976):86–93.

42. "Safety Shut-Off Device Reduces Heater Hazard," *CPSC Memo* (Washington, D.C.: Consumer Product Safety Commission, October 1979).

43. A. Chapanis and L.E. Lindenbaum, "A Reaction Time Study of Four Control-Display Linkages," *Human Factors* 1 (1959):1–7.

44. D. Shinar, "Control-Display Relationships on the Four-Burner Range: Population Stereotypes Versus Standards," *Human Factors* 20 (1978):13–17.

45. M.E. Stefl and J.J. Persensky, *An Evaluation of a Range-Top Warning Light System* (Washington, D.C.: National Bureau of Standards, U.S. Department of Commerce, Report NBSIR 75-797, 1975).

46. B.J. McGuire, J.R. Sorrels, and J.D. Moore, *Resistance of Human Skin to Puncture and Laceration* (Washington, D.C.: National Bureau of Standards, U.S. Department of Commerce, Report NBSIR 73-123, 1973).

47. *Hazard Analysis: Bottles for Carbonated Soft Drinks* (Washington, D.C.: Consumer Product Safety Commission, April 1975).

48. *Summary Analyses of Unpowered Coffeemakers and Teapots (0405)* (Washington, D.C.: Consumer Product Safety Commission, 23 March 1973).

49. "Refuse Bins," *NEISS News* 4(6) (April 1976) (Washington, D.C.: Consumer Product Safety Commission).

50. *Summary Analysis of Gasoline Rotary Power Mower (1418)* (Washington, D.C.: Consumer Product Safety Commission, 14 March 1973).

51. A.J. Thurston, "Foot Injuries Caused by Power Lawn Mowers," *New Zealand Medical Journal* 91 (1980):131–133.

52. R.M. Letts and A. Mardirosian, "Lawnmower Injuries in Children," *Canadian Medical Association Journal* 116 (1977):1151–1153.

53. J.L. Grosfeld, T.S. Morse, and E.J. Eyring, "Lawn Mower Injuries in Children," *Archives of Surgery* 100 (1970):582–583.

54. *Summarization of 55 In-Depth Investigations of Product-Related Injuries: Chain Saws (1411)* (Washington, D.C.: Consumer Product Safety Commission, 18 March 1974).

55. "Injuries Associated with Power Saws," *NEISS News* 1(5) (July 1973) (Washington, D.C.: Consumer Product Safety Commission).

56. C.D. Haynes, W.A. Webb, and C.R. Fenno, "Chain Saw Injuries: Review of 330 Cases," *Journal of Trauma* 20 (1980):772–776.

57. *Summarization of 100 In-Depth Investigations of Product-Related Injuries: Snow Throwers, Blowers (1406)* (Washington, D.C.: Consumer Product Safety Commission, September 1974).

58. J.A. Waller, "Snowblower Injuries," *Journal of Trauma* 17 (1977):122–125.

59. "Powered Hedge Trimmers," *NEISS News* 2(8) (April 1974) (Washington, D.C.: Consumer Product Safety Commission).

60. *Summarization of 23 In-Depth Investigtions of Product-Related Injuries. Step Ladders (0618) and Straight Ladders (0619)* (Washington, D.C.: Consumer Product Safety Commission, December 1973).

61. "Garden Tractor Injuries," *NEISS News* 2(8) (April 1974) (Washington, D.C.: Consumer Product Safety Commission).

62. "CPSC Moves Toward Chain Saw Standard," *CPSC Memo* (Washington, D.C.: Consumer Product Safety Commission, November 1980).

63. "Impact-Resistant Lenses to Be Required In Eyeglasses," *Hospital Tribune* 16 November 1970, p. 5.

Chapter 20

1. *Accident Facts, 1981 Edition* (Chicago, Ill.: National Safety Council, 1981).

2. *Report on the Fire/Burn Problem in the United States: Volume I. Analysis* (Virginia Beach, Va.: Systems Management Associates, Inc., Contract CPSC-C-76-0138, 1978).

3. G.S. Young and S.P. Baker, "Recent Trends in Childhood Burn Deaths," paper presented at the 1978 American Public Health Association Meeting (Baltimore, Md.: Johns Hopkins School of Hygiene and Public Health, 1978).

4. S.P. Baker, B. O'Neill, and R. Karpf, *Injury Fact Book* (Lexington, Mass.: Lexington Books, 1984).

5. J.I. Barancik and M.A. Shapiro, *Pittsburgh Burn Study* (Pittsburgh, Pa.: Graduate School of Public Health, University of Pittsburgh, 1972).

6. S. Ducic and H.R. Ghezzo, "Epidemiology of Accidental Home Fires in Montreal," *Accident Analysis and Prevention* 12 (1980):67–73.

7. M.N. Tempest, "A Survey of Domestic Burns and Scalds in Wales during 1955," *British Medical Journal* 1 (1956):1387–1392.

8. J.P. Bull, D.M. Jackson, and C. Walton, "Causes and Prevention of Domestic Burning Accidents," *British Medical Journal* 1 (1964):1421–1427.

9. "Accidents in the Home," *WHO Chronicle* 20 (1966):3–19.

10. J.D.F. Lockhart, G.I. Forbes, and R.K. Bowman, "A Survey of Domestic Accidents in Hong Kong during May 1966," *Canadian Journal of Public Health* 58 (1957):249–256.

11. M. Oddy and M. Humphrey, "Social Recovery during the Year Following Severe Head Injury," *Journal of Neurology, Neurosurgery and Psychiatry* 43 (1980):798–802.

12. M.S. Knudson-Cooper, "Adjustment to Visible Stigma: The Case of the Severely Burned," *Social Science and Medicine* 15B (1981):31–44.

13. M.S. Levine and E.P. Radford, "Fire Victims: Medical Outcomes

and Demographic Characteristics," *American Journal of Public Health* 67 (1977):1077–1080.

14. E.T. Takafuji, D.P. Driggers, and K.W. Leisher, "On Tap Water Burns," *American Journal of Public Health* 70 (1980):1300.

15. J.A. Waller, "Nonhighway Injury Fatalities: I. The Roles of Alcohol and Problem Drinking, Drugs and Medical Impairment," *Journal of Chronic Diseases* 25 (1972):33–45.

16. H. Wechsler, E.H. Kasey, D. Thum, and H.W. Demone, "Alcohol Level and Home Accidents," *Public Health Reports* 84 (1969):1043–1050.

17. J.A. Waller, "Emergency Care for Fatalities from Injury and Illness in the Nonhighway Setting," *Journal of Trauma* 12 (1973):54–60.

18. "Electric Blanket Fires," *New England Journal of Medicine* 268 (1963):1308.

19. E.W. Brown, "Space Heater Hazards," *New England Journal of Medicine* 265 (1961):794–795.

20. *Hazard Analysis: Space Heaters* (Washington, D.C.: Consumer Product Safety Commission, February 1975).

21. *Hazard Analysis: Television Sets* (Washington, D.C.: Consumer Product Safety Commission, October 1974).

22. *Summarization of 254 In-Depth Investigations of Product Related Injuries Associated with Cooking Ranges* (Washington, D.C.: Consumer Product Safety Commission, August 1974).

23. *Hazard Analysis: Aluminum Wiring* (Washington, D.C.: Consumer Product Safety Commission, April 1975).

24. P.M. Fulcomer, *Temperature Measurement on Operating Recessed Lighting Fixtures* (Washington, D.C.: National Bureau of Standards, Department of Commerce, Report NBSIR 79-1913, 1979).

25. R.D. Peacock, "Activities in Wood-Heating Safety," *Dimensions* (December 1980): 20–23 (Washington, D.C.: National Bureau of Standards, Department of Commerce).

26. L. Colebrook, V. Colebrook, J.P. Bull, and D.M. Jackson, "The Prevention of Burning Accidents," *British Medical Journal* 1 (1956):1379–1386.

27. J.A. Waller and D.I. Manheimer, "Nonfatal Burns to Children in a Well Defined Urban Population," *Journal of Pediatrics* 63 (1964):863–869.

28. J.A. Waller, "Testimony about Floor Furnace Burns before the National Commission on Product Safety," *Hearings, National Commission on Product Safety*, vol. 3B (1969), 655–681.

29. D. Shinar, "Control-Display Relationships on the Four-Burner Range: Population Stereotypes Versus Standards," *Human Factors* 20 (1978):13–17.

30. R.E. Bland, "To the Roof, Boys—To the Roof!" *Flame-Free '72: A Summary Report*, Flame-Free Design Conference, Houston, Tex., March 1972, 4–11.

31. W.V. White, "Flammable Fabrics and the Burn Problem: A Status Report," paper read at the American Public Health Association Meeting,

Houston, Tex., 28 October 1970 (Washington, D.C.: Consumer Product Safety Commission).

32. A Blum and B.N. Ames, "Flame-Retardant Additives as Possible Cancer Hazards," *Science* 195 (1977):17–23.

33. D. Bixler, "The Dilemma: How to Produce 'No Burn' Garments from 'Flame-Retardant' Fabrics," *Flame-Free '72: A Summary Report*, Flame-Free Design Conference, Houston, Tex., March 1972, 26–29.

34. J.B. Terrill, R.R. Montgomery, and C.F. Reinhardt, "Toxic Gases from Fires," *Science* 200 (1978):1343–1347.

35. R.E. Miller, K.S. Reisinger, M.M. Blatter, and F. Wucher, "Pediatric Counseling and Subsequent Use of Smoke Detectors," *American Journal of Public Health* 72 (1982):392–393.

36. V.J. Pezoldt and H.P. Van Cott, *Arousal from Sleep by Emergency Alarms: Implications from the Scientific Literature* (Washington, D.C.: National Bureau of Standards, Department of Commerce, Report NBSIR 78-1484 (HEW, 1978).

37. F.H. Rohles, Jr., "The Unfalse Alarm in Rochester," *Human Factors Society Bulletin* 24(12) (December 1981):2.

38. D. Canter and R. Matthews, *The Behaviour of People in Fire Situations: Possibilities for Research* (Borehamwood, Hertfordshire, U.K.: Building Research Establishment, Fire Research Station, Report CP11/76 January 1976).

39. J. Watts, "Systematic Methods of Evaluating Fire Safety: A Review," *Hazard Prevention* 18(2) (March/April 1982):24–27.

40. L.M. Garner, D.M. Love, and S.B. Jones, *A Community Action Approach for Prevention of Burn Injuries* (Washington, D.C.: Injury Control Branch, Public Health Service, U.S. Department of Health, Education and Welfare, DHEW Publication (HSM) 72-10008, 1972).

41. S.B. Jones, personal communication (Kansas City, Mo.: Accident Prevention Program, Missouri Division of Health, 26 June 1979).

Chapter 21

1. *Accident Facts, 1981 Edition* (Chicago, Ill.: National Safety Council, 1981).

2. J.A. Waller, "Falls Among the Elderly: Human and Environmental Factors," *Accident Analysis and Prevention* 10 (1978):21–33.

3. *Persons Injured and Disability Days by Detailed Type and Class of Accident. United States, July 1971–June 1972* (Washington, D.C.: National Health Survey, U.S. Department of Health, Education and Welfare, Series 10-No. 105, 1976).

4. J.E. Gordon, P.V. Gulati, and J.B. Wyon, "Traumatic Accidents in Rural Tropical Regions: An Epidemiological Field Study in Punjab, India," *American Journal of Medical Science* 243 (1962):158–178.

5. A.P. Iskrant and P.V. Joliet, *Accidents and Homicide* (Cambridge, Mass.: Harvard University Press, 1968).

6. M. Gyepes, M.Z. Mellins, and I. Katz, "The Low Incidence of Fracture of the Hip in the Negro," *Journal of American Medical Association* 181 (1962):133–134.

7. D.W. Anderson and R.L. McLaurin, "Report on the National Head and Spinal Cord Injury Survey," *Journal of Neurosurgery* 53 (1980):suppl. S1–S43.

8. J.F. Kraus, C.E. Franti, N.O. Borhani, and R.S. Riggins, "Survival With an Acute Spinal-Cord Injury," *Journal of Chronic Diseases* 32 (1979):269–283.

9. E.J. Gibson and R.D. Walk, "The Visual Cliff," *Scientific American* 202(4) (April 1960):64–71.

10. R.G. Snyder, M.L. Spencer, C.L. Owings, and L.W. Schneider, *Physical Characteristics of Children as Related to Death and Injury for Consumer Product Safety Design* (Ann Arbor, Mich.: Highway Safety Research Institute, University of Michigan, Final Report UM-HSRI-B1-75-5 31 May 1975).

11. J.A. Waller, "Nonhighway Injury Fatalities: I. The Roles of Alcohol and Problem Drinking, Drugs and Medical Impairment," *Journal of Chronic Diseases* 25 (1972):33–45.

12. H. Wechsler, E.H. Kasey, D. Thum, and H.W. Demone, "Alcohol Level and Home Accidents," *Public Health Reports* 84 (1969):1043–1050.

13. R. Honkanen, L. Ertama, P. Kuosmanen, M. Linnoila, and T. Visuri, "A Case-Control Study on Alcohol as a Risk Factor in Pedestrian Accidents," *Modern Problems of Pharmacopsychiatry* 11 (1976):1–5.

14. H. Honkanen and T. Visuri, "Blood Alcohol Levels in a Series of Injured Patients with Special Reference to Accident and Type of Injury," *Annales Chirurgiae et Gynaecologia* (Helsinki) 65 (1976):287–294.

15. M.N. Tempest, "A Survey of Domestic Burns and Scalds in Wales during 1955," *British Medical Journal* 1 (1956):1387–1392.

16. D.O. Maisels and B.V.M. Corps, "Burned Epileptics," *Lancet* 1 (1964):1298–1301.

17. J.H. Sheldon, "On the Natural History of Falls in Old Age," *British Medical Journal* 1 (1960):1685–1690.

18. P.W. Overstall, J.W.P. Hazell, and A.L. Johnson, "Vertigo in the Elderly," *Age and Aging* 10 (1981):105–109.

19. D. Wild, U.S.L. Nayak, and B. Isaacs, "How Dangerous Are Falls in Old People at Home?," *British Medical Journal* 282 (1981):266–268.

20. H. Droller, "Falls among Elderly People Living at Home," *Geriatrics* 10 (1955):239–244.

21. M.D. Blumenthal and J.W. Davie, "Dizziness and Falling in Elderly Psychiatric Outpatients," *American Journal of Psychiatry* 137 (1980):203–206.

22. D. Prudham and J.G. Evans, "Factors Associated with Falls in the Elderly: A Community Study," *Age and Aging* 10 (1981):141–146.

23. P.W. Overstall, "Prevention of Falls in the Elderly," *Journal of the American Geriatric Society* 28 (1980):481–484.

24. R.M. Guimaraes and B. Isaacs, "Characteristics of the Gait in Old People Who Fall," *International Rehabilitation Medicine (Basle)* 2 (1980):177–180.

25. B.E. Nilsson and N.J. Abdon, "Episodic Cardiac Arrhythmia and Accident Rate," *Acta Medica Scandinavica (Stockholm)* 208 (1980):69–71.

26. R. Over, "Possible Visual Factors in Falls by Old People," *Gerontologist* 6 (1966):212–214, 236.

27. B.L. Riggs, S.F. Hodgson, D.L. Hoffman, P.J. Kelly, K.A. Johnson, and D. Taves, "Treatment of Primary Osteoporosis with Fluoride and Calicum," *Journal of the American Medical Association* 243 (1980):446–449.

28. N.S. Weiss, C.L. Ure, J.H. Ballard, A.R. Williams, and J.R. Daling, "Decreased Risk of Fractures of the Hip and Lower Forearm with Postmenopausal Use of Estrogen," *New England Journal of Medicine* 303 (1980):1195–1198.

29. T.P. Eddy, "Deaths from Domestic Falls and Fractures," *British Journal of Preventive and Social Medicine* 26 (1972):173–179.

30. L. Hiatt Snyder, R. Rupprecht, J. Pyrek, S. Brekhus, and T. Moss, "Wandering," *Gerontologist* 18 (1978):272–280, and personal communication, L. Hiatt.

31. W. Haddon, Jr., E.A. Suchman, and D. Klein, *Accident Research: Methods and Approaches* (New York: Harper & Row, Publishers, 1964).

32. R.L. Sieben, J.D. Levitt, and J.H. French, "Falls as Childhood Accidents: An Increasing Urban Risk," *Pediatrics* 47 (1971):886–892.

33. E. Nemy, "Fashion Is Usually Harmless Enough—But This Is a Menace," *New York Times* 24 August 1973, p. 38.

34. J.H. Sheldon, "Accidents in the Home," *Journal of the Royal Institute of Public Health and Hygiene* 26 (1963):41–44.

35. J.A. Waller, "Emergency Care for Fatalities from Injury and Illness in the Nonhighway Setting," *Journal of Trauma* 12 (1973):54–60.

36. D. Sudnow, "Dead on Arrival," Trans-Action 5 (1967):36–43.

37. M. deC. Hinds, "Window Guards: For a Child's Safety," *New York Times*, 16 August 1979, p. C3.

38. F.J. Prial, "Landlords Resisting City Mandate for Window Guards for Children," *New York Times*, 14 March 1978, p. 39.

39. M. Weinstein, "Estrogen Use in Postmenopausal Women: Costs, Risks, Benefits," *New England Journal of Medicine* 303 (1980):308–316.

40. L.A. Jason, "Modifying Snow Shoveling Behaviors in An Urban Area," *American Journal of Public Health* 71 (1981):861.

Chapter 22

1. B.M. Barraclough, "Poisoning Cases: Suicide or Accident," *British Journal of Psychiatry* 124 (1974):526–530.

2. *Accident Facts, 1981 Edition* (Chicago, Ill.: National Safety Council, 1981).

3. F.E. Russell, "Injuries by Venomous Animals in the United States," *Journal of the American Medical Association* 177 (1961):903–907.

4. "Poisoning by Venomous Animals," *American Journal of Medicine* 42 (1967):107–128.

5. E.M. Backett, *Domestic Accidents* (Geneva, Switzerland: World Health Organization, Public Health Papers 26, 1965).

6. *Types of Injuries: Incidence and Associated Disability, United States July 1965–June 1967* (Washington, D.C.: National Center for Health Statistics, Department of Health, Education and Welfare, Series 10 No. 57, 1969).

7. H.L. Verhulst and J.J. Crotty, "Childhood Poisoning Accidents," *Journal of the American Medical Association* 203 (1968):1049–1050.

8. N. Wright, "An Assessment of the Unreliability of the History Given by Self-Poisoned Patients," *Clinical Toxicology* 16 (1980):381–384.

9. D.T. Teitelbaum, J. Morgan, and G. Gray, "Nonconcordance between Clinical Impression and Laboratory Findings in Clinical Toxicology" *Clinical Toxicology* 10 (1977):417–422.

10. P.A. Palmisano, "Hospitalization as a Measure of Clinical Toxicity," *Clinical Toxicology* 16 (1980):377–380.

11. *Survey of the Most-Frequently Accidentally Ingested Products* (Washington, D.C.: National Clearinghouse for Poison Control Centers, Department of Health, Education and Welfare, 1963).

12. R.A. Stallones and L. Corsa, Jr., "Epidemiology of Childhood Accidents in Two California Counties," *Public Health Reports* 76 (1971):25–36.

13. D.I. Manheimer, J. Dewey, G.D. Mellinger, and L. Corsa, Jr., "50,000 Child-Years of Accidental Injuries," *Public Health Reports* 81 (1966):519–533.

14. L. Corsa, Jr., and R.A. Stallones, "Epidemiology Study of Childhood Poisonings in Two California Counties," *Pediatrics* 28 (1961):480–489.

15. A.R. Temple and K. Stremming, "Taste as a Deterrent in Pediatric Poisonings, *Clinical Toxicology* 8 (1975):541–546.

16. J.R. Sibert and R.G. Newcombe, "Accidental Ingestion of Poisons and Child Personality," *Postgraduate Medical Journal* 53 (1977):254–256.

17. M.A. Stewart, B.T. Thach, and M.R. Freidin, "Accidental Poisoning and the Hyperactive Child Syndrome," *Diseases of the Nervous System* 31 (1970):403–407.

18. J.A. Margolis, "Psychosocial Study of Childhood Poisoning: A 5-Year Follow-up," *Pediatrics* 47 (1971):439–444.

19. R. Sibert, "Stress in Families of Children Who Have Ingested Poisons," *British Medical Journal* 3 (1975):87–89.

20. R. Sobel, "The Psychiatric Implications of Accidental Poisoning in Childhood," *Pediatric Clinics of North America* 17 (1970):653–685.

21. H.A. Carithers, "Accident Prevention in Childhood: The Kerosene Hazard," *Journal of the American Medical Association* 159 (1959):109–111.

22. R.J. Meyer, "Acetylsalicylic Acid (Aspirin) Poisoning," *American Journal of Diseases of Children* 102 (1961):47–54.

23. F.J. DeCastro and J.L. Kocur, "Child Poisoning: Importance of Early Rising," *Pediatrics* 51 (1973):589.

24. G.H. Maragos, C.A. Greene, and J.R. Mitchell, "Accidental Poisoning of Children in Transit," *Journal of Pediatrics* 79 (1971):125–126.

25. J. Pach, L. Colewa, K. Prochowska, and A. Koczur, "The Epidemiology of Acute Poisoning in the Krakow Region," *Acta Pharamcologica et Toxicologica (Copenhagen)* (suppl.) 41 (1977):528–533.

26. A.J. McBay and P. Hudson, "Drug Deaths in North Carolina: A Brief Survey of Deaths Attributed to Drugs in North Carolina, 1973," *North Carolina Medical Journal* 35 (1974):542–544.

27. H.L. Taylor and R.P. Hudson, Jr., "Acute Ethanol Poisoning: A Two-Year Study of Deaths in North Carolina," *Journal of Forensic Science* 22 (1977):639–653.

28. J. Ipsen, M. Moore, and L. Alexander, "Prevalence of Alcoholism in the Population and among Suicides and Accidents from Poisoning, Massachusetts 1938–1948," *Quarterly Journal of Studies on Alcohol* 13 (1952):204–214.

29. P.Schernitski, J.L. Bootman, J. Byers, K. Likes, and J.H. Hughes, "Demographic Characteristics of Elderly Drug Overdose Patients Admitted to a Hospital Emergency Department," *Journal of the American Geriatric Society* 28 (1980):544–546.

30. D. Schwartz, M. Wang, L. Zeitz, and M.E.W. Goss, "Medication Errors Made by Elderly, Chronically Ill Patients," *American Journal of Public Health* 52 (1962):2018–2029.

31. H.M. Cann, A.P. Iskrant, and D.S. Neyman, "Epidemologic Aspects of Poisoning Accidents," *American Journal of Public Health* 50 (1960):1914–1924.

32. H. Jolly and T.R.W. Forrest, "Accident Poisoning in Childhood," *Lancet* 1 (1958):1308–1309.

33. F.D. Burg and J.M. Douglass, "In Cold Gas," *Clinical Pediatrics* 8 (1969):590–593.

34. F.B. Oglesbay, Jr., and J.L. Morgan, "The Carbon Monoxide, Fire, and Explosion Problem in Travel Trailers and Pickup Campers," paper presented at the 33d Annual Educational Conference, National Association of Sanitarians, Houston, Tex., 22–29 June 1969.

35. "The Dangers of 'Safe' Solvents," *Journal of the American Medical Association* 208 (1969):1484.

36. S.P. Baker, R.S. Fisher, W.C. Masemore, and I.M. Sopher, "Fatal Unintentional Carbon Monoxide Poisoning in Motor Vehicles," *American Journal of Public Health* 62 (1972):1463–1467.

37. N. Kreitman, "The Coal Gas Story," *British Journal of Preventive and Social Medicine* 30 (1976):86–93.

38. N. Sadan and B. Soroker, "Observations on the Effects of the Bite of a Venomous Snake on Children and Adults," *Journal of Pediatrics* 76 (1970):711–715.

39. J.A. Cimino and H. Raybin, "Semantics of Pesticides," *New England Journal of Medicine* 277 (1967):1152.

40. J.M. Arena, "Safety Closure Caps," *Journal of the American Medical Association* 169 (1959):1187–1188.

41. C.S. Hoskins and A.M. Williamson, "The Ability of Children to Obtain Tablets From Different Containers," *Medical Journal of Australia* 2 (1969):793–794.

42. C.E. Stracener and R.G. Scherz, "Experiences with Safety Containers for Prevention of Accidental Childhood Poisoning," *Northwest Medicine* 69 (1970):334–339.

43. M.S. McIntire, C.R. Angle, K. Sathees, and P.S.T. Lee, "Safety Packaging: What Does the Public Think?" *American Journal of Public Health* 67 (1977):169–171.

44. M.S. McIntire, C.R. Angle, and M.L. Grush, "How Effective Is Safety Packaging?," *Clinical Toxicology* 9 (1976):419–425.

45. "Child-Resistant Safety Caps Are Paying Off," *CPSC Memo* (Washington, D.C.: Consumer Product Safety Commission, August/September 1979).

46. H.C. Mofenson and J. Greensher, "Keeping Up with the Changing Trends in Childhood Poisonings," *Clinical Pediatrics* 14 (1975):621.

47. R.H. Godwin, "Child-Resistant Locks in Poison Control," *Pediatrics* 61 (1978):750–752.

48. L. Fisher, J. Van Buren, J.L. Nitzkin, R.A. Lawrence, and R. Swackhamer, "Highlight Results of the Monroe County Poison Prevention Demonstration Project," *Veterinary and Human Toxicology* 22 (supp. 2) (1980):15–17.

49. B.T. Braden, "Validation of a Poison Prevention Program," *American Journal of Public Health* 69 (1979):942–944.

50. E.P. Krenzelok and R.J. Garber, "Teaching Poison Prevention to Preschool Children, Their Parents and Professional Educators through Child Care Centers," *American Journal of Public Health* 71 (1981):750–752.

51. B. de la Burdé and B. Reames, "Prevention of Pica, The Major Cause of Lead Poisoning in Children," *American Journal of Public Health* 63 (1973):737–743.

52. M. Thebaut, "Prize Case," *Bulletin* (November 1963):33–34 (Oakland, Calif.: Alameda-Contra Costa County Medical Association).

Chapter 23

1. *Accident Facts, 1981 Edition* (Chicago, Ill.: National Safety Council, 1981).

2. *Accident Prevention Can Be Learned* (New York: Metropolitan Life Insurance Co., 1962).

3. S.E. Leard, "Clinical Aspects of the College Student's Health," *Archives of Environmental Health* 8 (1964):846–849.

4. G. Scheffler, "Student Accidental Injury Experience," *Journal of the American College Health Association* 16 (1967):85–90.

5. O.P. Arya and C.B. Bosa, "Injury in the University Environment," *East African Medical Journal* 48 (1971):420–426.

6. D. Hughes, "Radiation Accidents in University Laboratories, *Accident Analysis and Prevention* 2 (1970):29–34.

7. J.A. Waller and J.K. Worden, "Strategies for Safety Program Planning and Evaluation: Lessons from the Vermont Alcohol and Highway Safety Campaign," *Proceedings of a Symposium on Traffic Safety Effectiveness (Impact) Evaluation Projects, Chicago, Ill., 19–20 May 1981* (Chicago, Ill.: National Safety Council, 1981), 117–131.

8. J.A. Waller, J.K. Worden, and I.W. Maranville, *Baseline Data for Public Education about Alcohol and Highway Safety in Vermont* (Waterbury, Vt.: Project CRASH, Vermont Department of Mental Health, 1972, CRASH Report I-1, NHTSA Contract FH-11-7543, 1972).

9. B. Preston, "Statistical Analysis of Child Pedestrian Accidents in Manchester and Salford," *Accident Analysis and Prevention* 4 (1972):323–332.

10. W.M. Bartholomew, "Pedestrian Accidents in Service Areas of Selected City Recreation Facilities," *Traffic Safety Research Review* 11 (1969):117–120.

11. *NEISS Data Highlights* 5(4) (October–December 1981) (Washington, D.C.: Consumer Product Safety Commission).

12. J.A. Waller, *Injuries Involving Playground Equipment* (Burlington, Vt.: University of Vermont, Final Report on Grants 1 RO1 FD 00003 of the Food and Drug Administration and CPSC 00003 of the Consumer Product Safety Commission, 1976).

13. *Public Playground Equipment: HIA Hazard Analysis Report* (Washington, D.C.: Consumer Product Safety Commission, 1979).

14. W.B. Beine and J.R. Sorrells, *Soil Impact Attenuation Performance: A Field Study* (Washington, D.C.: National Bureau of Standards, Department of Commerce, Report NBSIR 80-2106, 1980).

15. T.E. Reichelderfer, A. Overbach, and J. Greensher, "Unsafe Playgrounds," *Pediatrics* 64 (1979):962–963.

16. P. Werner, "Playground Injuries and Voluntary Product Standards for Home and Public Playgrounds," *Pediatrics* 69 (1982):18–29.

17. Playground Fun May Be Hazardous," *CPSC Memo* (Washington, D.C.: Consumer Product Safety Commission, June 1979), 4.

18. L. Fisher, V.G. Harris, J. Van Buren, J. Quinn, and A. De Maio, "Assessment of a Pilot Child Playground Injury Prevention Project in New York State," *American Journal of Public Health* 70 (1980):1000–1002.

19. R.B. Sleight, K.G. Cook, and P.J. Verhoven, *Investigation of Youth*

Camp Safety (Arlington, Va.: Century Research Corp. and National Recreation and Park Association, Final Report on Contract HSM 99-73-37, 1974).

20. R.S. Asnes, B. Feldman, W.M. Gersony, S. Morrison, and M. Weiss, "The Medical Care of Children at Summer Camps," *American Journal of Diseases of Children* 128 (1974):64–66.

21. R. Meyer, A.K. Kibrick, S. Kibrick, M.P. Ryan, R. Godbout, and E. Brown, "Epidemiology of Summer Camp Accidents," *Archives of Environmental Health* 7 (1963):325–330.

22. P.B. Stanilonis and R.J. Meyer, "Health and Safety in Summer Camps," *Public Health Reports* 81 (1966):305–310.

23. M.E. Cosand, *Accidents and Illnesses in Summer Camps Serving 85,000 Southern California Children* (San Bernadino, Calif.: San Bernadino County Health Department, 1964).

24. H.S. Barrett, "Summer Residential Camp Accidents, Injuries and Emergencies," *Connecticut Medicine* 33 (1969):521–523.

25. J.A. Waller and C.E. Gettinger, "Rural EMS: The Other Pickwickian Syndrome and the Pooh Bah Dilemma," *EMT Journal* 1(3) (September 1977):31–35.

26. Education Committee, *Emergency Department Nurses Association Core Curriculum, 2d ed.* (Chicago, Ill.: Emergency Department Nurses Association, 1980).

27. M.A. Weiner, C.E. Gettinger, J.A. Waller, D.B. Pilcher, and J.R. Goss, "In-Service Training for Rural Nurses in Emergency Care Concepts and Skills," *Journal of Emergency Nursing* 1 (March/April 1975):16–23.

28. R. Halloran, "Campaign by Father Who Lost Son Improves Safety in National Parks," *New York Times,* 28 February 1977, p. 16.

29. S. Herrero, "Human Injury Inflicted by Grizzly Bears," *Science* 170 (1970):593–598.

Chapter 24

1. A.J. Ryan, "Recreational Accidents: Prevention and Management," *Archives of Environmental Health* 13 (1966):507–510.

2. E.L. Lehr, "Recreation Safety," *Proceedings of the 1st Conference on Recreation Sanitation and Safety, Little Rock, Ark., 25–26 May 1966,* 45–51.

3. *NEISS Data Highlights* 5(4) (October–December 1981) (Washington, D.C.: Consumer Product Safety Commission).

4. B. Zaricznyj, L.J.M. Shattuck, T.A. Mast, R.V. Robertson, and G.D'Elia, "Sports-Related Injuries in School-Aged Children," *American Journal of Sports Medicine* 8 (1980):318–324.

5. A.P. Millar, "Sporting Injuries: Counting the Cost," *Medical Journal of Australia* 2 (26 August 1978):188.

6. J.F. Kraus, C.E. Franti, R.S. Riggins, D. Richards, and N.O.

Borhani, "Incidence of Traumatic Spinal Cord Lesions," *Journal of Chronic Diseases* 28 (1975):471–492.

7. K.W. Lindsay, G. McLatchie, and B. Jennett, "Serious Head Injury in Sport," *British Medical Journal* 281 (1980):789–791.

8. G.F. Rowbotham, I.N. Maciver, and J. Dickson, "Analysis of 1,400 Cases of Acute Injury to the Head," *British Medical Journal* 1 (1954):726–730.

9. J.F. Kraus, C.E. Franti, N.O. Borhani, and R.S. Riggins, "Survival with an Acute Spinal-Cord Injury," *Journal of Chronic Diseases* 32 (1979):269–283.

10. R.J. Burdge, "Levels of Occupational Prestige and Leisure Activity," *Journal of Leisure Research* 1 (1969):262–274.

11. J.A. Waller and D. Klein, "Society, Energy, and Injury: Inevitable Triad?" *Research Directions toward Reduction of Injury in the Young and the Old* (Bethesda, Md.: National Institute of Child Health and Human Development, Department of Human Services, DHEW Publication (NIH) 73-124, 1973).

12. J. Huberman, *A Psychological Study of Participants in High-Risk Sports* (Vancouver, B.C.: University of British Columbia, 1968).

13. T.D. Orlick, "Sport Participation: A Process of Shaping Behavior," *Human Factors* 16 (1974):558–561.

14. L. Martin, *Effects of Competition upon the Aggressive Responses of College Basketball Players and Wrestlers* (Cortland, N.Y.: Department of Physical Education, State University College at Cortland, 1976).

15. F.R. Eastwood, "Hazards to Health: Athletic Injuries," *New England Journal of Medicine* 271 (1964):411–413.

16. G.R. McLatchie, "Equestrian Injuries: A One Year Prospective Study," *British Journal of Sports Medicine* 13 (1979):29–32.

17. K.S. Clarke and W.E. Buckley, "Women's Injuries in Collegiate Sports," *American Journal of Sports Medicine* 8 (1980):187–191.

18. D.L. MacIntosh, T. Skrien, and R.J. Shephard, "Physical Activity and Injury," *Journal of Sports Medicine* 12 (1972):224–237.

19. W.A. Grana, "Summary of 1978–79 Injury Registry for Oklahoma Secondary Schools," *Oklahoma State Medical Association Journal* 72 (1979):369–372.

20. R.N. Marshall and H. Sandes, "Dunedin Sports Injuries 1974–1976," *New Zealand Medical Journal* 86 (1977):423–427.

21. "Sports Hazards," *Statistical Bulletin* 60(3) (July–September 1979):2–5 (New York: Metropolitan Life Insurance Co.).

22. J.P. Sparks, "Half a Million Hours of Rugby Football," *British Journal of Sports Medicine* 15 (1981):30–32.

23. D.S. Jackson, W.K. Furman, and B.L. Berson, "Patterns of Injuries in College Athletes: A Retrospective Study of Injuries Sustained in Intercollegiate Athletics in Two Colleges over a Two-Year Period," *Mt. Sinai Journal of Medicine* 47 (1980):423–426.

24. R.E. Hogue, "Principles for the Prevention of Sports Injuries in the Eight to Seventeen Year Old Age Group," *Progress in Physical Therapy* 1 (1970):118–123.

25. C.S. Blyth and F.O. Mueller, *An Epidemiologic Study of High School Football Injuries in North Carolina* (Chapel Hill, N.C.: Department of Physical Education, University of North Carolina, Final Report CPSC-C-74-18, 1974).

26. G. Snively, Statement before National Commission on Product Safety, 18 February 1969, *Hearings, National Commission on Product Safety, Washington, D.C., January–February 1969,* vol. 3A (New York: Law-Arts Publishers, Inc., 1970), 432–442.

27. "Skateboarding, New Nationwide Fad, Brings Fear of Injuries to Come," *Medical Tribune* 6(59) (17 May 1965):1, 22.

28. S.H. Schuman, "Skateboard Injuries in a Campus Community," *Clinical Pediatrics* 6 (1967):252–254.

29. R.L. Allum, "Skateboard Injuries: A New Epidemic," *Injury* 10 (1978):152–153.

30. "Skateboarding: Study Points Out Injuries and Hazards," *CPSC Memo* (Washington, D.C.: Consumer Product Safety Commission, May 1978), 1, 6.

31. "Skate-Boarding Curbed by Cities," *New York Times,* 13 June 1976, p. 43.

32. W.J. Morgan, D.J. Galloway, and A.R. Patel, "Prevention of Skateboard Injuries," *Scottish Medical Journal* 25 (1980):39–40.

33. Commission Denies Request to Ban Skateboards," (Washington, D.C.: Consumer Product Safety Commission, press release, 25 June 1979).

34. "Roller Skates Pass Skateboards as Major Cause of Recreational Injury," (Washington, D.C.: Consumer Product Safety Commission, press release, 15 April 1980).

35. R.D. Ferkel, L.L. Mai, K.C. Ullis, and G.A.M. Finerman, "An Analysis of Roller Skating Injuries," *American Journal of Sports Medicine* 10 (1981):24–30.

36. *Summary Analysis of Toy Cars and Trucks (1305)* (Washington, D.C.: Consumer Product Safety Commission, 8 August 1973).

37. "Toy Boxes and Chests," *NEISS News* 3(1) (July 1974):3 (Washington, D.C.: Consumer Product Safety Commission).

38. "Toys: Ingestions and Aspirations," *NEISS News* 4 (2) (October 1975):3 (Washington, D.C.: Consumer Product Safety Commission).

39. "Fact Sheet No. 47: Toys" (Washington, D.C.: Consumer Product Safety Commission, 1974).

40. Y.C. Ching, J.D. Huitt, and G.I. Magao, "The Dangerous Toy Balloon," *Pediatrics* 50 (1972):476–477.

41. G. Rutherford, Jr., *Injuries Associated with Projectile Toys* (Washington, D.C.: Consumer Product Safety Commission, 1979).

42. W.H. Mosberg and J.O. Sharrett, "Penetrating Wounds of Skull

Due to Metal Axle of Collapsible Toy Cars," *Journal of the American Medical Association* 173 (1960):804–805.

43. S.N. Sesser, "News From Toyland," *New Republic,* 20 December 1969, pp. 11–13.

44. H. Saha and V.J. Rama Rao, "Accidental Deaths among Children," *Indian Journal of Pediatrics* 36 (1969):103–111.

45. V.D. Plueckhahn, "The Aetiology of 134 Deaths Due to 'Drowning' in Geelong during the Years 1957 to 1971," *Medical Journal of Australia* 2 (1972):1183–1186.

46. P.E. Dietz and S.P. Baker, "Drowning: Epidemiology and Prevention," *American Journal of Public Health* 64 (1974):303–312.

47. E. Press, J. Walker, and I. Crawford, "An Interstate Drowning Study," *American Journal of Public Health* 58 (1968):2275–2289.

48. *Accident Facts, 1981 Edition* (Chicago, Ill.: National Safety Council, 1981).

49. J.H. Pearn, R.D. Bart, and R. Yamaoka, "Neurologic Sequelae after Childhood Near-Drowning: A Total Population Study from Hawaii," *Pediatrics* 64 (1979):187–191.

50. R. Eriksson, H. Fredin, P. Gerdman, and J. Thorson, "Sequelae of Accidental Near-Drowning in Childhood," *Scandinavian Journal of Social Medicine* 1 (1973):3–6.

51. J.H. Modell, S.A. Graves, and E.J. Kuck, "Near-Drowning: Correlation of Level of Consciousness and Survival," *Canadian Anaesthetists Society Journal* 27 (1980):211–215.

52. A.W. Conn, J.E. Montes, G.A. Barker, and J.F. Edmonds, "Cerebral Salvage in Near-Drowning Following Neurological Classification by Triage," *Canadian Anesthetists Society Journal* 27 (1980):201–210.

53. S.H. Schuman, J.R. Rowe, H.M. Glazer, and J.S. Redding, "Risk of Drowning: An Iceberg Phenomenon," *Journal of the American College of Emergency Physicians* 6 (1977):139–143.

54. J.H. Pearn, J. Brown III, R. Wong, and R. Bart, "Bathtub Drownings: Report of Seven Cases," *Pediatrics* 64 (1979):68–70.

55. J.H. Pearn and J. Nixon, "An Analysis of the Causes of Freshwater Immersion Accidents Involving Children," *Accident Analysis and Prevention* 11 (1979):173–178.

56. J. Thorson, H. Fredin, P. Gerdman, and R. Wiklund, "Accidental Drowning Among Children in Sweden 1958–1967," *Acta Socio-Medica Scandinavica* 2–3 (1970):149–159.

57. S. Walker and J.N. Middelkamp, "Pail Immersion Accidents," *Clinical Pediatrics* 20 (1981):341–343.

58. I. Mackie, "Alcohol and Aquatic Disasters," *Medical Journal of Australia* 1 (1978):652–653.

59. "Alcohol and Drowning," *Medical Journal of Australia* 1 (1981):157–158.

60. M.I.Rowe, A. Arango, and G. Allington, "Profile of Pediatric Drowning Victims in a Water-Oriented Society," *Journal of Trauma* 17 (1977):587–591.

61. "Notion of Not Eating before Swimming May be Altered by Swimming Pool Test," *Medical Tribune,* 27 May 1963, p. 29.

62. J.W. Nixon, J.H. Pearn, and R. Wells, "Child Safety and the Public Media: An Analysis from the Brisbane Drowning Study," *Australian Paediatric Journal* 16 (1980):166–168.

63. J.H. Pearn and J. Nixon, "Swimming Pool Immersion Accidents," *Medical Journal of Australia* 1 (1977):432–437.

64. D. Crum, "Beware of 'Drowning' Equipment," *Family Safety* (Chicago, Ill.: National Safety Council, Summer 1962), 25–27.

65. "Swimming Pool Injuries: A Summary Report," *NEISS News* 1 (6) (August 1973):2 (Washington, D.C.: Consumer Product Safety Commission)

66. *Summarization of 39 In-Depth Investigations of Product Related Injuries: Swimming Pools and Associated Equipment (Above Ground) (1262)* (Washington, D.C.: Consumer Product Safety Commission, 1974).

67. L.S. Kewalramani and J.F. Kraus, "Acute Spinal-Cord Lesions from Diving: Epidemiological and Clinical Features," *Western Journal of Medicine* 126 (1977):353–361.

68. "CPSC Discloses Pool Injury Study," (Washington, D.C.: Consumer Product Safety Commission, press release, 22 June 1978).

69. O.W. Albrand and J. Walter, "Underwater Deceleration Curves in Relation to Injuries from Diving," *Surgical Neurology* 4 (1975):461–464.

70. D.C. Burke, "Spinal Cord Injuries from Water Sports," *Medical Journal of Australia* 2 (1972):1190–1194.

71. U. Mennen, "A Survey of Spinal Injuries from Diving," *South African Medical Journal* 59 (1981):788–790.

72. R.H. Allen, B. Eiseman, C.J. Straehley, and B.G. Orloff, "Surfing Injuries at Waikiki," *Journal of the American Medical Association* 237 (1977):668–670.

73. M. Kennedy and G. Vanderfield, "Medical Aspects of Surfcraft Usage," *Medical Journal of Australia* 2 (1976):707–709.

74. "Water Skiing Hailed as Safe, Careless Athletes the Peril," *Medical Tribune* 7 July 1969, p. 28.

75. R.J. Mann, "Propeller Injuries Incurred in Boating Accidents," *American Journal of Sports Medicine* 8 (1980):280–284.

76. P.G. Landsberg, "South African Underwater Diving Accidents, 1969–1976," *South African Medical Journal* 50 (1976):2155–2159.

77. M.K. Denney and R.C. Read, "SCUBA-Diving Deaths in Michigan," *Journal of the American Medical Association* 192 (1965):220–222.

78. P.R.F. Lewis, "Skin Diving Fatalities in New Zealand," *New Zealand Medical Journal* 89 (1979):472–475.

79. P.G. Landsberg, "Decompression Sickness in South African Sport Divers," *South African Medical Journal* 55 (1979):213–217.

80. J.A. Waller, P. Caplan, and A.E. Lowe, *Skin and SCUBA Diving as a Health Problem* (Berkeley, Calif.: California Department of Public Health, Technical Bulletin, 1964).

81. M.J. Nemiroff, L.H. Somers, and R.E. Anderson, "A Five-Year Study of Prevention of SCUBA-Diving Morbidity in a University Training Program," *Journal of the American College Health Association* 24 (1975):95–97.

82. B.W. Halstead, *Dangerous Marine Animals* (Cambridge, Md.: Cornell Maritime Press, 1959).

83. F.E. Russell, "Stingray Injuries," *Public Health Reports* 74 (1959):855–859.

84. D.H. Davies and G.D. Campbell, "The Aetiology, Clinical Pathology and Treatment of Shark Attack," *Journal of the Royal Naval Medical Service* 48 (3) (Summer 1962):3–28.

85. S. Nilsson and A. Roaas, "Soccer Injuries in Adolescents," *American Journal of Sports Medicine* 6 (1978):338–361.

86. D.A. Lingard, N.E. Sharrock, and C.E. Salmond, "Risk Factors of Sports Injuries in Winter," *New Zealand Medical Journal* 83 (1976):69–73.

87. W.C. McMaster and M. Walter, "Injuries in Soccer," *American Journal of Sports Medicine* 6 (1978):354–357.

88. J.W. Pritchett, "Cost of High School Soccer Injuries," *American Journal of Sports Medicine* 9 (1981):64–66.

89. T.E. Durkin, "A Survey of Injuries in a 1st Class Rugby Union Football Club from 1972–1976," *British Journal of Sports Medicine* 11 (1977):7–10.

90. D. Alexander, M. Kennedy, and J. Kennedy, "Injuries in Rugby League Football," *Medical Journal of Australia* 2 (1979):341–342.

91. R.M. Davies, D. Bradley, R.W. Hale, W.R.E. Laird, and P.D. Thomas, "The Prevalence of Dental Injuries in Rugby Players and Their Attitude to Mouthguards," *British Journal of Sports Medicine* 11 (1977):72–74.

92. J.G. Morton and J.F. Burton, "An Evaluation of the Effectiveness of Mouthguards in High-School Rugby Players," *New Zealand Dental Journal* 75 (1974):151–153.

93. E. Davies and T. Gibson, "Injuries in Rugby Union Football," *British Medical Journal* 2 (1978):1759–1761.

94. *Hazard Analysis: Football Activity and Related Equipment* (Washington, D.C.: Consumer Product Safety Commission, 1974).

95. J.F. Kraus and G. Colberg, "Some Epidemiologic Factors Associated with Intramural Football Injuries on a Rural College Campus," *Journal of the American College Health Association* 20 (1971):106–114.

96. J.F. Kraus, B.C. Anderson, and C.E. Mueller, "The Quality of Officiating as an Injury Prevention Factor in Intramural Touch Football," *Medicine and Science in Sports* 3 (1971):143–147.

97. E. Marshall, "Drugging of Football Players Curbed by Central Monitoring Plan, NFL Claims," *Science* 213 (1979):626–628.

98. "Mouth Protectors: 11 Years Later," *Journal of the American Dental Association* 86 (1973):1365–1367.

99. J.S. Garrick, G.S. Collins, and R.K. Requa, "Out of Bounds in Football: Player Exposure to Probability of Collision Injury," *Journal of Safety Research* 9 (1977):34–38.

100. W.W. Kundelin, G.S. Krahenbuhl, and C.A. Schacht, "Athletic Field Microclimates and Heat Stress," *Journal of Safety Research* 8 (1976):106–111.

101. J.S. Keene, "Environmental Factors in Early Season Practice," *Wisconsin Medical Journal* 76 (1977):S85–S87.

102. R. Morrow, "Grass for Player Safety," *Turf-Grass Times* (September/October 1967) (Jacksonville Beach, Fla.: Turf-Grass Publications, Inc.).

103. J.W. Adkison, R.K. Requa, and J.G. Garrick, "Injury Rates in High School Football," *Clinical Orthopedic and Related Research* 99 (1974):131–136.

104. J.S. Keene, R.G. Narechania, K.M. Sachtjen, and W.G. Clancy, "Tartan Turf on Trial," *American Journal of Sports Medicine* 8 (1980):43–47.

105. K.D. Bowers, "Ankle and Knee Injuries at West Virginia University before and after Astro Turf," *West Virginia Medical Journal* 69 (1973):1–3.

106. C.L. Stanitski, J.H. McMaster, and R.J. Ferguson, "Synthetic Turf and Grass: A Comparative Study," *Journal of Sports Medicine* 2 (1974):22–27.

107. B.R. Cahill and E.H. Griffith, "Effect of Preseason Conditioning on the Incidence and Severity of High School Football Knee Injuries," *American Journal of Sports Medicine* 6 (1978):180–184.

108. W.B. Beine, *Risks Associated with Certain Sports Activities* (Washington, D.C.: Center for Consumer Product Technology, National Bureau of Standards, Department of Commerce, Report NBSIR 77-1218, 1977).

109. T. Ryan, "Study Assessed Influence of Movies on Hockey Players," *Burlington (Vt.) Free Press,* 20 January 1982, pp. 1D, 4D.

110. Z. Hornof and C. Napravnik, "Analysis of Various Accident Rate Factors in Ice Hockey," *Medicine and Science in Sports* 5 (1973):283–286.

111. T.J. Pashby, "Eye Injuries in Hockey," *International Ophthalmology Clinics* 21 (4) (1981):59–81.

112. "Questions, Not Count, Called Best Guide to Boxer's State," *Medical World News* 3 (10) (11 May 1962):9.

113. J.C. Elia, "Head Injuries in Boxing," *International Surgery* 56 (1971):334–343.

114. A.L. Whiteson, "Injuries in Professional Boxing: Their Treatment and Prevention," *Practitioner* 225 (1981):1053–1057.

115. I.A. McCown, "Protecting The Boxer," *Journal of the American Medical Association* 169 (1959):1409–1413.

116. "Precareer, Prefight Exams Held Key to Reducing Injury," *Medical Tribune,* 9 July 1962, pp. 28–29.

117. T. Rogers, "Canadian Boxer Dies after Fight Injury," *New York Times,* 8 July 1980, p. B10.

118. G.A. Snook, "Injuries in Intercollegiate Wrestling," *American Journal of Sports Medicine* 10 (1982):142–144.

119. J.W. Powell, "National Athletic Injury/Illness Reporting System: Eye Injuries in College Wrestling," *International Ophthalmology Clinics* 21 (4) (1981):47–58.

120. J.J. Estwanik, J. Bergfeld, and T. Canty, "Report of Injuries Sustained during the United States Olympic Wrestling Trials," *American Journal of Sports Medicine* 6 (1978):335–340.

121. G.R. McLatchie, "Analysis of Karate Injuries Sustained in 295 Contests," *Injury* 8 (1977):132–134.

122. G.R. McLatchie, J.E. Davies, and J.H. Caulley, "Injuries in Karate: A Case for Medical Control," *Journal of Trauma* 20 (1980):956–958.

123. G.R. McLatchie and M.B. Morris, "Prevention of Karate Injuries: A Progress Report," *British Journal of Sports Medicine* 11 (1977):78–82.

124. K.K. Klein, "The Martial Arts and the Caucasian Knee," *Journal of Sports Medicine* 3 (1975):44–47.

125. "Fact Sheet No. 49: Sleds, Toboggans and Snow Disks," (Washington, D.C.: Consumer Product Safety Commission, 1974).

126. R.K. Requa, J. M. Toney, and J.G. Garrick, "Parameters of Injury Reporting in Skiing," *Medicine and Science in Sports* 9 (1977):185–190.

127. J.G. Garrick and L. Kurland, "The Epidemiologic Significance of Unreported Ski Injuries," *Journal of Safety Research* 3 (1971):182–187.

128. E. Eriksson and R.J. Johnson, "The Etiology of Downhill Ski Injuries," *Exercise and Sport Science Reviews* 8 (1980):1–17.

129. J.T. Weston, S.M. Moore, and T.H. Rich, "A Five-Year Study of Mortality in a Busy Ski Population," *Journal of Forensic Science* 22 (1977):222–230.

130. J.A. Waller, R.J. Johnson, and M.H. Pope, paper in progress (Burlington, Vt.: University of Vermont).

131. R.J. Johnson, C. F. Ettlinger, R.J. Campbell, and M.H. Pope, "Trends in Skiing Injuries," *American Journal of Sports Medicine* 8 (1980):106–113.

132. N.E. Westlin, "Injuries in Long Distance Cross Country and Downhill Skiing," *Orthopedic Clinics of North America* 7 (1976):55–58.

133. J. Sandelin, O. Kiviluoto, and S. Santavirta, "Injuries of Competitive Skiers in Finland: A Three Year Survey," *Annals Chirurgiae et Gynecologiae (Helsinki)* 69 (1980):97–101.

134. " 'Hotdogging' Increases Risk of Spinal-Cord Injury in Skier," *Medical Tribune*, 22 May 1974, p. 23.

135. M. Strauss, "Safety on Ski Lifts Being Upgraded," *New York Times*, 3 December 1976, p. 8.

136. E.B. Whorton, Jr., letter to Bolton Valley Ski Lodge, Bolton Valley, Vt., 21 March 1969.

137. Unpublished investigations (Burlington, Vt.: Epidemiology Unit, Vermont Department of Health, 1982).

138. E.C. Percy, "The Snowmobile: Friend or Foe?," *Journal of Trauma* 12 (1972):444–446.

139. R.E. Dewar, "A Review and Critique of Snowmobile Accident Reports," *Journal of Safety Research* 5 (1973):36–44.

140. B. Rice, "The Snowmobile Is an American Dream Machine," *New York Times Magazine*, 13 February 1972, pp. 14, 15, 26–33.

141. J.A. Waller, "A Survey of Snowmobiling in Vermont," *Accident Analysis and Prevention* 7 (1975):207–212.

142. J.A. Waller and K.R. Lamborn, "Snowmobiling: Characteristics of Owners, Patterns of Use and Injuries," *Accident Analysis and Prevention* 7 (1975):213–223.

143. W.L. Carlson and D. Klein, "Behavioral Patterns of Snowmobile Operators: A Preliminary Report," *Journal of Safety Research* 3 (1971):150–156.

144. G.A. Peters, "Snowmobiles and the New Standards," *Journal of Products Liability* 1 (1977):107–114.

145. "Snowmobiles" *CPC Memo* (Washington, D.C.: Consumer Product Safety Commission, February 1979), pp. 3, 6.

146. M.B. Habal, M.M. Meguid, and J.E. Murray, "The Long Scarf Syndrome: A Potentially Fatal and Preventable Hazard," *Journal of the American Medical Association* 221 (1972):1269–1270.

147. *Snowmobile Collisions on Highways and Roads in Ontario* (Toronto: Ontario Department of Transport, 1970).

148. "Snowmobile Trails Said to Need Built-In Safety to Reduce Accident Rate," *Medical Tribune*, 16 February 1970, p. 22.

149. "Sleds, Toboggans and Snow Disks," *NEISS News* 2 (4) (3 December 1973) (Washington, D.C.: Consumer Product Safety Commission).

150. L.D. Hensley and D.C. Paup, "A Survey of Badminton Injuries," *British Journal of Sports Medicine* 13 (1979):156–160.

151. D.N. Kulund, F.C. McCue III, D.A. Rockwell, and J.H. Gieck, "Tennis Injuries: Prevention and Treatment," *American Journal of Sports Medicine* 7 (1979):249–253.

152. C.A. Soderstrom and M.T. Doxanas, "Racquetball: A Game with Preventable Injuries," *American Journal of Sports Medicine* 10 (1982):180–183.

153. P.F. Vinger, and D.W. Tolpin, "Racket Sports: An Ocular Hazard," *Journal of the American Medical Association* 239 (1978):2575–2577.

154. M. Easterbrook, "Eye Injuries in Racket Sports," *International Ophthalmology Clinics* 21 (4) (1981):87–119.

155. G.V. Barrell, P.J. Cooper, A.R. Elkington, J.M. MacFadyen, R.G. Powell, and P. Tormey, "Squash Ball to Eye Ball: The Likelihood of

Squash Players Incurring an Eye Injury," *British Medical Journal* 283 (1981):893–895.

156. F.L. Allman, "The Prevention and Treatment of Orthopedic Problems Related to an Adult Exercise Program," *Journal of Occupational Medicine* 13 (1971):573–576.

157. G. Mirkin, "The Prevention and Treatment of Running Injuries," *Journal of the American Podiatry Association* 66 (1976):880–884.

158. D.B.Clement and J.E. Taunton, "A Guide to the Prevention of Running Injuries," *Australian Family Physician* 10 (1981):156–164.

159. M.E. Blazina, R.S. Watanabe, and E.C. Drake, "Fatigue Fractures in Track Athletes," *California Medicine* 97 (1962):61–62.

160. A.F. Williams, "When Motor Vehicles Hit Joggers: An Analysis of 60 Cases," *Public Health Reports* 96 (1981):448–451.

161. R.L. Hughson, H.L. Green, M.E. Houston, J.A. Thomson, D.R. MacLean, and J.R. Sutton, "Heat Injuries in Canadian Mass Participation Runs," *Canadian Medical Association Journal* 122 (1980):1141–1144.

162. "Prevention of Heat Injuries during Distance Running: Statement of the American College of Sports Medicine," *Journal of Sports Medicine and Physical Fitness* 16 (1976):345–346.

163. G.M. O'Donoghue and K.C. Condon, "Facial Injuries in Hurlers," *Journal of the Irish Medical Association* 72 (1979):448–449.

164. "Pole Vaulting Champ Remains Quadriplegic after a 17-Foot Fall," *Medical Tribune,* 19 August 1963, p. 29.

165. J.G. Garrick and R.K. Requa, "Epidemiology of Women's Gymnastics Injuries," *American Journal of Sports Medicine* 8 (1980):261–264.

166. A. Hammer, A.L. Schwartzbach, and P.E. Paulev, "Trampoline Training Injuries: One Hundred and Ninety-Five Cases," *British Journal of Sports Medicine* 15 (1981):151–158.

167. A.B. Lipscomb, "Baseball Pitching Injuries in Growing Athletes," *Journal of Sports Medicine* 3 (1975):25–34.

168. J.J. Gugenheim, R.F. Stanley, G.W. Woods, and H.S. Tullos, "Little League Survey: The Houston Study," *American Journal of Sports Medicine* 4 (1976):189–200.

169. R.L. Larson, K.M. Singer, R. Bergstrom, and S. Thomas, "Little League Survey: The Eugene Survey," *American Journal of Sports Medicine* 4 (1976):201–209.

170. R.L. Larson, "Pre-High School Baseball Injuries," *American Medical Association Proceedings of the 3d National Conference on Medical Aspects of Sports, Denver, Colo., 26 November 1961,* 4–7.

171. "Complaints Issued to Amusement Firms," *CPSC Memo* (Washington, D.C.: Consumer Product Safety Commission, October 1980), 1–8.

172. G.G. Youngson and R. Baker, "Go-kart Injuries," *Injury* 9 (1978):212–215.

173. S.S. Miller and D. Proctor, "Go-kart Injuries at a Fairground," *British Medical Journal* 3 (1973):685–686.

174. S.B. Seager, L. Jui-Aenile, and N. Faux, "The Urban Cowboy Syndrome," *Annals of Emergency Medicine* 10 (1981):252–253.

175. J. Gierup, M. Larsson and S. Lennquist, "Incidence and Nature of Horse-Riding Injuries," *Acta Chirurgica Scandinavica (Stockholm)* 142 (1976):57–61.

176. L.G. Danielsson and N.E. Westlin, "Riding Accidents," *Acta Orthopaetica Scandinavica (Copenhagen)* 44 (1973):597–603.

177. J.A.I. Grossman, D.N. Kulund, C.W. Miller, R. Winn, and R.H. Hodge, Jr., "Equestrian Injuries: Results of a Prospective Study," *Journal of the American Medical Association* 240 (1978):1881–1882.

178. P. Edixhoven, S.C. Sinha, and D.J. Dandy, "Horse Injuries," *Injury* 12 (1981):279–282.

179. T.L. Hanna and L.A. Selby, "Characteristics of the Human and Pet Populations in Animal Bite Incidents Recorded at Two Air Force Bases," *Public Health Reports* 96 (1981):580–584.

180. A.M. Beck, H. Loring, and R. Lockwood, "The Ecology of Dog Bite Injury in St. Louis, Missouri," *Public Health Reports* 90 (1975):262–266.

181. D.R. Berzon, "The Animal Bite Epidemic in Baltimore, Maryland: Review and Update," *American Journal of Public Health* 68 (1978):593–595.

182. R. Lockwood, A.M. Beck, and K. Hornberger, "Dog Bites among Letter Carriers in St. Louis," *Public Health Reports* 90 (1975):267–269.

183. J.S. Marr, A.M. Beck, and J.A. Lugo, Jr. "An Epidemiologic Study of the Human Bite," *Public Health Reports* 94 (1979):514–521.

184. M. Heins, R. Kahn, and J. Bjordnal, "Gunshot Wounds in Children," *American Journal of Public Health* 64 (1974):326–330.

185. S.P. Baker and P.E. Dietz, *Injury Prevention* (Baltimore, Md.: Johns Hopkins School of Hygiene and Public Health, background paper for a *Report to Surgeon General of the United States on Disease Prevention and Health Promotion,* 1 November 1978).

186. N.B. Rushforth, C.S. Hirsch, A.B. Ford, and L. Adelson, "Accidental Firearm Fatalities in a Metropolitan County," *American Journal of Epidemiology* 100 (1975):499–505.

187. D. Klein, M.S. Reizen, G.H. Van Amburg, and S.A. Walker, "Some Social Characteristics of Young Gunshot Fatalities," *Accident Analysis and Prevention* 9 (1977):177–182.

188. J.A. Waller and E.B. Whorton, "Unintentional Shootings, Highway Crashes and Acts of Violence: A Behavior Paradigm," *Accident Analysis and Prevention* 5 (1973):351–356.

189. *Hazard Analysis: Fireworks Injuries* (Washington, D.C.: Consumer Product Safety Commission, 1973).

190. "Despite Strict Rules Fireworks Injuries Are Up," *CPSC Memo* (Washington, D.C.: Consumer Product Safety Commission, June 1981), 1–2.

191. G. Wakely and P. Richards, "Accidents from Fireworks," *New Zealand Medical Journal* 79 (1974):918–920.

192. B.Collins and D. Karsner, *Special Report: Fireworks Injuries, 1978 Independence Day Period* (Washington, D.C.: Consumer Product Safety Commission, 1979).

193. R.S. Wilson, "Fireworks Blindness in Arkansas," *Journal of the Arkansas Medical Society* 72 (1976):357–359.

194. "Federal Government Warns of Annual Hazard from Fireworks" (Washington, D.C.: Consumer Product Safety Commission, press release 18 June 1979).

195. "Hazardous Avocations," *Statistical Bulletin* 51 (June 1970):2–4 (New York: Metropolitan Life Insurance Co.).

196. B.G. Ferris, Jr., "Mountain-Climbing Accidents in the United States," *New England Journal of Medicine* 268 (1963):430–431.

197. B.G. Ferris, Jr., "Mountain-Climbing Safety," *New England Journal of Medicine* 268 (1963):662–664.

198. I.A. Olson and R.O. Ward, "Accidents on Mountains: Letters to Editor," *British Medical Journal* 2 (1964):1462.

199. "Portable Camping Equipment," *NEISS News* 5 (2) (September 1976):1,2,6,7 (Washington, D.C.: Consumer Product Safety Commission).

200. B. Eiseman, "Hang Gliding," *Journal of the American Medical Association* 233 (1975):171–172.

201. G.M. Yuill, "Icarus's Syndrome: New Hazards in Flight," *British Medical Journal* 1 (1977):823–825.

202. J.R. Tongue, "Hang Gliding Injuries in California," *Journal of Trauma* 17 (1977):898–902.

203. W.B. Krissoff, "Follow-Up On Hang Gliding Injuries in Colorado," *American Journal of Sports Medicine* 4 (1976):222–229.

204. W.B. Krissoff and B. Eiseman, "Injuries Associated with Hang Gliding," *Journal of the American Medical Association* 233 (1975):158–160.

205. T. Hallel and L. Naggan, "Parachuting Injuries: A Retrospective Study of 83,718 Jumps," *Journal of Trauma* 15 (1975):14–19.

206. A.J. Ryan and C.L. Thomas, "Sport Parachuting and Sky Diving," *Journal of the American Medical Association* 194 (1965):259–263.

207. "Sport-Parachutist Injuries Cut to 1:1,000 in Few Years," *Hospital Tribune,* 6 May 1968, p. 20.

208. F.W. Kiel, "Parachuting for Sport," *Journal of the American Medical Association* 194 (1965):264–268.

209. M.I. Bullock, "Ripcord Release Capability of Female Parachutists," *Aviation, Space and Environmental Medicine* 49 (1978):1177–1183.

210. N.A. Marcus, E.R. Sweetser, and R.W. Benson, "Hot-Air Ballooning Injuries," *American Journal of Sports Medicine* 9 (1981):318–321.

211. Flying in Balloons, Blimps, Gliders, and Kites," *Statistical Bulletin* 56 (September 1975):5–7 (New York: Metropolitan Life Insurance Co.).

212. W. Haddon, Jr., "Principles in Research on the Effects of Sports on Health," *Journal of the American Medical Association* 197 (1966):885–888.

Chapter 25

1. L.R. Schauer, *Work Injuries and Work Injury Rates in Hospitals* (Washington, D.C.: U.S. Department of Labor, BLS Report 340, 1968).

2. R.G. Lee, "Health and Safety in Hospitals," *Medicine, Science and the Law* 19 (1979):89–103.

3. M. Oliva, "Safety in Hospitals," *Modern Hospital* 105 (July 1965):91–93.

4. F. Grubel, "Falls: A Principal Patient Incident," *Hospital Management* 88 (November 1959):37–38, 137.

5. T.P. Weil, J.J. Freysinger, and H.M. Parrish, "Epidemiology of Patient Accidents," *Industrial Medicine and Surgery* 31 (1962):186–190.

6. W.R. Williams, "The Patients' Accident Pattern," *Hospitals: Journal of the American Hospital Association* 22 (December 1948):39–41.

7. W.E. Snell, "Accidents to Patients in Hospitals," *Lancet* 2 (1956):1202–1203.

8. I.D. Fagin and M. Vita, "Who? Where? When? How? An Analysis of 868 Inpatient Accidents," *Hospitals: Journal of the American Hospital Association* 39 (16 August 1965):60–65.

9. T.P. Weil and H.M. Parrish, "How Did It Happen? An Analysis of the Causes of 2,036 Patient Accidents at New York's Mt. Sinai Hospital," *Hospitals: Journal of the American Hospital Association* 32 (1 September 1958):43–48.

10. I. Margulee, G. Librach, and M. Schadel, "Epidemiological Study of Accidents Among Residents of Homes for the Aged," *Journal of Gerontology* 25 (1970):342–346.

11. B.R. Ballinger and A.C. Ramsay, "Accidents and Drug Treatment in a Psychiatric Hospital," *British Journal of Psychiatry* 126 (1975):462–463.

12. J. Foerster, "A Study of Falls: The Elderly Nursing Home Resident," *Journal of the New York State Nurses Association* 12 (2) (June 1981):9–17.

13. I.B. Corless, "A Critique," *Journal of the New York State Nurses Association* 12(2) (June 1981):30–36.

14. E.F. Morris and B. Isaacs, "The Prevention of Falls in a Geriatric Hospital," *Age and Aging* 9 (1980):181–185.

15. L. Hiatt Snyder, "Environmental Changes for Socialization," *Journal of Nursing Administration* 8(1) (January 1978):44–50.

16. L. Hiatt Snyder, "Living Environments, Geriatric Wheelchairs and Older Persons' Rehabilitation," *Journal of Gerontological Nursing* 1(5) (November/December 1975):17–20.

17. K.N. Barker and W.E. McConnell, "How to Detect Medication Errors in Hospitals," *Modern Hospital* 99 (July 1962):95–106.

18. A.K. Byrne, "Errors in Giving Medication," *American Journal of Nursing* 53 (1953):829–831.

19. C.I. Corcoran, *An Analysis of Recorded Errors in the Administration of Medications* (Boston, Mass.: Boston University School of Nursing, submitted for partial fulfillment of requirements for the masters degree, June 1954).

20. E. Schlossberg, "16 Safeguards against Medication Errors," *Hospitals: Journal of the American Hospital Association* 32 (1 October 1958):62–70.

21. M. Lodge, *A Study of the Frequency of Reported Medication Errors Among Practical Nurses in a General Hospital* (Detroit, Mich.: Wayne State University, submitted in partial fulfillment of requirements for the master of science in nursing degree, 1958).

22. A. Chapanis and M.A. Safren, "Of Misses and Medicines," *Journal of Chronic Diseases* 12 (1960):403–408.

23. W. Whitcomb, "Patient Medications and Dosage Accuracy," *American Professional Pharmacist* 24 (1958):316–322.

24. H.L. Hartley, "Medication Errors in Hospitals," *Northwest Medicine* 57 (1969):239–242.

25. D.V. Sheehan, J. O'Donnell, A. Fitzgerald, L. Hervig, and H. Ward, "Psychosocial Predictors of Accident/Error Rates in Nursing Students: A Prospective Study," *International Journal of Psychiatry in Medicine* 11 (1981):125–136.

26. M.A. Safren and A. Chapanis, "A Critical Incident Study of Hospital Medication Errors," *Hospitals: Journal of the American Hospital Association* 34 (1 May 1960):32–34, 57–66.

27. M. MacRostie, "You're Not a Pharmacist," *RN* 21(5) (May 1958):44–47, 80–85.

28. W.E. McConnell, K.N. Barker, and L.F. Garrity, "Centralized Unit: Dose Dispensing," *American Journal of Hospital Pharmacy* 18 (1961):531–541.

29. K.N. Barker, "The Effects of an Experimental Medication System on Medication Errors and Costs. Part One: Introduction and Errors Study," *American Journal of Hospital Pharmacy* 26 (1969):324–333.

30. K.N. Barker, "The Effects of an Experimental Medication System on Medication Errors and Costs. Part Two: The Cost Study," *American Journal of Hospital Pharmacy* 26 (1969):388–396.

31. S.M. Schultz, S.N. White, and C.J. Latiolais, "Medication Errors Reduced by Unit-Dose," *Hospitals: Journal of the American Hospital Association* 47 (16 March 1973):106–112.

32. "Hospital Fatalities Blamed on Faulty Diagnosis Aids," *AMA News, 3 March 1969, p. 10.*

33. V. Chernick and M.B. Raber, "Electrical Hazards in the Newborn Nursery," *Journal of Pediatrics* 77 (1970):143–147.

34. J.M.R. Bruner, S. Aronow, and R.V. Cavicchi, "Electrical Incidents in a Large Hospital: A 42 Month Register," *Journal of the Association for the Advancement of Medical Instrumentation* 6 (1972):222–230.

35. "Use of Electric Instruments Increases Hospital Hazards," *Medical Tribune* 25 November 1968, p. 10.

36. B. Parker and S.A. Ritterman, "An Inspection Procedure for Hospital Room Electrical Systems," *Medical Instrumentation* 9 (1975):108–111.

37. M.J. Schaeffer, J.C. Rios, and C.H. Klingenmaier, "Instrumentation Performance Testing: A Prerequisite for Hospital Safety," *American Heart Journal* 91 (1956):819–820.

38. J.J. Fauceglio, "Preventive Maintenance Program at Lutheran Hospital of Maryland," *Journal of Clinical Engineering* 1 (October–December 1976):29–45.

39. M.T. Banner, "Engineering," *Hospitals: Journal of the American Hospital Association* 49 (1 April 1945):145–149.

40. J.A. Burgun, "Fire Safety in Health Care Institutions," *Hospitals: Journal of the American Hospital Association* 48 (1 May 1974):91–95.

41. R.L. Davis, "A Review of Accreditation Requirements For Hospital Safety," *Hospital and Community Psychiatry* 24 (1973):341–342.

42. T.M. Barry, "Safety and Environmental Factors in Accreditation of Facilities," *Hospital and Community Psychiatry* 27 (1976):796–799.

43. M. Heyman, "Fire Safety for Health Care Facilities: Cutting Costs without Cutting Corners," *Dimensions/NBS* (Washington, D.C.: National Bureau of Standards, Department of Commerce, July/August 1979), 4–11.

44. H.V. Fineberg, L.A. Pearlman, and R.A. Gabel, "The Case for Abandonment of Explosive Anesthetic Agents," *New England Journal of Medicine* 303 (1980):613–617.

45. K.J. Cruickshank, "Fire and Evacuation Planning in Hospitals," *Australasian Nurses Journal* 8(1) (September 1978):7–14.

46. T.H. Rockwell, D. Nameche, and W.E. Tarrants, *Work Injuries and Accident Causes in Hospitals* (Washington, D.C.: U.S. Department of Labor, BLS Report 341, 1968).

47. M.J. Smith, M.J. Colligan, I.J. Frockt, and D.L. Tasto, "Occupational Injury Rates among Nurses as a Function of Shift Schedule," *Journal of Safety Research* 11 (1979):181–187.

48. G.M. Ederer and B. Tucker, "Accident Surveys and Safety Programs in Two Hospital Clinical Laboratories," *American Journal of Medical Technology* 26 (1960):219–227.

49. A.H. Shaikh, "Safety Procedures in Clinical Laboratories," *American Journal of Medical Technology* 45 (1979):793–796.

50. J.D. Ramsey, B.A. Rowley, and M.D. Vaugn, "Occupational Safety and Health in Hospitals and Institutions (Lubbock, Tex.: Texas Tech University, Institute for Ergonomics Report 34–76, 1976).

Chapter 26

1. B.W. Carnow, A.L. Miller, B.M. Boulos, B.Z. Lebovitz, and J. Roumain, "A Bookshelf on Occupational Health and Safety," *American Journal of Public Health* 65 (1975):503–520.

2. S.P. Baker, J.S. Samkoff, and R.S. Fisher, "Fatal Occupational Injuries," *Journal of the American Medical Association* 248 (1982):692–697.

3. N.R. Brown, M. Corn, and E.B. Sansone, "Problem Severity Model and Implementation Plan for Occupational Health and Safety," *American Industrial Hygiene Association Journal* 33 (1972):813–821.

4. T.K.W. Ng, "Some Observations on the Needs of Ergonomics in Industries in Hong Kong," *Journal of Human Ergology* 5 (1976):149–159.

5. *Accident Facts, 1981 Edition* (Chicago, Ill.: National Safety Council, 1981).

6. J.P. Mitchell, Speech presented at the President's Conference on Occupational Safety, Washington, D.C., 4 June 1952 (Washington, D.C.: U.S. Department of Labor, 1952).

7. J.M. Howard, "The History of Occupational Injuries in the United States (1776–1976)," *Journal of Trauma* 17 (1977):411–418.

8. "Golden Anniversary," *National Safety News,* May 1963, pp. 33–92 (Chicago, Ill.: National Safety Council).

9. E. Pochin, "Estimates of Industrial and Other Risks," *Journal of the Royal College of Physicians* 12 (1978):210–218.

10. *Occupational Injuries and Illnesses in the United States by Industry, 1978* (Washington, D.C.: Bureau of Labor Statistics, Department of Labor, BLS Bulletin 2078, 1978).

11. J.F. Coyne, "Hidden Injuries in Industry," *Journal of Occupational Medicine* 4 (1962):20–22.

12. D.G. Harper, E.G. Lister, and M. Middleton, "A Study of Regional Variation in Workdays Lost through Accidents," *Accident Analysis and Prevention* 3 (1971):229–236.

13. J.E. Gordon, P.V. Gulati, and J.B. Wyon, "Traumatic Accidents in Rural Tropical Regions: An Epidemiological Field Study in Punjab, India," *American Journal of Medical Science* 243 (1962):158–178.

14. S.P. Datta and P.S. Verma, "A Study of Rural Accidents in Pondicherry, South India," *Indian Journal of Public Health* 13(1) (January 1969):25–29.

15. J.T. Saari and J. Lahtela, "Characteristics of Jobs in High and Low Accident Frequency Companies in the Light Metal Working Industry," *Accident Analysis and Prevention* 11 (1979):51–60.

16. R.H. Simonds and Y. Shafai-Sahrai, "Factors Apparently Affecting Frequency in Eleven Matched Pairs of Companies," *Journal of Safety Research* 9 (1977):121–127.

17. W.N. Cooke and M.W. Blumenstock, "The Determinants of Occupational Injury Severity: The Case of Maine Sawmills," *Journal of Safety Research* 11 (1979):115–120.

18. R.B. Sleight, K.G. Cook, et al., *Problems in Occupational Safety and Health: A Critical Review of Select Worker Physical and Psychological Factors,* vol. 1 (Arlington, Va.: Century Research Corp., Contract HS M-99-72-043 for the National Institute for Occupational Safety and Health, 1974).

19. A. Akman, M. Brooks, and J. Gordon, "Use of Work Injury Rate Tables in Estimating Disabling Work Injuries," *American Journal of Public Health* 62 (1972):917–923.

20. N.F. Burov and V.P. Bizyayev, "The Effect of Workers' Age and Length of Employment on Industrial Injuries," *Bezopasnost Truda v Promyshlennosti* (May 1967):11–13, as quoted by C. Fried, V.M. Forbes, K.P. Giles, S.J. Mumford, et al., *The Miner, His Job and His Environment: A Review and Bibliography of Selected Recent Research on Human Performance* (Washington, D.C.: National Bureau of Standards, Department of Commerce, NBS Report 10 868 for Bureau of Mines, Department of Interior, Working Fund Agreement HO 122019, April 1972).

21. J.W. Freymoyer, M.H. Pope, J.H. Clements, D.G. Wilder, B. MacPherson, and T. Ashikaga, "Risk Factors in Low-Back Pain," *Journal of Bone and Joint Surgery* 65A (1983):213–218.

22. M.A. Persinger, W.J. Cooke, and J.T. Janes, "No Evidence for Relationship Between Biorhythms and Industrial Accidents," *Perceptual and Motor Skills* 46 (1978):423–426.

23. S. Folkard and T.H. Monk, "Shiftwork and Performance," *Human Factors* 21 (1979):483–492.

24. A.J. Tilley, R.T. Wilkerson, P.S.G. Warren, W.B. Watson, and M. Drud, "The Sleep and Performance of Shift Workers," *Human Factors* 24 (1982):629–641.

25. P. Lavie, S. Kremerman, and M. Wiel, "Sleep Disorders and Safety at Work in Industrial Workers," *Accident Analysis and Prevention* 14 (1982):311–314.

26. B.B. Morgan, P.S. Winne, and J. Dugan, "The Range and Consistency of Individual Differences in Continuous Work," *Human Factors* 22 (1980):331–340.

27. M. Shain, "Alcohol, Drugs and Safety: An Updated Perspective on Problems and Their Management in the Workplace," *Accident Analysis and Prevention* 14 (1982):239–246.

28. R. Honkanen, "Alcohol Involvement in Accidents" (Helsinki: Department of Public Health Science, University of Helsinki, 1976).

29. H. Wechsler, E.H. Kasey, H.W. Demone, and D. Thum, *Alcohol Level and Some Home Injuries: Final Report to U.S. Public Health Service on Grant 5 RO1 UI-00022* (Boston, Mass.: The Medical Foundation, 1969).

30. R. Honkanen and T. Visuri, "Blood Alcohol Levels in a Series of Injured Patients with Special Reference to Accident and Type of Injury," *Annales Chirurgiae et Gynaecologia (Helsinki)* 65 (1976):287–294.

31. R. Honkanen and J. Ottelin, "Blood Alcohol Levels in Injury Victims at the Emergency Station of a Rural Central Hospital," *Annales Chirurgiae et Gynaecologia (Helsinki)* 65 (1976):282–286.

32. Observer and M. Maxwell, "A Study of Absenteeism, Accidents and Sickness Payments in Problem Drinkers in One Industry," *Quarterly Journal of Studies on Alcohol* 20 (1959):302–308.

33. P.M. Roman and H.M. Trice, "Deviance and Work: The Influence

of Alcohol and Drugs on Job Behaviors," *Reviews on Environmental Health* 1 (1972):9–51.

34. R.C. Behan and A.H. Hirschfeld, "Current Concepts of Accident Proneness," *Archives of Environmental Health* 13 (1966):462–466.

35. P. Verhaegen, B. Vanhalst, H. Derijcke, and M. Van Hoecke, "The Value of Some Psychological Theories on Industrial Accidents," *Journal of Occupational Accidents* 1 (1976):39–45.

36. D.J. Murphy, "Farm Safety Attitudes and Accident Involvement," *Accident Analysis and Prevention* 13 (1981):331–337.

37. A. Kowalski, "Production Pressures Put Lives of Polish Miners at Risk," *Occupational Health* 32 (1980):145–147.

38. O. Östberg, "Risk Perception and Work Behavior in Forestry: Implications for Accident Prevention Policy," *Accident Analysis and Prevention* 12 (1980):189–200.

39. D.F. Jones, "Back Injury Research: Have We Overlooked Something?," *Journal of Safety Research* 14 (1983):53–64.

40. A. Garg and U. Saxena, "Container Characteristics and Maximum Acceptable Weight of Lift," *Human Factors* 22 (1980):487–495.

41. M. Tolonen and J. Hassi, "Arrangement of Municipal Occupational Health Services for Small Workplaces," *Scandinavian Journal of Work Environment and Health* 5(supp.2) (1979):50–59.

42. S.M. Gadalla, *Selected Environmental Factors Associated with Farm and Farm Home Accidents in Missouri* (Columbia, Mo.: University of Missouri Agricultural Experimental Station, Research Bulletin 790, 1962).

43. F.C. Jackson, "Farm and Ranch Injuries in West Texas" paper presented at a conference on *Control and Prevention of Injury,* Galveston, Tex., 26–28 May 1982 (Lubbock, Tex.: Texas Tech University School of Medicine, 1982).

44. N. Nachlas and J.D. Schlenker, "The Mechanical Cornpicker," *Illinois Medical Journal* 159 (1981):371–374.

45. R. Booth, "Design for Machinery Safety," *Occupational Health* 27(1) (January 1975):24–26.

46. C.M. Vira and W.W. Cloe, *Occupational Fatalities Related to Fixed Machinery as Found in Reports of OSHA Fatality/Catastrophe Investigations* (Washington, D.C.: Office of Statistical Studies and Analysis, Directorate of Technical Support, Occupational Safety and Health Administration, Department of Labor, Report OSHA/RP-80/001, 1978).

47. A. Pekkarinen, K. Ukkola, M. Tolonen, and J. Hassi, "Occupational Safety and Accident Prevention in Small Workplaces with Special Reference to Occupational Health Services," *Scandinavian Journal of Work Environment and Health* 5(supp.2) (1979):45–49.

48. R.A. McFarland, "Human Factors in Industrial Safety," *Journal of the American Society of Safety Engineering* (August 1957):39–48.

49. S.W. Meagher, "ANSI: An Imperfect Arbiter," *Occupational Health and Safety* 50(9) (1981):77–79.

50. M.C. Kaplan, "Task and Tool Design: It's a 'Man's World'," *Occupational Health and Safety* 50(2) (1981):29–34.

51. M.J. Brooks, "Barriers" (letter to the editor) *Human Factors Society Bulletin* 20(6) (June 1977):10.

52. J.D. Ramsey, "Identification of Contributory Factors in Occupational Injury," *Journal of Safety Research* 5 (1973):260–267.

53. C.M. Vira, *Occupational Fatalities Related to Ladders as Found in Reports of OSHA (Occupational Safety and Health Administration) Fatality/Catastrophe Investigations* (Washington, D.C.: Occupational Safety and Health Administration, Department of Labor, Report OSHA/RP-80/004, 1979).

54. L. Tarnopol, "Origins of Industrial Safety Engineering," *Hazard Prevention* 14(4) (March/April 1978):27–30.

55. L. Ellis, "Workman's Compensation and Occupational Safety: A Review and Evaluation of Current Knowledge," *Journal of Occupational Medicine* 18 (1976):418–425.

56. C.A. Olson, *Trade Unions, Wages, Occupational Injuries, An Empirical Analysis* (Madison, Wis.: University of Wisconsin, thesis in partial fulfillment of requirements for the Ph.D. in Industrial Relations, 1979).

57. A.I. Glendon, "Safety Economics," *Occupational Health* 27 (1975):488–490.

58. R.S. Smith, "The Impact of OSHA Inspections on Manufacturing Injury Rates," *Journal of Human Resources* 14 (1979):145–170.

59. L. Greenberg, "A National Policy in Occupational Safety and Health," *Hazard Prevention* 16(10) (May/June 1980):8–11.

60. S.R. Concha, "What Is Wrong with Industrial Safety and Health Programs in the U.S.?," *Hazard Prevention* 17(5) (November/December 1981):4–5, 31.

61. E.K. Jarasunas, "Safety Programs in Diversified Industry," *Hazard Prevention* 17(5) (November/December 1981):7, 32.

62. J.M. Gleason and D.T. Barnum, "Effectiveness of OSHA Sanctions in Influencing Employer Behavior: Single and Multi-Period Decision Models," *Accident Analysis and Prevention* 10 (1978):35–49.

63. J.L. Weeks and M. Fox, "Fatality Rates and Regulatory Policies in Bituminous Coal Mining, United States, 1959–1981," *American Journal of Public Health* 73 (1983):1278–1280.

64. E.D. Heath, "Worker Training and Education in Occupational Safety and Health (pt. 1)," *Hazard Prevention* 18(2) (March/April 1982):4–10.

65. E.D. Heath, "Worker Training and Education in Occupational Safety and Health: A Report on Practice in Six Industrialized Western Nations," *Hazard Prevention* 18(3) (May/June 1982):4–9, 31.

66. R.J. Cunitz, "Psychologically Effective Warnings," *Hazard Prevention* 17(3) (May/June 1981):5–7.

67. A. Cohen, M.J. Smith, and W.K. Anger, "Self-Protective Measures against Workplace Hazards," *Journal of Safety Research* 11 (1979):121–131.

68. G.M. Fraser, "Industrial Accidents and Their Prevention," *Australian Family Physician* 9 (1980):79–83.

69. B. Sulzer-Azaroff and M.C. deSantamaria, "Industrial Safety Hazard Reduction through Performance Feedback," *Journal of Applied Behavioral Analysis* 13 (1980):287–295.

70. K. Walker and M. Shain, "Employee Assistance Programming: In Search of Effective Interventions for the Problem-Drinking Employee," *British Journal of Addiction* 78 (1983):291–303.

71. G.E. Leyshon and H.W.S. Francis, "Lifting Injuries in Ambulance Crews," *Public Health, London* 89 (1975):71–75.

72. A.D. Swain, "Design of Industrial Jobs a Worker Can and Will Do," *Human Factors* 15 (1973):129–136.

73. S.P. McKenna, "First Aid Training and Its Effect on Safety," *Occupational Health* 29 (1977):426–431.

Chapter 27

1. I. Burton, R.W. Kates, and G.F. White, *The Environment as Hazard* (New York: Oxford University Press, 1978).

2. "Catastrophic Accidents: A 35-Year Review," *Statistical Bulletin* 58 (March 1977):2–4 (New York: Metropolitan Life Insurance Co.).

3. R.I. Glass, R.B. Craven, D.J. Bregman, B.J. Stoll, N. Horowitz, P. Kerndt, and J. Winkle, "Injuries from the Wichita Falls Tornado: Implications for Prevention," *Science* 207 (1980):734–738.

4. R.I. Glass, J.J. Urrutia, S. Sibony, H. Smith, B. Garcia, and L. Rizzo, "Earthquake Injuries Related to Housing in a Guatemalan Village," *Science* 197 (1977):638–643.

5. P. Slovic, H. Kunreuther, and G.F. White, "Decision Processes, Rationality, and Adjustment To Natural Hazards," in G.F. White (ed.), *Natural Hazards: Local, National, Global* (New York: Oxford University Press, 1974), 187–205.

6. J.H. Sims and D.D. Baumann, "The Tornado Threat: Coping Styles of the North and South," *Science* 176 (1972):1386–1392.

7. D. Wright and P.H. Rossi (ed.), *Social Science and Natural Hazards* (Cambridge, Mass.: Abt Books, 1981).

8. N.J.H. Smith, "Colonization Lessons from a Tropical Forest," *Science* 214 (1981):755–761.

9. S. Nichols and J. Mansfield, *The Fragile Mountain* (film) (Boston, Mass.: Television Station WGBH, Nova Production 912, 1982).

10. K. Frazier, *The Violent Face of Nature* (New York: William Morrow and Co., 1979).

11. W.R. McCann, O.J. Pérez, and L.R. Sykes, "Yakataga Gap,

Alaska: Seismic History and Earthquake Potential," *Science* 207 (1980):1309–1314.

12. D.H. Harlow, R.A. White, and I.L. Cifuentes, "Quiet Zone within a Seismic Gap near Western Nicaragua: Possible Location of a Future Large Earthquake," *Science* 213 (1981):648–651.

13. D.G. Herd, T.L. Youd, H. Meyer, J.L. Arango, W.J. Person, and C. Mendoza, "The Great Tumaco, Colombia Earthquake of 12 December 1979," *Science* 211 (1981):441–445.

14. *The Assessment and Mitigation of Earthquake Risk* (Paris: UNESCO, United Nations, 1978).

15. C.B. Raleigh, J.H. Healy, and J.D. Bredehoeft, "An Experiment in Earthquake Control at Rangely, Colorado," *Science* 191 (1976):1230–1237.

16. "Avalanches Reveal Their Inner Workings," *New York Times,* 29 December 1981, pp. C1, C3.

17. B.K. Hartline, "Snow Physics and Avalanche Prediction," *Science* 203 (1979):346–348.

18. *Snow Avalanche* (Washington, D.C.: Forest Service, U.S. Department of Agriculture, Report 551-826, 1974).

19. C.C. Bradley, "The Location and Timing of Deep Slab Avalanches," *Journal of Glaciology* 9 (1970):253–261.

20. "Specially Designed Florida Beach Weathered the Hurricane's Blast," *New York Times,* 1 September 1979, p. A22.

21. R. Lindsey, "Property Owners on Coast Block Measure on Safety in Earthquakes," *New York Times,* 12 December 1976, p. 36.

22. R.A. Kerr, "Doppler Radar: New Look into Violent Weather," *Science* 202 (1978):1172–1174.

23. R.A. Kerr, "Tidal Waves: New Method Suggested to Improve Prediction," *Science* 200 (1978):521–522.

24. R.A. Kerr, "Mount St. Helens: An Unpredictable Foe," *Science* 208 (1980):1446–1448.

25. *Mount St. Helens: Why They Died* (film) (San Diego, Calif.: KPBS-TV, San Diego State University, 1982).

26. D. Shapley, "Chinese Earthquakes: The Maoist Approach to Seismology," *Science* 193 (1976):656–657.

27. D. Shapley, "Earthquakes: Los Angeles Prediction Suggests Faults in Federal Policy," *Science* 192 (1976):535–537.

28. A.L. Hammond, "Earthquakes: An Evacuation in China, A Warning in California," *Science* 192 (1976):538–539.

29. R.A. Kerr, "Quake Prediction by Animals Gaining Respect," *Science* 208 (1980):695–696.

30. H. Wakita, Y. Nakamura, K. Notsu, M. Noguchi, and T. Asada, "Radon Anomaly: A Possible Precursor of the 1978 Izu-Oshima-Kinkai Earthquake," *Science* 207 (1980):882–883.

31. R.A. Kerr, "Earthquakes: Prediction Proving Elusive," *Science* 200 (1978):419–421.

32. R.A. Kerr, "Prospects for Earthquake Prediction Wane," *Science* 206 (1979):542–545.

33. E.F. Loftus, "Words That Could Save Your Live," *Psychology Today* 13(6) (November 1979):102–110, 136–137.

34. D. Robinson, *The Face of Disaster* (Garden City, N.Y.: Doubleday and Co., 1959).

35. L. Plommer, "The Disaster Game," *New York Times,* 17 November 1978, p. A29.

36. C. deVille de Goyet, E. del Cid, A. Romero, E. Jeannée, and M. Lechat, "Earthquake in Guatemala: Epidemiologic Evaluation of the Relief Effort," *PAHO Bulletin* 10 (1976):95–109.

37. L.S. Jiménez, "Planning Health Services for Emergency Situations," *PAHO Bulletin* 11 (1977):31–40.

38. S.R. Mohler, A.C. Webb, J. Pixley, J. Butcher, L. Star, and L. Abelson, "Panel: The Modern View of Airport Disaster Medical Management," *Aviation, Space and Environmental Medicine* 51 (1980):1256–1269.

39. "Cairo's Housing Crisis: 100,000 Live in Cemetery," *Montreal Gazette,* 27 September 1978, p. 32.

40. L.L. Philipson, "An Assessment of Risk Assessment Methodologies and Its Application to Hazardous Materials Transportation," *Hazard Prevention* 18(1) (January/February 1982):19–25.

41. R.K. Mark and D.E. Stuart-Alexander, "Disasters as a Necessary Part of Benefit-Cost Analyses," *Science* 197 (1977):1160–1162.

42. C. Hohenemser, R. Kasperson, and R. Kates, "The Distrust of Nuclear Power," *Science* 196 (1977):25–34.

43. E. Marshall, "A Preliminary Report on Three Mile Island," *Science* 204 (1979):280–281.

44. "Atomic Plants Had 2835 Incidents in '78," *New York Times,* 15 April 1979, p. 26.

45. E. Marshall, "Reactor Safety and the Research Budget," *Science* 214 (1981):766–768.

46. R.P. Hummel and C.M. McConnell, "Jailhouse Burns," *Journal of Trauma* 16 (1976):232–234.

47. C.O. Miller, "Safety Management Factors Germane to the Nuclear Reactor Accident at Three Mile Island, March 28, 1979," *Hazard Prevention* 16(special issue) (Summer 1980):1213–1245.

48. Engineers Committee on Three Mile Island, "Review of the President's Commission Report on the Accident at Three Mile Island," *Hazard Prevention* 16(9) (March/April 1980):16–18.

49. "Study Faults Kansas City Building Inspection," *New York Times,* 21 March 1982, section i, p. 29.

50. J.W. Schmidt and D.L. Price, "The Flow of Hazardous Materials on Virginia Highways," *Journal of Safety Research* 11 (1979):109–114.

51. J.E. Haas, R. Kates, and M.J. Bowden, *Reconstruction Following Disaster* (Cambridge, Mass.: MIT Press, 1977).

52. K.T. Erikson, "Trauma at Buffalo Creek," *Society* 13(6) (September/October 1976):58–65.

53. R. Stuart, "Coping with Great Disasters Through Revenge," *New York Times*, 23 December 1979, p. 14E.

54. J.N. Logue, H. Hansen, and E. Struening, "Emotional and Physical Distress Following Hurricane Agnes in Wyoming Valley of Pennsylvania," *Public Health Reports* 94 (1979):495–502.

55. J.N. Logue, H. Hansen and E. Struening, "Some Indications of the Long-Term Health Effects of a Natural Disaster," *Public Health Reports* 96 (1981):67–79.

56. M.E. Melick, "Life Change and Illness: Illness Behavior of Males in the Recovery Period of a Natural Disaster," *Journal of Health and Social Behavior* 19 (1978):335–342.

57. B. Boman, "Behavioral Observations on the Granville Train Disaster and the Significance of Stress for Psychiatry," *Social Science and Medicine* 13A (1979):463–471.

58. T.S. Kilijanek and T.E. Drabek, "Assessing Long-Term Impacts of a Natural Disaster: A Focus on the Elderly," *Gerontologist* 19 (1979):555–566.

59. G. Caplan, *Principles of Preventive Psychiatry* (New York: Basic Books, 1964).

Chapter 28

1. M. Greenwood and H.M. Woods, *The Incidence of Industrial Accidents upon Individuals with Special Reference to Multiple Accidents* (Industrial Fatigue Research Board, Report 4, 1919).

2. E.J. Bernacki, "Accident Proneness or Accident Liability: Which Model for Industry?," *Connecticut Medicine* 40 (1976):535–538.

3. F.A. Haight, "Accident Proneness: The History of an Idea," *Automobilismo et Automobilisoma Industriale*, Estratto dal Num 4, Lug-Agos, 1964.

4. F. Dunbar, *Mind and Body* (New York: Random House, 1955).

5. K. Menninger, *Man against Himself* (New York: Harcourt Brace Publishing Co., 1937).

6. F. Alexander, "The Accident Prone Individual," *Public Health Reports* 64 (1949):357–362.

7. A.T. Rawson, "Accident Proneness," *Psychosomatic Medicine* 6 (1944):88–94.

8. R.C. Behan and A.H. Hirschfeld, "Current Concepts of Accident Proneness," *Archives of Environmental Health* 13 (1966):462–466.

9. A.G. Arbous and J.E. Kerrich, "The Phenomenon of Accident Proneness," *Industrial Medicine and Surgery* 22 (1953):141–148.

10. G.D. Mellinger and D.I. Manheimer, "An Exposure-Coping Model of Accident Liability among Children," *Journal of Health and Social Behavior* 8 (1967):96–106.

11. J.A. Waller and E.B. Whorton, "Unintentional Shootings, Highway Crashes, and Acts of Violence: A Behavioral Paradigm," *Accident Analysis and Prevention* 5 (1973):351–356.

12. J.A. Waller, "Accidents and Violent Behavior: Are They Related?," in D.J. Mulvihill, M.M. Tumin, and L.A. Curtis (eds.), *Crimes of Violence: A Staff Report to the National Commission on the Causes and Prevention of Violence,* vol. 13 (Washington, D.C.: U.S. Government Printing Office, 1969), app. 33, pp. 1525–1558.

13. J.A. Waller and K.R. Lamborn, "Snowmobiling: Characteristics of Owners, Patterns of Use and Injuries," *Accident Analysis and Prevention* 7 (1975):213–224.

14. H.M. Vernon, *Accidents and Their Prevention* (New York: Cambridge University Press, 1936).

Chapter 29

1. S.P. Baker, "The Man in the Street: A Tale of Two Cities," *American Journal of Public Health* 65 (1975):524–525.

2. H. Marcusson and W. Oehmisch, "Accident Mortality in Childhood in Selected Countries of Different Continents, 1950–1971," *World Health Statistics Report* 30 (1977):57–92.

3. R.J. Meyer, H.A. Roelofs, J. Bluestone, and S. Redmond, "Accidental Injury to the Preschool Child," *Journal of Pediatrics* 63 (1963):95–105.

4. D.I. Manheimer and G.D. Mellinger, "Personality Characteristics of the Child Accident Repeater," *Child Development* 38 (1967):491–513.

5. J. Langley, P.A. Silva, and S. Williams, "A Study of the Relationship of Ninety Background, Developmental, Behavioral and Medical Factors to Childhood Accidents," *Australian Paediatric Journal* 16 (1980):244–247.

6. G.D. Mellinger and D.I. Manheimer, "An Exposure-Coping Model of Accident Liability among Children," *Journal of Health and Social Behavior* 8 (1967):96–106.

7. G.W. Brown and S. Davidson, "Social Class, Psychiatric Disorder of Mother, and Accidents to Children," *Lancet* 1 (1978):378–381.

8. E.M. Backett and A.M. Johnston, "Social Patterns of Road Accidents to Children," *British Medical Journal* 1 (1959):409–413.

9. K. Dalton, "Children's Hospital Admissions and Mother's Menstruation," *British Medical Journal* 2 (1970):27–28.

10. M.N. Tempest, "A Survey of Domestic Burns and Scalds in Wales during 1955," *British Medical Journal* 1 (1956):1387–1392.

11. J.P. Bull, D.M. Jackson, and C. Walton, "Causes and Prevention

of Domestic Burning Accidents," *British Medical Journal* 2 (1964):1421–1427.

12. S.H. Schuman, D.C. Pelz, N.J. Ehrlich, and M.L. Selzer, "Young Male Drivers," *Journal of the American Medical Association* 200 (1967):1026–1030.

13. D. Klein, "Body-Contact Sports: Catharsis or Reinforcement?" *Accident Analysis and Prevention* 6 (1974):85–91.

14. R. Berfenstam, "Prevention of Childhood Accidents in Sweden," *Acta Paediatrica Scandinavica (Stockholm)* (supp.275) (1970):88–95.

15. S.H. Sheldon, "Unintentional Trauma Prevention and Injury Control: Curriculum Design for Resident Training," *27th Annual Proceedings, American Association for Automotive Medicine, San Antonio, Tex., 3–6 October 1983* (Morton Grove, Ill.: American Association for Automotive Medicine), 303–309.

16. E.R. Schlesinger, D.G. Dickson, J. Westaby, et al., *Rockland County Child Injury Prevention Project 1960–1963* (New City, N.Y.: Rockland County Department of Health, 1964).

17. R.A. Dershewitz and J.W. Williamson, "Prevention of Childhood Household Injuries: A Controlled Clinical Trial," *American Journal of Public Health* 67 (1977):1148–1153.

18. S.P. Baker, "Prevention of Childhood Injuries," *Medical Journal of Australia* 1 (1980):446–470.

19. B. Sorenson, "Prevention of Burns and Scalds in a Developed Country," *Journal of Trauma* 16 (1976):249–258.

20. K.N. Durrani and S.K. Raza, "Studies on Flammability of Clothing of Burn Victims, Changes Therein and Their Wearability after a Borax Rinse," *Journal of the Pakistan Medical Association* 25 (1975):99–102.

21. S.P. Baker and R.S. Fisher, "Childhood Asphyxiation by Choking or Suffocation," *Journal of the American Medical Association* 244 (1980):1343–1346.

22. P.J. Hletko, J. Hletko, A. Shelness, and J. Nyberg, "The Effect of a Toddler/Child Restraint Device Rental Program on Observed Correct Use," *27th Annual Proceedings, American Association for Automotive Medicine, San Antonio, Tex., 3–6 October 1983* (Morton Grove, Ill.: American Association for Automotive Medicine), 115–125.

23. D. Shinar, "Control-Display Relationships on the Four-Burner Range: Population Stereotypes versus Standards," *Human Factors* 20 (1978):13–17.

24. G.S. Young and S.P. Baker, "Recent Trends in Childhood Burn Deaths," paper presented at the 1978 American Public Health Association Meeting, Baltimore, Md., Johns Hopkins School of Hygiene and Public Health, 1978.

25. S.O. Oduntan, "Pattern of Disease and Accidents in Nigerian Children of School Age," *Journal of Tropical Medicine and Hygiene* 76 (1973):28–35.

26. P.F. Agran and D.E. Dunkle, "A Comparison of Police Accident

Reports versus Hospital Monitoring Systems in the Study of Noncrash Events," *27th Annual Proceedings, American Association for Automotive Medicine, San Antonio, Tex., 3–6 October 1983* (Morton Grove, Ill.: American Association for Automotive Medicine), 159–168.

27. R.D. Blomberg, D.F. Preusser, A. Hale, and W.A. Leaf, *Experimental Field Test of Proposed Pedestrian Safety Messages,* vol. 1–3 (Norwalk, Conn.: Dunlap and Associates East, Contract DOT-HS-4-00952, 1983).

28. M.W. Bartholomew, "Pedestrian Accidents in Service Areas of Selected City Recreation Facilities," *Traffic Safety Research Review* 11 (1967):117–124.

29. J. Pearn, "Aquatics for Epileptic Children," *Australian Paediatric Journal* 18 (1982):255–256.

30. S. Livingston and W. Berman, "Participation of Epileptic Patients in Sports," *Journal of the American Medical Association* 224 (1973):236–238.

31. R.L. McLaurin, "Epilepsy and Contact Sports," *Journal of the American Medical Association* 225 (1973):285–287.

Chapter 30

1. J.L. Fozard, E. Wolf, B. Bell, R.A. McFarland, and S. Podolsky, "Visual Perception and Communication," in J.E. Birren and K.W. Schaie, *Handbook of the Psychology of Aging* (New York: Van Nostrand Reinhold Co., 1977), 497–534.

2. A. Burg, *The Relationship between Vision Test Scores and Driving Record: General Findings* (Los Angeles, Calif.: Institute of Transportation and Traffic Engineering, University of California at Los Angeles, Report 67-24, 1967).

3. J.F. Corso, "Auditory Perception and Communication," in J.E. Birren and K.W. Schaie, *Handbook of the Psychology of Aging* (New York: Van Nostrand Reinhold Co., 1977), 535–553.

4. A.T. Welford, "Motor Performance," in J.E. Birren and K.W. Schaie, *Handbook of the Psychology of Aging* (New York: Van Nostrand Reinhold Co., 1977), 450–496.

5. L.G. Hiatt, "Environmental Design and Older People: Pre- and Post-Presentation Questions" (New York: Consultant on Aging to American Foundation for the Blind, material presented at a workshop, Brattleboro, Vt., 11 April 1980).

6. L.G. Hiatt, "Architecture for the Aged: Design for Living," *Inland Architect* (November/December 1978):6–17, 41.

7. A.T. Welford, "Sensory, Perceptual and Motor Processes in Older Adults," in J.E. Birren and R.B. Sloane, *Handbook of Mental Health and Aging* (Englewood Cliffs, N.J.: Prentice-Hall, Inc., 1980), 192–213.

8. K.A. Conrad and R. Bressler (eds.), *Drug Therapy for the Elderly* (St. Louis, Mo.: C.V. Mosby Co., 1982).

9. D.R. Kenshalo, "Age Changes in Touch, Vibration, Temperature,

Kinesthesis and Pain Sensitivity," in J.E. Birren and K.W. Schaie, *Handbook of the Psychology of Aging* (New York: Van Nostrand Reinhold Co., 1977), 562–579.

10. F.I.M. Craik, "Age Differences in Human Memory," in J.E. Birren and K.W. Schaie, *Handbook of the Psychology of Aging* (New York: Van Nostrand Reinhold Co., 1977), 384–420.

11. D. Arenberg and E.A. Robertson-Tchabo, "Learning and Aging," in J.E. Birren and K.W. Schaie, *Handbook of the Psychology of Aging* (New York: Van Nostrand Reinhold Co., 1977), 421–449.

12. J.A. Mortimer and L.M. Schuman (eds.), *The Epidemiology of Dementia* (New York: Oxford University Press, 1981).

13. J.H. Sheldon, "On the Natural History of Falls in Old Age," *British Medical Journal* 2 (1960):1685–1690.

14. J.A. Waller, "Transportation Patterns of Persons with Recent Hospitalization for Heart Disease" (Burlington, Vt.: University of Vermont, Final Report to NRTA-AARP Andrus Foundation, 1981).

15. R. Zylman, "Age Is More Important Than Alcohol in the Collision-Involvement of Young and Old Drivers," *Journal of Traffic Safety Education* 20(1) (October 1972):7–8, 34.

16. E.S. Parker and E.P. Noble, "Alcohol and the Aging Process in Social Drinkers," *Journal of Studies on Alcohol* 41 (1980):170–178.

17. J.A. Waller, "Chronic Medical Conditions and Traffic Safety, Review of California Experience," *New England Journal of Medicine* 273 (1965):1413–1420.

18. A. Crancer and L. McMurray, "Accident and Violation Rates of Washington's Medically Restricted Drivers," *Journal of the American Medical Association* 205 (1968):272–276.

19. A. Crancer and D.L. Quiring, "The Mentally Ill as Motor Vehicle Operators," *American Journal of Psychiatry* 126 (1969):807–813.

20. J.A. Waller and T.J. Naughton, Jr., "Driving and Crash Experience and Ischemic Heart Disease: Implications for Countermeasures," *27th Proceedings of the American Association for Automotive Medicine, San Antonio, Tex. 3–6 October 1983* (Morton Grove, Ill.: American Association for Automotive Medicine), 249–261.

21. L. Ysander, "The Safety of Physically Disabled Drivers," *British Journal of Industrial Medicine* 23 (1966):173–180.

22. J.A. Waller, "Cardiovascular Disease, Aging, and Traffic Accidents," *Journal of Chronic Diseases* 20 (1967):615–620.

23. J.A. Waller, T.J. Naughton, Jr., T.C. Gibson, and J.W. Eberhard, "Methodologic and Other Issues Concerning Medical Impairment to Driving," *25th Annual American Association for Automotive Medicine Proceedings, San Francisco, Calif., 1–3 October 1981* (Morton Grove, Ill.: American Association for Automotive Medicine), 189–200.

24. J.D. Ramsey, "Product Safety and Liability Considerations for Home Furnishings," *Proceedings of the 6th Congress of the International Ergonomics Association, College Park, Md., 11–16 July 1976*, 498–506.

25. L. Hiatt Snyder, "Living Environments, Geriatric Wheelchairs and Older Persons' Rehabilitation," *Journal of Gerontological Nursing* 1(5) (November/December 1975):17–20.

26. D. Shinar, "Control-Display Relationships on the Four-Burner Range: Population Stereotypes versus Standards," *Human Factors* 20 (1978):13–17.

27. M. Halpern, Statement presented at meeting of the International Association for Accident and Traffic Medicine, Paris, 12 September 1972.

28. C.L. Popkin, "An Examination of the Driving Performance of Medically Evaluated Drivers," *27th Proceedings of the American Association for Automotive Medicine, San Antonio, Tex., 3–6 October 1983* (Morton Grove, Ill.: American Association for Automotive Medicine), 263–274.

29. J.A. Waller, *Medical Impairment to Driving* (Springfield, Ill.: Charles C. Thomas, Publisher, 1973).

Chapter 31

1. "ABC Laws," *Alcohol Health and Research World* 4(2) (Winter 1979–80) (Washington, D.C.: Alcohol, Drug Abuse and Mental Health Administration, Department of Health, Education and Welfare).

2. M. Keller, "The Great Jewish Drink Mystery," *British Journal of Addiction* 64 (1970):287–296.

3. *1968 Alcohol and Highway Safety Report* (Washington, D.C.: U.S. Department of Transportation, Report from the Secretary of Transportation to the U.S. Congress, 1968).

4. J. Cohen, E.J. Dearnaley, and C.E.M. Hansel, "The Risk Taken in Driving under the Influence of Alcohol," *British Medical Journal* 1 (1958):1438–1442.

5. S.E. Gitlow, "The Disease of Alcoholism," *Cancer Research* 39 (1979):2836–2839.

6. J.E. Barmack and D.E. Payne, "Injury-Producing Private Motor Vehicle Accidents among Airmen," *Bulletin No. 285* (Washington, D.C.: Highway Research Board, 1961).

7. T.A. Loomis and I.C. West, "The Influence of Alcohol on Automobile Driving Ability," *Quarterly Journal of Studies on Alcohol* 19 (1958):30–46.

8. I.M. Rabinowitch, "Medico-Legal Aspects of Chemical Tests of Alcohol Intoxication," in H. Elliot (ed.), *Medical Aspects of Traffic Accidents* (Montreal: Traffic Accident Foundation for Medical Research and Sun Life Assurance Co. of Canada, 1955), 205–252.

9. B.B. Coldwell (ed.), *Report on Impaired Driving Tests* (Ottawa: Crime Detection Laboratory, Royal Canadian Mounted Police, 1957).

10. L. Goldberg, "Tolerance to Alcohol in Moderate and Heavy Drinkers and Its Significance to Alcohol and Traffic," *Proceedings of the First*

International Conference on Alcohol and Road Traffic, Stockholm, 1950 (Stockholm: Kugelbergs Boktrycheri, 1951), 85–106.

11. M.M. Hyman, "Accident Vulnerability and Blood Alcohol Concentrations of Drivers by Demographic Characteristics," *Quarterly Journal of Studies on Alcohol 29* (supp. 4) (1968):34–57.

12. R. Zylman, "Age Is More Important Than Alcohol in the Collision-Involvement of Young and Old Drivers," *Journal of Traffic Safety Education* 20(1) (October 1972):7–8, 34.

13. R.F. Borkenstein, R.F. Crowther, R.P. Shumate, W.B. Ziel, and R. Zylman, *The Role of the Drinking Driver in Traffic Accidents* (Bloomington, Ind.: Department of Police Administration, Indiana University, 1964).

14. R. Zylman, "The Variability of Collision Involvement at Low Blood Alcohol Concentrations: The Grand Rapids Curve Explained," *Butalkohol* 9(1) (January 1972):25–32.

15. P.W. Wright and L.S. Robertson, "Priorities for Roadside Hazard Modification: A Study of 300 Fatal Roadside Object Crashes," *Traffic Engineering* 46(8) (August 1976):24–30.

16. J.A. Waller, "Accidents and Violent Behavior: Are They Related?," in D.J. Mulvihill, M.M. Tumin, and L.A. Curtis, *Crimes of Violence: A Staff Report to the National Commission on the Causes and Prevention of Violence,* vol. 13 (Washington, D.C.: U.S. Government Printing Office, 1969), 1525–1558.

17. A.C. Wagenaar, *Alcohol, Young Drivers, and Traffic Accidents* (Lexington, Mass.: Lexington Books, 1983).

18. I. Colon and H.S.G. Cutter, "The Relationship of Beer Consumption and State Alcohol and Motor Vehicle Policies to Fatal Accidents," *Journal of Safety Research* 14 (1983):83–89.

19. H.L. Ross, *Deterring the Drinking Driver* (Lexington, Mass.: Lexington Books, 1981).

20. J.A. Waller and J.K. Worden, "Strategies for Safety Program Planning and Evaluation: Lessons from the Vermont Alcohol and Highway Safety Campaign," *Proceedings of Symposium on Traffic Safety Effectiveness (Impact) Evaluation Projects, Chicago, Ill., 19–21 May 1981* (Chicago, Ill.: National Safety Council, 1981), 117–131.

21. K.B. Bjerver, L. Goldberg, and P. Linda, "Blood Alcohol Levels in Hospitalized Victims of Traffic Accidents," *Proceedings of the 2d International Conference on Alcohol and Road Traffic, Toronto, 1953* (Toronto: Garden City Press Cooperative, 1955), 92–102.

22. K. Handel, "Die Persönlichkeit Alkoholbeeinflusster Verkehrsteilnehmer," *Proceedings of the 3d International Conference on Alcohol and Road Traffic, London, 1962* (London: BMA House, 1963), 61–65.

23. J.A. Waller, "Identification of Problem Drinking among Drunken Drivers," *Journal of the American Medical Association* 200 (1967):114–120.

24. Criteria Committee, National Council on Alcoholism, "Criteria for the Diagnosis of Alcoholism," *American Journal of Psychiatry* 129 (1972):127–135.

25. C. Ringer, H. Küfner, K. Antons, and W. Feuerlein, "The N.C.A. Criteria for the Diagnosis of Alcoholism," *Journal of Studies on Alcohol* 38 (1977):1259–1273.

26. R.E. Mann, G. Leigh, E.R. Vingilis, and K. deGenova, "A Critical Review on the Effectiveness of Drinking-Driving Rehabilitation Programmes," *Accident Analysis and Prevention* 15 (1983):441–461.

27. H.H. Holder and J.B. Hallan, *Medical Care and Alcoholism Treatment Costs and Utilization: A Five Year Analysis of the California Pilot Project to Provide Health Insurance Coverage for Alcoholism, December 1981* (Washington, D.C.: Alcohol, Drug Abuse, and Mental Health Administration, Department of Health and Human Services, National Institute on Alcohol Abuse and Alcoholism Health Insurance Resource Kit RPO 392, 1981).

28. K. Walker and M. Shain, "Employee Assistance Programming: In Search of Effective Interventions for the Problem-Drinking Employee," *British Journal of Addiction* 78 (1983):291–303.

29. E.M. Pattison, "A Critique of Abstinence Criteria in the Treatment of Alcoholism," *International Journal of Social Psychiatry* 14 (1968):268–276.

30. R.E. Kendell and M.C. Staton, "The Fate of Untreated Alcoholics," *Quarterly Journal of Studies on Alcohol* 27 (1966):30–41.

31. F. Lemere, "What Happens to Alcoholics," *American Journal of Psychiatry* 109 (1953):674–676.

32. D. Cahalan, *Problem Drinkers* (San Francisco, Calif.: Josey-Bass, Inc., 1970).

33. D. Cahalan, I.H. Cisin, and H.M. Crossley, *American Drinking Practices* (New Brunswick, N.J.: Rutgers Center of Alcohol Studies, 1969).

34. L.R.H. Drew, "Alcoholism as a Self-Limiting Disease," *Quarterly Journal of Studies on Alcohol* 29 (1968):956–967.

35. G. Caplan, *Principles of Preventive Psychiatry* (New York: Basic Books, 1964).

36. R.E. Hagen, R.L. Williams, E.J. McConnell, and C.W. Fleming, *An Evaluation of Alcohol Abuse Treatment as an Alternative to Drivers License Suspension or Revocation* (Sacramento, Calif.: California Department of Motor Vehicles, Report CAL-DMV-RSS-78-68, 1978).

37. J.A. Waller, "Drugs and Highway Crashes: Can We Separate Fact from Fancy?" *Journal of the American Medical Association* 215 (1971):1477–1482.

38. K.B. Joscelyn and R.P. Maickel, *Drugs and Driving: A Research Review* (Bloomington, Ind.: Indiana University, Report DOT-HS-4-00994-2, 1975).

39. D.C.G. Skegg, S.M. Richards, and R. Doll, "Minor Tranquillisers and Road Accidents," *British Medical Journal* 1 (1974):917–919.

40. J.A. Waller, "Chronic Medical Conditions and Traffic Safety: A Review of California Experience," *New England Journal of Medicine* 273 (1965):1413–1420.

41. K.W. Terhune, "An Evaluation of Crash Culpability to Assess Alcohol and Drug Impairment Effects," *26th Proceedings of the American*

Association for Automotive Medicine, Ottawa, Canada, 4–6 October 1982 (Morton Grove, Ill.: American Association for Automotive Medicine, 1982), 329–341.

42. J.A. Waller, "Response to 'An Evaluation of Crash Culpability to Assess Alcohol and Drug Impairment Effects'," *26th Proceedings of the American Association for Automotive Medicine, Ottawa, Canada, 4–6 October 1982* (Morton Grove, Ill.: American Association for Automotive Medicine, 1982), 342–346.

Chapter 32

1. "Recommended Undergraduate Medical School Curriculum for Emergency Medicine and Services: A Joint ACEP and UA/EMS Position Paper," *Journal of the American College of Emergency Physicians* 5 (1976):377.

2. M.A. Weiner, C.E. Gettinger, J.A. Waller, D.B. Pilcher, and J.R. Goss, "In-Service Training for Rural Nurses in Emergency Care Concepts and Skills," *Journal of Emergency Nursing* 1 (March/April 1975):16–23.

3. N.M. Holloway (ed.), *Core Curriculum, 2d ed.* (Chicago, Ill.: Emergency Department Nurses Association, 1980).

4. J.A. Waller, "Education of Medical Students about Injury Control," *Proceedings of 22d Conference of the American Association for Automotive Medicine and 7th Conference of the International Association for Accident and Traffic Medicine, Ann Arbor, Mich., 10–14 July 1978* (Morton Grove, Ill.: American Association For Automotive Medicine), 12–20.

5. W. Haddon, Jr., "On The Escape of Tigers: An Ecologic Note," *American Journal of Public Health* 60 (1970):2229–2234.

Final Words

T.M. Fraser, "Recreation, Technology and System Safety," *Human Factors* 16 (1974):447–453. Copyright 1974 by The Human Factors Society, Inc., and reproduced by permission.

Index

Abbreviated Injury Scale (AIS), 74–75, 528
Abdomen, impact tolerance, 28
Accident, definition, 7
Accident Facts, 199
Accident proneness, 435, 467–471
Acetyl salicylic acid. *See* Aspirin
Acids, 3
Acute care facilities, 408
Adelaide, 479
Adobe homes, 455
Advertising, 292
Aerodynamic turbulence and vehicles, 169
Africa, 93, 108
Age: and air accidents, 251–252, 253; and alcohol effects, 98, 115, 116, 118; and bicycle injuries, 199, 200; and boating facilities, 240; and burns, 301–302, 303; and disaster injury, 449; and drowning, 371; and falls, 409; and fatalities from injuries, 3, 98; and fatigue of drivers, 167; and firearm injuries, 397–398; and fractures, 24, 25; and highway injuries, 66, 110, 113, 115, 116–118, 119, 126, 128, 165–166, 473; and home injuries, 265, 266, 267; and impact tolerance, 27; and injury rates, 93, 98; and motorcycle injuries, 186, 187, 188; and occupational injuries, 427–430, 473; and pedestrian injuries, 212, 213–215, 473; and poisoning, 332; and reporting of injuries, 69; and sport injuries, 380; and suicide, 103; and truck injuries, 165–166; *see also* Children; Elderly; Teenagers; Young adults
Aggression and sports, 362–363, 378, 382
Aging. *See* Elderly
Agriculture, occupational illness, 423, 437–438
Aikido, 386
Air controllers, 248, 249–250, 254, 257–258, 260
Air guns, 320
Air pollution, 451
Air Safety Reporting System, 254
Air transport, 245–261; and age, 251–252, 253; alarm devices, 44; and alcohol, 250–251, 260; and children, 258; crash rates, 245–246, 255–256, 449; emergency service, 259, 260, 261; exposure measurement, 259; fatalities, 245, 246, 259, 260; and fire, 258, 259, 260; and inexperience, 248–249, 251; investigation of crashes, 78, 230; licensing, 42; reporting of accidents, 67–68, 246; runways, 257; and weather, 246–248, 249, 258
Airbags, 82, 151, 155
Alarm systems, 44, 45; carbon monoxide, 345; fire, 316, 401, 480, 501; smoke, 316, 480, 501
Alcohol, 19, 469–470, 471, 511–523; absorption rate, 512; and age of fatalities, 98, 115, 116, 118; and air transport, 250–251, 260; arrest programs, effectiveness, 81; and bicycle injuries, 206–207; and bleeding, 26; and boating accidents, 238; and college students, 349–351; concentration, 115, 116, 514, 518–519; congeners, 512; countermeasures,

40, 147–149; and developing countries, 115; and diving injuries, 375; and drowning, 238, 250, 372, 373, 491, 515; and drugs, 338, 512; and education, 517–518; and elderly, 323–324, 497, 498, 514; and falls, 220, 323–324, 328, 329; and firearms, 469; and hang gliding, 402; and highway injuries, 11, 37, 77, 115–116, 118, 119, 126, 129, 145, 147–149, 165, 180, 207, 219, 491, 498, 514–515, 521; and home injuries, 266, 267–268; impairment, 513–514; and law enforcement, 145, 146, 148–149, 517; metabolic and physiological factors, 511–514; and motorcycles, 186, 187; and occupational injuries, 430, 433–434, 444; and passengers, 37, 115; and pedestrians, 215–216, 219, 222–223, 226; as poison, 30–32, 334, 338; programs, 140, 148–149, 519–522; and railroad injuries, 226–227, 433; and sex, 324; and skiing, 388; and smoking, 306, 515; and snowmobiling, 391; and teenagers, 477, 514, 515; testing for, 77, 79–80, 141, 519; and tolerance to injury, 25–26, 29, 328, 513; and trucks, 165; and vision, 513, 514
Alcohol Safety Action Program (ASAP), 148–149
Allegheny Co., Pa., 421
Alternating current, 33–34
Aluminum wiring, 279–284, 309
Alzheimer disease, 496, 509
Amber traffic signal, 120–121
Ambulances, 178–180; and camps, 357–358; design, 159, 180–181; and hospitals, 182
American Association of Motor Vehicle Administrators, 161–162
American Hospital Association, 527
American National Standards Institute, 438–439
Ammonia poisoning, 334
Amphetamines, 116, 435, 522
Amputees and highway injuries, 117
Analysis of injury, 3–4
Andersen, J.H., 200, 203
Anelid worms, 376
Anger, W.K., 443
Angina, 507
Animals, 269–270; bites, 357, 376–378, 396, 483; and highway injuries, 107, 169, 189; and occupational injuries, 437; and parks, 359–360; poisonous, 332–333, 340–341, 357
Antiflashback devices, 240
Antigua, Guatemala, 463
Appliances, 283, 287–292, 294–297, 304, 309; and carbon monoxide poisoning, 296, 339–340
Arabian Gulf countries, 68, 137
Arbous, A.G., 468
Archery, 361, 370
Arsenic, 333, 341
Arthritis, 19, 36, 267; and falls, 324, 325; and highway injuries, 142, 499; and seat belts, 80–81
Ash trays, 317
Asher, J.W., 83
Asogwa, S.E., 197
Asphalt, impact attenuation, 353
Asphyxiation, 476, 482, 491; countermeasures, 482, 486, 488
Aspirin, 41, 333, 334, 337, 339, 341, 342, 343
Athletics. *See under individual activities*
Attractive nuisance, 296
Australia: alcohol, 116; diving, 375; highway injuries, 109, 115, 130, 186–187; motorcycles, 186–187; seat belts, 154; shark attacks, 376; falls, 321
Automobile injuries: and bicycles, 200, 201, 203, 205, 206, 208, 210; braking systems, 121, 123, 150; costs of safety standards, 55–56; countermeasures, 149–160; and defects, 121–125, 129–133, 149; and disasters, 455; fatalities, 162–163; and joggers, 394; manufacturers and safety programs, 48–49, 82, 121, 149; and medical impairment, 251–253, 260; and motorcycle accidents, 21, 185; number of automobiles, 161;

and pedestrians, 215, 216–220; and railroad injuries, 226, 227, 228; recalls, 121, 152–153, 180; reporting of, 67–69; rollovers, 129, 130, 133, 151; and size of vehicle, 124, 132, 155, 158, 159; and teenagers, 43; and trailers, 163–165, 167, 170, 171, 176; and trucks, 163–164, 173, 176, 177; and visibility, 21, 122–123, 124, 150; *see also* Highway injuries
Autopsies, 66–67, 528; records, 74
Avalanches, 387, 392, 447, 455; prediction, 456

Baby carriages, 327
BAC. *See* Alcohol, concentration
BAC 1-11, crash rate, 255
Back pain, 432–433, 437
Back-sliding effect, 87
Backett, E.M., 477
Bacteria, 16
Badminton, 393
Baker, S.P., 26, 48, 74–75, 119, 163, 187, 211, 218, 220, 238, 241, 302, 340, 371, 399, 422, 437, 473, 479, 482
Bako, G., 215
Ballinger, B.R., 408
Balloons, 370, 486
Baltimore: alcohol, 434; fires, 317; pedestrians, 212, 218, 220–221
Bangkok, 218
Bangladesh, 450, 453
Banisters, 271, 326, 328, 329; and children, 482
Bar stools, 292
Barancic, J.I., 303, 314
Barbiturates, 41, 116; and alcohol, 338, 512
Barker, K.N., 411–412, 413–414
Barmack, J.E., 513
Barraclough, B.M., 331
Barrett, H.S., 357
Barry, P.Z., 186
Bartholomew, W.M., 223
Bauer, K.H., 191
Baseball, 393, 395
Basketball, 362–363; injury rate, 378, 382
Bathing suits, 488–489
Bathroom injuries, 278–279, 327, 329; and elderly, 228; and electricity, 278, 283; and nursing homes, 408, 409
Battered children. *See* Children, assaults on
Bed disability and injury rate, 93
Beds: falls from, 265, 293, 327, 329; fires, 314; hospitals, 41, 112, 408, 410, 414
Bee stings, 333
Beer, 511–512, 517
Behan, R.C., 435–436, 468
Behavior modification and safety, 48–50, 81; and highway injuries, 147
Bell bottom trousers, 317
Benner, L., Jr., 11, 14, 20, 77, 526
Benson, D.A., 50, 56–57
Berfenstam, R., 478
Berg, W.D., 228
Bernaki, E.J., 467–468, 470
Bicycles, 199–210, 361; and adults, 206–207; and age, 199, 200; and alcohol, 206–207; and automobiles, 200, 201, 203, 205, 206, 208, 210; and children, 199, 200–207, 487, 489; countermeasures, 207–210, 489; design, 199, 208–209; and developing countries, 113, 207, 208, 209; and education, 207–208, 489; and elderly, 43; fatalities, 72, 199–200; and helmets, 209–210, 487; high-rise, 204; injury phase, 205; licensing, 207–208; number of, 200; passengers, 201, 204, 209; paths, 194, 209, 489, 491; and pedestrians, 209; and sex, 200–201, 202–203, 206; stability, 205, 207; and visibility, 205
Bigson, T., 379
Biljani, M.G., 242
Biologic rhythms, 433; *see also* Circadian rhythms
Birds, airplane collisions with, 257, 260
Bites: cats, 396; dogs, 396; human, 396–397; rats, 269–270, 396, 483
Bizyayev, V.P., 429–430
Blacks: burns, 302; drownings, 241–242, 372, 373; and firearms, 397,

398; hip fractures, 326; pedestrian injuries, 212
Blatnick, John, 126
Bleeding and alcohol, 26
Block trains, 227
Bloomberg, R.D., 223
Blue Cross Immunization Record, 343
Blum, Henrick, 463
Boarding houses, fires, 310
Boating. *See* Recreational boating
Body contact sports: and aggression, 362–363; individual, 383–386; team, 377–383
Boeing 707, 257
Boeing 727, 246, 255
Bombay, India, 270
Bone mass loss, 44, 325, 494
Booze, C.F., 253
Boston: citations, 71; kerosene space heaters, 309; occupational injuries, 434
Bothwell, P.W., 190–191, 193, 196
Botswana, 111, 122
Bottles: broken, 485; lamps, 311–314
Boxing, 7, 44, 366, 383–385
Boy Scout camp, 356, 357
Brakes: airplanes, 249; automobiles, 121, 123, 150; bicycles, 204, 208; motorcycles, 189, 193, 195; and pedestrian injuries, 219; railroad, 227, 232–233; trucks, 168, 169, 172, 175
Brazil, poisonous bites, 333
Brezina, E., 204, 205
Bricklayers, 430
Bridges, 128, 133, 158
Brodner, R.A., 26
Brooks, M.J., 439
Brown, G.W., 172, 178
Brown, I.D., 167
Brown, R.A., 51
Brown, T.C., 259
Bruner, J.M., Jr., 414
Buchanan, L.S., 190
Bucking mechanical bull, 395–396
Buffalo, N.Y., window injuries, 273–278
Buffalo Organization for Social and Technological Innovation (BOSTI), 272, 278
Buildings, 269–286; codes, 42, 271, 272, 278, 283, 284–286, 317–318, 485; collapse, 266, 269; and disasters, 455, 456–457; falls from, 326; and fatalities, 269
Buley, L.E., 252–253
Bull, J.P., 74, 291–292, 309
Bullock, M.I., 256
Bumpers, 56, 224
Bunks. *See* Beds
Burdge, R.J., 362
Bureau of Motor Carrier Safety, 527
Burke, D.C., 375
Burlington, Vt., 200
Burns: and age, 301–302, 303; and alcohol, 305, 306–308; and appliances, 296–297, 304, 309; and camping, 401; and camps, 356; and children, 301–302, 305–306, 309–310, 476, 480, 484; countermeasures, 41, 43, 44, 317–319, 480, 484, 488; and developing countries, 304; and elderly, 498, 501; and electricity, 34, 279; emergency treatment, 316, 480; and energy sources, 16–17; fatalities, 263, 301–302, 303; and medical impairment, 78; nonfatal, 302–303; and sex, 302, 304; social adjustment after, 304–305; and stoves, 265, 304, 308, 317, 484, 501; and teenagers, 490; and temperature tolerance, 30; and toys, 370, 488; *see also* Fire; Scalds
Burov, N.F., 429–430
Burton, I., 447, 449–450, 453, 454
Buses: crash impacts, 173; crash rates, 163; and developing countries, 108, 176; fatalities, 111, 163, 211; fatigue of driver, 166–167; overcrowding, 37, 108, 111, 113, 168, 175–176; size, 158; windows, 177; *see also* School buses

Cab drivers, 119
Cabinet makers, 430
Cabinets, child-resistant, 342, 479
Cable cutters, 439
Cahalan, D., 519–520

Cairns, H., 191
Cairo, housing, 269, 459
Caisson's disease, 375
Calcium therapy, 329
California: alcoholism, 519; boating, 235–236; camps, 356; earthquakes, 457; highway crashes, reporting of, 68, 69; highway improvements, 153; motorcycles, 185, 191, 194, 195–196; pedestrian programs, 222, 223; poison information center, 333; traffic citations, 71–72
CALSPAN CRASH computer, 76
Campbell, B.J., 107
Campbell, D.T., 84
Campers, 170, 173, 175, 401–402
Camps, 355–359
Canada: air crashes, 249; alcohol, 115, 116; basketball, 382; electricity, 279; fire evacuation study, 416; fireworks, 400; highway injuries, 36, 67, 107, 109, 115, 116; poisoning, 265; railroads, 228, 233; snowmobiling, 390
Cancer, 36, 103
Cann, H.M., 338
Cannabinols, 116; *see also* Marihuana
Canoes, 237
Caplan, G., 464
Carbon monoxide, 19, 30; alarms, 345; and appliances, 296, 339–340; countermeasures, 344–345, 489; and fires, 316; incidence, 339–340; and motor vehicles, 124, 176, 180, 340, 489; and SCUBA, 376
Carbon tetrachloride, 41, 341
Carbonated beverages, explosions, 297
Cardiac arrhythmias, 325
Cardiopulmonary resuscitation, 528
Cardiovascular disease, 494, 495, 497; and driving, 507–508; *see also* Heart attack
Cargo vessels, 235–236, 238–243
Caribbean, 183
Carithers, H.A., 337
Carlson, W.L., 391
Carnival amusements, 395
Carpenters, 430
Carr, R.W., 26
Carter, L.J., 239
Cataracts, 36, 325
Cats: alcohol and injuries, 25–26; bites, 396; causing falls, 327
Causation of injury event, information validity, 76–78
Cause the Effect: Effect the Cause, 527
Caustics, 333
Central America, 108
Centralized Traffic Control (railroads), 227
Cerebral palsy, 142, 308, 477
Ceylon: burns, 265, 304, 309; kerosene poisoning, 333
Chain grocers, injuries, 431
Chain saws, 297, 298
Chairs, 293; falls from, 329, 500
Chapanis, A., 296, 413
Chapman, P.J.C., 252–253, 260
Cheekbones, impact tolerance, 27
Chemical energy, 8, 16–17, 30–33; countermeasures, 41, 43, 44, 45; with kinetic energy, 25–26
Chicago: poison information center, 333; railroad injuries, 229; snow removal, 329
Child-care centers, 483
Children, 469, 473–491; air crashes, 258; appliances, 295, 296; asphyxiation, 476, 482, 486; assaults on, 69, 483; and bicycles, 199, 200–207, 487, 489; and burns, 301–302, 305–306, 309–310, 476, 480, 484; in developing countries, 473; and doors, 277; drowning, 372, 373–374, 476, 482, 488–489; and drugs, 41, 43, 339, 341–342, 485; and electricity, 283, 483; falls, 267, 321, 323, 326, 352–354, 480–481, 484, 488; and firearms, 266, 397–398, 487; and fires, 476; and fireworks, 400, 487; and highway injuries, 482–483, 487, 489; and home injuries, 267, 272, 277, 283; hyperactivity, 336, 357, 477; injury rate, 98; locomotion, 267, 323; medical impairment, 477; as pedestrians, 177, 473, 483, 487; poisoning,

333, 334, 336–339, 343–344, 469, 479, 481, 485–486, 488; and railroads, 229; and recreational activities, 361–362; risk factors, 476–478; and sharp objects, 28–29; and skiing, 387; socioeconomic class, 289–290; and stairs, 272; taste sense, 336; and visual cues, 214; *see also* Age; Toys
Chile, 98, 331
Chimney fires, 311
China, 93, 457–458
Chittenden Co., Vt., 390
Chlapecka, T.W., 202
Chlorinated hydrocarbons, 45
Cholera, 16
Cholinesterase, 251
Christmas tree bulbs, 296
Chrysler, 180
Circadian cycles, 19; and occupational injuries, 433; and pilots, 254; and psychophysiological response, 167; and severity of injury, 24
Circuit breakers, 279
Cirrhosis, 36
Clacker balls, 370
Clark, C.C., 291
Clayton, A.B., 127–128
Cleaning and polishing agents, poisoning, 334, 340, 484
Clear air turbulence (CAT), 258
Cleveland, firearms, 397
Climate and occupational injury, 436–437
Climbing apparatus, 352–353, 354
Climbing irons, 439
Clothes dryers, 296
Clothing: and falls, 327; and fire, 302, 309, 314–316, 484, 501, 529; *see also* Protective clothing
Coaches, 367–368, 380
Cocker spaniels, 396
Coconut Grove fire, 461
Code of Hummarabi, 271
Coffeepots, 295–296, 297, 309, 480
Cohen, A., 443
Cold: and injury threshold, 30; *see also* Hypothermia
Cold water and burns, 316, 480
Colebrook, L., 314
College students: and alcohol, 349–351; and bicycles, 206; injuries, 348–351; and motorcycles, 187, 349; sport injuries, 363
Collies, 396
Colorado, 196
Commercial vessels, 235, 236–240, 241
Concha, S.R., 441
Conduction and burns, 30
Congenital malformation, 36
Conger, J.J., 82
Connecticut: camps, 357; speeding enforcement, 82, 87
Construction, occupational injuries, 423, 425
Construction zones, warning signs, 125
Consumer Product Safety Commission, 327; and amusement ride injuries, 395; and fireworks, 400; and furniture, 292–293, 482; investigations, 78; and ladders, 298, 490; and playgrounds, 351, 354–355; and poison, 485; and toys, 481
Consumer Reports, 241
Containers, 297; and poisoning, 43, 338–339, 341–342, 343, 485–486
Contra Costa Co., Calif., 463
Contrast effect, 88
"Control" population and evaluations, 83–84
Convection and burns, 30
Cook, K.G., 427, 430
Cook, T.D., 84
Coppin, R.S., 144
Corless, I.B., 409
Corn picker, 438
Corsa, L., Jr., 334, 336, 337, 339
Corvair, 124
Cosand, M.E., 356
Cosmetics, poisoning, 334
Cost/benefit analysis and safety programs, 50–57, 81
Countermeasures against injuries, 4, 39–45; assessment of, 47–58, 79–89; simultaneous, 88–89; and time, effect of, 87–88
Coupling devices: railroads, 230–231, 232, 233; trailers, 171, 176

Cribs, 267, 292–293, 305–306, 481, 482; *see also* Sudden infant death
Crisis intervention, 464
Crop dusting. *See* Pesticides, air crashes
Cross, K.D., 205, 206–207, 209
Cross country skiing, 388–389
Crosswalks, 120–121, 218, 224
Crotty, J.J., 334
Cummings, V., 229
Cyanide, 30
Cycling Proficiency Training Program, 207
Cyclones, 449, 451–452
Cypress, 111, 218
Czechoslovakia: hockey, 383; poisoning, 33

Dallas, 71
Dams, 447, 456, 459–460
Danaher, J.W., 254
Darts, 370
Dashboards, impact with, 129–130
Data, accuracy of, 56, 65
Datta, S.P., 425
Davies, E., 379
DC-10, 255
Deadman's switch, 298
Deafness. *See* Hearing
De Castro, F.J., 337–338
Deceleration forces, 26
Decompression, 371, 375
Defensive Driving Course, 143–144
Defibrillators, 414
Definitions of injury, 7–9, 66
Deforestation and disaster, 455
De Haven, H., 25, 258
Delhi, India, 165
Denmark: alcohol, 116; ambulances, 178–179; children, 98; highway injuries, 116
Depression, 508–509
Depth perception, 494
Design and occupational injuries, 438–439, 445
Desjardins, S.P., 260
Detroit, 397
Developing countries, 3; and alcohol, 115; and bicycles, 113, 207, 208, 209; and burns, 304; and children, 473; disasters, 447–449, 457; elderly fatalities, 308; emergency services, 137; highway injuries, 108, 109, 111–113, 115, 120, 122, 128–129, 137, 153, 170, 447; housing, 263, 269, 308; motorcycles, 113, 185–186; occupational injuries, 445; pedestrians, 113, 212; railroads, 229; reporting of injuries, 69; roadways, 128–129, 158; transportation, 37; vehicle inspection programs, 153
Dewar, R.E., 208, 390
Diabetes, 16, 19; and driving, 508; and elderly, 495–496, 498, 499, 508; and highway injuries, 117, 174; and vision, 496, 508
Dials, 42–43, 438
Dietz, P.E., 238, 241, 371, 399
Dille, J.R., 250–251, 253
Diphtheria, 44, 483
Diplopia, 506
Direct current, 33–34
Disasters, 447–464; countermeasures, 450, 454, 456–459; and developing countries, 447–449, 453; fatalities, 447, 449, 454–455; magnitude, 450–452; and parks, 366; planning, 160, 463, 464; prediction, 457–458; and sex, 449
Distance judgment, children, 476
Diuretics, 408–409
Diving, 370, 371, 374–375
Dizzy spells, 324, 496
Dog bites, 396
Dolls, 369–370
Door locks: automobiles, 129–130, 149, 151, 154; and children, 487
Doors, 272–277
Doppler radar, 457
Driessen, G.J., 206
Driver education, 42, 138, 139; and developing countries, 120, 129; effectiveness, 140–141, 143–144; evaluation of programs, 82–83; and motorcycles, 190, 193–194; and rehabilitation, 142–144; and sex, 143–144
Drought, 449, 451–452
Drowning, 25, 371–374, 404; and alcohol, 238, 250, 372, 373, 491,

515; and boating accidents, 237, 241–243, 371; and children, 372, 373–374, 476, 482, 488–489; countermeasures, 482, 486–487, 488–489, 491; near, 371–372; as occupational injury, 437; and parachuting, 403; rate, 263; and sex, 371; and wells, 265, 371, 476
Drug store injuries, 431
Drugs, 522–523; and air accidents, 251; and alcohol, 338, 512; and children, 41, 43, 339, 341–342, 485; and education, 523; and elderly, dosage, 326, 329, 338, 344, 497, 498; and falls, 323, 326, 329, 338, 408–409, 497, 498; and highway injury, 116, 491, 498, 509, 522–523; and occupational injuries, 435; and poisoning, 333, 338; and sports, 381; and students, 351; and suicide, 41, 331; and teenagers, 477, 491; *see also* Medication
Ducic, S., 303, 306
Duffy, J.C., 259
Duration of impact and severity, 26
Dyson, R.B., 54–55
Dyspnea, 508

Earthquakes, 37–38, 447, 449; and building design, 456–457; countermeasures, 42, 44, 455–456, 457–458; magnitude, 451, 452
Ebneter, A., 251
Education and injuries, 39, 42; and alcohol, 517–518; and appliances and furniture, 287–291; and bicycle riders, 207–208, 489; and camps, 358–359; and children, 478–479; and drugs, 523; effectiveness of, 140–141, 143–144; and emergency personnel, 44–45, 159; evaluation of, 80; and fire prevention, 318–319; and health care professionals, 525–529; and highway injuries, 140, 141, 529; and occupational injuries, 427, 441–444; and pedestrians, 222, 223; and poisoning, 342–344, 486; and seat belts, 80–81, 85, 141; and socioeconomic factors, 287–288
Egypt, 160, 301
Eiseman, B., 402–403
Elderly, 469, 493–510; and alcohol, 323–324, 497, 498, 514; and bathroom injuries, 278; and bicycles, 43; bone fragility, 44, 325, 329; and burns, 303, 308, 498, 501; and chairs, 293; in developing countries, 308; and disaster, 465; and driving evaluation, 116–117, 503–510; and drugs, 326, 329, 338, 497, 498; and falls, 68, 103, 267, 270, 271, 308, 323–325, 327, 328, 329, 497–498, 499–501; fatalities, 98, 103, 324; and fires, 269, 310, 501; and glare, 327, 329, 409, 494, 500; hearing, 215, 316, 494, 506; and highway injuries, 116–117, 119, 123, 129, 497, 498–499, 502–503; and hypothermia, 242, 308, 501; injury rate, 98; locomotion, 267, 325, 494, 496; medical impairment, 493–510; as pedestrians, 214–215, 216, 222–223, 226, 498, 502; and poisoning, 498, 501; and railroads, 226–227; vision, 215, 267, 271, 308, 324, 325, 493–494, 496, 498, 500, 506, 508; *see also* Age
Electric blankets, 295, 309
Electric mixers, 41, 295
Electric heaters, 295–296
Electrical energy, 8, 16, 265, 296; and bathrooms, 278, 283; and burns, 34, 229; and children, 283, 483; chronic exposure, 36; countermeasures, 41–42, 479; and hang gliding, 402; and home and maintenance equipment, 298; and hospital injuries, 414–415; receptacle closures, 43, 283; tolerance thresholds, 33–34; and toys, 370
Elevators, 461
Elia, J.C., 384
Ellis, L., 440
Emergency Department Nurses Association, 358–359

Emergency services: air crashes, 259, 260, 261; camps, 357–359; developing countries, 137; and highway injuries, 36–37, 137, 140, 159–160; parks, 359; shark attacks, 376–377; training, 44–45, 159
Emergency vehicles, 159, 178–182
EMT-A certification, 159
Energy and injury, 8, 16–17; acute vs. chronic exposure, 35–36; and countermeasures, 40–45; massing of and severity of injury, 17–18, 23, 43; rate of release, 23–24; spreading out of, 24, 25
Enzymes: defects, 16, 25; and poison, 25, 30
Epidemiological studies of injuries, 13–14, 16–17
Epilepsy, 19, 42, 260, 267, 477; and driving, 498, 506–507; and drowning, 489; and highway injuries, 117, 166; *see also* Seizures
Equestrian activities, 363
Eriksson, E., 387, 388
Erwin, R.D., 169
"Escape of Tigers" (Haddon), 528
Escape ramps, 176–177
Eskimos, 320
Estrogen therapy, 329
Evacuation: airplanes, 259; disasters, 458–459; fires, 416
Evaluation of programs, 79–89
Evans, Stanley, 519
Exhaust systems, 44, 45
Explosions: appliances, 295, 309; carbonated beverages, 297; and ocean transport, 239, 240
Explosives, 37, 174
Exposure and injury, 69–72, 139
Extension cords, 279, 305, 480
Eyeglasses, impact-resistant, 44, 299, 349, 440
Eyes: and fireworks, 400; and hockey, 383; and toys, 29

Face guards, 381
Fagan, I.D., 406, 407
Failure Model and Effects analysis (FMEA), 13
Falls, 4, 321–329; and age, 409; and alcohol, 220, 323–324, 328, 329; from beds, 265, 293, 327, 329; and burns, 308, 324; camps, 356; and children, 267, 321, 323, 326, 352–354, 480–481, 484, 488; and drugs, 323, 326, 329, 338, 408–409, 497, 498; and elderly, 68, 103, 267, 270, 275, 308, 323–325, 327, 328, 329, 497–498, 499–501; emergency treatment, 328; fatalities, 263, 321, 325; and floors, 293, 325, 327, 328, 329; and glass, 328, 329; and hospitals, 407–410; and lighting, 329, 500; and medical impairment, 324–326, 328, 497–498; and occupational injuries, 437, 439–440; and pets, 327–328; and playgrounds, 352–353, 354–355; and railroads, 229, 233; and sex, 321, 322, 324; and stairs, 270–272, 322, 325, 326; survival, 25; from vehicles, 111, 113, 168; and vision, 324, 500
Fans, 295, 340
Fatal Accident Reporting System (FARS), 162
Fatigue, 166–167
Fault tree, 12–14
Federal Aviation Agency, 248, 255–256, 258, 259, 527
Federal Bureau of Motor Carrier Safety, 174
Federal Housing Administration, 278
Federal Railroad Administration, 227–228
Ferris, B.G., Jr., 401
Field hockey, 378
55 MPH speed limit, 84–85, 109, 146, 221
Fiji, 111
Finance/insurance industry, injuries, 423
Fineberg, H.V., 416
Finland: motorcycles, 184; occupational injuries, 426, 434, 437, 438; water fatalities, 238
Fire: and air crashes, 258, 259, 260; alarms, 316, 461, 480, 501; and appliances, 295; and boating, 240, 241; and cargo vessels, 239; and clothing, 302, 309, 314–315, 484,

501, 529; countermeasures, 44, 151, 317–319, 480, 484, 488; and education, 318–319; and elderly, 269, 310, 501; evacuation, 416; fatalities, 263, 301, 306, 318; and furniture, 302, 315, 316; and highway injuries, 137, 151, 173–174; and hospitals, 415–416; and ocean transport, 239, 240, 241; and power equipment, 298; residential, 302, 303; safety codes, 317–318; and sex, 313; and smoking, 306–308, 311; toxic fumes, 306–308, 316, 461; wiring, 284; *see also* Burns
Fire escape falls, 326
Fire Safety Evacuation System, 415–416
Fire trucks, 178, 180
Firearms, 265–266, 291, 397–400; and accident proneness, 468–469; and alcohol, 469; and children, 266, 397–398, 487; control legislation, 399–400; fatalities, 266, 397; reporting of injuries, 67; and sex, 398; spinal injuries, 362; and suicide, 266, 397
Fireplace guards, 291–293
Fireworks, 400
First aid: and athletic staff, 368; and burns, 316, 480; and camp counselors, 358; and occupational injuries, 445; and ship's crew, 242, 243; *see also* Emergency services
Fisher, G., 205, 206–207, 209
Fisher, R.S., 187, 482
Fishing, 236, 237, 361
Fishing vessels, 235, 236
Flame-retardant materials, 315–316; and airplanes, 259, 260; and automobiles, 151; and boating, 241; and clothing, 302, 480; and elderly, 501; tents, 402
Flamm, E.S., 25–26
Flammable materials, 266–267; clothing, 314–315, 484; furniture, 294, 314; transport, 177, 230–231
Flannelette, flammability, 314
Floods, 37–38, 321, 447, 449, 450, 455; human response, 452–454; magnitude, 450–451, 452; and retaining walls, 453–454, 456
Flooring, 268; and falls, 293, 325, 327, 328, 329
Florida, hurricanes, 456
Flotation devices, 241, 242–243, 358, 374; and parachuting, 403
Fluoride treatment, 329
Foerster, J., 408–409
Fog, 451
Folding furniture, 292
Food chain distribution, injuries, 432
Food poisoning, 7, 8
Football, 362, 363, 366, 377, 378, 379–382; equipment, 380; fatalities, 379; touch, 381
Ford, 180
Forestry, injuries, 423
Forrest, T.R.W., 339
Fort Ord, Calif., 306
Foundrymen, 430
Fractures, 44; and age, 24, 25; and bicycles, 201; greenstick, 24, 25; and motorcycles, 187, 197; and nursing homes, 409; and falls, 321, 326, 328, 352, 353, 409; and impact tolerance, 27; and skiing, 388
France: alcohol, 434; children, 98; drowning, 371; falls, 321; highway safety expenditures, 50; railroads, 231
Frankfurters, choking on, 482
Freeways, 133
Frequency of injury events: determination of, 13–14; prediction of, 11–12
Freymoyer, J.W., 437
Fuel tanks, 44, 137, 191–192; and air crashes, 248; and motorcycles, 191–193; standards, 151; and trucks, 177
Furnace grates, 309–310
Furniture, 287–294; falls, 329, 501; fires, 302, 315, 316
Fuses, 279

Gadalla, S.M., 437–438
Garden tools, 291, 297–299
Garden tractors, 298
Garrick, J.G., 394

Garrick, J.S., 381–382, 387
Gas heaters, 339
Gas stoves, 295
Gas tanks. *See* Fuel tanks
Gasoline sales and driving exposure, 70
Gasoline shortage and highway injuries, 84–85, 109
Gastrointestinal problems: and pilots, 253; and alcohol, 512
Gastropods, 376
Gatekeepers and countermeasures, 81–82
Gear shifting, 121, 150, 170
Geelong, Australia, 237, 371
General Services Administration, 151
Genital injuries and bicycles, 205, 209
Georgia, 133–137
German shepherds, 396
Germany: alcohol, 116, 434; children, 98; highway injuries, 116, 122; trampoline injuries, 394
Ghana, 122
Ghezzo, H.R., 303, 306
Gibson, E.J., 323
Gibson, J.J., 16
Girl Scout camps, 357
Glare and elderly, 325, 327, 329, 409, 494, 500
Glass: broken, 193, 377, 485; and falls, 328, 329
Glasses. *See* Eyeglasses
Glaucoma, 325, 496
Gliders. *See* Sailplanes
Glider kits, 170
Go-karts, 395
Goldberg, L., 514
Golf, 361, 366
Gonski, L., 205
Gordis, L., 79
Gordon, J.E., 93, 322, 425, 437
Graham, J.W., 187
Green, C.H., 51
Green, J.A., 227
Green, L.W., 87–88
Greenberg, L., 44
Greenwood, M., 467–468
Grizzly bears, 359–360
Ground fault circuit interrupter (GFCI), 279, 284
Grubel, F., 407
Guardrails, 158
Guards and machinery, 438, 440
Guatemala, 449, 455, 463
Guns. *See* Firearms
Gustafson, J., 175, 478
Gym mats, 353, 385
Gymnastics, 393

Haas, J.E., 463
Haddon, W., Jr., 16, 40–41, 70–71, 211, 214–215, 279, 326, 404, 526, 528
Haight, F.A., 109, 218, 468
Hakim, H.A., 168
Hallel, T., 403
Halpern, Milton, 503
Hand tools, 439
Handball, 361
Handler, Philip, 255
Handrails, 271
Hang gliding, 363, 366, 402–403
Harano, R.M., 143–144
Hard hats, 44
Harnett, R.M., 242
Harper, C.R., 250, 251
Harper, D.G., 425
Hartley, H.L., 412–413
Hartunian, N.S., 103
Hashish, 116
Havard, J.D.J., 212–214
Hazard analysis, 12–14
Hazardous materials: disaster plans, 177–178, 230; ocean transport, 240, 241, 242; railroads, 230–231; transport, 37, 44, 173–174, 175, 177, 459, 462
Head injuries, 25, 304; and air crashes, 259; and automobiles, 322; and bicycles, 201, 207, 209–210; and burns, 305; costs, 322; and equestrian activities, 396; and falls, 322, 328; and motorcycles, 191, 195–196; and recreational activities, 362, 369, 489; and skiing, 388–389; and tolerance to impact, 27
Head restraints, 150, 152
Headway between vehicles, 120
Health professionals and injury, 3, 40, 141, 525–529

Hearing: and driving, 506; and elderly, 215, 316, 494, 506; and fires, 316; and occupational injuries, 166, 494
Heart attacks, 98; airline pilots, 252, 250; and falls, 321; and highway injuries, 66, 117, 174, 497; and swimming, 371
Heat stress and sports, 379, 382
Heat stroke, 394
Heating systems, 284, 310, 339; *see also* Space heaters; Wood stoves
Hedge trimmers, 297
Heimlich maneuver, 528
Heins, M., 399
Helicopters, 256
Helmets, 529; and bicycles, 209–210, 487; and equestrian activities, 396; and hang gliding, 402, 403; and motorcycles, 191, 193, 195–197, 367; and skateboards, 369; and sports, 366, 367, 380–381, 388
Helsinki, Finland, occupational injuries, 426, 434
Hemiplegia, 325
Hensley, L.D., 393
Hepatitis, 16
Herrera, S., 359
Hess, Robert, 118
Hiatt, L., 293, 409–410
High chairs, 41, 292, 327, 480
Highway injuries: and age, 66, 110, 113, 115, 116–118, 119, 126, 128, 165–166, 473; and alcohol, 11, 37, 77, 115–116, 118, 119, 126, 129, 145, 147–149, 165, 180, 207, 219, 491, 498, 514–515; and animals, 107, 169, 189; and children, 479, 482–483, 487, 489; and college students, 349; countermeasures, 138–160, 174–178, 479, 482–483, 487, 489, 502–503; data validity, 65–66, 67–68, 111–112; and developing countries, 108, 109, 111–113, 115, 120, 122, 128–129, 137, 153, 170, 447; and disaster, 447–449; and drugs, 116, 491, 498, 509, 522–523; economic costs, 103, 110, 113; and education of health care professionals, 140, 141, 529; and ejection, 129–130, 151, 154; and elderly, 116–117, 119, 123, 129, 497, 498–499, 502–503; and emergency care, 36–37, 137, 140, 154–160, 193; and exposure, measurement of, 70–71; fatalities, 65–66, 109–110, 112, 130–131; fatalities, international, 107, 111–113; and fires, 137, 151, 173–174; and heart attack, 66, 117, 174; and inexperience, 118, 119, 167–168, 186, 190; injury phase, 129–137, 173, 177; inspection programs, 139, 153, 176; laws and obedience, 118–121, 141, 144–149; and lighting, 271–272; and medical impairment, 116–117, 142, 166, 174, 498; and occupational injury, 437; patterns, 109–113; and physician-to-population ratio, 112; and population per vehicle, 108–109; post-injury phase, 137, 159–160, 173–174, 177–178; pre-injury phase, 113–129; and productivity losses, 52; property damage, 75–76, 110; reporting of, 67–69, 111–112; and roadway system, 113, 119, 125–129, 133–137, 155–158; and rural areas, 69, 107, 110, 130, 133, 137, 153; and sex, 110, 113, 118, 123, 143–144; and speed, 120, 128, 132, 144–146, 168, 175; and stability of vehicles, 113, 169–170, 187–188; and stopping distance, 169; and task demands, 19–20, 21; and teenagers, 117–118 473, 491, 504; and time of day, 110; and vehicle defects, 121–125, 129–133, 149; and visibility, 21, 113, 122–123, 124; and warning signs, 125–126, 127, 176; *see also* Automobile injuries; Bicycles; Motorcycles; Pedestrians; Trucks
Highway Safety Act, 149–150
Highway Users Federation for Safety and Mobility (HUFSAM), 139
Hiking, 356, 359–360, 401
Hippocrates, 24
Hiroshima, 460
Hirshfeld, A.H., 435–436, 468

Hitching mechanism, 171, 176; *see also* Coupling devices
Hoffman, M.A., 253–254
Hogue, E.E., 367
Hoists, 439
Home injuries, 263–268
Homeostasis and injury event, 12, 14–16, 24, 35–36
Homicide, 98, 254; and accident proneness, 468–469; and firearms, 266, 397
Hong Kong: beds, falls from, 265, 293, 327; employment, 421
Honkanen, R., 324, 433–434
Hoods: latches, 150; ornaments, 221
Horses. *See* Equestrian activities
Horseshoes, 361
Hospital beds, 41; electric, 414; falls from, 408, 410
Hospitals, 405–421; and ambulances, 182; and electrical injuries, 414–415; employee injuries, 416–420; falls, 407–410; fires, 415–416; and highway injuries, 159–160; medication errors, 405, 408–409, 410–414; and motorcycle victims, 193; poisonings, 343; psychiatric, 417
Hot-air ballooning, 403–404
Hot dogs, choking on, 482
Hot water heaters: and carbon monoxide, 296; temperature, 297, 306, 480, 501
Hotel industry, injuries, 439
Hricko, A.R., 251
Huberman, J., 362
Huelke, D.F., 152
Human bites, 396–397
Human Factors, 254
Humidifiers, 295–296, 480
Hunter, W.W., 184
Hunting, 398–399
Hurlers, 394
Hurricanes, 453, 456, 457
Hurt, H.H., 184–185, 189–190, 191, 193, 194–195
Hyperactivity, 477; and camp injuries, 357; and poisoning, 336
Hypertension, 499, 508
Hypodermic needles, puncture by, 7, 8
Hypothermia: and alcohol, 308; and elderly, 242, 308, 501; and homeless, 263, 308; and skiing, 389; and snowmobiling, 392; and water accidents, 242
Hypoxia and airplane pilots, 252

Iatrogenic illness, 45, 405
Ice, falls on, 324
Ice cream trucks, 220, 224
Ice hockey, 366, 382–383
Ice skating, 361, 368
Ignition locks, 43
Illinois, 69
ILO, 235
Immunization, 483
In the Crash, 528
India: adobe homes, 455; burns, 265, 304; drownings, 265, 371; floods, 38; highway injuries, 112; injury rate, 93; mopeds, 183; occupational injuries, 525
Indiana, vehicle defects, 121, 122
Individual assessment of safety, 58
Indonesia: crosswalks, 218; highway injuries, 112, 121
Induced exposure, 71
Inexperience and accidents, 19, 476–477; and airplane crashes, 248–249, 251; and camps, 356; and highway injuries, 118, 119, 167–168, 186, 190; and home injuries, 266, 267; and motorcycle injuries, 186, 190; and occupational injuries, 428–430
Infants: countermeasures, 479–483; pedestrian casualties, 212; restraints, 154–155, 479, 480, 482–483, 487
Information processing, 18
Injury phase of injury event, 12, 23–36; and education of health care professionals, 527–528
Injury Severity Score (ISS), 74–75, 528
Innocent bystanders, 37–38
Ischemic heart disease, 497, 498–499
Insect stings, 48, 333, 357
Ishkrant, A.P., 322
Inspection programs and highway injuries, 139, 153, 176

Instrument panels: airplanes, 256–257; automobiles, 149; clearness of, 42–43, 123; padding, 44, 150
Insulation, 283, 284, 296
International Air Transportation Association, 252–253
International Civil Aviation Organization, 245
International Ice Patrol, 240
Interstate Commerce Commission, 233
Interviews: and driver rehabilitation, 143; with victims, 70–71, 73–74
Intoxication, 513–514; *see also* Alcohol
Ionizing radiation, 8, 16; countermeasures, 44; remote control handling, 24; tolerance to, 25, 35
Iowa, motor vehicle crashes, 77
Irons, 295–296
Israel: nursing home injuries, 407; roadway improvements, 158; vehicle defects, 122
Israeli Armed Forces parachuting, 403

Jacobs, G.D., 111, 112–113, 168, 218
Jails, 461, 462
Jamaica: crosswalks, 218; highway injuries, 120–121
Japan: burns, 304; drowning, 371; motorcycles, 193; railroads, 225, 231
Jellyfish, 376
Jet blasts, 257
Job market, entry into, 98
Joggers, 394
Johnson, R.J., 387, 388
Joint Commission on Accreditation of Hospitals, 415
Joliet, P.V., 322
Jolly, H., 339
Jones, D.F., 437
Jones, R.D.H., 227
Jones, R.K., 51
Joscelyn, K.B., 51
Judo, 386

Kangri pot tumors, 36
Kansas, 196; tornadoes, 449
Kansas City, Mo., balcony collapse, 286
Kaolin, 32
Karate, 383, 386
Karlson, T.A., 163
Keating, W.R., 242
Keith-Wagner retinopathy, 508
Kelley, A.B., 55
Kennedy Airport, crash, 248
Kenya: crosswalks, 218; highway injuries, 66, 113, 120–121, 163, 168
Kerosene: bottle lamps, 309, 313–314; poisoning, 265, 333, 334, 337; space heaters, 289, 295, 309
Kerrich, J.E., 468
Kewalramani, L.S., 374
Kinetic energy, 8, 16, 17, 26–29; with chemical energy, 25–26; countermeasures, 41, 43, 44; tolerance to, 25–26; and toys, 370
Klein, David, 49, 138–139, 287–289, 362, 391, 398, 399–400
Knives, 29
Knoblauch, R.L., 215, 216–218, 222
Knowledge of environment and injury, 17–18, 19
Kocur, J.L., 337–338
Krakow, Poland, alcohol poisoning, 338
Kramer, M., 204, 205
Kraus, J.F., 374, 381
Krissoff, W.B., 402–403
Kung fu, 386
Kurland, L., 387
Kuwait, 109, 113, 211

L-188 crash rate, 255
Laboratories: and injury analysis, 13, 14; hospitals, 420; infections, 7, 44, 420; school, 348, 349
Lacefield, D.J., 251
Ladders, 298–299, 326–327, 490; and occupational injuries, 439–440
Lahtela, J., 426
Lakonia, 242
Lamborn, K.R., 391–392
Lane, J.C., 252–253, 259
Law enforcement: and alcohol, 145, 146, 148–149, 517; and highway

injuries, 144–149, 218; and reporting of injuries; and systems analysis of injury, 13
Lawnmowers, 287, 298, 299
Lead poisoning, 341, 342, 343, 481
Leard, S.E., 348
Lederer, J., 246
Lehr, E.L., 361
Leighton-White, R.C., 260
Leukemia, 30, 460
Levine, M.S., 306
Lewis, F.J., Jr., 181–182
Li, L.K., 169
Liberia, 238, 239
Licensing, 471; airplane pilots, 42; bicycles, 207–208; costs, 140; effectiveness of programs, 141–142; and elderly, 116–117, 503–510; motorcycles, 190, 194; recreational vehicles, 174; revocation, 144; trucks, 166, 168, 174
Life, value of, 51–57
Life jackets. *See* Flotation devices
Lifting, 437
Lighting, 266; and falls, 325, 329, 500; and highway injuries, 126, 128; and insulation, 284; and motorcycles, 194–195; and stairs, 271–272
Limited rationality, theory of, 51
Lind, M.G., 200, 209–210
Lindenbaum, L.E., 296
Lindgard, D.A., 377, 378
Linoleum cement, 314
Lip cancer, 36
Little League, 187, 395
Liver: and drugs, 333, 344, 494, 500; failure, 7, 8, 36, 41
Lockhart, J.D.F., 304
Locks, automobile, 43, 129–130, 149, 150, 151, 154
Locomotion: children, 267, 323; elderly, 267, 325, 494, 496; and nursing home injuries, 409
Locomotive Grade Crossing Attenuation Device, 57
Logic tree, 12–14
Logue, J.N., 463–464
Lomotil, 342
London: highway injuries, 184; pedestrian crosswalks, 218
Longshoremen, injuries, 236
Lowrance, W.W., 48
LSD, 116, 323
Lung cancer, 36
Lye, 30

M151 quarter-ton tank, 170
McAllister, J.F., 287
McConnell, W.E., 411–412
McFarland, R.A., 170, 438
McLatchie, G.R., 386
McMaster, W.C., 377
MacRostie, M., 413
Maintenance and repair equipment, 297–299
Malaysia, 211
Males. *See* Sex
Malik, M.A.O., 168
Mandibles, impact tolerance, 27
Manheimer, D.I., 334, 468, 470, 477
Manufacturers and safety, 48–49, 82, 121, 149; and appliances and furnishing, 291–292, 296; and fires, 314–315; and highway injuries, 195
Manufacturing, occupational injuries, 423
Maoris, 370
Margolis, J.A., 336
Margulee, I., 409
Marihuana, 116, 435
Martial arts, 383, 386
Maryland: drowning, 371; motorcycles, 189–190
MAST trousers, 159
Matches, 305, 311, 484; and elderly, 498, 501
Maximum tolerable disability, 51
Maxwell, M., 603
Meagher, S.W., 438–439
Meals-on-wheels program, 223
Measles, 16, 17
Meat processing, injuries, 431
Medial meniscus, 386
Medical examination: and highway injuries, 142; and pilots, 252
Medical impairment, 78; and air transport, 251–253, 260; and burns, 305, 308; and children, 477; and elderly, 493–510; and falls, 324–326, 328, 497–498; and highway injuries, 116–117, 142, 166, 174, 498; and home injuries,

266, 268; and pedestrians, 214–215; and truck crashes, 166, 174
Medical records and injury statistics, 74
Medication: and hospital errors, 405, 408–409, 410–414; *see also* Drugs
Medicine bottles, child-proof closures, 43, 339, 341–343, 485
Mela, D.F., 130–132
Mellanby phenomenon, 513
Mellinger, G.D., 468, 470, 477
Memory and aging, 495, 508–509
Memphis, Tenn., and gas heaters, 339
Men. *See* Sex
Menninger, K., 468
Mennon, U., 375
Menopause, 494
Menstrual cycle, 431, 432, 433; *see also* Premenstrual tension
Mental illness, 19
Merrill, S.A., 48–49, 50
Metal fabrication, injuries, 426, 431–432
Metal-toed shoes, 44, 299, 440, 445
Methane, 41
Mexico: drownings, 371; fireworks, 400
Meyer, R.J., 337, 356, 357
Michigan: firearms, 397–398; motorcycles, 186; railroad injuries, 221
Michigan Alcoholism Screening Test, 519
Mihalasky, J., 22–23
Miners, 430
Minibikes, 183, 187, 291
Mining and quarrying, occupational injuries, 423, 425, 441, 449
Mirrors: and highway injuries, 123, 124, 150, 188, 220; and pedestrian injuries, 220, 224; and trucks, 170, 220
Mississippi, highway crashes, 69
Mr. Yuk labels, 342, 343–344
Mitchell, James, 422
Mobile homes, 167, 269, 455
Modified Mercalli scale, 451
Modified Richter scale, 451
Molnar, G., 229
Monroe Co., N.Y., 342–343, 344
Montreal, residential fires, 303, 306, 310, 311
Mopeds, 183, 184–185, 188, 194, 195, 203–204, 491
Morality and safety programs, 49–50
Mordant, 316
Morgan, W.J., 369
Morganstein, D., 52, 55–56
Mortimer-Filkins test, 519
Moscow, pedestrian injuries, 215
Moslem countries and alcohol, 115, 148, 518
Motor Vehicle Safety Act, 140, 149–150
Motorcycles, 107, 183–197, 203–204, 362; and alcohol, 186, 187; and automobiles, 21, 185; countermeasures, 193–197, 491; and developing countries, 113, 185–186; and driver education, 190, 193–194; fatalities, 111, 184–186, 211; and helmets, 191, 193, 195–197, 367; and inexperience, 186, 190; licensing, 190, 194; and lighting, 194–195; and passengers, 188, 191; and police, 178; pre-injury phase, 186–187; and property damage, 184; reporting of accidents, 68; size of machines, 188–189, 191; and visibility, 21, 186–187, 188, 189–190, 194–195, 196
Mount Pelee, 463
Mount St. Helens, 457
Mountain climbing, 363, 401
Mouth guards, 366, 378–379, 381
Mouth-to-mouth resuscitation, 489
Muller, A., 196
Multidisciplinary Accident Investigation teams (MDAIs), 78
Multilinear events sequencing model, 14–15
Multiple factor model of injury events, 11–12, 17
Multiple sclerosis, 324, 496
Munden, J.M., 188–189, 191
Muscle mass, 44; and falls, 325–326, 494, 497, 499–500; and sport injuries, 366
Myocardial infarction, 36, 372; and driving, 507; *see also* Heart attack

Nader, Ralph, 121, 124, 129, 414
Naggar, N., 403
NASA, 254
Natal, 376–377
National Accident Sampling System, 78
National Advertising Review Board, 292
National Building Code, 272–273
National Bureau of Standards, 28–29, 270, 316, 415
National Clearinghouse for Poison Control Centers, 334, 345
National Commission on Product Safety, 286
National Council on Alcoholism, 519
National Crash Severity Study (NCSS), 132–133
National Fire Protection Association, 415
National Head and Spinal Cord Injury Survey, 322
National Health Survey, 67, 93, 185, 235, 333, 422, 425
National Highway Safety Advisory Committee, 123–124
National Highway Traffic Safety Administration: cost/benefit studies, 52, 55; and motorcycles, 189; standards, 56, 149–152, 169, 175, 177, 195
National Rifle Association, 265–266, 399
National Safety Council, 77, 143, 235, 422, 441–442
National Transportation Safety Board, 57, 123–124, 173, 229; and air crashes, 246, 248, 455
Natural gas, 41
Near midair collisions (NMACs), 254
Neck injuries: and helmets, 196; and impact tolerance, 27–28
Needle punctures, 7, 8, 44
Netherlands, drownings, 371
New Amsterdam, 317
New Orleans, pedestrians and alcohol, 216
New South Wales, 186
New York City: ambulance crashes, 180; falls, 326; homeless, 263; human bites, 396–397
New York state: ambulance crashes, 179; boxing, 384
New Zealand, 314, 370; fireworks, 400; rugby, 378–379; soccer, 377
Newcombe, R.G., 336
Nicholi, A.M., 187
Nigeria: highway injuries, 112, 166, 167, 172, 197; pedestrians, 211
Nilsson, S., 377
Nixon, J., 372, 373–374
No-fault automobile insurance, 48
"No Siop!" program, 343
North Carolina: alcohol poisoning, 338; driver licenses, 144; football injuries, 374–381; motorcycles, 186; vehicle defects, 170–171
Norway, drownings and alcohol, 238
Nose, impact tolerance, 27
Notice of disaster, ignoring of, 38
Nuclear power, 14, 460–461, 462
Nurses: injuries, 417–418; medication errors, 411, 413
Nursing homes, 405–421; and drugs, 326, 409–410; and falls, 407–410, 500–501; and fires, 315, 415–416; and floors, 325, 409
Nylon, flammability, 314, 315
Nystagmus, 506

Occupational illness, 8, 35–36
Occupational injuries, 421–445, 494; and absenteeism, 435–436; and alcohol, 430, 433–434, 444; countermeasures, 440–445; and developing countries, 445; and education, 427, 441–444; exposure measurement, 70; fatalities, 422–425; and inexperience, 428–430; reporting of, 67, 422–423, 425; and sex, 430–434, 439, 445; and teenagers, 422, 473, 477–478
Occupational Safety and Health Act, 44
Occupational Safety and Health Administration, 235, 422, 424, 441
Ocean tankers, 44, 241
Oceania, 473
O'Day, J., 152
Oil spills, 240, 241, 242
Oklahoma, 196
Olsen, R.A., 125, 218

O'Neill, B., 55
Open-registry vessels, 238, 239, 240
Opiates, 116
Oppenlander, J.C., 228
OPSKARBO, 79–82
Oral injuries, 378–379, 381
Oregon, 143
Orlick, T.D., 362
Osteoporosis, 44, 325, 494
Owasina, F.A.O., 128, 166, 172

Pacemakers, 414, 508
Pain threshold, 30, 494
Paint, poisoning, 339, 341, 342, 481
Pakistan: crosswalks, 218; fatalities, 93; traffic signal response, 121
Panama, 238, 239
Panic and highway injury, 127, 128
Papermakers, 430
Parachuting. *See* Sky diving
Paralysis agitans, 325
Parasympathetic nervous system, 496, 497
Parathion, 30
Parker, G.B., 249
Parkinsonism, 308, 408, 495, 496, 500, 522
Parks, 359–360
Parrish, H.M., 406–407
Pascarella, E.A., 202
Passenger restraints, 44, 129–130, 153–154; airplanes, 258–259; costs, 138; and infants, 154–155, 479, 480, 482–483, 487; *see also* Airbags; Seat belts
Patrick, L.M., 26
Paup, D.C., 393
Pavement sensors, 44
Payne, D.E., 513
PCB, 116
Pea gravel, 353, 354
Pearn, J.H., 372, 373–374
Peck, R.C., 143–144
Pedestrians, 211–214; and alcohol, 215–216, 219, 222–223, 226; and ambulance crashes, 180; and automobiles, 215, 216–220; and bicycles, 209; and children, 177, 473, 483, 487; countermeasures, 222–224, 483; in developing countries, 113, 212; and education, 222, 223; and elderly, 214–215, 216, 222–223, 226, 498, 502; fatalities, 110, 211–212, 215; and medical impairment, 214–215; and playgrounds, 221, 223, 351; and railroads, 226–227; and sex, 212–221
Peking, 107
Penttila, A., 238
Pep pills, 165; *see also* Amphetamines
Peru: fires, 311; railroad injuries, 229
Pesticides: and air crashes, 245, 251, 256; poisoning, 334, 339, 341; transport, 174
Peters, G.A., 260
Petroleum products poisoning, 334, 341
Pets: bites, 396, 487; and falls, 327–328
Pezoldt, V.J., 316
Phenylketonuria, 16
Philipson, L.I., 459
Phillips, D.P., 254
Phosphorus, 30
Physical education injuries, 347–348, 362
Pica, 344, 481
Pierson, K.L., 161
Pilot Health Center, 235
Pilot light, 309
Pinch points, 266; and furniture, 292–293; and playgrounds, 352, 353; and toys, 369
Plasterers, 430
Plastic sheets, 293, 482, 486
Platt, F.N., 21
Playgrounds: equipment, 351–355, 484, 485; and pedestrian injuries, 221, 223, 351
Playpens, 267, 292, 293, 305–306, 369, 482
Plumbers, 430
Pochin, E., 423
Poison Prevention Packaging Act, 341
Poisoning, 4, 25, 331–345; and alcohol, 30–32, 334, 338; and children, 333, 334, 336–339, 343–344, 469, 479, 481, 485–486, 488; containers, 43, 338–339, 341–342, 343; countermeasures, 341–345,

481, 485–486, 501; and education, 342–344, 486; and elderly, 498, 501; information centers, 333, 334, 345, 481; labeling, 267; rate, 265, 331–333; and sex, 332, 334; and suicide, 331; threshold of injury, 30–33; toxicity scale, 32–33; and water animals, 371
Pole vaulting, 394
Police: auto chases, 125, 181; enforcement of highway laws, 144–149; records, 74; vehicles, 178, 179, 180, 181
Poliomyelitis, 16, 39–40
Politics and safety programs, 48, 49
Polyurethane, 316
Popliteal tendon, 386
Post-injury phase of injury event, 12, 16, 36–37; and education of health professionals, 528
Potholes, 19
Power mower. *See* Lawnmower
Power saws, 297, 298
Powerboats, 237, 291, 362
Prediction of accident events, 9, 11–12, 74–75
Pre-injury phase of injury event, 12, 18–23; and countermeasures, 39–45
Premenstrual tension, 19, 117; and occupational injury, 431, 432
Press, E., 371
Pressure cookers, 43
Preston, B., 221
Prevention model of injury, 12
Pritchard, J.W., 378
Problem-solving ability and elderly, 495
Productivity losses, 3, 54–55, 103
Property damage: assessment of, 75–76; and disaster, 447; and highway injury, 75–76, 110; and motorcycles, 184; reporting criteria, 68; and snowmobiles, 390
Protective clothing, 44; and bicycles, 209; and laboratories, 349; and motorcycles, 195–196, 197; and occupational injuries, 440, 445; and sports, 366
Prothero, J.C., 144
Public utilities, occupational injuries, 423
Pulmonary edema, 401
Punjab, 93, 322; occupational injuries, 425, 437

Qatar, 113
Quaaludes, 116
Quadriplegia, 374–375, 394, 402

Rabies, 357, 396, 487
Racket sports, 393–394
Radford, E.P., 306
Railroads, 225–233; alcohol and employees, 226–227, 433; and automobiles, 226, 227, 228; collisions, 225, 227–231; countermeasures, 233; derailments, 231–232; developing countries, 229; and elderly, 226–227; falls, 229, 237; fatalities, 178, 225, 232; grade crossings, 225–226, 228; and pedestrians, 226–227
Ramsay, A.C., 408
Rats: bites, 269–270, 396, 483; wiring fires, 284
Rattles, 369–370
Rawson, A.T., 468
Rayon, flammability, 314–315
Reaction response, 18; and alcohol, 512; and elderly, 494, 498; and highway injury, 119; and occupational injury, 430; and warning signs, 126
Reading, 218
Rear pillars of automobiles, 21, 122–123, 188
Recreational boating, 235–243, 358, 361; and alcohol, 238; and drowning, 237, 241–243, 371; fatalities, 236, 241–242; and fires, 240, 241; and weather, 236, 237, 240
Recreational vehicles, 161, 170, 173, 175; crash rates, 163; and inexperience, 167; licensing, 174; *see also* Minibikes; Motorcycles; Mopeds; Snowmobiles
Red Cross, 459
Red light, right turn on, 223
Reflectors: and bicycles, 205, 208; and railroad crossings, 228, 229; and pedestrians, 223–224, 483, 502
Refrigerators, abandoned, 296, 476, 486

Regression toward the mean, 85–87
Regulations and safety, 441, 449, 461–462
Reinschmidt, A.J., 231–232
Renal/hepatic disease: drugs, 338, 344, 500; and elderly, 494
Reporting of accidents, variation in, 66, 67–69
Requa, R.K., 394
Ribicoff, Abe, 87
Richter scale, 451
Right-of-way, railroad, 229
Rio de Janeiro, pedestrians, 212, 218, 220–221, 473
Risk assessment, 51
Risk taking, 470–471
Riveters, 430
Roaas, A., 377
Roadways: and developing countries, 128–129, 158; and highway injuries, 113, 119, 125–129, 133–137, 155–158; and motorcycles, 189–191, 194; and pedestrians, 219–220; and trucks, 171–172, 176–177
Robertson, L.S., 119
Rockwell, T.H., 418
Rodents. *See* Rats
Rohles, F.H., Jr., 316
Rollover: ambulances, 180, 181; automobiles, 129, 130, 133, 151; trucks, 163, 169–170, 177
Roman, P.M., 434–435
Ross, Lawrence, 146
Rossi, P.H., 454, 463
Royal Canadian Mounted Police, 514
Rugby, 363, 366, 378–379, 381
Rugby School, 378, 382
Rugs, 293, 294; and falls, 326, 327; and fires, 315
Running, 394
Rural areas: emergency personnel, 160; fires, 69; highway injuries, 69, 107, 110, 130, 133, 137, 153; pedestrian injuries, 212; railroads, 228, 229
Russell, F.E., 376
Ryan, A.J., 403

Saari, J.T., 426
Sabey, B., 109, 128
Sadan, N., 341
Safety glass, 277, 278
Safety programs. *See* Education
Safren, M.A., 413
Sailing, 236, 237, 240, 362
Sailplanes, 402, 404
St. Helena, 111
Saint-Pierre, Martinique, 463
San Diego, pedestrian injuries, 219
San Francisco, 453
Sand, absorbency, 354, 355
Sanders, M.G., 253–254
Sarawak, 111
Satisficing, 51, 291
Saunders, A.B., 50, 56–57
Sawmills, injuries, 427
Sayer, I.A., 168
Scaffolding, 439–440
Scalds, 267, 306, 311; *see also* Burns
Scandinavia, drinking laws, 145
Schauer, L.R., 416–418
Scheffey, C.F., 138
Schizophrenia, 508–509
School buses, 163, 172, 174; and carbon monoxide, 176, 489; defective equipment, 170, 171; standards, 177, 489; warning devices, 224
Schools, 347–351
Schuman, S.H., 371–372, 373
Schupack, S.A., 206
Scooters, 183, 188; and college students, 349; fatalities, 111, 184
Scotoma, 506
Scottish games, 386
SCUBA, 363, 366, 371, 375–376
Sea anemones, 376
Sea urchins, 376
Seat belts, 491; and airplanes, 258–259; and automobile manufacturers, 149; and children, 487; compliance, 154; compulsory use, 153–155; and driver controls, 123; and education, 80–81, 85, 141; effectiveness, 130–132, 154; and elderly, 503; interlock, 82, 151; *see also* Passenger restraints
Segregated ballast tanks (SBT), 241, 242
Seizures, 469, 496; and burns, 308, 324; and drowning, 371, 372; and

driving, 504, 506–507; *see also* Epilepsy
Semi-trailer trucks, 111
Senile dementia, 19, 142, 496; and driving, 499, 508–510; and falls, 324
Service and government, injuries, 423
Service stations: certification of personnel, 153; diagnosis of defects, 122
Sesame Street, 222
Sesser, S.N., 370
Severity of injury events, 73–76
Sex: and alcohol, 324; and bicycle injuries, 200–201, 202–203, 206; and burns, 302, 304; and disaster injuries, 449; and driver education effectiveness, 143–144; and drowning, 371; and falls, 321, 322, 324; and fatalities, 98; and fires, 313; and firearms, 398; and highway injuries, 110, 113, 118, 123, 143–144; and home injuries, 265, 302; and hospital injuries, 406; and nursing home injuries, 409; and occupational injury, 422–423, 425, 430–432, 439, 445; and pedestrian injuries, 212, 221; and poisoning, 332, 334; and school injuries, 347–348, 349, 351–352; and sport injuries, 363, 387; and window injuries, 277
Shafai-Sahrai, Y., 426–427
Shain, M., 444
Shapiro, M.A., 303, 314
Sharks, 376–377
Sharp edges, 266, 328, 481; and bathroom, 278–283; and furniture, 294; and playgrounds, 352, 353, 354; and toys, 370
Sheldon, J.H., 325–326, 327–328
Shelves, 293–294
Shinar, D., 296
Showers, 278–283
Sibert, J.R., 336–337, 338
Signs. *See* Warning signs
Simon, Herbert, 51, 291
Simonds, R.H., 426–427
Simulation and injury analysis, 14
Singapore, open registry, 239
Single cause model of injury event, 11
Sirens, audibility, 125, 179–180, 181
Skandia Report, 214
Skateboards, 83, 361, 366, 368–369
Skates, 361, 368–369
Ski jumping, 388
Skiing, 42, 361, 366, 387–390; and alcohol, 388; and safety bindings, 43
Skin: cancer, 36; temperature threshold, 30; tensile strength, 28; thickness, 27
Skin diving, 366
Sky diving, 363, 366, 402, 403
Sledding, 387, 390, 392–393
Sleeper effect, 87
Sleight, R.B., 427, 430
Slides, 353, 354
Slovic, P., 452
Smart, C.N., 103
Smeed, R.J., 211–212, 219
Smith, M.J., 443
Smoke alarms, 316, 480, 501
Smoking: and alcohol, 306, 515; and back pain, 433; and fires, 306–308, 311
Snake bite, 332–333, 340–341, 357, 376
Snell, W.E., 407
Snively, G., 367
Snook, G.A., 385
Snow discs, 387, 392–393
Snowblowers, 297, 298
Snowmobiles, 291, 362, 387, 390–392; reporting of damage, 68
Snowstorm, 452
Snyder, M.B., 215, 216–218, 222
Snyder, R.G., 258–259
Sobel, R., 337, 345
Soccer, 363–366, 377–378
Socioeconomic factors, 37, 469; and alcohol, 268; and education, 287–288; and furniture and appliances, 287–291; and housing, 269–270; and recreational activity, 362; and traffic citations, 71–72
Softball, 361, 367
Solomon, D., 120
Somers, R.L., 26, 74–75
Soroker, B., 341
South Africa: diving, 375; sharks, 376–377
South America, 93; highway injuries, 108; poisonous bites, 333
South Carolina, 372

South Dakota, 196
Soviet Union, 97
Space heaters, 284, 289, 295, 309, 310, 480; toxic gases, 296
Spare capacity, 20, 22
Speed limits, 84–85, 109, 146; and pedestrians, 221; and railroads, 228
Spelunking, 366, 402
Spider bites, 333
Spinal cord injuries, 25; and diving, 370, 373–374; economic costs, 103, 322; and falls, 322, 362; and firearms, 362; and skiing, 389, 404; survival rate, 362; and trampoline, 394
Sports. *See under individual sports*
Spot improvement of highways, 155–158
Squash, 393–394
Sri Lanka: crosswalks, 218; and highway injuries, 112
Stability: and appliances, 295–296; and bicycles, 205, 207; and furniture, 292; and highway injuries, 113, 169–170, 187–188; and repair and maintenance equipment, 297–298
Stairs, 268, 270–272, 322, 325, 326
Stake trucks as transportation, 37, 108, 177–178
Stallones, R.A., 334, 336, 337, 339
Stapp, J.P., 25
Starr, Chauncey, 459
States, John, 74
Statistical analysis, 56, 65–78; and countermeasure evaluation, 85–87; and education of health care professionals, 526
Stature: and automobile design, 123; and occupational injury, 439
Steel-tipped shoes. *See* Metal-tipped shoes
Steering column, impact with, 129–130, 150–151, 152
Stewart, M.A., 336
Sting ray, 376
Stockholm, bicycles, 200
Stoll, A.M., 30
Stop signs, 144
Stoves: burns, 265, 304, 308, 317, 484, 501; ceramic tops, 42, 296–297; controls, 266, 296–297, 308, 310
Streib, V.L., 144
Stremming, K., 336
Stress: and falls, 325; and occupational injury, 435–436
Strokes, 267, 496; and burns, 308; and diving, 508
Strollers, 292
Strychnine, 333, 341
Student Health Service, 348
Stutts, J.C., 184
Sudan, 120, 140, 168
Sudden infant death, 7, 66–67, 98, 265
Suffocation. *See* Asphyxiation
Suicide: and accident proneness, 468–469; and age, 103; and air transport, 254; data validity, 67; and drugs, 41, 331; and firearms, 266, 397; and poisoning, 331
Sundowning, 509
Surfing, 371, 375
Suspension systems, 149, 175
Swain, A.D., 445
Sweden, 98, 141; and aftereffects of injury, 103; bicycles, 200, 207; motorcycles, 197; pedestrian injuries, 211, 214
Swimming, 356; *see also* Drowning
Swimming pools, 283, 371, 373; alarms, 486; fencing, 373–374, 486
Swings, 352, 353, 354
Synthetic turf, 353, 382
Syria, falls, 321
Systems-analysis, model of injury event, 12–14, 526

Table tennis, 361
TAD vehicle damage scale, 76
Tailpipes, short, 124, 180, 340
Takafuji, E.T., 306
Talc, 32
Tank cars, 230–231
Tanker trucks, 44
Target shooting, 398, 399
Task demand, 18–23; and countermeasures, 42–43; and elderly, 493; and highway injuries, 19–20, 21

Taste sense and children, 336, 476
Taxicabs, crash rate, 163
Teapots, 295–296, 297, 309, 480
Tectonic plates, 42, 455–456, 458
Teenagers, 469; and alcohol, 477, 514, 515; and burns, 490; and drugs, 477, 491; and falls, 490; fatalities, 103; and highway injuries, 117–118, 473, 491, 504; and occupational injuries, 422, 473, 477–478; and pedestrians, 473
Television, 287, 295, 309
Temperature, sensitivity to, 494
Tempest, M.N., 308
Temple, A.R., 336
Tennis, 361, 393–394
Tents, 402
Tetanus, 44, 48, 483
Texas: derailment, 231; truck crashes, 178; vehicle defects, 171
Textile workers, injuries, 432
Thailand: children, 98; crosswalks, 218; traffic signal response, 121
THC, 116
Thermal energy, 8, 16–17, 25, 30; countermeasures, 41, 42, 43; tolerance to, 30; *see also* Burns; Fires; Hypothermia; Scalds
Third New International Dictionary, 8
Third rails, electrified, 229, 233
Thomas, C.L., 403
Thompson, M.S., 103
Thorson, J., 77–78, 103, 200, 207, 372
Three Mile Island, 460, 462
Thromboangiitis obliterans, 36
Tibial fractures and skiing, 388
Tile cement, 314
Time of day: and highway injuries, 110; and hospital injuries, 408; and pedestrian injuries, 219; *see also* Circadian rhythms
Time of year and poisoning, 339
Time period of injury, 8
Time-sequence techniques, 84–87
Tires: blowouts, 19; defects, 121–122, 150, 171, 176; load capacity, 123; motorcycles, 189, 193; standards, 176; trucks, 170, 176
Titanic, 240
Tobogganing, 387, 392–393
Tokuhata, G.K., 291
Tokyo, earthquakes, 453
Tolerance to injury: and alcohol, 25–26, 129, 328, 513; and deceleration, 26–28
Tongue, J.R., 402, 403
Tooth injuries and sports, 378–379
Tornadoes, 447, 451, 452, 454–455
Toxic fumes: and air crashes, 260; and appliances, 296; and fires, 306–308, 316, 461; and furniture, 294
Toy chests, 293, 369, 476, 482
Toys, 368–370; and burns, 370, 488; and eyes, 29; fatalities, 361; projectile, 29, 368, 488; standards, 481
Trachoma, 496
Track and field, 393, 394
Tractors, 298
Trade, occupational injuries, 423
Trade unions: and building codes, 285; and occupational injuries, 440–441
Traffic citations: and bicycles, 208; and driver education, 144; and drugs, 523; and highway injuries, 71–72, 118–119; and motorcycles, 186; outcomes, 146
Traffic signals, obedience to, 120–121; and pedestrians, 223
Trail bikes, 185, 187, 190, 194
Trailers, 163–165, 167, 170; coupling failures, 171, 176; crash design, 173
Trampolines, 366, 394
Tranquilizers, 116, 326, 331, 522; and alcohol, 512
Transport industry, occupational injury, 423, 425
Transverse ligament, 386
Trice, H.M., 434–435
Tricycles, 43, 368, 369
Trigger effect, 87
TRIS, 315
Trucking industry, taxes, 78
Trucks: and alcohol, 165; and automobile collision, 163–164, 173, 176, 177; brakes, 168, 169,

172, 175; defective equipment, 170–171; definitions, 161–162; fatalities, 162–163, 178; licensing, 166, 168, 174; and medical impairment, 166, 174; and pedestrians, 224; and roadways, 171–172, 176–177; rollovers, 113, 169–170, 177; size of, 158, 168–169, 172, 175; and speed, 168, 175; and visibility, 172, 176; and weather, 172, 176; and weight, 175, 224
Tsunamis, 457
Tubs, 278–283; drownings, 371, 372, 482; scalds, 306
Turkey: crosswalks, 218; traffic signals, 121
Turpentine, poisoning, 334, 343
Two-by-two evaluation design, 87, 88–89
Tyworth, J.E., 231–232

Uganda: highway fatalities, 66; school injuries, 349
Underwriters Laboratories, 296, 309
Uniform Driver Improvement School, 144
Uniform Vehicle Code, 181
Unintentional injuries, definition of, 7–9
United Airlines, 252
United Kingdom: air transport, 253; alcohol, 115; burns, 304; drownings, 237; electrocution, 265; expenditures for safety, 50–51; firearms, 266; go-kart injuries, 395; highway injuries, 65, 111, 115, 120–121, 130; hospital fires, 416; hospital injuries, 406; motorcycles, 183, 196; natural gas, 41, 333, 340, 341; occupational injuries, 440; pedestrians, 211, 214, 218, 223; poisoning, 265; skateboards, 369; toxic gases, 296
U.S. Coast Guard, 235–236, 240, 241
U.S. Department of Housing and Urban Development, building codes, 272, 273, 278, 284–285
U.S. Department of Transportation, 78, 148, 153–154, 527; testing, 173
U.S. Food and Drug Administration, 299
U.S. Highway Safety Standards, 139–140
U.S. Navy, diving tables, 375
U.S. Supreme Court, 196
University of Vermont, 349, 381
Urban areas: fires, 69; highway injuries, 107, 110, 130; pedestrian injuries, 212; railroads, 228, 229

Van Cott, H.P., 316
Vehicle identification number, 150
Venter, F.T., 285–286
Verhulst, H.L., 334
Verma, P.S., 425
Vermont: camps, 357; firearms, 398, 399; highway deaths, 81, 88–89; playground injuries, 353
Vernon, H.M., 469
Vertebrae, impact tolerance, 26, 27
Vertigo, 325
Vilardo, F.J., 200, 203
Vinje, M.P., 214
Visibility: and automobile accidents, 21, 122–123, 124, 150; and bicycles, 205; and highway injuries, 21, 113, 122–123, 124; and motorcycle injuries, 21, 186–187, 188, 189–190, 194–195, 196; and trucks, 172, 176
Vision: and alcohol, 513, 514; and diabetes, 496, 508; and elderly, 215, 267, 271, 308, 324, 325, 493–494, 496, 498, 500, 506, 508; and falls, 324, 500; and furniture injuries, 294; and pilots, 253, 257
Visual flight capability (VFR), 249
Volcanoes, 37–38, 447, 451; prediction, 457
Volkswagen, 124, 129
Volley ball, 361
Volunteers in studies, bias of, 82–83
Vita, M., 406, 407

Wagar, I.J., 193
Wagons, children's, 368, 369
Wakeland, H.H., 57, 221
Walk, R.D., 323
Walker, K., 444
Waller, J.A., 49, 200, 216, 226, 306, 362, 391–392, 398, 468

Waller, P.F., 169, 186, 188
Walls, 268
Walter, M., 377
Warning signs, 125–126, 127, 176
Washing machines, 295, 485
Wasp stings, 333
Watch makers, 430
Water skiing, 361, 371, 375
Water sports, 361, 370–377
Water temperature, regulation, 41, 297, 306, 480, 501
Water transportation. *See* Commercial vessels; Recreational boating
Watts, J., 317–318
Weather: and air accidents, 246–248, 249, 258; and boating accidents, 236, 237, 240; and housing, 269; and railroad injury, 227; and school buses, 176; and truck crashes, 172, 176
Webster's Twentieth Century Dictionary, 7, 8
Wechsler, H., 323
Weil, T.P., 406–407
Weiner, E.L., 222–223
Wells, drowning in, 265, 371, 476
Werner, P., 354
Wheelchairs, 409–410; motorized, 43
Whitcomb, W., 412
White, M.V., 314–315
Whorton, E.B., 398, 468
Wick, R.L., 248
Wigglesworth, E.C., 227
Williams, A.F., 141–142, 201
"Willie Whistle," 222
Windows, 268, 273–278; and buses, 177; and children, 481, 485; and elderly, 502; and falls, 326, 328–329
Windshields, 151; cleaning fluid, poisoning, 342; defoggers, 150; impact with, 129–130; wipers, 149, 150
Wine, 511–512
Winter sports, 361, 387–393
Wiring, 279–284, 309
Wisconsin, occupational injury, 422
Wollin, S., 207, 209–210
Women. *See* Sex
Wood stoves, 80, 284, 309, 310–313
Woods, H.M., 467–468
Woodworking tools, 291
Wool, flammability, 314, 480
Workers compensation, 422, 440
World Health, 139
World Health Organization, 65–66, 103; Pilot Health Center, 236
World Health Satistical Annual, 93
Wrestling, 362–363, 383, 385–386
Wright, D., 454, 463
Wu, Y.C., 33, 34

Y.5-11, crash rate, 255
Yellowstone National Park, 359
Young, G.S., 302
Yugoslavia, roadways, 128–129, 220
Yuill, G.M., 402
Young adults, 473–491

Zalinger, D.A., 228
Zariczny, B., 382
Zohar, D., 294

About the Author

Julian A. Waller, M.D., M.P.H., is professor of medicine at the University of Vermont and formerly chairman, Department of Epidemiology and Environmental Health, at that institution. His activities in injury control research, programs, and program evaluation span twenty-five years and include medical and environmental aspects of highway and home safety, injury to children and the elderly, product safety, recreational injury, emergency medical services, and alcohol and drug abuse. Dr. Waller is a member of the National Academy of Sciences Committee on Trauma Research, and a past president of the American Association for Automotive Medicine and has been advisor on injury control to the World Health Organization, presidential appointee to the National Highway Safety Advisory Committee, and an evaluator for the Consumer Product Technology Center, National Bureau of Standards. As one of the few physician members of the Human Factors Society and the System Safety Society he is in a unique position to bridge the gaps that often exist between the health practitioner and other professionals, such as psychologists, engineers, legal specialists, and educators working in the field of injury control.